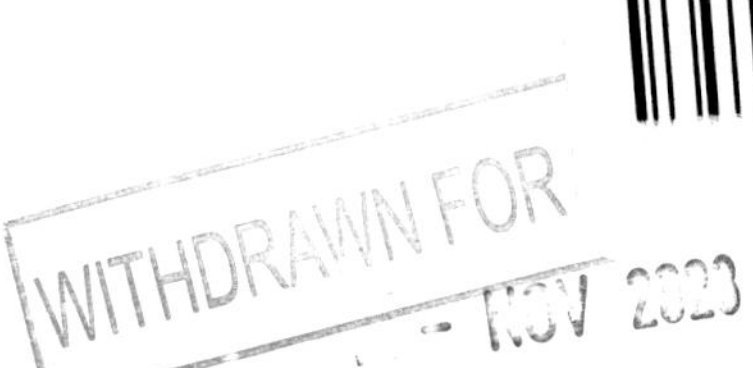

OXFORD CLINICAL NEPHROLOGY SERIES

Mechanisms and Clinical Management of Chronic Renal Failure

Oxford Clinical Nephrology Series

Analgesic and NSAID-induced kidney disease
Edited by J. H. Stewart

Dialysis amyloid
Edited by Charles van Ypersele and Tilman B. Drüeke

Infections of the kidney and urinary tract
Edited by W. R. Cattell

Polycystic kidney disease
Edited by Michael L. Watson and Vicente E. Torres

Treatment of primary glomerulonephritis
Edited by Claudio Ponticelli and Richard J. Glassock

Inherited disorders of the kidney
Edited by Stephen H. Morgan and Jean-Pierre Grünfeld

Complications of long-term dialysis
Edited by Edwina A. Brown and Patrick S. Parfrey

Rapidly progressive glomerulonephritis
Edited by C. D. Pusey and A. J. Rees

Lupus nephritis
Edited by Edmund Lewis, Melvin Schwartz, and Stephen Korbet

Nephropathy in type 2 diabetes
Edited by Eberhard Ritz and Ivan Rychlík

Hemodialysis vascular access
Edited by Peter J. Conlon, Michael Nicholson and Steve Schwab

Mechanisms and clinical management of chronic renal failure (Second edition; formerly *Prevention of progressive chronic renal failure*)
Edited by A. Meguid El Nahas with Kevin P. G. Harris and Sharon Anderson

Mechanisms and Clinical Management of Chronic Renal Failure

Second Edition

Edited by

A. MEGUID EL NAHAS
Professor of Nephrology, University of Sheffield, UK

And Associate Editors

KEVIN P. G. HARRIS
Senior Lecturer/Honorary Consultant Nephrologist, University of Leicester, UK

SHARON ANDERSON
Professor of Medicine, Division of Nephrology and Hypertension, Oregan Health Sciences University, Portland, USA

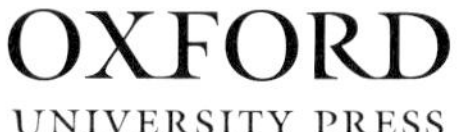

OXFORD
UNIVERSITY PRESS

Great Clarendon Street, Oxford OX2 6DP

Oxford University Press is a department of the University of Oxford.
It furthers the University's objective of excellence in research, scholarship,
and education by publishing worldwide in

Oxford New York

Athens Auckland Bangkok Bogotá Buenos Aires Calcutta
Cape Town Chennai Dar es Salaam Delhi Florence Hong Kong Istanbul
Karachi Kuala Lumpur Madrid Melbourne Mexico City Mumbai
Nairobi Paris São Paulo Singapore Taipei Tokyo Toronto Warsaw

with associated companies in Berlin Ibadan

Oxford is a registered trade mark of Oxford University Press
in the UK and in certain other countries

Published in the United States
by Oxford University Press, Inc., New York

First published 1993 (as Prevention of progressive chronic renal failure)

Second edition published 2000

British Library Cataloguing in Publication Data

Mechanisms and clinical management of chronic renal failure / edited by Meguid El
Nahas, and associate editors, Kevin Harris, Sharon Anderson.—2nd ed.
p. ; cm.—(Oxford clinical nephrology series)
Rev. ed. of: Prevention of progressive chronic renal failure / edited by A. Meguid El
Nahas, Netar P. Mallick, and Sharon Anderson. 1993.
Includes bibliographical references and index.
1. Chronic renal failure. I. El Nahas, A. Meguid. II. Harris, Kevin P. G., 1957–
III. Anderson, Sharon, 1949– IV. Series.
[DNLM: 1. Kidney Failure, Chronic—physiopathology. 2. Kidney Failure,
Chronic—therapy. WJ 342 M4855 2000]
RC918.R4 P68 2000 616.6′14—dc21 99-042841

Library of Congress Cataloging in Publication Data

1 3 5 7 9 10 8 6 4 2

ISBN 0 19 262933 6

Typeset by Best-set Typesetter Ltd., Hong Kong
Printed in Great Britain on acid free paper by
Bookcraft (Bath) Ltd
Midsomer Norton, Avon

CONTENTS

CONTRIBUTORS

S. Anderson Division of Nephrology and Hypertention, Oregan Health Sciences University, Portland, USA

R. S. Barsoum Department of Internal Medicine, Cairo University, Cairo, Egypt

G. A. Coles Institute of Nephrology, University of Wales College of Medicine, Cardiff, UK

G. D'Amico Divisione di Nefrolgiea e Dialisi, Milan, Italy

L. Del Vecchio Department of Nephrology, Lecco Hospital, Lecco, Italy

L. D. Dworkin Department of Medicine, Brown University, Providence, USA

A. A. Eddy Division of Nephrology, Children's Hospital and Regional Medical Center, University of Washington, Seattle, USA

A. M. El Nahas Sheffield Kidney Institute, Sheffield, UK

K. P. G. Harris Department of Medicine and Therapeutics, University of Leicester, UK

S. M. Jernigan Division of Nephrology, Children's Hospital and Regional Medical Center, University of Washington, Seattle, USA

E. Jones European Dialysis and Transplant Association Registry, St Thomas' Hospital, London, UK

B. L. Kasiske Department of Medicine, University of Minnesota, USA

F. Locatelli Department of Nephrology, Lecco Hospital, Lecco, Italy

C. E. Mogensen Medical Department, Aarhus Kommunehospital, Aarhus, Denmark

J. E. Scoble Guy's Hospital, London, UK

R. M. Smith Department of Renal Medicine, Southmead Hospital, Bristol, UK

S. K. Swan Department of Medicine, Hennepin County Medical Center and University of Minnesota, USA

C. R. V. Tomson Department of Renal Medicine, Southmead Hospital, Bristol, UK

M. R. Weir Department of Medicine, University of Maryland, Baltimore, USA

A. J. Wing St George's Hospital, London, UK

1

Epidemiology of end-stage renal failure: a global perspective

A. J. Wing and E. Jones

Introduction

The ultimate problem resulting from progressive renal disease is end-stage renal failure (ESRF). Many diseases and the interplay of a spectrum of mechanisms result in damaged kidneys which are doomed to be incapable of maintaining the integrity of the internal environment on which life depends. Description of the numbers of patients suffering from these conditions is the business of epidemiology. The tool of its trade is the classification and nomenclature of renal diseases.

Epidemiology

Epidemiology is the platform from which we must consider the scope of the problem. The scale of ESRF is probably the best documented account of a fatal chronic disease in economically developed countries. The financial burden of providing renal replacement therapy (RRT) has made it inevitable that information about numbers of patients would be well known in individual renal centres and throughout different countries and regions.

Statistics are expressed as numbers maintained on treatment, otherwise known as the prevalence of the illness or the 'stock' of the patients; and the numbers presenting over time, usually the annual incidence or 'flow'. Prevalence is usually given as a point prevalence that is the number of patients on a particular therapy on a certain date—a 'snap shot', but is sometimes the period prevalence which denotes the number of patients on that treatment at any time during the period defined, for example, 1 month or 1 year. Likewise incidence should always be defined in terms of the period which is being described, for instance, a weekly, monthly or (most usually) annual incidence. Prevalence and incidence statistics are best linked to a population denominator, expressed by 100 000 or 1 million, either of total population (crude) or of age- and sex-specific population (Fig. 1.1).

Classification of end-stage renal failure

Fortunately, the need for accurate information on numbers of patients and the causes of their ESRF was recognized early in the history of dialysis and transplantation and

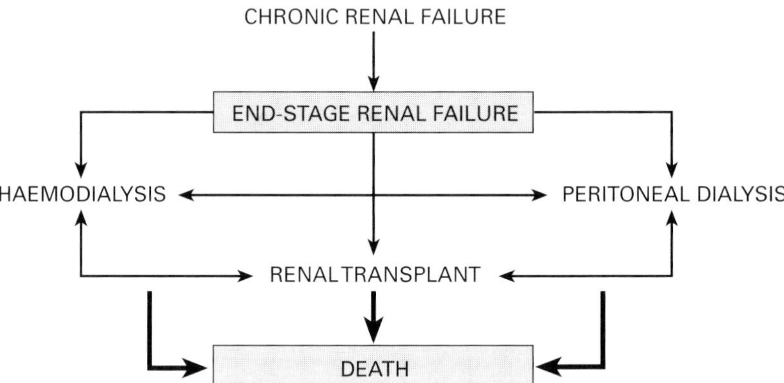

Fig. 1.1 Complementary treatments for end-stage renal failure. For each of the arrows a rate can be determined. The net effect of the rates (flow) results in the number of patients on each modality (stock).

in Europe a registry of patients was set up almost from the outset of the treatments [1]. The Registry of the European Dialysis and Transplant Association (EDTA), later the European Renal Association (ERA) [2] was established by practising clinicians who sought the best advice available in the early 1960s concerning the classification of the causes of progressive renal diseases. This classification, now with 60 coded diagnoses, has proved useful and has been followed or adapted by other registries [3,4]. There has been resistance to changing it despite increasing sophistication of diagnostic skills because changes would invalidate historic comparisons. It was appreciated that with growth in facilities and clinical skills a broader selection policy would come into effect permitting the treatment of older patients and those with multisystem diseases and significant co-morbid factors. Changes in the classification of renal diseases causing ESRF would have obscured comparisons of the demography of the treated patients and would have undermined comparison of outcomes.

The recently established United States Renal Data System (USRDS) has followed an interactive method to derive its present classification of primary categories of renal disease [5]. Early versions of the medical evidence form required the diagnosis to be written out and this was then translated by the Health Care Finance Administration (HCFA) into one of 130 possible causes. The new version of the form requires providers to enter a primary cause of end-stage renal disease (ESRD) from a relatively complete and contemporary coded list of 72 diagnoses. These diagnoses can be aggregated into major diagnostic groups for comparison with early data. Continued evolution of the diagnostic classification is anticipated [5].

The full classification used by the ETD–ERA Registry is displayed in Table 1.1. This is resolved under 10 groups in Figures 1.3 and 1.5. The classification into primary categories used by the USRDS is shown in Figure 1.6. Most renal centres adopt the practice of classifying the causes of ESRF according to these coded listings. This has the advantage of facilitating inter-centre and historic comparisons. It is also a secure basis for multicentre collaborative work on the assessment of outcomes.

Provided with facilities to carry out a full work up of the individual patient including modern imaging and histological interpretation, the nephrologist will have little difficulty in selecting an appropriate diagnostic label. However, failure to investigate fully and skilfully, as often happens when patients are referred too late, will result in the choice being more speculative. It is common experience in London that about one-third of all ESRF patients present with advanced renal failure and have a history no longer than 3 months before they require dialysis. About 50% of these have no antecedent history, proteinuria of less than 1.0 g/24 h and imaging reveals bilateral shrunken kidneys with smooth outlines. In such cases the aetiology of chronic renal failure is 'uncertain' [6].

Diagnostic criteria in general usage have not always been evaluated for their specificity. A commendable example of diagnostic objectivity has recently been provided in defining the investigatory findings in analgesic nephropathy [7]. This avoids misunderstanding between clinicians as to which features constitute the disease. Another approach has been that of a consensus conference to agree the subdivisions of a group of related diseases. This approach is exemplified by the Chapel Hill consensus conference on systemic vasculitides [8].

Interpretation of apparent differences

Apparent historical or geographical differences in the frequencies of renal diseases causing ESRF must be interpreted with caution [9].

First, an apparent geographical variation could be produced by the selection of patients. In countries with restricted dialysis facilities there is consequent rationing of treatment. Usually this results in younger patients with fewer co-morbid factors being accepted and older patients with multisystem diseases, most importantly hypertension and diabetes, being rejected. This effect of patient selection is evident in the early stages of evolution of a national programme of RRT.

Secondly, apparent differences may be an artefact of diagnostic fashion. For example, analgesic nephropathy is more frequently recognized in Belgium and Switzerland where clinicians are familiar with its presentation, but its diagnosis may be missed in other territories where awareness is lower. Of greater numerical importance are physician attitudes about attributing small scarred kidneys to a diagnosis of pyelonephritis, glomerulonephritis or hypertension. Fashion has certainly swung through these major categories in the last three decades [10]. Alternatively, some clinicians are more prepared to admit uncertainty and where scientific agnosticism is fashionable more will elect for a category of 'chronic renal failure, aetiology uncertain'. The end-stage kidney is a tombstone, not an historic document [6].

Ample illustration of wide variation between these two major categories will be presented in this chapter to make the point that it is probable that not all nephrologists faced with an identical clinical presentation will give the same diagnostic label to the patient.

Thirdly, apparent differences may represent true geographical variation in clinical pathology. They may, therefore, be the first clues of either environmental or genetic factors influencing the frequency of individual diseases. Analgesic nephropathy was identified because of early observation [11] of areas of high frequency of renal papillary necrosis [12] and the ultimate result of high analgesic consumption was documented in the earlier reports of the EDTA–ERA Registry [13]. Balkan nephropathy appears to be another example of an environmentally determined disease, although its cause is not yet identified [14]. High incidence of diabetic nephropathy as a cause of ESRF in young adults in Scandinavian countries has been suggested to result from a high frequency of HLA-DR3 and DR4 and its association with type I diabetes [15]. A genetic factor has long been suggested for the high incidence of ESRD in black people and a recent report suggests that this may be mediated through a hyperexpression of transforming growth factor (TGF)-β1 which has been identified in African-American ESRD patients [16]. TGF-β1, a multifunctional cytokine, can induce renal fibrosis and insufficiency in experimental models and can also stimulate endothelin-I and angiotensin-II production and so may be involved in the pathogenesis of hypertension. The authors of this report offer the hypothesis that heightened TGF-β1 expression is a mechanism for the increased prevalence of ESRD in the US black population.

Epidemiology of end-stage renal failure

Description of the causes and proportional contribution of these causes to ESRF is based on reports of the major international registries supplemented by some local reports where relevant.

The Registry of EDTA–ERA has used the same coded list of primary renal diseases since 1970. There have been some additions but no major alterations since then. In particular, there has been no change in the 10 major groups [1]. Codes used by the Australia–New Zealand Registry [3] and also by the Canadian Registry [4] are similar. The Japanese society has followed its own pattern [17]. The US renal data system has evolved its version of the classification but the present pattern of diseases reported is not grossly dissimilar [5]. None of these registries has adopted the WHO classification, finding the clinically based approach to be more in harmony with the nosological conventions of their practising colleagues. The greatest advantage is that the registries are known to be run by physicians for physicians [1].

Historical (Tables 1.1, 1.2; Figures 1.2–1.4)

In order to present an historical perspective for this review we have analysed the proportional distribution (%) of causes of ESRF in patients starting RRT in Europe in three periods: 1973–4, 1983–4, and 1993–4. During the two decades encompassed by these years facilities for treatment have expanded and criteria for acceptance have been progressively liberalized. New centres and new countries have been recruited to report to the Registry with consequent expansion in the population covered.

Table 1.1 Proportional distribution (%) of causes of end-stage renal failure in patients starting renal replacement therapy in the period 1993–4 according to age at start of therapy (total Registry)

Causes of end-stage renal failure	Age at start of renal replacement therapy 1993–4 (years)				
	<15	15–34	35–54	55–64	>65
Chronic renal failure, aetiology uncertain	9.1	14.2	13.6	14.9	19.8
Glomerulonephritis					
Histologically not examined	4.7	17.7	17.5	10.3	6.7
Histologically examined	16.9	19.6	11.6	6.3	3.8
Pyelonephritis/interstitial nephritis					
Cause not specified	1.1	4.7	6.1	6.9	7.2
Associated with neurogenic bladder	0.9	0.9	0.3	0.2	0.1
Due to congenital obstructive uropathy with or without vesicouretic reflux without obstruction	8.8	4.1	0.7	0.3	0.2
Due to acquired obstructive uropathy	0.7	0.6	0.7	1.4	2.7
Due to vesicoureteric reflux without obstruction	5.7	4.4	1.0	0.4	0.3
Due to urolithiasis	0.7	0.7	1.7	2.7	2.3
Due to other cause	0.4	0.4	0.8	0.7	0.6
Tubulo interstitial nephritis (not pyelonephritis)	0.9	0.4	0.6	0.8	0.5
Toxic nephropathy					
Caused by drugs or nephrotoxic agents—cause not specified	0.0	0.4	0.5	0.3	0.2
Due to analgesic drugs	0.1	0.2	0.8	2.1	2.1
Cystic kidney disease—type unspecified	0.7	0.5	1.5	1.4	0.8
Polycystic kidneys—Adult type	1.5	1.4	10.1	7.6	3.7
Infantile and juvenile types	2.1	0.4	0.2	0.1	0.1
Medullary cystic disease, including nephronophthisis	3.6	0.9	0.1	0.1	<0.1
Hereditary/familial nephropathy—type unspecified	20.4	3.5	0.9	0.4	0.2
Hereditary nephritis with nerve deafness (Alport's syndrome)	1.2	2.3	0.4	0.1	0.1
Cystinosis	2.7	0.1	<0.1	0.1	<0.1
Oxalosis	1.1	0.2	<0.1	0.1	<0.1
Fabry's disease	0.0	<0.1	<0.1	0.0	<0.1
Renal vascular disease					
Type unspecified	1.0	0.5	1.9	3.9	8.2
Due to malignant hypertension (no primary renal disease)	0.0	1.2	1.8	1.0	0.9
Due to hypertension (no primary renal disease)	1.5	1.3	4.2	6.9	10.4
Due to polyarteritis	0.2	0.2	0.3	0.4	0.8
Wegener's granulomatosis	0.2	0.2	0.4	0.4	0.6

Table 1.1 *(Continued)*

Causes of end-stage renal failure	Age at start of renal replacement therapy 1993–4 (years)				
	<15	15–34	35–54	55–64	>65
Diabetes					
Insulin-dependent (type I)	0.9	9.4	11.8	10.8	7.5
Non-insulin dependent (type II)	1.0	0.3	3.5	11.9	12.5
Multisystem diseases					
Myelomatosis	0.0	0.1	0.6	1.3	1.9
Amyloid	0.6	1.5	1.4	1.8	1.5
Lupus erythematosus	0.2	3.0	1.1	0.4	0.1
Henoch-Schönlein purpura	0.7	0.7	0.1	0.1	0.1
Goodpasture's syndrome	0.0	0.6	0.2	0.2	0.2
Scleroderma	0.0	<0.1	0.2	0.2	0.1
Hemolytic uraemic syndrome	5.0	1.1	0.3	0.1	0.1
Multisystem diseases—other	0.4	0.2	0.3	0.3	0.4
Other diseases					
Cortical or tubular necrosis	1.0	0.3	0.4	0.3	0.3
Tuberculosis	0.0	0.1	0.4	0.4	0.5
Gout	0.1	0.1	0.3	0.6	0.2
Nephrocalcinosis and hypercalcaemic nephropathy	0.1	0.3	0.2	0.2	0.1
Balkan nephropathy	0.0	<0.1	0.1	0.1	<0.1
Kidney tumour	0.6	0.1	0.3	0.8	0.8
Traumatic or surgical loss of kidney	0.5	0.1	0.2	0.4	0.3
Other identified renal disorders	2.2	1.3	0.8	0.8	0.9
Total patients with diagnosis available	804	5464	12710	10829	17719
% Patients with recorded Primary Renal Disease	95.8	96.4	96.9	97.3	93.5

Age of patients

Figure 1.2 summarizes the number of new patients entering treatment for the first time in each of these three 2-year periods and gives their age distribution. Numbers increased threefold over the 20 years. Age distribution showed an increasing proportion of elderly patients; in 1973–4 more than eight of every 10 patients was aged less than 55 but by 1993–4 this was halved, and the proportion aged over 65 had risen more than 10-fold. Despite the increase in total new patients those aged less than 55 decreased in 1993–4 compared with 1983–4.

Renal diseases

Table 1.1 presents a detailed analysis of the primary renal diseases reported for 47 526 patients who started RRT in the 2 years, 1993–4. The proportional

Table 1.2 Histologically examined glomerulonephritis (GN) in new pediatric and adult patients commencing renal replacement therapy in 1993–4

	Children <15	Adults 15≥	Total (%)
Severe nephrotic syndrome with focal sclerosis (pediatric patients only)	65	185	250 (6.2)
IgA nephropathy (proven by immunofluorescence, not Henoch–Schönlein purpura)	6	1012	1018 (25.2)
Dense deposit disease, membranoproliferative GN, type II (proven by immunofluorescence or electron microscopy)	3	116	119 (2.9)
Membranous nephropathy	2	362	364 (9.0)
Membranoproliferative GN, type I (proven by immunofluorescence or electron microscopy, not lupus erythematosus or multisystem disease)	7	417	424 (10.5)
Rapidly progressive GN without systemic disease (crescentic, histologically confirmed, not coded elsewhere)	17	222	239 (5.9)
GN, histologically examined	36	1586	1622 (40.2)
Total, histologically examined GN	136	3900	4036

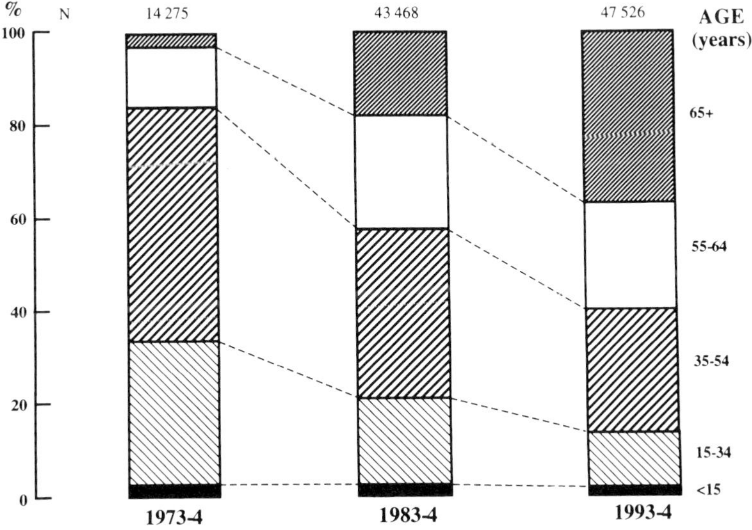

Fig. 1.2 Distribution of new patients who were registered as commencing treatment in 1973–4, 1983–4, and 1993–4 according to their age showing absolute numbers (n) and percentages in each age group. EDTA data.

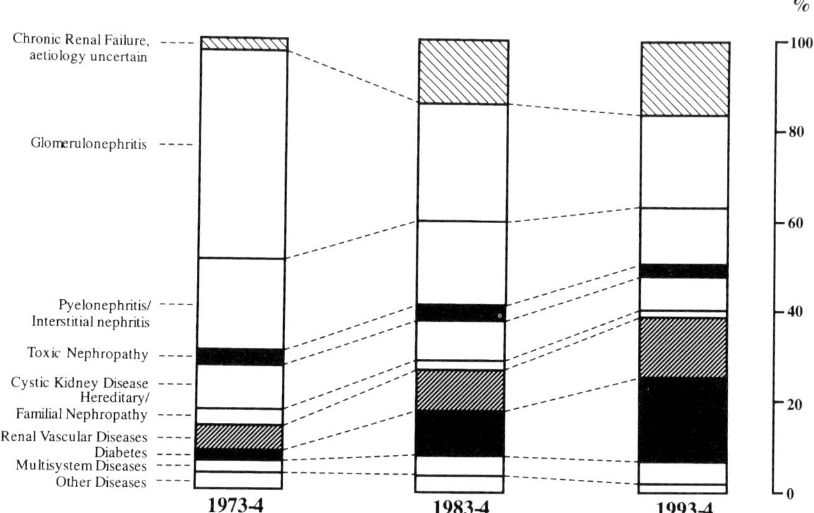

Fig. 1.3 Proportional distribution (%) of causes of end-stage renal failure in patients commencing renal replacement therapy in 1973–4, 1983–4, and 1993–4. EDTA data.

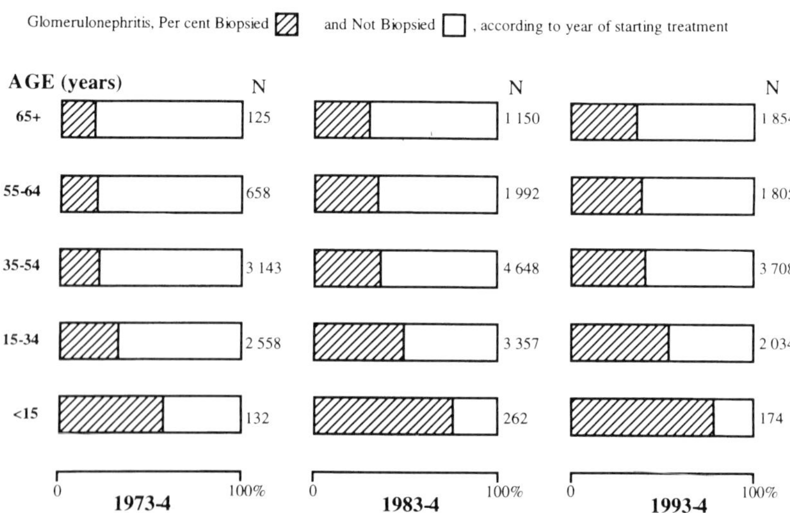

Fig. 1.4 The diagnosis of glomerulonephritis and the proportion of patients in whom histological examination was carried out according to year of first treatment and age. EDTA data.

distribution (%) is shown in columns according to five age groupings. The response rate for reporting the primary renal diseases was excellent, at best 97.3% in the 55–64 age group and at worst 93.5% in the 65 plus age group. Diseases are shown under 10 groups and in subsequent tables the data has been summarized under these groups. However, before describing the broader view than this summarized information gives, it may be useful to draw attention to the finer details available in Table 1.2. It is gratifying that the proportion of patients with analgesic nephropathy and renal tuberculosis has decreased, compared with earlier reports [6], interesting that those with renal tumour has increased. Overall, it is remarkable that there is a fairly constant recognition rate for rare multisystem and other identified diseases, and in this respect this table is very similar to one published in 1992 with data from 1985 to 7 [6].

Comparison with the proportional distribution of primary renal diseases for 1973–4, 1983–4 shows changes which would be expected in the light of the growing liberalisation towards acceptance of patients of older age and with multisystem diseases (Figure 1.3). Thus on the one hand the proportions with glomerulonephritis histologically examined or not histologically examined and of those with pyelonephritis/interstitial nephritis have progressively diminished in parallel with the decreased proportion of younger patients. However, there is also in 1993–4 an absolute decrease in the numbers of patients with these two diagnoses of 22% and 30% respectively compared with the numbers predicted from figures for 1983–4 taking account of the larger overall numbers commencing treatment in the later period. On the other hand the proportion with diabetes or renal vascular causes of ESRF has grown with the rising acceptance of older patients for treatment. There was also in 1993–4 an increase in the absolute numbers of patients with these two diagnoses of 91% and 50% respectively compared with the numbers predicted from figures for 1983–4 taking account of the larger numbers commencing treatment in the later period.

These trends must also be influenced by the changing demography of patients reported to the Registry. Not only has the proportion of younger patients diminished but the numbers reported has also gone down between 1983–4 and 1993–4. Numbers predicted from the overall increase in new patients were down by 30% for those aged under 15, by 37% for those aged 25–34 and by 27% for those aged 35–54. In patients aged less than 55 there was a 34% fall in cases of glomerulonephritis and a 47% fall in pyelonephritis/interstitial nephritis in 1993–4 compared with predictions based on 1983–4 returns. These reductions were replaced by an increase of over 100% above predicted numbers in patients aged 65 and over. This increase was supported by a 200% rise in patients with renal vascular disease and a 350% rise in those with diabetes compared with 1983–4.

Registry data therefore appears to reinforce the impression of many nephrologists that fewer young patients are presenting with ESRF nowadays compared with 10 years ago. That there is no lack of patients coming forward for treatment is entirely due to the increase of those accepted from the 65 plus age band, and implies a swing towards a population heavily disadvantaged by vascular disease and hypertension and by diabetes.

Uncertain diagnosis

'Chronic renal failure, aetiology uncertain' is the diagnosis placed first in Table 1.1. This is for historic reasons. In the early 1970s this diagnosis was placed at the bottom of the listing of codes, assigned code 99. In those years returns showed a low percentage of patients with this diagnosis, 2.9% for 1973–4, presumably because the form fillers encountered this option only after they had worked through 50 coded alternatives. In the late 1970s the listing of codes was reordered placing 'chronic renal failure, aetiology uncertain' at the top and immediately a higher percentage was coded for this diagnosis. This experience alerted us to an unexpected pitfall in data collection for the results had been changed by reordering the list of codes without altering the phraseology or any other aspect of the printed words. We therefore conclude that both low and high percentages may be influenced by bias arising from data collection instruments and any change in those instruments may invalidate historic comparisons. Fortunately, for the purposes of this review, no other changes have been made in the Registry's methods for data acquisition concerning primary renal diseases, with the exception of the addition of codes for some rare histological types of glomerulonephritis, for tubulo-interstitial nephritis (not pyelonephritis) and for Fabry's disease.

Chronic renal failure, aetiology uncertain accounted for 16.4% of all 1993–4 patients and for one-fifth of those in the 65 plus age group. The increase in percentage of patients with this diagnosis is due largely to the swing to older patients among whom the precise cause of 'end-stage kidney' is not easy to elucidate.

Biopsy rate

The diagnosis of glomerulonephritis (Figure 1.4) was made on 6616 patients in 1973–4. In 1717 (26%) of these the diagnosis was confirmed by histological examination. Of 11 409 patients diagnosed with glomerulonephritis in 1983–4, 4471 (39%) had histological proof and of 9575 in 1993–4, 4051 (42%). Biopsy rate has thus increased over the years. It is higher in children, over three quarters of whom had histological diagnoses in 1983–4 and 1993–4 and in young adults. Over one-third of patients aged over 64 and diagnosed with glomerulonephritis were biopsied in 1983–4. Registry codes for histological diagnoses (Table 1.2) had been driven by research interests rather than an attempt to be comprehensive, and because of this 40% of patients who were histologically examined were classified under the code for glomerulonephritis, histologically examined (specify if you wish). One-quarter of 4036 patients with ESRF who were biopsied had immunoglobulin A (IgA) nephropathy, and 10.5% had membranoproliferative glomerular nephritis type I and 9.0% had membranous nephropathy.

Geographical (Figures 1.5–1.6; Table 1.3)

Europe

There are geographical differences in the pattern of causes of ESRF recorded in Europe. We have illustrated these in Figure 1.5 in which the returns from six

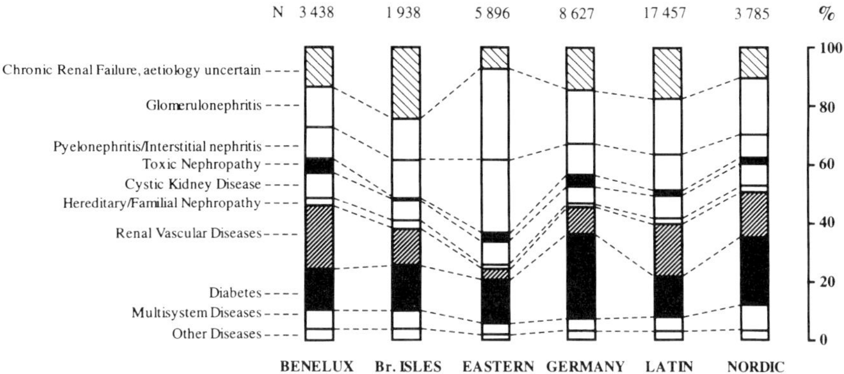

Fig. 1.5 Proportional distribution (%) of causes of end-stage renal failure in patients commencing renal replacement therapy in 1993–4 in six geographic regions: *Benelux* = Belgium, Netherlands, Luxembourg; *British Isles* = U.K., Ireland; *Eastern* = Bulgaria, Czechoslovakia, Hungary, Poland; *Germany* = previously East and West Germany; *Latin* = France, Italy, Portugal, Spain; *Nordic* = Denmark, Finland, Iceland, Norway, Sweden. EDTA data.

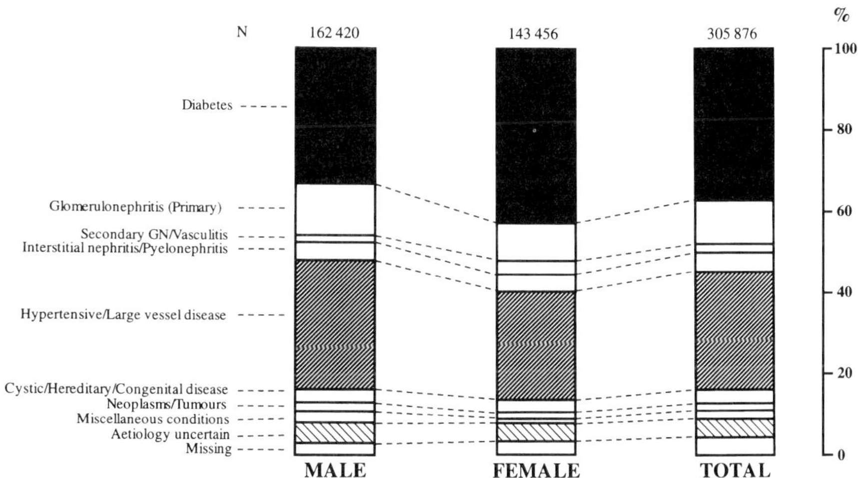

Fig. 1.6 From USRDS 1997 Annual Data Report. Proportional distribution (%) of 10 primary disease categories causing end-stage renal disease in 305 876 patients incident in 1991–5.

geographical regions are shown—Benelux (Belgium, Netherlands, Luxembourg), British Isles (UK, Ireland), Eastern (Bulgaria, Czechoslovakia, Hungary, Poland), Germany (East and West), Latin (France, Italy, Portugal, Spain), Nordic (Denmark, Finland, Iceland, Norway, Sweden). These six regions differ not only in their geography, climate and foodstuffs, but also in ethnic background and economic, and

Table 1.3 Causes (%) of chronic renal failure in India (after ref. 39). Clinical diagnoses in 4837 patients seen in Madras over 10 years, and autopsy diagnoses in 300 patients in Chandigarth

	Madras	Chandigarth
Diabetic nephropathy	30.29	14.04
Chronic glomerulonephritis	11.03	17.70
Systemic diseases including collagen diseases	—	10.00
Focal and segmental glomerulosclerosis	3.58	—
Chronic interstitial nephritis	23.05	12.30
Obstructive uropathy	—	13.04
Chronic pyelonephritis	9.45	—
Nephrosclerosis	10.09	22.07
Polycystic kidney disease	2.27	4.01
Amyloidosis	—	12.04
Renal tuberculosis	—	1.30

therefore health services development. Therefore, differences in the causes of ESRF are likely to be multifactorial.

The high percentage of cases assigned to the diagnosis of chronic renal failure, aetiology uncertain in the British Isles could be influenced by a large proportion of elderly patients and inadequate facilities for investigation allied to cynical scientific realism. The low percentage in eastern European countries suggests that negative selection is important, and the large proportion of cases with glomerulonephritis is typical of a treatment programme in its early years when younger patients predominate. There has been a rapid expansion in facilities in Italy, Portugal, and Spain in the last 20 years and the proportion with glomerulonephritis has fallen from 45% to 19% in Latin countries in that time.

Pyelonephritis/interstitial nephritis is also found more frequently in national programmes at an early stage of development. However, it is possible that there is a variation in diagnostic practice. Among Latin countries in 1993–4 the reported percentage of pyelonephritis/interstitial nephritis ranged between 9% and 12%. This is a narrow band compared with Eastern bloc countries where the proportions spanned 15% to 43%.

Belgium and Germany are known to have a high incidence of analgesic nephropathy and it is therefore not surprising to find that the regions with the highest proportions of toxic nephropathy are Benelux and Germany. Cystic kidney disease presents a clear diagnosis and contributes similar percentages of patients in each of the regions. Heredo-familial nephropathies would not be expected to account for more than a minimal percentage in these programmes dominated by adult patients.

Influenced presumably by the intake of older patients and also possibly by changing diagnostic fashions, renal vascular disease has risen from 7% in 1973–4 to 18% in 1993–4 in Latin countries and from 5% to 22% in Benelux countries. A low proportion is reported from the Eastern bloc. Developments in clinical practice have made it possible to accept more patients with diabetes and in Germany the percentage has risen from 3% in 1973–4 to 29% in 1993–4. In Nordic countries, where there is a high frequency of insulin-dependent diabetes mellitus, it has risen from 6% to 24%.

United States

The USRDS 1998 Annual Data Report [5] contains tabulated information which may be crudely compared with European data (Figure 1.6). The ratio of male to female patients shows a slight preponderance in favour of males, 1.17 : 1.0 which is not so marked as in Europe where it is 1.42 : 1.0 [6].

The treated ESRD population in the USA, with a mean age at incidence of 60 in 1996 is older than the European. In keeping with this, the proportional contributions through the years 1991–5 of diabetes in particular and of hypertensive/large vessel disease are greater than in Europe and that of glomerulonephritis is less. Diabetes has a high frequency in Asian patients (41.6%) and particularly in native Americans (63.2%). As in Europe, glomerulonephritis accounts for a larger proportion of young patients, 31.7% of those aged less than 20 but it is not clear whether all of these are biopsy proven. Interstitial/pyelonephritis is also commoner in the young, 10.8% of those aged less than 20. Polycystic kidney, adult (dominant) accounts for only 2.6% of all new patients in the US, a markedly smaller proportion than that in Europe.

Among the secondary vasculitides, lupus erythematosus, polyarteritis, Wegner's granulomatosis, Henoch–Schönlein syndrome, and scleroderma all appear to be seen at similar frequencies in the USA to those in Europe. Hypertensive/large vessel disease is diagnosed as the primary disease in a larger proportion of ESRD patients in all age groups in the USA and is particularly noted in black people among whom this group of conditions accounts for 35.9% of patients. There is a striking difference in the apportionment to 'miscellaneous conditions', only 2.6% of all cases being placed in this category compared with the European returns of 16.4% for 1993–4. Possibly clinical diagnostic practice differs between the two sides of the Atlantic with a tendency to attribute ESRD to hypertension (no primary renal disease) which accounts for 94% of all hypertensive/large vessel disease cases in the USA, rather than to aetiology uncertain. Our experience with the EDTA–ERA Registry prompts us to draw attention to the fact that in Europe we put chronic renal failure, aetiology uncertain at the head of the code list, whereas in the USA it appears as a final choice.

Australia

In Australia [3] glomerulonephritis has always been the commonest cause of primary renal disease (34%) in patients on RRT, but 24% of the cases were diagnosed without biopsy. IgA mesangial proliferative glomerulonephritis was the most common histologically proven form of glomerulonephritis (32% of biopsy proven glomerulonephritis). Diabetic nephropathy has risen from 12% to 18% over the past 6 years and is the second commonest cause. There was a much higher incidence of diabetic nephropathy among non-Caucasoid patients, particularly Aboriginals, Maoris, and Pacific Islanders many of whom had type II diabetes. Analgesic nephropathy has historically been a significant contributor to ESRD in Australia [12] but, although it still features particularly among older patients, the proportion of all new patients with this condition has fallen from 11% in 1990 to 7% in 1996. Experience of polycystic kidney disease is similar to the European with 7% new cases.

Hypertension is given as the cause of ESRD in 12% of Australian patients but it is pointed out [3] that it is a frequent concomitant observation, but not necessarily the prime causative factor. Therefore, due to altered diagnostic practice and fashion, no otherwise meaningful comment can be based on changes in the reported incidence of hypertensive renal failure among the middle-aged and elderly patients. 'Uncertain diagnosis' comes at the bottom of the list of primary renal diseases in the Australian report [3] and 7% of patients were classified under this in 1996.

Japan

The Japanese Society for Dialysis Therapy has recently reported on the most frequent causes of chronic renal failure in 22 622 patients commencing hemodialysis (or allied treatments) and 1372 commencing continuous ambulatory peritoneal dialysis (CAPD) therapy in 1994 [17]. There was a more marked preponderance of male to female patients, 1.59 : 1.0, than in the other registries. The mean ages at the end of the year for patients who began treatment in 1994 was 61.3 years for hemodialysis patients and 54.1 for CAPD patients.

The commonest cause of chronic renal failure for all new dialysis patients in 1994 in Japan was chronic glomerulonephritis with 40.5%. There has been a progressive rise in the proportion of the stock of dialysed patients who had diabetes from 8.4% in 1984 to 18.2% in 1994 and diabetic nephropathy was the second commonest disease among new patients in 1994 with 30.7%. It is therefore expected that diabetes will someday approach the US level. What is well documented is the excellent survival among Japanese dialysis patients and that this appears unlikely to be due to differences in the case mix of primary renal diseases [18]. Polycystic kidney disease is similar to US rather than European experience with 2.5%.

The diagnosis of nephrosclerosis is used by the Japanese Society without any implication that this is attributed to hypertension. A moderate proportion of 6.1% of 1994 patients had this diagnosis. Systemic lupus erythematosus caused chronic renal failure in 1.4% of patients accepted for CAPD treatment, surprisingly not dissimilar to the European experience. The Society has an equivalent to 'aetiology uncertain' in patients accorded the diagnosis 'nephritis which is impossible to categorize', but unfortunately does not publish its proportional contribution. It is also not clear what proportion of patients diagnosed as having glomerulonephritis had this diagnosis proven by biopsy.

Latin America

The Latin American Registry collects data from 21 countries with a total population of 468.56 million and a wide variation in value of the per capita GNP ($220–8060) and in human development index [19]. The most frequent causes of renal failure in the 10 countries with registered dialysis patients were glomerulopathies (22.6%), vascular nephropathy (20.9%), and diabetes (16.9%). Diabetes was particularly prominent in Puerto Rico and Paraguay whereas glomerulonephritis accounted for a large proportion of patients in Brazil, Panama, and Peru.

Eastern Europe

The Polish Registry has recently recounted its experience of RRT in an era of socio-economic changes following the implosion of the Soviet Bloc [20]. Because of the shortage of dialysis facilities treatment had been restricted for many years to patients below the age 60–65 and with primary nephropathies. Now, with a centralized purchasing arrangement, facilities are expanding and there has been a dramatic increase in the number of patients with diabetic nephropathy, from 4.1% in 1992 to 9.1% in 1995.

Third World

Information on the causes of chronic renal failure in India are available for two large single centres. An analysis of patients seen over 10 years at Madras in southern India has been contrasted with a series of 300 autopsies in patients dying of renal failure in Chandigarth in the north [21]. Diabetic nephropathy, glomerulonephritides, and interstitial/pyelonephritis (including obstructive nephropathy) were encountered with similar frequencies in the two centres. More than 1 in 10 patients in Chandigarth died of amyloidosis, thought to be associated with the high prevalence of tuberculosis. Nephrosclerosis was a particularly frequent pathological diagnosis in Chandigarth. Hypertension has a high prevalence (reported at 8.2%) in urban communities of India, a country of 900 million people predicted to overtake China as the world's most populous country [21]. The scale of the problem appears to be vast.

Ethnic

Non-white Americans are over-represented in the ESRD programme in the USA [22]. In 1995 white people contributed 61.3% of a total of 71 875 new patients, but black people with 29.5% and native Americans with 1.6% and Asian/Pacific Islanders with 3.2% accounted for higher percentages than in the general population. The age-, sex-, and ethnic-specific incidence was 831 p.m.p. for black people, 757 p.m.p. for Native Americans, and 383 p.m.p. for Asian/Pacific Islanders but with 191 p.m.p. white people had a relatively low incidence [5]. The difference in the incidence is attributed to a higher frequency of hypertensive renal disease, particularly in black people [23] and of diabetes in all non-white people.

The non-white populations of European countries represent smaller proportions of their total populations, the result of historic colonial links, and are mostly concentrated in urban areas. Of 771 patients with ESRD treated in one London centre over 26 years the racial distribution showed 79.0% Caucasian, 12.7% Indian subcontinent, 5.6% Caribbean, 1.6% African, and other Asian 1.2% [24]. The contribution of ethnic minorities to renal failure treatment programmes in London were studied throughout the capital by Roderick *et al.* [25]. Incidence was linked to the varying distribution of ethnic minorities in different areas. The observed increment of patients was converted into a factor to predict the incidence of ESRF according to the ethnic mix of the various areas. This work was then extended to a national survey [26]. It is relevant to note that immigrant minorities have a lower age distribution than host populations and therefore with the increasing incidence of renal disease in older age, their contribution to renal failure will increase with the passing of years.

The motive for these studies has been to predict clinical need and to strengthen the case for funding. However, ethnic variations in susceptibility to renal failure are important epidemiological clues in researching the causes of renal diseases and their progression. The possibility that hyperexpression of TGF-β1 occurs in black people and makes renal sclerosis more likely has recently been advanced [16].

Race-specific new acceptances are reported from Australia and New Zealand [3]. In 1996 acceptance of Caucasoid patients in Australia was 69 p.m.p., but from the small Aborigine population it was 288 p.m.p. In New Zealand caucasoid patients were accepted at the rate of 55 p.m.p., but Pacific Islanders at 149 p.m.p. and Maoris at 194 p.m.p. This ethnic effect probably accounts for the fact that diabetic nephropathy was the commonest cause of renal failure (36%) in New Zealand.

Reports from South Africa suggest that IgA nephropathy is rare in black people [27,28]. However, its frequency in series of renal biopsies will be influenced by clinical indications for biopsy, as it is so often found as the cause of renal haematuria and accounts for only a small proportion of cases presenting with the nephrotic syndrome. Similar findings are reported from the Caribbean [29].

In London relatively more patients from the Indian subcontinent presented in terminal renal failure with smooth small kidneys [24] and it has been suggested that tuberculosis may contribute to this excess of cases [30].

The prevention of end-stage renal failure

The epidemiological surveys presented in this chapter show that a progressive change is occurring in the spectrum of patients entering RRT.

Spontaneous change in young patients

The numbers of young patients are diminishing and are being replaced by the acceptance of an increasing number of old patients. Reduction in young patients is occurring mostly because of a reduction in the number of patients with glomerulonephritis reaching ESRF. This could be due to more effective treatment. However, it seems more likely to reflect a change in the impact of infectious agents in developed countries because of improved living standards and nutrition. This would be in keeping with experience over a longer time scale. Deaths due to nephritis in Great Britain have decreased progressively since the beginning of the century. This spontaneous change did not await the availability of antibiotics and was interrupted only by the First World War.

Challenge among the elderly

Increasing numbers of old patients accepted for RRT have renal vascular/hypertension or diabetes as their diagnosis. Dialysis units are becoming geriatric renal care centres. The patients have important co-morbidities which determine ultimate prognosis. More than half of all deaths are due to cardiovascular causes. Both hypertension and diabetes could be ameliorated by better care in earlier years. Classical protocols and methods are already available. Early identification of patients at risk is the advised starting point. The care of blood pressure must be implemented at primary care level to be effective on any important scale. The identification of patients with proteinuria both in the hypertension clinic and the diabetic clinic is important. It is especially so if there are many black patients attending these clinics. Therefore, there is a greater opportunity to make an impact on incidence of ESRF in the inner city and socially deprived areas where most high-risk patients are found.

The mystery of the end-stage kidney

In a large proportion of patients the precise diagnosis is uncertain. We are learning more about progressive loss of renal function in damaged kidneys. There is encouragement that certain hypotensive agents notably angiotensin-converting enzyme inhibitors may slow progressive impairment of function, certainly in diabetics, possibly in other patients. If the scarring process can be slowed by interrupting cytokine actions then it will become urgent to improve screening for patients at an early stage of renal disease.

Acknowledgements

We are grateful to Dr Douglas Briggs for permission to quote data from the EDTA–ERA Registry and to all our colleagues who worked with ourselves on the preparation of reports from the registry. We are all indebted to the clinicians in over 2000 renal centres in Europe on whose returns these are based.

Key references

Disney APS (ed.). *The twenty first report of the Australia and New Zealand Dialysis and Transplant Registry*. The Queen Elizabeth Hospital, Woodville South, Adelaide, South Australia, 1998.

US Renal Data System. *USRDS 1998 Annual Data Report.* National Institues of Health, National Institutes of Diabetes and Digestive and Kidney Diseases, Bethesda, MD, 1998. *Am J Kidney Dis*, 1998; **32** (Suppl 1). S1–S162.

Berthoux F, Bernheim J, Gellet R, Valderrabano F, Carrera F, Cambi V, Mendel S, Saker L,

Jones E. The project of the European Renal Association (ERA-EDTA) for a European nephrological network. *Nephron Dial Transplant*, 1998; **13** (Suppl 1): 30–33.

Jennette JC, *et al.* Nomenclature of systemic vasculitides: proposals of an International Consensus Conference. *Arthritis Rheumatism*, 1994; **37**: 187–192.

Shinzato T, *et al.* Current status of renal replacement therapy in Japan: results of the annual survey of the Japanese Society for Dialysis Therapy. *Nephrol Dial Transplant*, 1997; **12**: 889–898.

References

1. Wing AJ, Brunner FP. Twenty-three years of dialysis and transplantation in Europe: experiences of the EDTA Registry. *Am J Kidney Dis*, 1989; **14**: 341–346.
2. Berthoux F, Bernheim J, Gellet R, Valderrabano F, Carrera F, Cambi V, Mendel S, Saker L, Jones E. The project of the European Renal Association (ERA-EDTA) for a European nephrological network. *Nephron Dial Transplant*, 1998; **13** (Suppl 1): 30–33.
3. Disney APS (ed). *The twenty first report of the Australia and New Zealand Dialysis and Transplant Registry*. The Queen Elizabeth Hospital, Woodville South, Adelaide, South Australia, 1998.
4. Canadian Renal Failure Register. *1988 Report*. Kidney Foundation of Canada, Ottowa, Canada, Ottowa Civic Hospital, 1989.
5. US Renal Data System. *USRDS 1998 Annual Data Report*. National Institues of Health, National Institutes of Diabetes and Digestive and Kidney Diseases, Bethesda, MD, 1998. *Am J Kidney Dis*, 1998; **32** (Suppl 1). S1–S162.
6. Wing AJ. Causes of end stage renal failure. In *Oxford Textbook of Clinical Nephrology*. (ed. S Cameron, AM Davison, J-P Grünfeld, D Kerr and E Ritz), pp. 1227–36. Oxford University Press, Oxford, 1992.
7. Elseviers MM, Waller I, Nenov D, *et al.* Evaluation of diagnostic criteria for analgesic nephropathy in patients with end-stage renal failure: results of the ANNE study. *Nephrol Dial Transplant*, 1995; **10**: 808–814.
8. Jennette JC, *et al.* Nomenclature of systemic vasculitides: proposals of an International Consensus Conference. *Arthritis Rheumatism*, 1994; **37**: 187–192.
9. Challah S, Wing AJ. The epidemiology of genito-urinary disease. In *Oxford Textbook of Public Health*, Vol. 4. (ed. WW Holland, R Detels, and G Knox), pp. 181–202. Oxford University Press, Oxford, 1985.
10. Heptinstall RH. The limitations of the pathological diagnosis of chronic pyelonephritis. In *Renal Disease*, 2nd edn. (ed. DAK Black), pp. 350–81. Blackwell Scientific Publications, Oxford; 1967.
11. Spühler O, Zollinger HU. Die chronische interstielle Nephritis. *Z Klin Med*, 1953; **151**: 1–50.
12. Nanra RS, *et al.* Analgesic nephropathy: aetiology, clinical syndrome and clinico pathologic correlations in Australia. *Kidney Int*, 1978; **13**: 79–92.
13. Wing AJ, *et al.* Contribution of toxic nephropathies to end stage renal failure in Europe: a report from the EDTA registry. *Toxicol Lett*, 1989; **46**: 281–292.
14. Polenakovic MH, Stefanovic V. Blakan nephropathy. In *Oxford Textbook of Clinical Nephrology*. (ed. S Cameron, AM Davison, J-P Grünfeld, D Kerr and E Ritz), pp. 857–66. Oxford University Press, Oxford, 1992.
15. Brunner FP. End stage renal failure due to diabetic nephropathy: data from the EDTA Registry. *J Diabetic Complications*, 1989; **3**: 127–135.

16. Suthanthiram M, Khanna A, Cukram D, Adhikarla R, Sharma VK, Singh T, August P. Transforming growth factor-β_1 hyperexpression in African American end stage renal disease patients. *Kidney Int*, 1989; **53**: 639–644.
17. Shinzato T, *et al.* Current status of renal replacement therapy in Japan: results of the annual survey of the Japanese Society for Dialysis Therapy. *Nephrol Dial Transplant*, 1997; **12**: 889–898.
18. Held PJ, Brunner FP, Odaka M, Garaia JR, *et al.* Five year survival for end stage renal disease patients in the United States, Europe and Japan, 1982–1987. *Am J Kidney Dis*, 1990; **15**: 451–457.
19. Mazzuchi N, Schwedt E, Fernandez JM, *et al.* Latin American Registry of dialysis and renal transplantation: 1993 annual dialysis data report. *Nephrol Dial Transplant*, 1997; **12**: 2521–2527.
20. Rutkowski B, *et al.* Renal replacement therapy in an era of socio economic changes—report from the Polish Registry. *Nephrol Dial Transplant*, 1997; **12**: 1105–1108.
21. Mani MK. The aetiology of end stage renal disease: its implications for the patient and the profession. *Saudi J. Kidney Dis Transplant*, 1997; **8**: 405–409.
22. Rostand SG, Kirk KA, Rutsky EA, Pate BA. Racial differences in the incidence of treatment for end stage renal disease. *N Engl J Med*, 1982; **306**: 1276–1279.
23. Rostand SG, Brown G, Kirk KA, Rutsky EA, Dustan HP. Renal insufficiency in treated essential hypertension. *N Engl J Med*, 1989; **320**: 684–688.
24. Pazianas M, Eastwood JB, MacRae KD, Phillips ME. Racial origin and primary renal diagnosis in 771 patients with end stage renal disease. *Nephrol Dial Transplant*, 1991, **6**: 931–935.
25. Roderick PJ, Jones I, Raleigh VS, McGeown M, Mallik NP. Population need for renal replacement therapy in Thames regions: ethnic dimension. *Br Med Journal*, 1994; **309**: 1111–1114.
26. Roderick PJ, Raleigh VS, Hallam L, Mallik NP. The need and demand for renal replacement therapy in ethnic minorities in England. *J Epidemiol Community Health*, 1996; **50**: 334–339.
27. Seedat YK, Nathoo BC, Parag KB, Naiker PI, Ramsaroop R. IgA nephropathy in Blacks and Indians of Natal. *Nephron*, 1988; **50**: 137–141.
28. Swanepoel CR, Madaus S, Cassidy MJD, *et al.* IgA nephropathy—Groote Schuur Hospital experience. *Nephrology*, 1989; **53**: 61–64.
29. Alleyene GAO. Renal disease in Africa and Caribbean: an overview. *Transplant Proc*, 1987; **19** (Suppl 2): 9–14.
30. Eastwood JB, Zaidi M, Maxwell JD, Wing AJ, Pazanias M. Tuberculosis as primary renal diagnosis in end stage uremia. *J Nephrol*, 1994; **7**: 290–293.

2

Natural history and factors affecting the progression of human renal diseases

Francesco Locatelli and Lucia Del Vecchio

Introduction

Following renal injury, a progressive deterioration in renal function generally occurs, regardless of the nature of the original nephropathy. In some patients, the disease process responsible for the initial renal injury may remain active throughout the progression of renal failure. However, in the majority of cases, renal failure progresses after a well-defined initiating process has remitted spontaneously or has been therapeutically controlled.

The mechanisms involved in the progression of chronic renal failure (CRF) have been extensively investigated and are fully discussed in Chapters 3–6. It has been found that a number of physiological and metabolic changes may contribute towards progressive renal destruction and that various intercurrent events may accelerate the deterioration of renal function. The detection and correction of these events may slow the progression of CRF and delay the need for dialysis. For that, a better understanding of the natural history of CRF and that of the underlying nephropathies as well as the factors that influence their progression is crucial. This chapter aims to define the natural history of chronic renal diseases and discuss some of the factors known to influence their progression.

Assessment of renal function in progressive renal diseases

Although CRF usually progresses towards end-stage renal disease (ESRD) in the majority of cases, the rate of decline in the glomerular filtration rate (GFR) varies between groups of patients with different nephropathies, but also among patients with the same disease.

It is generally believed that renal function is lost at a constant rate, suggesting a continuous process. In the late seventies Rutherford *et al.* [1] and Mitch *et al.* [2] described the rate of progression of patients with CRF from various diseases and found straight line relationships between time and the reciprocal of the serum creatinine (1/Cr) concentration. However, it was already clear from these original observations that some patients displayed a non-linear rate of progression, independently of any therapeutic intervention. Rutherford *et al.* [1]

reported non-linearity for 10 of 63 sequences, whereas Mitch *et al.* [2] considered three of 34 sequences to be non-linear. Subsequent studies found that the non-linear rate of progression is a common feature of the 'natural history' of CRF [3–5]. By linear regression analysis, Shah and Levey [3] searched for spontaneous changes in the slope (breakpoints) of 77 patients with an apparent constant rate of decline and identified significant changes in one-third to one-half of the patients. These changes could be either spontaneous or related to intercurrent events, such as infections, dehydration, or insufficient blood pressure control. Furthermore, in immunologically mediated glomerular disease, the pathophysiological mechanisms that initiate and perpetuate renal damage may act during the course of the disease in a discontinuous fashion.

Assessing the rate of progression of CRF is useful not only for prognostic purposes, but also for establishing the effect of therapy on the natural history of renal disease. However, most of the clinical studies to evaluate the progression of CRF have been widely criticized for being inadequate and statistically misleading. Main problems are linked to the large variability of patient sample due to the different individual progression rates and to the very long time necessary to establish the progression rates with sufficient likelihood. Furthermore, a great debate exists on the appropriate method to measure renal function and the progression rate. A number of markers, which can be divided into direct and indirect ones, have been proposed to assess renal function. 'Direct' markers (i.e. true GFR, creatinine clearance, serum creatinine and reciprocal of serum creatinine) reflect renal function itself and are not time-related, whereas 'indirect' markers (i.e. need of RRT, doubling of serum creatinine, and halving of GFR) indicates the time up to a certain degree of renal functional impairment is reached [6].

True glomerular filtration rate

Repeated measurements of the renal clearance of inulin or radioisotopes are generally accepted as the 'gold standard' for measuring true GFR in patients with CRF. The advantages of the use of true GFR as an index of severity and progression of renal failure is that it is a direct measure of renal function [7], it is reduced early in the course of renal disease, and it also correlates with the severity of renal histological findings, such as tubulo-interstitial scarring [8].

Inulin is an ideal filtration marker because it is freely filtered by the glomeruli and it is not secreted, reabsorbed, synthesized, or metabolized by the tubule. The classical inulin clearance method include continuous intravenous infusion of inulin, urine collection by bladder catheterization, and measurements under standard conditions [7]. Therefore, this method is not practical for clinical practice or research. As a consequence, alternative filtration markers have been developed. In the US, the most widely used markers are ^{125}I-iothalamate and ^{99m}Tc-diethylenetriaminepenta-acetic acid (DPTA), whereas in Europe ^{51}Cr-ethylenediaminetetra-acetic acid is also available. Radionucleotide labeling permits accurate detection of minute doses of these markers in plasma and urine with minimal radiation exposure. Simultaneous measurements of renal inulin clearance and plasma clearance of these three markers have yielded similar results [9,10]. However, these methods require expensive and time-consuming laboratory techniques and many difficulties arise when they are used in large-scale, long-term, multicentre trials requiring renal function measurements every 2–3 months. Furthermore, large circadian and day-to-day variations of GFR have been observed [11,12], leading to some concern about reproducibility of sequential determination of GFR.

Simplified techniques for estimating GFR have been proposed to determine accurately and safely the level of renal function at reasonable cost. After a single intravenous injection of minute doses of non-radioactive iothalamate [13] or iohexol [14], plasma clearance of these markers is estimated by multiple blood samples. It seems that the renal clearance of these two X-ray tracers is similar to inulin clearance in normal subjects and in patients with CRF [15,16].

Serum creatinine

The measurement of serum creatinine (S_{Cr}) is the simplest and most commonly used measure of renal function in every-day clinical practice. However, in patients with early renal failure, large decrements in GFR produce only small increases in S_{Cr}, whereas in patients with advanced renal failure, small changes in GFR produce large changes in S_{Cr}. Furthermore, S_{Cr} level is determined by its rate of production, its volume of distribution, and its rate of excretion. With the onset of CRF, creatinine production and volume of distribution may not be stable, creatinine secretion may be significant, and extrarenal excretion of creatinine may occur [17]. It must also be remembered that dietary and blood pressure control interventions can affect creatinine secretion and excretion, as well as GFR [18]. It has been shown that restricting protein intake reduces creatinine secretion and excretion, whereas lowering blood pressure preserves creatinine secretion. These factors can lead to misleading results if the rate of progression is assessed by means of endogenous creatinine clearance or serum creatinine measurements. These tests are all the more unreliable determinants of renal function in unstable patients with muscular mass and changes in protein and caloric intakes.

Although S_{Cr} is not considered an accurate marker of renal function, repeated measurements of S_{Cr} levels over a long period of follow-up have been used for the assessment of the rate of progression. Indeed, some authors have found a good correlation between S_{Cr} and radioisotopic measurements of GFR [19,20]. Interestingly enough, it has also been demonstrated that the coefficient of variation of radioisotopic clearance in advanced CRF is 12%, whereas that of S_{Cr} is 6.3%; thus suggesting that serial measurements of S_{Cr} may be more precise than radioisotopic clearance when comparing renal function variations in the same patient [21].

De Santo *et al.* [22] also showed that creatinine clearance (C_{Cr}) (calculated using the Cockcroft and Gault formula [23]) correlated closely with true GFR measured by inulin clearance in patients with impaired renal function, and provided a better correlation with inulin clearance than the use of measured C_{Cr} based on 24-h urine collection.

Creatinine clearance

The most commonly used method to estimate GFR in clinical practice is the measurement of creatinine clearance. However, it has been shown that the measurements of C_{Cr} are highly variable in the individual patients, mainly because of difficulties to obtain a proper collection of urine [24]. Furthermore, as serum creatinine levels, C_{Cr} is influenced by creatinine production and elimination. When renal function is impaired, C_{Cr} tend to overestimate the GFR, perhaps up to 15%, and this percentage tends to increase as GFR decreases and tubular secretion of creatinine accounts for larger proportions of creatinine in the urine. Cimetidine competitively inhibits tubular secretion of creatinine, without influencing GFR, thereby reducing the overestimation of GFR by C_{Cr}. It has been shown that, after the administration of cimetidine, C_{Cr} can equal inulin clearance [25]. However, even with a daily maximal cimetidine dose of 2000 mg, in some patients, it was not possible to maintain complete inhibition of tubular creatinine secretion during 24 h [11].

Donadio *et al.* [26] recently proposed a method to predict C_{Cr} from S_{Cr} and from the values of body cell mass obtained by means of bioimpedance data, thus avoiding urine collection. This method showed a better agreement with GFR (measured as renal clearance of ^{99m}Tc-DPTA) and a lower variability of its measurements than C_{Cr}. Indeed, the coefficient of variation of duplicate measurements of C_{Cr} by means of body cell mass was 6.2%, whereas the coefficient of variation of C_{Cr} ,calculated by means of 24-h urine collection, was 20.8%.

Reciprocal of serum creatinine and the logarithm of serum creatinine versus time

As reported above, Mitch *et al.* [2] and Rutherford *et al.* [1] initially observed that in the majority of individual patients with CRF, the rate of change in S_{Cr} was quite orderly and that rate could be quantitated using simple linear regression analysis of plotted data as logarithm of S_{Cr} (log Cr) or 1/Cr versus time. If creatinine excretion ($U_{Cr} \times V$) remains constant, a linear decline in 1/Cr with time indicates a linear decrease in C_{Cr} with time, suggesting that nephrons are lost at a constant rate, whereas the straight line relationship between log Cr and time suggests that nephrons are lost at a constant fractional rate [1]. More patients had courses of the disease described by a single straight line on the reciprocal plot than on the logarithm plot [1]. Thereafter, the slope of the inverse of serum creatinine versus time has been extensively used to quantify the progression of chronic renal diseases [27,28]. However, this model has been widely criticized, because it assumes a constant ratio of the tubular secretion and glomerular filtration of creatinine, stable extra-renal metabolism and an unchanged lean body mass, which is not usually the case in patients with long-lasting CRF [21,29]. It has been demonstrated that creatinine excretion declines in advanced renal failure. As 1/Cr decreases linearly even in severe CRF, the rate of decline in C_{Cr} should accelerate at the end-stage of CRF [2]. Consequently, there should be a greater chance of encountering patients with a faster decline in renal function at higher serum creatinine levels, regardless of the nature of the underlying nephropathy. As the reciprocal of a large number is a small fraction, in those patients with two apparent rates of progression, the second slope may be hardly detected on the reciprocal plot [1]. Therefore, to predict the time when transplantation or dialysis would be required, the plot of log Cr versus time might be more useful, allowing to detect more easily the second slope [1].

The slope of 1/Cr versus time may also be inadequate to evaluate the efficacy of a therapeutic trial: the apparent straight line of the reciprocal plot may lead to interpret an ineffective regimen as being beneficial [1]. Furthermore, the analysis of data derived from large clinical trials have shown different results when rates of progressions were considered as single or double slopes. In the Modification of Diet in Renal Disease (MDRD) study [30], a large trial aimed at examining the effects of low protein intake and strict blood pressure control in 840 patients with various renal diseases, a non-linear slope of 1/Cr versus time was found in the group of patients with moderate CRF who received both low protein diet and strict blood pressure control. A small but statistically significant reduction in GFR was found during the first 4 months of follow-up; thereafter a significant reduction in the steepness of the GFR slope was observed ($p = 0.009$ and $p = 0.006$, respectively). Using a single-slope model, the low protein diet and strict blood pressure control did not show any beneficial effect on CRF progression while analysis relying on a two-slope model did.

In the Angiotensin-converting Enzyme Inhibition in Progressive Renal Insufficiency (AIPRI) study [32], a similar behaviour of the rate of CRF progression was observed in the patients who had been randomized to benazepril, who displayed an initial faster decline in renal function in comparison with the placebo. Analysing the findings of this study, it was evident that the average time needed to demonstrate a beneficial effect of this angiotensin-converting enzyme (ACE) inhibitor on the rate of progression increases as patients with more slowly progressive disease are considered, whereas the initial apparent negative effect of benazepril persisted over different times. Considering the curve of renal survival after 6 months, the apparent negative effect of benazepril lasted all over this period and the beneficial effect in slowing down the rise in serum creatinine was not evident; in the cohorts that did not reach an end-point at 12, 24, and 36 months, the apparent negative effect lasted respectively 4, 9, and 25 months and the beneficial effect of treatment on serum creatinine became evident thereafter. This means that in some patients not only a very long time is needed to establish the true progression, but also that any spontaneous or therapeutically induced modification of the course of their disease could take years before reaching the previous slope of progression. Subsequently, there could be again a different ratio of progression in comparison with the placebo regression line (slower in case of a positive therapeutic intervention). Therefore, without the knowledge of this pathophysiological behaviour, one could consider negative the effect of some therapeutic intervention able to improve renal survival in the long term. Thus, caution is warranted in analysing the effects of any treatment on renal function in studies with a follow-up period that do not take into account the extreme variability of the rate of progression in CRF and that the effect of spontaneous or therapeutic-induced modification in renal function deterioration could last for a long time.

The 'breakpoint' analysis

The statistical problem of estimating whether or not a series of data depart from a linear model at an unknown point (breakpoint) is an important issue in the analysis of the effect of factors influencing CRF progression. The 'breakpoint' test was proposed to identify one or more breakpoints of a line which suddenly changes slope [32]. This test was based on a four-parameter linear regression involving three linear parameters and one non-linear parameter: the breakpoint was identified as the value of the non-linear parameter that minimized the residual sum of squares and the hypothesis that the broken line was a significantly better fit than the straight line was then tested with an F-test based on the extra-sum of square principle. Zoccali *et al.* [4] applied this method to retrospectively study the progression of CRF and found that, although 1/Cr was significantly better fitted by a single straight line in 11 patients, in the remaining six cases the progression was non-linear.

The advantage of this method is that it allows variable levels of significance to be attributed to the effect of intervening factors in individual patients.

Interestingly, a re-analysis of studies of the efficacy of the low-protein diet by means of the breakpoint test has shown that in about 26% of cases the favourable effect attributed to a low-protein diet may simply reflect a fluctuation due to the variability of the data, rather than a true slowing in the progression rate [4].

Renal end-points and their evaluation

Usually the end-point of a patient with CRF is the need for dialysis. However, many patients display a slow rate of progression and many years are then needed to reach this 'hard' end-point. Consequently, in clinical trials lasting no more than 4–5 years, many patients may never reach ESRD. For this reason other 'surrogate' end-points have been proposed, such as the doubling of S_{Cr} from baseline or the decline (or increase in S_{Cr}) of 25% or 50% over baseline. However, considering the 11% coefficient of variation (i.e. the ratio of the standard deviation to the mean) of serum creatinine in subjects with normal renal function [33], a 25% increase of S_{Cr} does not seem adequate to detect true modifications of renal function. There are several advantages of using time to doubling of S_{Cr} instead of the slope of GFR with time [34]. Using time to doubling of S_{Cr}, it is not necessary to assume the decline of renal function to be linear. Furthermore, the slope of GFR with time needs of several measurements of renal function over a period of time, preferentially years, and therefore patients dropping out of a study after shorter periods of follow-up are not eligible for evaluation. In contrast, all patients with at least two measurements of S_{Cr} are eligible in an analysis of time to doubling of S_{Cr}.

In the AIPRI study [31], only two of the 583 enrolled patients (0.34%) reached the need for dialysis after a 3-year follow-up, whereas the most common outcome event was the doubling of the baseline serum creatinine level ($n = 86$, 14%). The proportion of patients reaching the primary end-point (the need for dialysis or the doubling of the baseline serum creatinine) was lower in the benazepril group than in the placebo group ($n = 31$, 10% and $n = 57$, 20% respectively). An extension of the AIPRI study has been performed to identify the number of patients reaching the need of dialysis or renal death during a longer follow-up (median total follow-up of 6.6 years) [35]. Interestingly, considering the whole follow-up, 31% of the patients reached the need for dialysis or had a renal-related death ($n = 79$, 26.3% in the benazepril group; $n = 102$, 36% in the placebo group). Although caution is needed in evaluating these findings, as during the extension period treatment was not randomized but left to the discretion of physicians, the former end-point may be considered as a good and useful marker of CRF progression.

In patients with normal GFR, the onset of CRF or the fall in urine protein excretion of 50% or 100% compared with baseline may also be considered as end-points.

The simplest way of evaluating the efficacy of a treatment modality is by counting the number of end-points reached in each group. These counts may be evaluated by a χ^2 test. However, this approach neglects the time of occurrence of end-points, which could be of importance if there are significant time-related effects [6].

Thus, data of studies on CRF progression have often been analysed with survival analysis, to describe time to any well-defined end-point [36]. The likelihood of renal survival is usually expressed with the actuarial method which is based on the question, applied for each day of observation time, 'which is the actual chance of surviving *N* days after you have survived *N*–1 days?'. This is a rather accurate method of description of a set of data, as it introduces a correction for the number of patients exposed to the risk of reaching the renal end-point [37]. Furthermore, this approach allows to build the survival curves, which are a good graphical and easy-to-understand way of presenting results. These curves may show whether there are major subgroups, which usually result in a plateau formation or a change in the slope of the curve. As a summary of the survival experience, the median survival is available. Survival analysis requires completeness of follow-up (sometimes practical difficulties are met in making the period of observation as complete as possible) and an initial event that must be clearly established and identifiable in all patients. Therefore, this analysis is better used in prospective studies.

Comparing surviving of different groups can be done by parametric and non-parametric analyses [36]. The log-rank test [38] is based on the comparison between the number of observed and expected events in a group being analysed under the null hypothesis that there should be no difference in event rate between the different groups of patients. The rationale of log-rank test is that the number of events (whatever the time of observation) should be equally divided among the various groups and it should be proportional to the number of patients exposed to the risk of reaching the end-point.

The quantitative impact of confounding factors, such as age, gender, hypertension, on the progression of the renal disease can be assessed by the Cox regression analysis [39]. This model is a way to look at the effect of each prognostic factor, considered to remain constant over time, adjusted for all the others [40]. It allows to identify those covariates that independently and significantly influence renal survival. The major advantage of this approach is that it takes into account patient drop-outs with different follow-up duration. However, it should be noted that comparing survival curves is only valid if about 70% of the patients have reached an end-point [41]. This is all too often neglected in the survival analyses of clinical trials.

Artificial neural networks

Artificial neural networks (ANNs) are layers of interconnected computer processors (nodes) whose structure and function are historically based on biological neural networks. ANNs are able to generalize from the input data to patterns inherent in the data, and to use these patterns to make predictions or to classify. In medicine they have been applied to a number of problems, including classification of EEG patterns, early diagnosis of myocardial infarction, and treatment of hypertension. Recently, ANNs have also been used to predict outcome in some renal diseases, trying to assess the role of various risk factors. Cattran *et al.* [42] have described a model to predict outcome in a semiquantitative fashion in patients with membranous nephropathy. After selecting the best potential predictors of CRF progression, such as the level of persistent proteinuria, the slope of creatinine clearance over time and the creatinine clearance at the start of the period of observation (6 months), they developed an algorithm, able to identify for each patient a risk score of progression to CRF. The overall accuracy of the model was 85%, compared with 52% using the nephrotic syndrome level of proteinuria at biopsy alone. Furthermore, when the patient's slope were varied by ±20% (the expected range of error in clinical practice), the mean change in the risk score was only 1.2%. An ANN was also able potentially to predict 7-year outcome for renal function in immunoglobulin A nephropathy (IgAN) more accurately than experienced nephrologists, thus allowing early identification of high-risk patients requiring close follow-up [43].

The effect of specific primary disease processes on the natural history of chronic renal failure

Over the last years, a number of studies have stressed the importance of the underlying disease as a factor determining the rate of progression of CRF, thus suggesting the possibility of disease-specific pathogenic mechanisms.

It seems that diabetic nephropathy (DN), polycystic kidney disease (PKD) and chronic glomerulonephritis (CGN) are more progressive than chronic interstitial nephritis (CIN), and hypertensive nephrosclerosis (HNS), although the results reported in the literature are equivocal. These differences can probably be explained by the fact that some of the authors only considered crude cumulative renal survival of the different nephropathies, without taking into account concomitant risk factors. Using the doubling of the baseline serum creatinine or the need for dialysis as primary end-points, and taking into account all of the known factors affecting the progression of CRF, Locatelli *et al.* [44] found that PKD and HNS had a relative renal death risk of 2.47 and 3.55 respectively in comparison with CIN. However, after taking into account the different baseline levels of renal function, multivariate analysis showed that PKD was as progressive as HNS (the 95% confidence intervals of renal death and relative risk were respectively 1.10–5.53 and 1.52–8.29 versus interstitial nephritis), whereas CGN had a statistically non-significant higher relative risk than CIN. After taking into account baseline 24-h proteinuria, the relative risk for progression in CGN patients was not significantly higher than in those with CIN (but proteinuria is a very frequent finding in CGN). It therefore seems difficult to analyse the importance of the underlying disease separately from the main risk factors for progression, by eliminating the influence of important determinants of CRF progression; multivariate analysis may also give misleading results.

Moreover, in these studies, the rate of decline in GFR was measured using different methods, not allowing comparisons [45]. Another confounding factor may be the degree of baseline CRF in the patients selected in these studies. Indeed, baseline S_{Cr} has been identified as an important factor associated with CRF progression, with a significantly higher rate of progression in the patients with more severe baseline CRF [44]. These findings have not been confirmed in the Ramipril Efficacy in Nephropathy (REIN) study [46], possibly because only patients with heavy proteinuria (more than 3 g/24 h), therefore fast progressive, have been analysed. By the way, no data were given in this study on rates of progression before randomization (run in = 1 month).

Jungers *et al.* [47] analysed retrospectively the effect of primary renal disease on the rate of renal function decline in patients with chronic renal disease. The slope

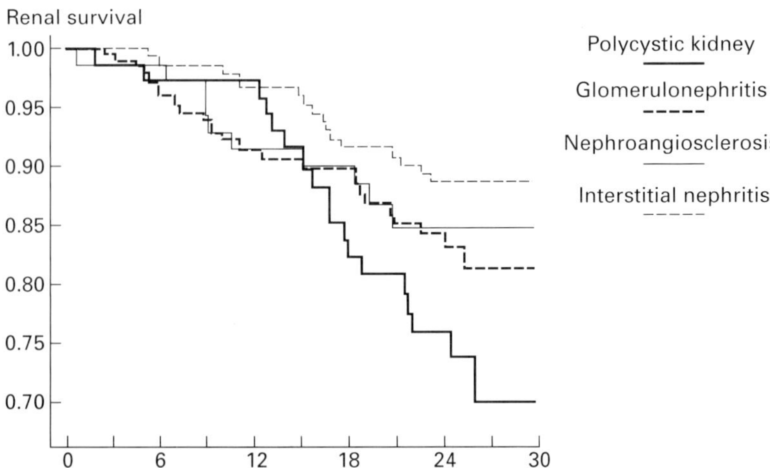

Fig. 2.1 Actuarial renal survival rates according to the underlying disease in 433 patients with CRF [45].

of the decline in creatinine clearance (ΔCcr) was 2.5 times higher in patients with CGN (mean ΔCcr 9.9 ± 6.5 ml/min per 1.73 m^2 per year) than in patients with CIN (mean ΔCcr 3.9 ± 2 ml/min per 1.73 m^2 per year), and 1.5 times higher than in those with PKD (mean ΔCcr 6 ± 2.5 ml/min per 1.73 m^2 per year) or HNS (mean ΔCcr 5.5 ± 2.4 ml/min per 1.73 m^2 per year). By multivariate analysis the type of nephropathy was the most significant factor affecting CRF progression among the nominal variables ($F = 4.25$, $p = 0.006$), while proteinuria was the only continuous variable identified as an independent factor. Interestingly, a considerably greater interindividual ΔCcr variability was found in patients with CGN; the distribution was more homogeneous in those with PKD, CIN, or vascular disease.

Other authors have reported a lower rate of progression in CIN and PKD than in glomerular or vascular kidney disease [48–50]. Even in the advanced phases of CRF, the rate of progression has been shown to be markedly influenced by the type of nephropathy: the ΔCcr is steeper in Alport's syndrome (AS) than in CGN and HNS, and steeper in HNS than in PKD and CIN [52].

Other studies have suggested that PKD is the most progressive chronic kidney disease.

By measuring the doubling in plasma creatinine levels in comparison with baseline, Locatelli *et al.* [44] found that the progression of CRF in patients with PKD, CGN, and CIN was respectively sevenfold (0.0704 mg/dl per month), threefold (0.0360 mg/dl per month), and twice (0.0203 mg/dl per month) as high as in patients with HNS (0.0102 mg/dl per month), regardless of their baseline renal function values.

On the basis of a univariate analysis of underlying renal diseases, the AIPRI Study also showed that only a small proportion of patients with HNS (2% in the benazepril group and 4% in the placebo group) or CIN (5% and 8%) reached an end-point, whereas the proportion was high in those with PKD (27% and 26%) or CGN (12% and 27%), and even higher in those with DN (17% and 47%) [31].

In the MDRD study, the rate of progression was higher in the patients with PKD than in those with all of the other conditions taken as a whole [30]. The rate of progression of PKD detected in this large trial was similar to that observed by Jungers *et al.* [47] (5.9 vs 6 ml/min per 1.73 m^2 per year), although the later study found that the rate of progression of PKD was less than that of the other renal diseases.

Wight *et al.* [52] retrospectively analysed the rate of CRF progression (ascertained from the slopes of $1/S_{Cr}$ versus time) in 102 patients with moderate to severe CRF, and obtained similar findings. Patients with CGN and PKD had faster rates of progression when compared with the other groups. HNS displayed the slowest rate of progression. When proteinuria and, to a lesser extent, hemoglobin, were taken into consideration, the rate of progression of CGN was comparable to the other diseases, while patients with PKD maintained a faster rate of progression compared with the other groups ($p = 0.0037$).

Franz and Reubi [53] analysed the course of PKD in 44 patients at different stages of affection and found that renal function did not decrease at a constant rate between birth and ESRD: it remained well preserved for many years but decreased rapidly at a later stage. These findings may partially explain the different rate of progression of PKD described in various studies. Indeed, after having taking in account the different risk factors for progression of renal function in the multivariate analysis, Locatelli *et al.* [46] found that patients with PKD had a relatively lower risk of renal death.

Factors influencing the progression of chronic renal diseases

Age

Elderly patients constitute an increasing segment of the ESRD population beginning renal replacement therapy (RRT) in Western countries, but there is still a lack of studies concerning CRF in the elderly.

The decline in renal function in the elderly

Although a number of past studies have demonstrated an inexorable decline in renal function in the elderly, it is now accepted that ageing is associated with more subtle changes in renal function indices, such as a reduction in effective renal plasma flow (ERPF) [55] and an increase in the filtration fraction (FF) [55,56].

It is assumed that a loss of renal mass occurs with ageing. Indeed at sonography, renal size decreases with age, almost entirely because of parenchymal reduction [57]. Tissue involution occurs primarily in the renal cortex, with relative sparing of the renal medulla [58]. Morphological studies have demonstrated sclerosis of 10–30% of the total glomerular population between the fourth and eight decade of life [59]. In addition, a high prevalence of renal vasculature abnormalities have been reported, such as a tapering of the interlobular and increased tortuosity of the intralobular arteries [62]. Increased dietary protein intake and atherosclerotic vascular disease have been mentioned as possible causes of age-related glomerulosclerosis [58]. Kasiske [61] reported that both age and intrarenal vascular disease were highly significantly and independently associated with glomerulosclerosis, and that individuals with more severe systemic atherosclerosis had a greater degree of intrarenal vascular disease. It was therefore suggested that arterial lumen narrowing may give rise to ischemia and/or thrombosis, causing subsequent glomerular damage.

In line with these morphological data, a number of studies reported that GFR and ERPF declined markedly with age even in the absence of renal disease [62–64], and it was assumed that, at the age of 80 years, the GFR is nearly 50% of the values recorded after puberty [62,65]. However, more recent studies have not confirmed the first reports concerning a marked reduction of GFR in the elderly. The Baltimore Longitudinal Study on Aging was the first to reveal that GFR, measured in terms of creatinine clearance, was not decreased at all in nearly one-third of apparently healthy elderly subjects [66]. The more recent Bronx Longitudinal Aging Study [67] also reached similar conclusions: renal function (evaluated by serum creatinine values) was stable over a 3-year period in the majority of the 500 subjects evaluated. Other studies have reported that GFR decreases from approximately 120 ml/min per $1.73\,m^2$ at the beginning of the fourth decade to about 90 ml/min per $1.73\,m^2$ in the sixth decade, and it remains virtually stable thereafter [68,69]. Fliser *et al.* [54] have very recently confirmed these findings: in healthy elderly individuals with a mean age of 68 years, the mean GFR was above 100 ml/min per 1.73 m^2 and remained within the normal range in two-thirds of the population studied. The Baltimore Longitudinal Study on Aging found that a decrease in GFR was primarily associated with cardiovascular diseases. GFR was significantly lower in elderly patients with mild compensated heart failure and hypertension than in normotensive healthy elderly subjects [70]. Fliser *et al.* [54] confirmed a lower GFR in subjects with heart failure. Multiple regression analysis showed that GFR was affected by age and heart failure, but not by mean arterial blood pressure (MAP). Hypertensive subjects were found to have a more marked decrease in ERPF and increase in FF than normotensives.

Ageing is also associated with changes in other indices of renal function. The ERPF is reduced proportionally more than GFR, and vasodilatation in response to an amino acid load (the so-called renal functional reserve) is diminished [55]. As a consequence, even in healthy elderly subjects the FF is increased [54]. Selective loss of cortical renal mass and preservation of juxtamedullary nephrons with higher FF may explain at least in part the rise in FF with age [55]. It would therefore seem that, by itself, age-related glomerulosclerosis poses no threat to the well-being of healthy subjects. But the finding of a well preserved GFR in the healthy elderly, despite the assumed decrease in renal mass with age, would imply that hyperfiltration takes place in the remaining nephrons. This, in the presence of systemic hypertension or an intrinsic renal disease, could accelerate the progression of underlying glomerulosclerosis.

Age and the progression of chronic renal failure

It has been shown that the incidence of renal failure from various renal diseases increases with age [71–73]. In a prospective study performed to determine the age-related incidence of advanced CRF in two areas of England, 51% of the 210 patients identified were over 70 years old. The age-related incidence rose from 58 patients/million population per year in those aged 20–49 to 588 patients/million population per year in those aged 80 or over [71]. Also in a prospective epidemiological study performed in a large French urban area, the overall annual incidence of CRF was nearly six times higher in patients aged 60–74 years (523/million population per year) and nearly seven times higher in those aged ≥75 years (619/million population per year), in comparison with a group aged less than 40 years (92/million population per year) [73]. This increase is most apparent in males, with an incidence peaking at 1124/million population per year in men aged over 75. Among this population, 251 patients were followed-up for 1 year. The proportion of patients who reached ESRD and started RRT was lower in the group aged ≥75 years than in younger patients (28% vs 48%, $p < 0.02$), while the proportion of patients who died before reaching ESRD was, as expected, higher in the older group (18% vs 5%, $p < 0.01$). In support of these observations, a growing incidence of ESRD in elderly patients has been observed in many countries [75–77].

Vascular disease and diabetes are the most frequent causes of ESRD in elderly patients, accounting for nearly 30–40% of the elderly subjects starting RRT in some

European countries [77] and for nearly 60% of the elderly subjects starting RRT in the US [74]. This is explained not only by a higher prevalence of these conditions with age, but also by an increased susceptibility to the development of renal complications.

Primary glomerulonephritis is also a common cause of ESRD in the elderly, accounting for nearly 12% of the elderly subjects starting RRT [77]. The incidence of primary glomerular diseases has been found to be similar to that observed in younger populations [78,79], but the prognosis is more severe. In a large series of 7086 patients who underwent renal biopsy between 1978 and 1990 [80], 825 of these patients (11.6%) were older than 65 years at the time of biopsy. Two hundred and seventy-one subjects (33%) of the elderly population were identified as having idiopathic glomerulonephritis, whereas 187 (23%) had glomerular involvement associated with a systemic disease; HNS accounted only for the 7% ($n = 58$) of the histological diagnosis. The mode of presentation was more severe in the elderly. Indeed, 52% of the patients aged >65 years presented with the nephrotic syndrome compared with 32% in the younger age group, whereas only 6% had asymptomatic urinary abnormalities compared with 38% in younger patients. Furthermore, the 34% of elderly patients had an impairment in renal function (either acute or CRF) compared with the 18% in the younger age group. However, it should be stressed that these differences may also be related to the criteria adopted to undertake renal biopsy in the elderly. Older patients with minimal change nephropathy seem to be particularly prone to developing acute renal failure and progressing towards CRF or death because of complications relating to renal failure or nephrotic syndrome [80]. Elderly patients with IgAN have a higher frequency of CRF, proteinuria, and hypertension at presentation, and a more severe prognosis. Of 13 patients aged ≥75 years reported by Caillette *et al.* [81], seven died and four reached end-stage renal failure within 38 months. About half of the older patients with focal segmental glomerular sclerosis (FSGS) present with renal insufficiency, and 70% with arterial hypertension [82]. Also in membranous glomerulonephritis older patients have a worse outcome, although with a slower rate of deterioration of renal function compared with younger subjects [83]. In this retrospective study, 88% of patients aged >60 ($n = 9$) developed CRF, while approximately 50% of patients aged ≤60 ($n = 53$) progressed towards renal failure.

Gender

ESRD from all causes considered together, or due to glomerulonephritis, diabetes (except perhaps type II disease) or hypertension, occurs more frequently in males than in females at most ages [75]. However, it is not certain to what extent this is due to males being more likely to suffer from the underlying disease, or more susceptible to the effects of this disease on kidney function.

Gender and the progression of chronic renal failure

Female gender confers some protection against the progression of renal disease in humans. Studies in patients with chronic non-diabetic renal disease suggest that the rate of progression to ESRD is more rapid in men than in women. However, caution should be used when evaluating studies that assess the rate of decline in renal function by measuring serum creatinine levels. Because they ingest more protein and have a larger muscle mass than women, men have an increased rate of creatinine generation. Thus differences in creatinine metabolism may influence apparently gender-related differences in renal disease progression [17].

In a prospective study of 62 men and 51 women with chronic renal disease Rosman *et al.* [84] found that creatinine clearance declined 50% more rapidly in men than in women.

In a retrospective study of patients with advanced CRF due to primary nephropathies, Hannedouche *et al.* [51] demonstrated that the rate of progression was nearly twice as fast in males than in females, and that the factors influencing the progression differed according to gender. In male patients, the slope of progression mainly correlated with MAP, whereas progression in females was significantly influenced by the type of nephropathy, with a more rapid progression being observed in the few women with Alport's syndrome than in the other groups. The MDRD study confirmed the deleterious effect of male gender on the progression of chronic renal disease [30]. In this prospective study of 840 subjects with chronic renal disease, male gender was identified as a risk factor for a more rapid decline in renal function [30]. Furthermore, women had lower rates of baseline proteinuria than men, even when adjusted for body size [85]. By means of multivariate analysis, other studies have not confirmed a statistically significant relationship between gender and renal survival [45].

Slower progression of renal failure in females has also been reported during the course of type 1 DN [86], PKD [87,88], hypertensive renal disease [89], and glomerulonephritis [47,85,90]. In membranous nephropathy, male gender is associated with a more rapid decline in renal function and a more frequent development of ESRD [91,92]. The data relating to IgAN are more conflicting. Although the univariate analyses performed in several studies have found that male gender is a risk factor for a negative outcome, multivariate analyses have failed to confirm this finding [93]. Interestingly, no gender difference has been noted in the progression of prepubertal subjects with nephronopthisis or cystinosis, thus indicating that the gender effect appears only after puberty, presumably via sex hormones [84]. On the other hand, an extremely high incidence of diabetic renal failure per million population has been described in postmenopausal African-American women [94].

In some hereditary kidney diseases, the faster rate of progression in males may be explained by genetic mechanisms. It is well known that most females with Alport disease have only microscopic haematuria and do not develop progressive renal failure, whereas a large number of affected males proceed to progressive renal failure by the third or fourth decade of life. The reason for this difference is probably an X-linked transmission of the disease in the majority of cases.

Race

In the US, African-Americans have a fourfold higher age-adjusted risk of treated ESRD compared with Caucasians [74]. Mexican-Americans have also been found to be at higher risk of developing ESRD than the general population [95]. These two high-risk groups make up over one-third of the dialysis patients in the US [96], although they account for only 14% of the total population. The incidence of ESRD is also higher in Native Americans and Asian/Pacific Islanders than in white people, although to a lesser extent than in African-Americans [74]. The two most common diseases responsible for the increased incidence of ESRD in these groups are hypertension and diabetes. When various known precursors are taken into account, including age, the prevalence and severity of hypertension, diabetes, and the level of education, black people still have a 4.5 times greater risk of developing ESRD than non-black people, thus suggesting the influence of genetic factors [98]. The yearly incidence of ESRD due to many other renal diseases (except PKD and vasculitis) is also significantly greater in black people than in white people [74,98].

Differences have also been found in the distribution of primary renal disease among patients from different racial groups attending a hospital in West London, whose catchment area contains large immigrant communities [100]. Patients from the Indian sub-continent had a significantly increased incidence of DN due to both insulin-dependent diabetes mellitus (IDDM) and non-insulin-dependent diabetes mellitus (NIDDM) when compared with Caucasians. Caribbean patients not only had a significantly increased incidence of DN due to IDDM, but also had a significantly higher incidence of hypertensive renal disease associated both to benign

Table 2.1 Incidence of ESRD by some primary diseases in different races in the US; years 1991–1995

Primary disease	White people (%)	Black people (%)	Asians (%)	Native Americans (%)
Diabetes	38.0	36.4	39.9	63.4
Type I diabetes	16.9	13.3	12.2	17.7
Type II diabetes	21.1	23.1	27.7	45.7
Nephrosclerosis	23.7	36.5	23.0	13.2
Glomerulonephritis	11.8	9.1	18.3	8.9
Focal segmental glomerular sclerosis	1.6	2.3	1.5	1.1
Membranous nephropathy	0.5	0.4	0.3	0.3
IgA nephropathy	0.2	0.1	0.7	0.3
Systemic lupus erythematosus nephritis	1.0	1.9	2.0	1.0
Wegener granulomatosis	0.4	0.0	0.1	0.1
Polycystic kidney disease	3.5	1.2	2.0	1.3
AIDS nephropathy	0.1	2.6	0.1	0.2
Other diseases	21.5	12.3	14.6	11.9

Source: US Renal Data System: USRDS 1997 Annual Data Report. (The interpretation and reporting of these data are the responsibility of the authors and in no way should be seen as an official policy or interpretation of the US government.)

and malignant hypertension, as in African patients. Adult PKD was almost entirely confined to Caucasians.

Socio-economic factors

Although minorities in the US are culturally and genetically different, one of the factor they have in common is that they share the lower rungs of the socio-economic ladder. As a consequence of their reduced educational and economical status, these people could have a greater burden of hypertension and poor glycaemic control for long periods, factors that may accelerate the rate of particularly diabetes and hypertension-induced renal deterioration. However, data of the Multiple Risk Factor Intervention Trial (MRFIT) show that the higher risk of ESRD in African-Americans than in white people is maintained at all levels of income [99].

Race and genetic factors

It has been suggested that genetic predisposition may explain some of the greater risk of ESRD in African-Americans [100]. In these subjects, a history of CRF in a first- or-second-degree relative is associated with an increased risk of ESRD [101], that becomes ninefold increased in the presence of a first-degree ESRD relative [102]. The familial clustering of ESRD in Caucasians is markedly weaker than that observed in African-Americans. As expected, family history appears to have a stronger relationship to ESRD due to hypertension and type II diabetes mellitus, than to ESRD due to CGN. However, it is still unknown to what extent such familial aggregation is influenced by genetic determinants, inherited life-style factors or social exposures. A biological cause of CRF susceptibility is further supported by close relatives having different aetiologies of ESRD in African-American multiplex renal failure families [103].

No clear linkage between CRF and candidate genes has yet been demonstrated in this population [104–106].

Race and hypertension

The incidence of hypertension among black people is reported to be at least twice that of white people for nearly every age and gender group [107], and it is associated with higher rates of morbidity and mortality. The age-adjusted prevalence of hypertension is also higher in Mexican-Americans than in the rest of the population. It has been suggested that the high prevalence of hypertension in these groups may contribute to the higher incidence of ESRD. It seems that black people at any given level of blood pressure do not suffer more vascular damage than non-black people, but they show a shift to the right of pressure distribution, thus yielding a higher overall prevalence and a higher proportion of severe disease [108]. It has been shown that ESRD associated with hypertension occurs as much as 17 times more often in American black people than in non-black people [109].

The pathogenesis of essential hypertension in black people differs from that observed in white people [110]. Several studies have documented a higher degree of blood pressure responsiveness to abrupt [111] and chronic [112] manipulations of sodium intake (defined as salt sensitivity) in African- and Mexican-Americans. In those who have a pressure response to a sodium load, the renal excretion of sodium is delayed and correlated with lower plasma renin levels. Such alterations are associated with a genetic disturbance of sodium cell membrane transport, which facilitates sodium retention and extracellular volume expansion [113]. Campese [114] hypothesized that, by raising glomerular pressure, salt may be a factor contributing to renal damage.

Racial differences have also been described in the prevalence of microalbuminuria in essential hypertension, with a significantly greater proportion of black patients having microalbuminuria [115]. Furthermore, microalbuminuria is a feature of salt-sensitive hypertension [116]. Altogether, these data seem to suggest a racial predisposition for end-organ damage susceptibility in black subjects.

Renal biopsies performed in black people with severe hypertension and varying degrees of renal function impairment have also revealed histopathological findings that are different from those found in white people with nephrosclerosis [117]. Blacks show an absence of fibrinoid necrosis, evidence of glomerular ischemia rather than proliferative glomerulonephritis and greater myointimal fibrodysplasia with mucopolysaccharide deposition. It has been proposed that these racial differences in nephrosclerosis may be due to an increased production of growth factors, such as transforming growth factor-β (TGF-β) and platelet-derived growth factor (PGDF), which promote renal scarring and fibrosis in a manner similar to that of keloids, which almost exclusively occurs in black people [118].

Analysing the MRFIT data after 16 years of follow-up, Klag *et al.* [99] found a higher incidence of all-cause ESRD in African-Americans than in white men at every level of blood pressure values. However, the strength of the association of blood pressure with the incidence of ESRD was similar in both groups. It has been shown that even when hypertensive African-Americans are treated as effectively as Caucasians, renal function in black people may continue to deteriorate whereas it remains stable or improves in non-black people [119]. A *post-hoc* analysis of the MDRD trial clearly demonstrated that, regardless of the origin of renal disease, African-Americans benefited only when their MAP was reduced to levels of less than 92 mmHg in comparison to 94 mmHg in Caucasians [120]. A prospective study of African-Americans with hypertensive, non-DN randomized to two different levels of blood pressure reduction, also demonstrated that a reduction in MAP to levels of less than 92 mmHg stopped the progression of renal disease [121]. These data suggest the importance of further reducing blood pressure values in this population in order to slow down the progression of CRF as much as possible.

Race and diabetes

The prevalence of diabetes mellitus in African-Americans is approximately double that in Caucasians. After adjusting for this increased prevalence, ESRD due to diabetes is three to six times more prevalent in African-Americans than in white people [122]. After adjustment for systolic blood pressure, income, age, and other potential risk factors, black people still have a 63% higher risk of developing ESRD [123].

Mexican-Americans have an ESRD rate ratio of 2.9–7 in comparison with white people [95,124]. However, after adjustment for the prevalence of diabetes, Mexican-Americans no longer have an excess risk [124]. The prevalence of NIDDM is also high and increasing rapidly in the American-Indian population, as is the risk of developing nephropathy and cardiovascular disease [125]. NIDDM is the leading cause of renal failure in Pima Indians, among whom the incidence of ESRD is 23 times that of the general US population. Familial factors seem to be related with the development of renal disease secondary to NIDDM in this population [126,127], thus suggesting that diabetes and renal disease may have independent determinants. However, little is known so far about the link between genetic and environmental influences in these subjects, that may explain the greater risk of developing ESRD.

Race and primary glomerulonephritis

Racial differences in the prevalence of glomerulonephritis have also been described [128,129]. It has been demonstrated that FSGS is the most common lesion in nephrotic black adults (occurring in 36–80% of cases), and that these subjects are four times more likely to have this nephropathy than white patients. The aetiology underlying this increased frequency of FSGS is unknown, although it is partially attributed to a possible genetic predisposition [130]. Black patients with FSGS also have a worse outcome than white people. On the other hand membranous and IgAN are more common in Caucasians [129]. This is also the case with idiopathic and antineutrophil-cytoplasmic-antibody (ANCA)-positive crescentic glomerulonephritis, with a ratio of 7 : 1 of Caucasians to African-Americans [131]. However, African-Americans were six times more likely to reach a renal end-point compared with Caucasians ($p = 0.0008$) [131].

Genetic factors

Familial factors

In recent years evidence has accumulated, suggesting that familial factors could influence both the development of DN and the progression rate of CGN.

A familial clustering of DN has been shown in patients with IDDM and NIDDM. In a large study of families with multiple IDDM siblings [132], the cumulative risk of nephropathy in siblings after 25 years of post-pubertal diabetes was 71.5% if the proband had persistent proteinuria, but only 25.4% if the proband had either normoalbuminuria or microalbuminuria. This difference of almost 50% in the risk of nephropathy is consistent with a major genetic effect that leads to a predisposition for advanced DN.

In addition to the familial clustering of DN, it has also been shown that in both IDDM [133,134] and NIDDM subjects [135], a predisposition for essential hypertension increases the risk of nephropathy. A recent case–control study has confirmed the fact that familial cardiovascular disease and familial hypertension are independently associated with an almost twofold and fourfold increased risk of nephropathy [136].

Parental hypertension may also be a risk factor for the progression of DN. In a collaborative study of the effects of captopril on DN, a parental history of hypertension was associated with an almost twofold increase in the risk of doubling serum creatinine levels [137]. An increased frequency of parental hypertension has also been reported in patients with glomerulonephritis [138]. This inherited predisposition for hypertension has also been shown to influence the progression towards CRF in patients with IgAN [139,140].

Family history of renal disease of any type has also been associated with an increased risk of ESRD [141]. The risk is even much higher when two or more first-degree relatives have renal disease. This familial aggregation of renal disease is in excess of that predicted by clustering of diabetes and hypertension within families, suggesting that either genetic susceptibility or environmental exposures shared within families increase the risk of developing ESRD.

Candidate genes

The approach so far used to detect the genes possibly involved in the progression of CRF is that of establishing 'candidate genes', by which is meant the genes coding for proteins that may play a part, which are tested in order to detect any differences in the frequency of the gene variant between patients with progressive chronic renal disease, and patients without progression or healthy subjects (case-control studies).

Genetically determined derangements of immune regulation may play a part not only in the genesis of primary glomerulonephritis and autoimmune disease, but also in CRF progression. The potentially associated immunogenetic abnormalities include inherited defects of the complement system, an increased prevalence of certain human leucocyte antigen (HLA) types, and altered frequencies in the polymorphism of immunoglobulins and T-cell receptor genes. Cytokines-related genes have also been recently proposed as candidate genes.

Given the important effects of hypertension and the renin–angiotensin system on CRF progression, together with the possible role of an inherited predisposition for hypertension, various authors have recently studied the polymorphism of the genes coding for components of the renin–angiotensin system in DN or chronic renal disease.

Immunogenetics and disease progression

Major histocompatibility complex

The data from the studies of experimental glomerulonephritis have suggested that the major histocompatibility complex (MHC) is involved in both organ specific and generalized autoimmunity. Therefore, detailed examination of the HLA complex has been performed in humans with glomerular disease by serologic detection and, more recently, by DNA hybridization and restriction fragment length polymorphism analysis, showing strong positive associations between particular HLA molecules and various types of nephritis [142–150]. Several associations have also been found between HLA antigens and negative outcome in various renal diseases.

Table 2.2 Major candidate genes in diabetic and non-diabetic nephropathies

Candidate gene	Insulin-dependent diabetes mellitus	Non-insulin-dependent diabetes mellitus	IgA nephropathy	Other nephropathies	End-stage renal disease
HLA antigens					
HLA-DR3	—	—	No*	Yes (MGN)*	Yes*
HLA-DR5	—	—	—	Yes	Yes
HLA-B35	—	—	Yes	—	—
HLA-B27	—	—	Yes	—	—
HLA-DR1	—	—	Yes	—	—
HLA-DQA1	—	—	Yes	—	—
HLA-DQalfa2	—	—	Yes	—	—
Complement factors					
C3fF	—	—	Yes	—	—
Bf gene	—	—	Yes	Yes	—
Immunoglobulin genes					
IgG switch region-α1 gene	—	—	Yes	—	—
Renin–angiotensin system genes					
ACE gene	Yes[†]	Yes[†]	Yes[‡]	Yes	No
Angiotensinogen gene	Yes/No	No	Yes/No	Yes (PKD)	—
AT_1R gene	No	No	No	—	—
Nitric oxide synthase gene	No	—	No	No	—
Renal failure genes	—	—	—	—	No*
Cytokines genes					
TNF-α gene	—	—	—	—	No*
TNF-β gene	Yes	—	Yes	Yes (MGN)	No*
Kallikrein gene	—	—	—	—	Yes*
IL-1 gene	Yes/No	Yes/No	—	—	—
IL-1RA gene	Yes	Yes	—	—	Yes*
TNF α and β genes	—	—	—	—	—
Growth factors genes					
TGF-β2 gene	—	—	—	—	Yes/no*[§]
TGF-β1 and β3 genes	—	—	—	—	No*
TNF α and β genes	—	—	—	—	No*
EGF and PDGF genes	—	—	—	—	No*
Insulin receptor gene	Yes	—	—	—	—
PAI-1 gene	No	—	—	—	—

* African-Americans, [†] mainly in Asiatics, [‡] small-size studies, [§] non-diabetic nephropathies.
TGF, transforming growth factor; TNF, tumor necrosis factor; EGF, epidermal growth factor; PDGF, platelet-derived growth factor; MGN, membranous glomerulonephritis; PKD, polycystic kidney disease, IL-1, interleukin-1, PAI-1, plasminogen activator inhibitor-1.

In an attempt to associate genetic markers with ESRD, a race-controlled investigation of HLA phenotype frequency associations in ESRD was performed using a large renal transplant registry. The most interesting finding was a consistent HLA-DR3 association in African-Americans with ESRD caused by hypertension, IDDM or membranous nephropathy, and in white people with ESRD caused by IDDM, systemic lupus erythematosus, or membranous nephropathy. Patients with ESRD caused by IgAN or FSGS did not show any association with HLA-DR3 [100].

In IgAN, the HLA-B35 antigen has been related to a poor prognosis [151]. This original finding has been then confirmed in an extensive study of 282 patients [152], in which the HLA-B35 antigen was found significantly related to the development of CRF by univariate analysis ($p = 0.0002$) and multivariate analysis (b/SE = +2.16, $p = 0.002$). In another study of 605 renal transplant recipients with ESRD due to IgAN, an increased frequency of HLA-B27 and HLA-DR1 and a decreased HLA-DR2 frequency were found compared with race-matched controls ($p < 0.004$) [153].

Other studies have reported an association between the frequency of HLA-DQ alleles and progression towards renal failure in IgAN. Raguenes *et al.* [154] identified a strong association between HLA DQB1*0301 and patients with an unfavourable outcome, whereas the DQA1 locus have been found to be associated with renal failure in an Italian cohort [150]. In a Chinese population, the DQalfa2 allele was found more frequently in the patients who progressed towards CRF (66.9%) than in those who maintained normal renal function (26.9%); the DQalfa2 allele did not correlate with the severity of the histopathological findings at renal biopsy [155]. In Japan, an association between IgAN and DR4 has also been described [156].

Considering membranous glomerulonephritis, HLA-DR3 and HLA-DR5 frequencies have been found increased in 250 renal transplant recipients with ESRD compared with race-matched controls ($p < 0.02$) [157]. The DR5 antigen seems also to influence the severity of microscopic polyarteritis with renal involvement [158].

In anti-glomerular basement membrane-antibody-mediated nephritis, the incidence of the HLA-DR2 antigen have been found greatly increased [142,144]. Interestingly, Rees *et al.* [142] have found an increased frequency of HLA-DR2 and HLA-B7 in 39 patients with anti- glomerular basement membrane -antibody nephritis compared with controls, but only the HLA-B7 antigen seemed to influence the severity of the disease. A subset of patients who inherited HLA-B7 together with DR2 had significantly higher plasma creatinine levels, a greater proportion of glomeruli surrounded by crescents, and a worse prognosis than the others.

Extended haplotypes are a combination of alleles that tend to occur together more frequently than would be expected by chance. Welch *et al.* [159] studied genetic markers for membranoproliferative glomerulonephritis within the MHC in 34 patients and their families and in 29 normal families. They found not only that the extended haplotype B8, DR3, SC01, GLO2 (glyoxalase I 2) was associated with susceptibility to this glomerulonephritis, but also that patients bearing this haplotype had a higher incidence of renal insufficiency than those without it ($p < 0.01$).

Gene polymorphisms associated with specific renal diseases

Complement factors

It is well known that the activation of the alternate and/or classic complement pathway plays a role in the pathogenesis of several glomerular diseases. The gene coding for C3 is located on chromosome 19 and it has two allelic isoforms: C3S and C3F. In patients with IgAN the homozygous genotype C3fF has been associated with an adverse clinical outcome [147]. It is unknown whether polymorphisms of C3 are associated with differences in complement function, although a higher capacity of C3F to bind to human mononuclear cells has been noted.

In IgAN, polymorphisms of the complement properdin factor Bf gene (located on the MHC region of chromosome 6) have been noted, with a significant excess of homozygosis for Bf-FF in patients with an adverse outcome [147]. An increased frequency of the Bf-F allele has also been found in patients with rapidly progressive glomerulonephritis [160] and in miscellaneous forms of glomerulonephritis [161].

The complement protein C4 exists in two isotypes C4A and C4B, encoded by separate genes within the MHC class III region. Both C4 genes are highly polymorphic with at least 31 alleles including null alleles of both loci [162]. A relatively high frequency of null alleles of C4A or C4B is found in the normal population (respectively 5–15% and 10–20%) and homozygosity or heterozygosity of C4 null alleles have been associated with immunological disease [163]. It has been suggested C4A deficiency may reduce solubilization of potentially nephritogenic immune complexes [164], possibly contributing to the development of more severe glomerular damage. Wyatt *et al.* [165] performed C4 phenotyping in 123 Caucasians IgAN patients: six subjects with total C4A deficiency were found and all had CRF, in contrast with 47% of the patients without C4A deficiency having CRF ($p = 0.001$). Similar findings were confirmed by Wopenka *et al.* [166].

Immunoglobulin genes

In IgAN, abnormalities of immunoglobulin production and characteristics have been reported.

In the switch region of the IgG-alpha1 gene (S-alpha 1), a significantly higher frequency of the homozygous 7.4/7.4 kb genotype has been observed in IgAN patients with negative outcome [147]. Ten years after renal biopsy, 36% of homozygous patients compared with 4% of the heterozygotes were in ESRD. Furthermore, homozygotes had a significantly higher prevalence of hypertension (62.1% vs 34.5% in heterozygotes, $p < 0.005$), and tended to have a higher frequency of interstitial fibrosis and more severe vascular lesions at renal biopsy than heterozygotes.

Angiotensin I converting enzyme gene

The human ACE gene is located on chromosome 17, and consists of 26 exons [167]. A 287 bp insertion/deletion (I/D) polymorphism in intron 16 of this gene has been associated with an increased risk of cardiovascular disease, early onset of essential hypertension [168], and blood pressure salt sensitivity [169,170]. Moreover serum ACE activity has been shown to be higher in subjects with the D allele than in those without [171]. In recent years, the role of I/D polymorphism has been tested in various renal diseases.

IgA nephropathy and primary glomerulonephritis

A number of authors have reported an association between the I/D polymorphism and a negative outcome in IgAN patients. After defining progression by determining the slope of the reciprocal of serum creatinine versus time, or creatinine clearance over time, they found that the DD genotype was more frequent in patients with a more rapid loss of renal function [172–175]. However, all of these studies involved a relatively small number of patients (fewer than 100 subjects). Schmidt *et al.* [176] studied a larger cohort of IgAN patients (122 subjects with stable renal function and 82 with ESRD) and found a tendency towards an increase in the frequency of the DD genotype in the ESRD group, but this difference was not statistically significant. A French study [177] also failed to confirm an association between the DD genotype and CRF progression in 157 IgAN subjects.

Interestingly, ACE gene polymorphism has been found to correlate with some histological features. The DD genotype has been associated with a larger glomerular planar area as determined in biopsy specimens [178], and with a higher percentage of sclerotic glomeruli [172,179].

ACE gene polymorphism possibly affects also the course of primary focal segmental glomerulosclerosis in children, with the II homozygotes significantly less likely to have progressive renal disease than patients with other genotypes [180]. The same may not be true for membranous nephropathy [181].

Diabetic nephropathy

The role of I/D polymorphism in IDDM and NIDDM patients with nephropathy is still controversial. Marre *et al.* [182] were the first to report an association between ACE polymorphism and DN in IDDM, with a reduced risk for DN in patients bearing the type II genotype, but although a number of reports confirmed this finding [183,184], others have failed to detect any association [185–187]. Doria *et al.* [188] not only confirmed a higher risk of DN in IDDM patients homozygous for the D allele, but they also found a stronger association with the polymorphism of the allele designated DdeI '=' in intron 7 of the ACE gene and the development of DN. Carriers of a susceptibility haplotype, defined by the deletion in intron 16 and the DdeI '=' in intron 7, had a fourfold risk of developing DN. However, this haplotype increased the risk of the onset of DN, but not of its progression. Freire *et al.* [189] also described an increased risk of nephropathy in patients homozygous for another allele in intron 7 detected with the restriction enzyme *Pst*I, with a nephropathy risk 2.3 times higher than that of the other genotypes (95% CI: 1.2–4.5). These findings suggest that several polymorphisms of the ACE gene could be involved in renal damage. Interestingly, it has been recently described that IDDM patients with the II genotype are resistant to glomerular changes induced by hyperglycemia, providing basis for their possible reduced risk of nephropathy [190].

Also in NIDDM patients, the relationship between ACE polymorphism and diabetic kidney disease has not been clearly established in either Caucasian [186,191,192] or Japanese [193,194] patients.

Recently, a systematic review of the studied performed between 1994 and 1997 in patients with IDDM or NIDDM ($n = 5336$) did not find any associations between the I/D polymorphism and nephropathy in Caucasians, whereas in Asian NIDDM patients the risk of nephropathy was increased in the presence of the DD or ID genotype (OR, 1.88; 95% CI, 1.42–2.85) [195]. This further underlines that ethnic differences may strongly affect the impact of the I/D polymorphism on both diabetic and non-diabetic nephropathies.

The conflicting results may also reflect the small number of patients studied in some reports and different definitions of DN (the presence of macroalbuminuria was more consistently associated with increased frequency of the D allele than that of microalbuminuria [182,186]. Indeed, the Genetique de la Nephropathie Diabetique study [183] found that the D allele frequency was significantly associated with both the presence of nephropathy and its severity in 494 IDDM patients, 47% of whom had advanced nephropathy with proteinuria or renal impairment. Thus ACE polymorphism may play mainly a part in the rate of progression of DN: in 168 Japanese patients with nephropathy secondary to NIDDM, Yoshida *et al.* [196] found a significantly higher incidence of the DD genotype in subjects with declining versus stable renal function, and a fourfold greater risk of progression to renal failure in the patients bearing the DD genotype. However, the decrease in GFR of IDDM patients was not found to be associated with I/D polymorphism in the study conducted by Tarnow *et al.* [197].

As in non-diabetic nephropathies [198], ACE gene polymorphism may also affect the response to ACE inhibitors [199,200]. In the EURODIAB Controlled Trial of Lisinopril [200] in 530 normotensive IDDM patients, a significant interaction between the II and DD genotype groups and treatment was found, with the II patients showing an enhanced response to lisinopril (at 2 years, albumin excretion rate was 51.3% lower on lisinopril than placebo). Conversely, the DD lisinopril-treated patients had only a 7.7% lower albumin excretion rate than those treated with placebo. However, the magnitude of the role of ACE gene polymorphism could have been partially influenced by the fact that the II placebo-treated patients had the fastest rate of albumin excretion rate progression, thus enhancing the effect of lisinopril.

Other renal diseases

Recent preliminary studies have reported an association between ACE gene polymorphism and renal artery stenosis [201], active lupus nephritis [202], and hypertensive renal disease [203], but no association has been found between this polymorphism and reflux nephropathy [204], PKD [205,206], and Henoch–Schönlein purpura [207].

Zoccali *et al.* [208] analysed I/D polymorphism in 226 patients with non-diabetic chronic nephropathies, but again the polymorphism was not predictive of disease progression.

End-stage renal disease

I/D polymorphism does not seem to be a *per se* risk factor for reaching ESRD because genotype frequencies have been found to be similar in dialysed patients with different renal diseases and in control populations [105,209,210]. Nevertheless, this result may be confounded by the fact that the DD genotype is a known risk factor for cardiovascular death, and this may lead to a low frequency in dialysed patients through the death of at-risk patients.

Angiotensinogen gene

A point mutation of the angiotensinogen (AGT) gene, resulting in an amino acid substitution of threonine for methionine at position 235 (M235T), has been associated with essential hypertension [211].

Only one study has so far found an association between AGT gene polymorphism and a negative outcome in IgAN [212]. The patients with the AGT MT and TT genotype not only had a faster rate of deterioration in terms of creatinine clearance than those with the MM genotype, but they also had higher maximal proteinuria values than those with the MM genotype. Interestingly, multivariate analysis detected an interaction between AGT and ACE gene polymorphism, with the presence of ACE/DD polymorphism adversely affecting disease progression only in patients with the AGT/MM genotype. Other authors failed to detect a role of AGT gene polymorphism in the progression of IgAN [177,208]. Preliminary data also suggest that the AGT 235T allele may play a protective part against the development of CRF in PKD [206].

In diabetic patients, the reports concerning an association between this polymorphism and DN have been conflicting. Fogarty *et al.* [213] found that the TT genotype was more common in IDDM patients with than in those without nephropathy. However, other studies have not confirmed this finding [214–215].

No association of M235T polymorphism with the development of DN has been found in NIDDM [214,217].

Angiotensin II receptor I gene

The ACE (DD) polymorphism has been shown to have synergy in its deleterious effects in myocardial infarction with a polymorphic locus in the angiotensin II type I receptor (AT1R) gene. This consists of an adenosine to cytosine transition at position 1166 (A1166C) in the 3′ untranslated region of the gene, which has also been associated with hypertension [218]. Although a 20-cM region around the AT1R gene possibly contains a major locus for susceptibility to DN [216], polymorphisms of this gene do not seem to influence the progression of IgAN [174,177] or the development of DN [216].

Nitric oxide synthase gene

The nitric oxide system has been implicated in the pathogenesis of glomerular inflammation and renal fibrosis. The nitric oxide synthase genotype does not seem to be involved in the progression of primary CGN [210,210] or IDDM DN [220].

Kallikrein gene

Kallikrein is a serine protease involved in blood pressure regulation and renal perfusion. Preliminary data suggest that polymorphisms in the human plasma kallikrein gene (alleles 7 and 9 of the KLK3b marker) may be involved in the pathogenesis of ESRD in African-Americans [106].

Renal failure genes

Two renal failure susceptibility genes, renal failure-1 (Rf-1) and renal failure-2 (Rf-2), have been identified in the Fawn-hooded rat, a model of hypertension and nephrosclerosis [221]. These two genes predispose to hypertensive renal injury, but have no apparent effect on blood pressure. The human homologue of the rodent Rf-1 gene has been localized to chromosome 10q. Yu *et al.* [222] have recently tested 129 African-American sibling pairs for genetic linkage between 21 polymorphic markers spanning chromosome 10 and ESRD due to diabetes, CGN or hypertension. Although two adjacent markers on 10p (D10S1435 and D10S249) approached significance for linkage to ESRD in sibling pairs with non-diabetic causes of ESRD, the human homologue of Rf-1 is unlikely to contribute substantially to renal failure susceptibility from common causes of kidney disease in black people.

Cytokine genes

Variations in disease severity have also been linked to polymorphisms in various proinflammatory cytokines, such as tumour necrosis factor (TNF) and the interleukins (IL). Differences in TNF-β gene polymorphism has been found in patients with IgAN, idiopathic membranous nephropathy and IDDM [223,224].

Preliminary reports suggested that genotypic alterations in the IL-1 gene cluster are associated with DN, but other studies have failed to find any associations with polymorphisms in the genes encoding IL-1β, the IL-1 receptor, and the natural antagonist of IL-1 [225]. Subsequently, Blakemore *et al.* [226] tested the association of the allele IL1RN*2 of the IL-1 receptor antagonist (IL-1RA) gene with complications of diabetes and found a significant association between carriage of this allele and DN ($p < 0.001$). The association was significant both in IDDM ($n = 128$) and NIDDM subjects ($n = 125$), but the increased frequency of the allele was higher in NIDDM. Further studies are needed to confirm these findings and to define if IL1RN*2 could be considered a genetic marker of severity of inflammatory complications of diseases rather than a marker of disease susceptibility.

Freedman *et al.* [104] have recently analysed the role of a number of cytokine-related candidate loci implicated in the pathogenesis of progressive renal disease in a high-risk African-American population. An association was found only between allele 2 of the IL-1RA gene and ESRD. TGF-β2 polymorphism approached significance for non-DN, but EGF, PGDF, TGF-β1, TGF-β3, TNF-α and TNF-β loci did not show any linkage to ESRD.

Insulin receptor gene

A number of studies have shown an association between insulin resistance, essential hypertension and DN [227,228]. It has been then proposed that functional or structural abnormalities in the insulin receptor gene may contribute to this phenomenon [229]. Interestingly, Krolewski *et al.* [230] found a significant difference in the distribution of polymorphisms located between exons 6 and 9 of the insulin receptor gene and IDDM patients who developed advanced DN (fast-progressors) or who developed only microalbuminuria during 15–20 years of diabetes (slow-progressors). At present the biological meaning of these associations is not clear.

Plasminogen activator inhibitor-1 gene

A 4/5-guanine tract polymorphism (4G/5G) in the promoter region of the plasminogen activator inhibitor-1 (PAI-1) gene is associated with the plasma activity of this substance which promotes antifibrinolysis and the accumulation of extracellular matrix. Although this polymorphism is not associated with DN, the interaction between the 4G4G PAI-1 genotype and the ACE DD genotype was positively associated with macrovascular disease in NIDDM [231].

Smoking

Increasing attention has recently been paid to the role of cigarette smoking and tobacco in the development and progression of renal diseases. Clinical evidence links smoking with the development of microalbuminuria in diabetic patients and its progression to overt proteinuria [232]. In non-diabetics, there appear to be a dose-dependent effect of cigarette consumption on the development of end-stage renal insufficiency with patients consuming 15 packs-year having a 5.8-fold increase risk [233]. Of interest, in these patients treatment with an ACE inhibitor attenuated the smoking-related risk. Such an association between smoking and progression of renal disease was also observed in the MRFIT study of hypertensive men [119]. The effect of smoking on progression may be related to the exacerbation of other risk factors such as systemic hypertension, proteinuria, or hyperlipidemia.

Effect of proteinuria on progression

It has recently been claimed that urinary protein excretion, which was originally thought to be merely an indicator of the degree of renal damage, plays a causal part in the progression of CRF in various renal diseases.

Proteinuria as marker of disease activity

In patients with FSGS, the presence of nephrotic syndrome carries a worse prognosis than sclerosis without nephrotic syndrome [234]. Similar observations have been reported in patients with membranoproliferative glomerulonephritis type 1 [235] and in patients with idiopathic membranous nephropathy [236,237]. In IgAN, proteinuria has also been found to be as a risk factor for a negative outcome by means of univariate and multivariate analyses [238,239]. A graded prognosis according to the degree of proteinuria has recently been shown in this nephropathy [240]: in patients with proteinuria >3 g/24 h, the cumulative probability of renal survival from the time of presentation was 0.36 at 15 years, whereas in those with proteinuria ranging from 1 to 3 g/24 h it was 0.43; on the contrary, the prognosis was excellent if urine protein loss was normal or below 1 g/24 h. Interestingly, proteinuria is a prognostic marker not only in glomerular diseases (in which it could be an index of disease activity), but also in tubulo-interstitial disorders or renovascular disease [47,241,242]. Indeed, according to Kincaid-Smith and Becker [241], proteinuria appeared as the worst prognostic factor in a cohort of patients with reflux nephropathy and pyelonephritic scarring. In a Japanese community-based screening of more than 100 000 subjects by dip-stick urinanalysis and blood pressure measurements, proteinuria was also found as the most potent predictor of ESRD over 10 years (adjusted odds ratio 14.9, 95% confidence interval 10.9–20.2) [243].

Proteinuria and the progression of chronic renal failure

In numerous clinical studies that have tried to identify the risk factors for progressive renal function loss, the severity of proteinuria has correlated with the rate of renal function decline [48,52]. Williams *et al.* [48] showed that in patients with linear progressive CRF, the mean 24-h urine protein excretion correlated strikingly with the linear rate of decline of renal function ($r = 0.75$, $p < 0.0001$). Furthermore, proteinuria was significantly less in patients with stable renal function than in patients who had progressive CRF ($p < 0.001$). By multiple regression analysis with backward elimination of variables, Wight *et al.* [52] found that only proteinuria was a significant predictor of the overall slope (regression coefficient = –0.1775, $p = 0.0075$, adjusted $r^2 = 0.1059$).

The MDRD study compared the rates of decline in GFR in 840 patients with a wide range of renal diseases, and found that baseline proteinuria was a strong predictor of a subsequent decline in GFR [30]. This finding has also been confirmed in a trial studying the effects of a low protein diet on the progression of renal disease in 456 patients with CRF [244]. A multivariate regression analysis of the differences between initial and final values of creatinine clearance and the factors potentially affecting the progression of CRF showed as statistically significant only the degree of proteinuria [244]. In a *post-hoc* analysis of this trial [44], the relationship between baseline proteinuria and renal survival was also evident at a descriptive analysis, with the probability of reaching an end-point (doubling of baseline serum creatinine or need for dialysis) becoming progressively higher from proteinuria levels of less than 1 g/24 h to more than 3 g/24 h. By multivariate analysis proteinuria was confirmed as a risk factor for CRF progression ($p < 0.001$, hazard ratio 1.5). In the AIPRI study, a multinational trial designed to investigate whether ACE inhibition can slow the progression of renal diseases of different aetiologies, the number of end-points (doubling of baseline serum creatinine or need for dialysis) increased progressively (in both the ACE inhibitor and the placebo group) in line with increasing proteinuria levels (from <1 g/24 h to >3 g/24 h during follow-up) [31]. These findings were confirmed in 177 patients with proteinuric non-diabetic renal diseases enrolled in the REIN study [46]. High baseline proteinuria was the only variable correlating significantly with a faster GFR decline. In a prospective randomized trial to investigate the effects of dietary protein restriction on CRF progression, D'Amico *et al.* [245] have also shown by multivariate stepwise analysis that the time-averaged values of proteinuria were the most powerful predictors of unfavourable outcome in 128 patients with different renal disease ($p = 0.000$). Similar findings have been found in children with CRF [246]. In these 191 patients aged 2–18 years, multivariate regression analysis showed again that proteinuria (≥50 mg/kg per 24 h) was the most important predictor of a decrease in creatinine clearance ($r = 0.42$, $p < 0.001$).

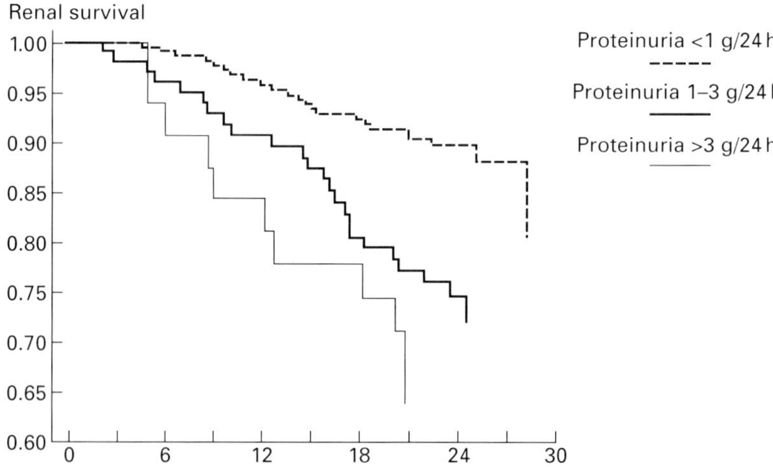

Fig. 2.2 Actuarial renal survival rates according to baseline 24-h proteinuria [45].

Reduction in proteinuria and better renal outcome

A reduction in urinary protein excretion correlates with better renal function outcome in diabetic and non-diabetic renal diseases [31,45,46,247]. In 1984 El Nahas *et al.* [50] described the effect of dietary protein restriction on proteinuria, observing a significant reduction in proteinuria in all the proteinuric patients receiving the low protein diet ($p < 0.025$). In patients with CGN a good correlation was found between the extent of the reduction in proteinuria and the improvement in creatinine slopes of individual patients ($r = 0.76$, $p < 0.01$), suggesting that the response of proteinuria to dietary restriction may identify the patients with a better chance of a favourable outcome in the long term. In recent years, numerous study have shown that a reduction in proteinuria by means of antihypertensive drugs may also influence the rate of decline in renal function.

In a *post-hoc* analysis of the MDRD study, a regression analysis was performed between the GFR slope and the change in proteinuria during 4 months of follow-up, to assess the effects of changes in proteinuria on the subsequent progression of renal disease. An initial reduction in proteinuria of 1.0 g/24 h was associated with a slower mean decrease in GFR [121]. Praga *et al.* [248] found that renal function (assessed as creatinine clearance) remained stable in a group of patients with nephrotic proteinuria in whom captopril induced a fall in proteinuria of at least 45%, whereas renal function deteriorated in the group with a less reduction in proteinuria. Gansevoort *et al.* [249] performed a retrospective study in 22 patients with proteinuria ≥3 g/24 h. Not only after 2 months of treatment with lisinopril proteinuria had fallen by 62%, but this antiproteinuric response remained stable during the next follow-up period of 1.5 years. A significant correlation was found between the initial antiproteinuric response and the 1/Cr slope over the follow-up period, with less deterioration in renal function in the patients with the most antiproteinuric response. Apperloo *et al.* [250] confirmed these data in a 2-year prospective study of 29 non-diabetic proteinuric patients treated with enalapril or atenolol: the per cent reduction in proteinuria after 12 weeks correlated with the slope of the long-term GFR decline (GFR was measured as the clearance of ^{125}I-iothalamate) ($r = 0.62$, $p < 0.0004$), such that the patients who responded with a marked fall in proteinuria had a relatively better preserved renal function during follow-up.

In the AIPRI study [31], a 3-year prospective trial involving 583 patients with renal failure caused by various disorders, the proportion of patients reaching the primary end-point (doubling of baseline serum creatinine or need for dialysis) was lower in the benazepril group than in the placebo group ($p < 0.001$). At the same time, urinary protein excretion significantly decreased after only 2 months of treatment in the benazepril group, whereas it increased slightly in the placebo group; the associated reduction in the relative risk of reaching the end-point was 53% in the ACE inhibitor group. Furthermore, the protective effect of benazepril on renal function was greatest in the patients with substantial proteinuria, (in patients with baseline proteinuria ≥3 g/24 h the reduction in risk was 66%) even after adjustments were made for diastolic blood pressure (DBP) over time (after adjustment reduction in risk, 56%). Anyway, benazepril seemed able to reduce the risk of reaching an end-point at all levels of baseline proteinuria: patients with a certain degree of baseline proteinuria had their risk of CRF progression reduced to that observed in the placebo group at a lower level of baseline proteinuria [251].

Similar findings have been shown by the REIN study [46]. In 78 patients randomized to ramipril with baseline proteinuria ≥3 g/24 h, the percentage reduction in urinary protein excretion from baseline in the first month of follow-up was inversely correlated with the long-term rate of GFR decline. On the other side, in the placebo group urinary protein excretion did not change significantly during follow-up and the mean rate of GFR decline was significantly higher than in the ramipril group.

Interestingly, a recent meta-analysis have found that baseline levels of urinary protein loss were not related to the subsequent antiproteinuric response [252].

The effect of the reduction in proteinuria on disease progression have also been shown in DN. In 20 hypertensive IDDM patients with nephropathy, Rossing *et al.* [253] found that the reduction in albumin excretion during the antihypertensive treatment (a beta-blocker plus furosemide in addition to the initial antihypertensive agent) in the first year of follow-up was the only parameter able to predict the subsequent fall in GFR.

Gansevoort *et al.* [254] analysed the combined effect of ACE inhibition and a low protein diet in non-diabetic patients with proteinuria exceeding 3 g/24 h. This combination was able to decrease proteinuria significantly more than each single treatment; however, the short time of follow-up (2 months for each phase of the study) do not allow to draw any conclusion about the combined effect of ACE inhibition and protein restriction on the long-term GFR decline. The AIPRI study did not find any interaction between protein intake and the effect of ACE inhibitors [31].

In the past few years, it has been shown that angiotensin II receptor antagonists are also able to reduce urinary protein excretion. According to Gansevoort *et al.* [255], after 4 weeks of treatment with losartan, an angiotensin II receptor antagonist, proteinuria was reduced of 20%, and the effect was further increased (–40%) after doubling the dosage of the drug. However, further studies are warranted to clarify if the reduction in proteinuria achieved with angiotensin II receptor antagonists may also be associated with a slower rate of CRF progression. Moreover, it has been suggested the possibility that these agents, by interfering with the renin–angiotensin system at a different level from that of ACE inhibitors, may allow a more complete counteraction of this system when used in association with ACE inhibitors. Although this hypothesis is extremely fascinating, caution is needed as we are still waiting confirmation of the clinical effects not only of the association but also of angiotensin II receptor antagonists alone. Altogether these data seems to suggest that proteinuria is not only a marker of disease activity, but also an important cause of glomerular injury. Reducing proteinuria may then help to prevent progressive renal function decline.

The role of proteinuria in CRF progression will be further discussed in another chapter.

Effect of hypertension on progression

Hypertension is an important presenting feature of renal disease, and is probably one of the most important factors contributing to progression.

The prevalence of hypertension in non-diabetic chronic renal disease

High blood pressure is a frequent finding even at the very early stages of glomerular disease. It has been shown that, at the time of renal biopsy, 10–50% of patients are hypertensive and about 5–25% become hypertensive during the course of CGN [256,257]. In a cohort of 374 IgAN patients, D'Amico *et al.* [238] found that the prevalence of hypertension was 63% after a mean follow-up of 5 ± 3.7 years, and that only 46% of these subjects had reduced renal function. This finding was subsequently confirmed. In 311 patients with CGN, the prevalence of hypertension was higher than in a comparable sample of the general population even in patients with serum creatinine levels of ≤1.1 mg/dl [256]. The prevalence was highest in patients with membranoproliferative glomerulonephritis and FSGS, intermediate in patients with membranous, mesangioproliferative or IgAN, and low in patients with minimal change nephropathy, thus suggesting that the presence of proliferative lesions may lead to systemic hypertension because of disturbed glomerular perfusion [256].

Considering patients with CRF with various renal diseases, it has been shown that nearly 80% are treated with antihypertensive drugs before the beginning of dialysis [31,243]. Patients with CGN and benign nephrosclerosis have significantly higher mean blood pressure levels than those with chronic pyelonephritis or PKD ($p < 0.05$) [31,244,259].

Hypertension and the progression of non-diabetic chronic renal disease

A number of retrospective longitudinal [260,261] and cross-sectional [89] studies have provided data showing that the higher the blood pressure, the faster the progression of renal disease. The results of the largest study, which included almost 7000 patients, indicated that the worsening in renal function correlated with blood pressure even within the normotensive range [89]; another study found that this observation was more evident for systolic blood pressure (SBP) than for DBP [262].

It seems that the rate of progression is a continuous function of MAP, which implies that renal protection is a continuous function of blood pressure down to the low end of the normal range. In individual patients, it has been shown in a retrospective study that hypertensive time periods (mean DBP 97 ± 2 mmHg) were associated with a significantly faster rate of decline in reciprocal creatinine versus time than normotensive periods (mean DBP 84 ± 1 mmHg) [261]. After having stratified patients in three main groups according to time-averaged MAP (first group MAP <100 mmHg, second group MAP between 100 and 110 mmHg, third group MAP >110 mmHg), Oldrizzi *et al.* [258] analysed renal survival after 10 years of follow-up in 544 patients and showed that the course of CRF was statistically worse in patients with MAP >110 mmHg than in those with MAP ≤110 mmHg, with a relative risk for the need of dialysis treatment of 5.3. Wight *et al.* [52] did not found a significant difference in the frequency of hypertension (defined as DBP >90 mmHg) between progressors (negative overall 1/Cr slope) and patients with stable or improving renal function. However, when only patients with non-linear progression rates were considered, blood pressure correlated inversely with the observed changes in breakpoint slopes (data points better fitted by a two-component line by using the breakpoint method proposed by Zoccali *et al.* [4]) (DBP: $r = -0.352$, $p = 0.003$; MAP: $r =$

−0.325, $p = 0.006$). Interestingly, the breakpoints showing an improvement in renal function were mainly associated with an intensification of antihypertensive therapy or to a better blood pressure control in the absence of change in therapy. Changes in slopes did not correlate with changes in SBP.

Other studies failed to show a significant relationship between the progression of CRF and blood pressure values during the course of the disease [47,48,263,264], except in patients with PKD [263,264]. Locatelli *et al.* [44,263] evaluated the role of blood pressure values as a prognostic factor for CRF progression. They found that the fast-progressive patients (defined as a significant plot of the reciprocal of serum creatinine against time together with a negative *b* value) or those who reached an end-point (doubling of baseline serum creatinine or need for dialysis) had significantly higher baseline blood pressure values than slowly-progressive patients (SBP: 157.8 vs 149.2 mmHg, $p < 0.01$; DBP: 98.2 vs 94.0 mmHg, $p < 0.05$). However, this relationship was not confirmed by a multivariate regression analysis [44]. During follow-up SBP, DBP, and MAP were not significantly different between slowly- and fast-progressive patients, only showing a statistically non-significant trend towards faster CRF progression for higher blood pressure values, possibly because a good blood pressure control was achieved with treatment and a low progression rate reduced the power of the analysis. Furthermore, no relationship was found between the number of antihypertensive drugs used during the follow-up and CRF progression [263,265]. Interestingly, Hannedouche *et al.* [51] found that the slope of progression was steeper in patients who required antihypertensive therapy than in patients who were spontaneously normotensive, even after adjustment for blood pressure values. This may suggest a better prognosis when blood pressure was spontaneously low than when a similar blood pressure level was achieved by antihypertensive treatment.

A number of trials have been performed to assess the degree of blood pressure reduction needed to achieve renoprotection. The MDRD study compared the effects of usual blood pressure control (defined as a MAP ≤107 mmHg or SBP/DBP ≤140/90 mmHg in subjects aged ≤60 years and MAP ≤113 mmHg or SBP/DBP ≤160/90 mmHg in subjects older than 60 years) and stricter blood pressure control (defined as a MAP ≤92 mmHg or SBP/DBP ≤125/75 mmHg in subjects aged ≤60 years and MAP ≤98 mmHg or SBP/DBP ≤145/75 mmHg in subjects older than 60 years) in 840 patients with CRF [30]. In study A (baseline GFR 25–55 ml/min) the mean decline in GFR was faster in the first 4 months of follow-up and slower thereafter in the strict than in the usual blood pressure group, while in patients with more advanced CRF (in study B baseline GFR 13–24 ml/min) the decline of GFR was linear and did not differ significantly between the two blood pressure groups. These data suggest that a stricter blood pressure control may be able to slow CRF progression only in the earlier phases of renal diseases. A secondary analysis compared the effects of blood pressure control in African-Americans and Caucasians who participated in the MDRD study [266]. In the usual blood pressure group, the mean rate of GFR decline after 4 months was 2.8 times greater in black people than white people ($p < 0.001$) and 2.0 times greater after 2 years ($p = 0.04$). In contrast, in the low blood pressure group, neither the rate of GFR decline after 4 months nor the

GFR after 2 years differed significantly between black people and white people. Furthermore, a sevenfold faster rate of decline of GFR was found in black people than white people at the same MAP achieved during follow-up ($p < 0.001$).

Considering all these findings, the authors have recommended a lower than usual blood pressure goal (MAP ≤92 mmHg or blood pressure ≤125/75 mmHg) for patients with moderate CRF and proteinuria >1g/24h, irrespective of race. In addition, attempts to achieve a blood pressure goal of MAP ≤98 mmHg or blood pressure ≤145/75 mmHg may be indicated for black people with moderate CRF, even if proteinuria is <1 g/24 h.

Another prospective study have demonstrated that in African-Americans with hypertensive non-DN, randomized to two different levels of blood pressure, a reduction in MAP to levels of less than 92 mmHg could stop the progression of renal disease [121]. This preservation of renal function seemed to be independent of the antihypertensive agents used.

Hypertension and diabetic nephropathy

Hypertension is a risk factor for the development of microvascular complications in diabetes, as well as for the progression of renal failure in patients with overt DN.

A positive linear correlation exists between the albumin excretion rate and arterial blood pressure in IDDM, but it is difficult to establish whether high blood pressure pre-dates the increase in albumin excretion: one prospective study found significant blood pressure elevation before the development of microalbuminuria [267], but another did not [268]. Not only do patients with microalbuminuria have higher blood pressure values than patients without [269], but also 24-h ambulatory blood pressure in normoalbuminuric IDDM subjects is lower in those with an albumin excretion rate of less than the median (5.8 μg/min) than in those with

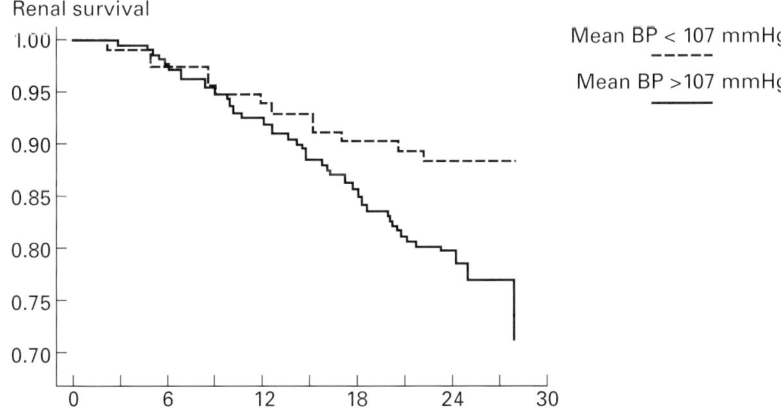

Fig. 2.3 Actuarial renal survival rates according to baseline blood pressure in 402 patients with CRF [45].

normoalbuminuria above this value [271]. Once persistent proteinuria develops in IDDM patients, SBP begins to rise at a rate that has been suggested to average about 1 mmHg/month [271].

The relationship seems to be different in NIDDM. An average 24-h blood pressure >130/80 mmHg was found in 60% of patients with a recent diagnosis of NIDDM; moreover, 94% of the untreated hypertensive patients had no micro-albuminuria, thus indicating that hypertension was not a result of nephropathy [272]. A high prevalence of hypertension (25.8%) in the pre-diabetic phase has also been documented in a large Hispanic population [273] as well as in Pima Indians [135].

A more rapid progression to ESRD has been documented in hypertensive diabetic patients with renal failure. According to Biesenbach [274], the rate of loss of creatinine clearance is higher in patients with SBP ≥160 mmHg. Walker *et al.* [275] found a progressive increase in serum creatinine only in individuals with stable SBP ≥140 mmHg while on therapy. When IDDM and NIDDM patients were examined separately, a more rapid decline in renal function was demonstrated in the hypertensive subjects of both groups. A significant difference was also found for DBP, even when the mean values were within the normal range.

Several studies of DN have also shown that a reduction in blood pressure induced by various antihypertensive drugs can slow the progression of renal failure [246,276–278].

Proteinuria and hypertension interaction

Many patients with progressive chronic renal disease suffer from both hypertension and proteinuria. Locatelli *et al.* [45] evaluated the possible relationship between proteinuria and hypertension in 456 patients. The hypertensive subjects (MAP >107 mmHg) had slightly lower renal survival rates than the normotensives (24-month cumulative survival 80% versus 89%), but the degree of proteinuria was more important than hypertension as a prognostic factor of renal death. The analysis of end-point renal survival according to baseline 24-h proteinuria and MAP found that patients with the higher level of MAP had a slightly worse renal survival in each 24-h proteinuria strata. By multivariate analysis proteinuria was again significantly related to renal survival, but MAP was not.

It has been suggested that the presence of proteinuria is a prerequisite for the occurrence of renal failure deterioration, whereas blood pressure becomes a relevant risk factor only in the presence of severe urinary protein loss [279]. Indeed, it has been shown that patients with greater proteinuria at baseline had higher MAP during follow-up ($p < 0.001$) [120].

In order to clarify the importance of reductions in both proteinuria and hypertension on CRF progression, Locatelli *et al.* [45] stratified proteinuric hypertensive patients (proteinuria ≥1 g/24 h and MAP ≥107 mmHg) according to the behaviour of 24-h proteinuria and mean blood pressure values during follow-up. It was shown that only the decrease in proteinuria affected renal survival, whereas a simultaneous decrease in proteinuria and mean blood pressure did not seem to give a further

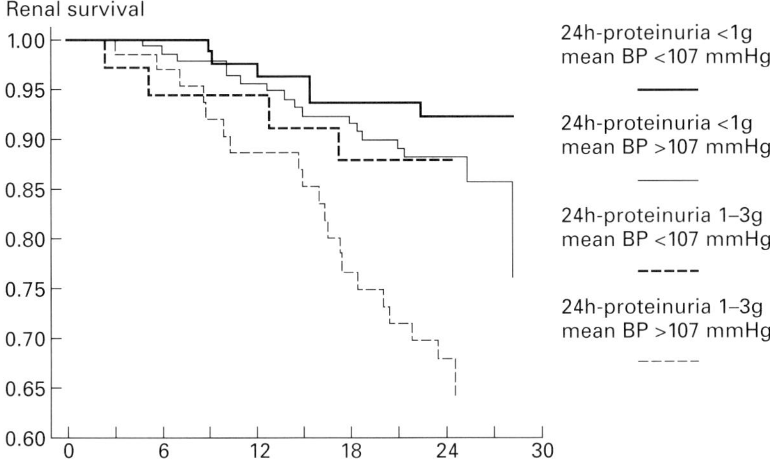

Fig. 2.4 Actuarial renal survival rates according to baseline proteinuria and blood pressure [45].

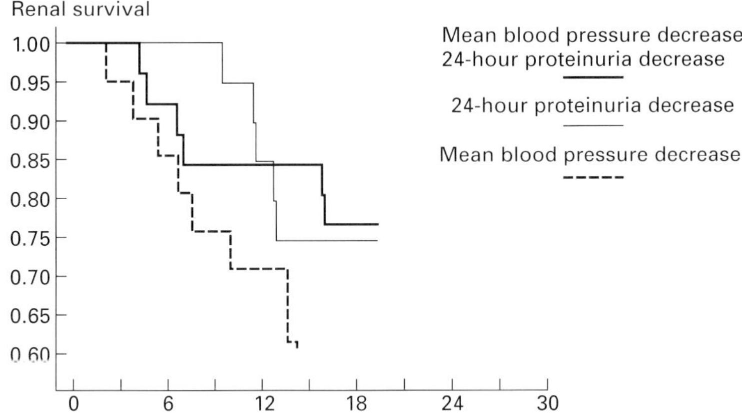

Fig. 2.5 Actuarial renal survival rates in patients with baseline proteinuria >1 g/24 h and mean blood pressure >107 mmHg ($n = 77$), stratified according to the behaviour of proteinuria and blood pressure during follow-up [45].

benefit, possibly because the good blood pressure control achieved with treatment and a low progression rate reduced the power of the analysis. Anyway, in a recent meta-analysis Maki *et al.* [281] found that long-term beneficial effects of antihypertensive agents on proteinuria and GFR were proportional to blood pressure reductions and were similar in diabetic and non-diabetic patients with renal disease. ACE inhibitors, and possibly non-dihydropyridine calcium antagonists, had additional beneficial effects on proteinuria that were independent of blood pressure reductions.

Proteinuria may identify renal disease patients who would benefit from stricter blood pressure control than that currently recommended. The MDRD study found that patients with higher levels of baseline proteinuria showed a faster decline in GFR and received greater benefits from being assigned to a low blood pressure target [30]. In patients with baseline GFR 25–55 ml/min (Study A) and baseline proteinuria of 0.25–3 g/24 h, the association of higher blood pressure with faster decline in GFR was apparent beginning at about a MAP of 98 mmHg, while in patients with proteinuria >3.0 g/24 h a greater decline in GFR was seen at a MAP ≥92 mmHg. The rate of decline of GFR was unrelated to follow-up blood pressure in the course of the study in patients with proteinuria of less than 0.25 g/24 h and assignment to a low blood pressure target did not affect the rate of progression in this group. In patients with more advanced CRF (in study B baseline GFR was 13–24 ml/min) and baseline proteinuria <1.0 g/24 h, the rate of decline of GFR was unrelated to follow-up blood pressure, whereas a faster decline in GFR was shown with higher follow-up blood pressure in the course of the study and baseline proteinuria >1.0 g/24 h [120]. In the strict blood pressure group of both studies, mean protein excretion was significantly reduced during follow-up ($p < 0.05$), with a percentage change in proteinuria similar for all levels of baseline proteinuria. However, it is worthwhile to underline that in patients with baseline proteinuria <1.0 g/24 h the difference in percentage change in proteinuria corresponds to a minimal difference in the magnitude of proteinuria. This may partially explain why patients with low baseline proteinuria seem not to benefit from a strict blood pressure control.

Considering these data, it has been suggested to consider the level of proteinuria before defining blood pressure goals in patients with CRF [120]. A MAP ≤92 mmHg (equivalent to a blood pressure of 125/75 mmHg) should be recommended in patients with proteinuria >1 g/24 h, while a MAP ≤98 mmHg (equivalent to a blood pressure of 130/80 mmHg) should be considered as a goal in patients with proteinuria 0.25–1 g/24 h. In patients with proteinuria <0.25 g/24 h, the target blood pressure of less than 138/82 mmHg, recently suggested to be achieved in essential hypertensives to reduce cardiovascular risk [281], seems to be adequate.

It should also be considered that antihypertensive agents are not all equally effective to reduce proteinuria. Despite similar blood pressure reductions, proteinuria tends to decrease more on ACE inhibitors (on average −45%) than on conventional therapy (on average −23%) or calcium channel blockers other than nifedipine (on average −35%) [282]. Furthermore, ACE inhibitors are able to reduce proteinuria of −28% without blood pressure changes and varied of 1.5% thereafter for each per cent of blood pressure change. On the other hand, on conventional therapy, proteinuria began to decrease only after a blood pressure reduction of 5% [282]. However, further reduction of proteinuria with progressive lowering of blood pressure is less with ACE inhibitors than with other antihypertensives. After a decrease of approximately 20 mmHg in blood pressure, the antiproteinuric effect becomes the same for all the drugs.

Calcium and phosphorus metabolism

Disordered calcium homeostasis, leading to intrarenal calcium deposition, is a characteristic feature of CRI. The calcium phosphate content of the kidney is increased both in experimental models of renal failure, as well as in patients with ESRD [283,284]. Gimenez *et al.* [285] documented increased calcium levels in renal biopsies obtained very early in the course of human renal disease, which were consistent with the hypothesis that increased renal calcium deposits may play a part in the progression of renal injury.

Laboratory animal studies also suggest a role for calcium and phosphorus precipitation in multiple intrarenal compartments, including the tubular lumen, parenchymal cell cytoplasm, and renal interstitium: the subsequent intracellular calcium intoxication could lead to disorders in cell function and eventually cell death, followed by interstitial inflammation and fibrosis [286].

An increased serum calcium phosphate product has been implicated in the pathogenesis of progressive renal failure in humans, with an improvement in the rate of decline of renal function in patients whose calcium phosphate product is reduced [287]. It has been suggested that phosphate absorbed in excess of the residual nephron excretory capacity leads to the precipitation and deposition of calcium phosphate microcrystals in the tubular lumen, peritubular space, capillaries, and interstitium, and thus causes progressive functional deterioration [286].

Williams *et al.* [48] found that the calcium phosphorus product was weakly correlated with the rate of decline of renal function only in patients with mild CRF (plasma creatinine <0.25 μmol/l) ($r = 0.74$, $p < 0.01$), and not in patients with more severe renal failure (plasma creatinine 0.25–0.55 μmol/l). In a prospective multicentre study to clarify the role of protein restriction in delaying CRF progression, Locatelli *et al.* [44] also found that serum calcium-phosphate product was significantly higher in the patients who reached an end-point (doubling of baseline serum creatinine or need for dialysis) ($p < 0.01$). However, by multivariate regression analysis the calcium-phosphate product correlated with 1/Cr ($p = 0.0337$), but not with C_{Cr} ($p = 0.65$). It seems to be more likely that the behaviour of the calcium-phosphate product is a consequence of progressive renal function deterioration rather than an important factor determining the progression of CRF and probably it may simply reflect the accumulation of phosphate that it is insufficiently controlled by diet or phosphate binders [41].

Dyslipidemia

The role of lipids in renal damage

CRF is accompanied by specific alterations in the lipoprotein metabolism. As the first observation that lipids accumulate within scarred kidneys [288,289], it has been suggested that dyslipoproteinemia contributes towards the progression of glomerular and tubular lesions, which leads to a subsequent deterioration in renal function. The possible mechanisms of damage include mesangial matrix accumulation, focal and segmental glomerulosclerosis and monocyte infiltration into pre-injured glomeruli [290]. Similarities have also been found between the processes of atherosclerosis and glomerular sclerosis, with lipids playing an important role in the pathogenesis of both [291,292].

Clinical trials on lipids and the progression of chronic renal failure

There are few prospective, randomized large-scale clinical trials concerning the relationship between lipids and worsening of CRF. In the diabetes cohort ($n = 131$) of the Longitudinal Diabetic Study, and in all of the participants in the MRFIT study [122,293], no statistical association was found between the level of cholesterol and evidence of progressive renal damage, even though the levels of serum cholesterol were higher in hypertensive subjects. In another group of IDDM patients with proteinuria, hypercholesterolemia was found to be an important independent predictor of the rate of loss of renal function [294]. In this study the prevalence of patients with rapid loss of renal function was found to rise with increasing level of serum cholesterol. About 26% of the patients with cholesterol levels <200 mg/dl had a rapid loss of renal function during follow-up, while this outcome was shown in 38% of those with levels ranging from 260 to 299 mg/dl, and in 48% of those with serum cholesterol ≥300 mg/dl. The Helsinki Heart Study found a 20% faster decline in renal function during the 5-year study period in subjects with a high LDL/HDL ratio (>4.4) than in those with a ratio of less than 3.2 [295]. A recent small prospective study of 73 non-diabetic patients with primary chronic renal disease found that lipoprotein abnormalities characteristic of renal dyslipoproteinemia (increased concentrations of intact or partially metabolized apolipoprotein (apo) B-containing lipoproteins and reduced concentrations of apoA-containing lipoproteins [296]) were significantly associated with the rate of progression of CRF [297]. In these patients, the initial total and low-density lipoprotein (LDL) cholesterol levels, together with the initial levels of apoB, correlated significantly with a more rapid decline of GFR, while no significant relation was found between triglycerides, very low-density lipoprotein (VLDL) cholesterol, apoC-III, apoE, or high-density lipoprotein (HDL)-related variables (HDL cholesterol, apoAI, apoAII, apoC-III-HS) and the rate of progression. Interestingly, the significant association between the initial total cholesterol, LDL cholesterol and apoB levels were independent of the GFR value at the entry in the study. By multiple linear regression analysis, LDL cholesterol, together with proteinuria and initial diastolic and systolic blood pressure values, remained significantly and independently associated with the rate of progression. ApoB levels did not reach the statistical significance ($p = 0.06$). When the patient population was divided into four groups using the median values of SBP (cut-off point 140 mmHg) and the median value of apoB (cut-off point 145 mg/dl), it was found that those with high SBP and a high plasma concentration of apoB had a four times higher progression rates than those with low SBP and apoB levels (−5.1 ml/min per 1.73 m^2 per year vs −1.4 ml/min per 1.73 m^2 per year; $p < 0.001$). Recently, a strong association was also observed between the plasma concentration of complex triglyceride-rich apoB-containing lipoproteins and the rate of CRF progression [298].

Conclusions

Following renal injury, a progressive deterioration in renal function generally occurs, regardless of the nature of the original nephropathy, even after the initiating process has remitted spontaneously or has been therapeutically controlled. In past years it was generally believed that renal function was lost at a constant rate, but thereafter it has became clear that non-linear rate of progression is a common feature of the 'natural history' of CRF. None of the proposed mathematics models aimed to describe the rate of CRF progression seem to be completely adequate.

Although the underlying disease is a determining factor able to influence the rate of progression of CRF by disease-specific pathogenic mechanisms, the results reported in the literature are equivocal. These differences can probably be explained by the fact that some of the authors only considered crude cumulative renal survival of the different nephropathies, without taking into account concomitant risk factors. On the other side, multivariate analyses testing the importance of the underlying disease after having eliminated the influence of important determinants of CRF progression, such as hypertension and, overall, proteinuria, may give misleading results. Another confounding factor may be the degree of baseline CRF, possibly because a selection of more progressive diseases at higher levels of renal function deterioration occurs. Furthermore, in these studies, the rate of decline in GFR was measured using different methods, not allowing easy comparisons.

Elderly patients constitute an increasing segment of the ESRD population beginning dialysis in Western countries. Although it was previously assumed that a loss of renal mass and an inexorable decline in renal function occur with ageing, in the few past years it has been demonstrated that in healthy elderly renal function remained within the normal range in two-thirds of cases and that a decrease in GFR was primarily associated with cardiovascular diseases, such as heart failure and hypertension. However, due to a reduction in ERPF and an increase in the FF, hyperfiltration may take place in the remaining nephrons, and, in the presence of systemic hypertension or an intrinsic renal disease, accelerate the progression of CRF.

As far as gender is concerned, ESRD occurs more frequently in males than in females at most ages. It is not certain whether males have a higher susceptibility to renal diseases or are more likely to develop the effects of this disease. Anyway, in chronic renal diseases the rate of progression seems more rapid in men than in women, whereas no gender difference has been noted in the progression of prepubertal subjects with nephronopthisis or cystinosis, indicating that the gender effect appears only after puberty, presumably via sex hormones.

African-Americans, Mexican-Americans and Native Americans are at higher risk of developing ESRD than the general population. The two most common diseases responsible for this higher incidence are hypertension and diabetes. It has been described that the pathogenesis of essential hypertension in black people differs from that observe in white people, with a higher prevalence of salt-sensitivity and a shift to the right of blood pressure distribution in the former, possibly leading to a rise of intraglomerular pressure and then to renal damage. African-Americans, Mexican-Americans and Native Americans have also a higher prevalence of diabetes and are at higher risk to develop DN. Although these minorities have a reduced educational and economical status, the MDRD study has shown that the higher risk of ESRD in African-Americans than in Caucasians is maintained at all levels of income, suggesting the important role of genetic factors. However, no clear linkage between CRF and candidate genes has yet been demonstrated in these populations.

As far as genetic factors are concerned, many studies have been performed to identify genes possibly involved in CRF progression. A number of associations have been found between HLA antigens and negative outcome in various renal diseases, but it seems that they may have a stronger influence on the susceptibility rather than on outcome of some immuno-mediated renal diseases. Data on a possible role of the ACE gene polymorphism are more promising. A number of authors have reported an association between the I/D polymorphism and the development of DN or a negative outcome in IgAN. However, not all the studies found a statistically significant higher frequency of the D allele in the patients with a more rapid loss of renal function and the I/D polymorphism does not seem to be a *per se* risk factor for reaching ESRD compared with control populations. The conflicting results may reflect the small number of patients studied in some reports, different definitions of 'progressive' nephropathy, and ethnic differences. Although the polymorphism of the AGT gene is the only one, together with α-adducin gene, that have been clearly associated with essential hypertension, only one study has so far found an association between this polymorphism and a negative outcome in IgAN. Also in IDDM the reports have been conflicting. Interestingly, the interaction between AGT and ACE gene polymorphism may adversely affect the disease progression in IgAN.

Cigarette smoking has been linked in the development and progression of diabetic and non-diabetic renal diseases. The effect of tobacco on CRF progression is possibly related to the exacerbation of other risk factors such as systemic hypertension, proteinuria, or hyperlipidemia.

Urinary protein excretion is not only a marker of disease activity, but it is probably the most important factor with a causal role in CRF progression. Baseline proteinuria is the strongest predictor of a subsequent decline in GFR and its mean value during follow-up correlates with the rate of decline in renal function. A reduction in urinary protein excretion is also associated with a better renal outcome in diabetic and non-diabetic renal diseases, with less deterioration in renal function in the patients with the most evident antiproteinuric response.

Hypertension is an important presenting feature of renal disease, and it is probably one of the most important factors, together with proteinuria contributing to progression. However, although a number of retrospective studies have confirmed that progression is faster with higher blood pressure values, other studies have failed to show a significant relationship between the rate of progression and blood pressure values during the course of the disease, except in patients with PKD. Perhaps a low progression rate and a certain degree of blood pressure control achieved anyway with treatment in all the patients may have reduced the power of the analysis. On the other side, a number of clinical trials have demonstrated that a strict blood pressure control may be able to slow CRF progression, especially in the earlier phases of renal diseases and in proteinuric patients.

However, it seems that only the decrease in proteinuria may affect renal survival, whereas a simultaneous decrease in proteinuria and mean blood pressure do not seem to give a further benefit. It should be considered that a reduction in blood pressure values leads to a contemporary reduction in proteinuria. Therefore, it may be difficult to separate the weight of the two effects on the rate of progression. Interestingly, after the reduction in blood pressure, a percentage change in proteinuria is observed for all levels of baseline proteinuria. This suggests that for low levels of baseline proteinuria the effect of blood pressure reduction may be small and not easily detectable, thus partially explaining why some patients seem not to benefit from a strict blood pressure control. It should also be considered that antihypertensive agents are not all equally effective in reducing proteinuria: despite similar blood pressure reductions, proteinuria tends to decrease more on ACE inhibitors than on conventional therapy or calcium channel blockers. Furthermore, ACE inhibitors are able to obtain this effect without blood pressure changes, whereas conventional therapy began to decrease proteinuria only after blood pressure reduction.

Although the calcium phosphate content of the kidney is increased in experimental models of renal failure and in patients with ESRD, the calcium and phosphorus metabolism seems not to play a major part in the progression of renal injury, at least in the early phases.

It has been found that total cholesterol, together with LDL-cholesterol levels and apoB, correlated independently and significantly with a more rapid decline of GFR in diabetic and non-diabetic proteinuric renal diseases. However, further studies enrolling larger numbers of patients with different degrees of proteinuria are needed to elucidate whether lipid abnormalities have a casual role in CRF progression or they are merely a consequence of metabolic derangements.

Interventions aiming to slow the progression of CRF will have to take into consideration the better understanding of the natural history of chronic renal diseases and the numerous factors, outlined in this chapter, that influence progressive renal insufficiency.

Acknowledgements

The authors would like to thank Professor Eberhard Ritz Editor-in-Chief of *Nephrology Dialysis Transplantation* for permission to reproduce published material in the paper: Locatelli F, Marcelli D, Comelli M, Alberti D, Graziani G, Buccianti G, Redaelli B, Giangrande A, and the Northern Italian Cooperative Study Group. Proteinuria and blood pressure as causal components of progression to end-stage renal failure. *Nephrol Dial Transplant* 1996; **11**: 461–467 (Figs 1, 2, 3, 4, 5).

They would like also to thank Mrs Castagna; librarian of the Azienda Ospedale di Lecco, for help with bibliographic research.

Key references

Klahr S, Levey AS, Beck GJ, Caggiula AW, Hunsicker LG, Kusek JW, Striker G, and the Modification of Diet in Renal Disease Study Group. The effects of dietary protein restriction and blood pressure control on the progression of renal disease. *N Engl J Med* 1994; **330**: 877–884.

Locatelli F, Marcelli D, Comelli M, Alberti D, Graziani G, Buccianti G, Redaelli B, Giangrande A, and the Northern Italian Cooperative Study Group. Proteinuria and blood pressure as causal components of progression to end-stage renal failure. *Nephrol Dial Transplant* 1996; **11**: 461–467.

Maschio G, Alberti D, Janin G, Locatelli F, Mann JFE, Motolese M, Ponticelli C, Ritz E, Zucchelli P, and the Angiotensin-Converting-Enzyme Inhibition in Progressive Renal Insufficiency Study Group. Effect of the Angiotensin-Converting-Enzyme inhibitor benazepril on the progression of chronic renal insufficiency. *N Engl J Med* 1996; **334**: 939–945.

Mitch WE, Walser M. A simple method of estimating progression of chronic renal failure. *Lancet* 1976; **ii**: 1326–1331.

Van Essen GG, Rensma PL, de Zeeuw D, Sluiter WJ, Scheffer H, Apperloo AJ. Association between angiotensin-converting-enzyme gene polymorphism and failure of renoprotective therapy. *Lancet* 1996; **347**: 94–95.

References

1. Rutherford WE, Blondin J, Miller JP, Greenwalt AS, Vavra JD. Chronic progressive renal disease: rate of change of serum creatinine concentration. *Kidney Int* 1977; **11**: 62–70.
2. Mitch WE, Walser M. A simple method of estimating progression of chronic renal failure. *Lancet* 1976; **ii**: 1326–1331.
3. Shah BV, Levey AS. Spontaneous changes in the rate of decline in reciprocal serum creatinine: errors in predicting the progression of renal disease from extrapolation of the slope. *J Am Soc Nephrol* 1992; **2** (7): 1186–1191.
4. Zoccali C, Postorino M, Martorano C, Salnitro F, Maggiore Q. The 'Breakpoint' Test, a new statistical method for studying progression of chronic renal failure. *Nephrol Dial Transplant* 1989; **4**: 101–104.
5. Fellin G, Gentile MG, Duca G, D'Amico G. Renal function in IgA nephropathy with established renal failure. *Nephrol Dial Transplant* 1988; **3**: 17–23.
6. Gretz NM. How to assess the rate of progression of chronic renal failure in children? *Pediatr Nephrol* 1994; **8**: 499–504.
7. Smith HW. Measurements of the filtration rate. In *The Kidney: Structure, Function in Health, Disease*. New York, Oxford University Press, 1951: 39–62.
8. Striker GE, Schainuck LI, Cutler RE, Benditt EP. Structural-functional correlations in renal disease. A method for assaying and classifying histopathological changes in renal disease. *Hum Pathol* 1970; **1** (4): 615–630.
9. Barbour GL, Crum CK, Boyd CM, Reeves RD, Rastogi SP, Pattersom RM. Comparison of inulin, iothalamate and ^{99m}Tc. DPTA for measurement of glomerular filtration rate. *J Nuclear Med* 1976; **17**: 317–320.
10. Rehling M, Moller ML, Thamdrup B, Lund JO, Trapjensen J. Simultaneous measurement of renal clearance and plasma clearance of ^{99}mTc-labelled diethylenetraminepenta-acetate, ^{51}Cr-labelled ethylenediaminetetra-acetate and inulin in man. *Clin Sci* 1984; **66**: 613–619.
11. Acker B, Koomen G, Koopman M, Krediet R, Arisz L. Discrepancy between circadian rhythms of inulin and creatinine clearance. *J Lab Clin Med* 1992; **120**: 400–410.
12. Schumann L, Wüstenberg P, Hortlan B, Kühnle H. Determination of glomerular filtration rate on two consecutive days using inulin in a single-sample plasma clearance method. *Clin Nephrol* 1993; **39**: 65–69.

13. Gaspari F, Mosconi L, Viganò G, Perico N, Torre L, Virotta G, Bertocchi C, Remuzzi G, Ruggenenti P. Measurements of GFR with a single intravenous injection of non radioactive iothalamate. *Kidney Int* 1992; **41**: 1081–1084.
14. Gaspari F, Guerini E, Perico N, Mosconi L, Ruggenenti P, Remuzzi G. Glomerular filtration rate determined from a single plasma sample after intravenous iohexol injection: it is reliable? *J Am Soc Nephrol* 1996; **7**: 2689–2693.
15. Brown SCW, O'Reilly PH. Iohexol clearance for the determination of glomerular filtration rate in clinical practice: evidence for a new gold standard. *J Urol* 1991; **146**: 675–679.
16. Holliday MA, Heilbro D, Al-Uzri A, Hidayat J, Uauy R, Conley S, Reisch J, Hogg RJ. Serial measurements of GFR in infants using the continuous iothalamate infusion technique. *Kidney Int* 1993; **43**: 893–898.
17. Levey AS, Berg RL, Gassman JJ, Hall PM, Walker WG. Creatinine filtration, secretion and excretion during progressive renal disease. Modification of Diet in Renal Disease (MDRD) study group. *Kidney Int* 1989; **27**: S73–S80.
18. Levey AS and the Modification of Diet in Renal Disease Study Group. Effects of diet and antihypertensive therapy on creatinine clearance and serum creatinine concentration in the Modification of Diet in Renal Disease Study. *J Am Soc Nephrol* 1996; **7**: 556–565.
19. Maschio G, Oldrizzi L, Rugiu C. Protein-restricted diet in early chronic renal failure. *Contrib Nephrol* 1989; **75**: 134–140.
20. Kamper AL, Strandgaard S, Nielsen SL. The validity of the reciprocal plasma creatinine to assess changes in renal function in severe chronic renal failure. [Abstract]. XXVIth Congress of European Dialysis and Transplant Society, 1989; 63.
21. Levey AS. Measurement of renal function in chronic renal disease. *Kidney Int* 1990; **38**: 167–184.
22. De Santo NG, Coppola S, Anastasio P, Coscarella G, Capasso G, Bellini L, Santangelo R, Massimo L, Siciliano A. Predicted creatinine clearance to assess glomerular filtration rate in chronic renal disease in humans. *Am J Nephrol* 1991; **11**: 181–185.
23. Cockcroft DW, Gault MH. Prediction of creatinine clearance from serum creatinine. *Nephron* 1976; **16**: 31–41.
24. Gabriel R. Time to scrap creatinine clearance? *Br Med J* 1986; **293**: 1119–1120.
25. van Acker BAC, Koomen GCM, Koopman MG, de Waart DR, Arisz L. Creatinine clearance during cimetidine administration for measurement of glomerular filtration rate. *Lancet* 1992; **340**: 1326–1329.
26. Donadio C, Lucchesi A, Tramonti G, Bianchi C. Creatinine clearance predicted from body cell mass is a good indicator of renal function. *Kidney Int* 1997; **52** (Suppl. 63): S166–S168.
27. Oldrizzi L, Rugiu C, Valvo E, Lupo A, Loschiavo C, Gammaro L, Tessitore N, Fabris A, Panzetta G, Maschio G. Progression of renal failure in patients with renal disease of diverse etiology on protein-restricted diet. *Kidney Int* 1985; **27**: 553–557.
28. Rosman JB, Ter Wee PM, Meijer S, Piers-Becht TPM, Sluiter WJ, Donker AJM. Prospective randomized trial of early dietary protein restriction in chronic renal failure. *Lancet* 1984; **ii**: 1291–1296.
29. Walser M. Progression of chronic renal failure in man. *Kidney Int* 1990; **37**: 1195–1210.
30. Klahr S, Levey AS, Beck GJ, Caggiula AW, Hunsicker LG, Kusek JW, Striker G and the Modification of Diet in Renal Disease Study Group. The effects of dietary protein restriction and blood pressure control on the progression of renal disease. *N Engl J Med* 1994; **330**: 877–884.

31. Maschio G, Alberti D, Janin G, Locatelli F, Mann JFE, Motolese M, Ponticelli C, Ritz E, Zucchelli P and the Angiotensin-Converting-Enzyme Inhibition in Progressive Renal Insufficiency Study Group. Effect of the angiotensin-converting-enzyme inhibitor benazepril on the progression of chronic renal insufficiency. *N Engl J Med* 1996; **334**: 939–945.
32. Jones RH, Molitoris BA. A statistical method for determining the breakpoint of two lines. *Anal Biochem* 1984; **141**: 287–290.
33. Brochner-Mortensen J. Routine methods and their reliability for assessment of glomerular filtration rate in adults. *Dan Med Bull* 1978; **25**: 181–202.
34. Rossing P. Doubling of serum creatinine: is it sensitive and relevant? *Nephrol Dial Transplant* 1998; **13**: 244–246.
35. Locatelli F, Carbarns IRI, Maschio G, Mann JFE, Ponticelli C, Ritz E, Alberti D, Motolese M, Janin G, Zucchelli P and the Angiotensin-Converting-Enzyme Inhibition in Progressive Renal Insufficiency Study Group. Long-term progression of chronic renal insufficiency in the AIPRI Extension Study. *Kidney Int* 1997; **52** (Suppl. 63): S63–S66.
36. Marthews DE, Farewell V. *Using and Understanding Medical Statistics*. Karger, Basel, 1985: 67–87, 148–157.
37. Kaplan EL, Meier P. Non parametric estimation from incomplete observations. *Am Stat Assoc J* 1958: 458–481.
38. Peto R, Pike MC, Armitage P, Breslow NE, Cox DR, Howard SV, Mantel N, McPherson K, Peto J, Smith PG. Design and analysis of randomized clinical trials requiring prolonged observation for each patient. *Br J Cancer* 1977; **35**: 1–38.
39. Kalbfleisch JD, Prentice RL. *The Statistical Analysis of Failure Time Data*.Wiley, New York, 1980.
40. Peduzzi P, Holford T, Detre K, Chan YK. Comparison of the logistic and Cox regression models when the outcome is determined in all patients after a fixed period of time. *J Chronic Dis* 1987; **40**: 761–767.
41. Gretz N, Strauch M. Low-protein diet and chronic renal failure. *Lancet* 1991; **338**: 442.
42. Cattran DC, Pei Y, Greenwood CMT, Ponticelli C, Passerini P, Honkanen E. Validation of a predictive model of idiopathic membranous nephropathy: its clinical and research implications. *Kidney Int* 1997; **51**: 901–907.
43. Geddes CC, Fox JG, Allison MEM, Boulton-Jones JM, Simpson K. An artificial neural network can select patients at high risk of developing progressive IgA nephropathy more accurately than experienced nephrologists. *Nephrol Dial Tranplant* 1998; **13**: 67–71.
44. Locatelli F, Alberti D, Graziani G, Buccianti G, Redaelli B, Giangrande A, Marcelli D, Francucci BM and the Northern Italian Cooperative Study Group. Factors affecting chronic renal failure progression: results from a multi-centre trial. *Miner Electrolyte Metab* 1992; **18**: 295–302.
45. Locatelli F, Marcelli D, Comelli M, Alberti D, Graziani G, Buccianti G, Redaelli B, Giangrande A and the Northern Italian Cooperative Study Group. Proteinuria and blood pressure as causal components of progression to end-stage renal failure. *Nephrol Dial Transplant* 1996; **11**: 461–467.
46. Gruppo Italiano di Studi Epidemiologici in Nefrologia (GISEN). A randomized placebo controlled trial of the angiotensin-converting-enzyme inhibitor ramipril on the decline of the glomerular filtration rate and end stage renal failure in proteinuric, non-diabetic chronic renal disease. *Lancet* 1997; **349**: 1857–1863.
47. Jungers P, Hannnedouche T, Itakura Y, Albouze G, Descamps-Latscha B, Man NK.

Progression rate to end-stage renal failure in non-diabetic kidney diseases: a multivariate analysis of determinant factors. *Nephrol Dial Transplant* 1995; **10**: 1353–1360.
48. Williams PS, Fass G, Bone JM. Renal pathology and proteinuria determine progression in untreated mild/moderate chronic renal failure. *Q J Med* 1988; **67**: 43–54.
49. Stenvinkel P, Alverstrand A, Bergström J. Factors influencing progression in patients with chronic renal failure. *J Intern Med* 1989; **226**: 183–188.
50. El Nahas AM, Masters-Thomas A, Brady SA, Farrington K, Wilkinson V, Hilson AJ, Varghese Z, Moorhead JF. Selective effect of low protein diets in chronic renal diseases. *Br Med J* 1984; **289**: 1337–1341.
51. Hannedouche T, Chauveau P, Kalou F, Albouze G, Lacour B, Jungers P. Factors affecting progression in advanced chronic renal failure. *Clin Nephrol* 1993; **39**: 312–320.
52. Wight JP, Salzano S, Brown CB, El Nahas AM. Natural history of chronic renal failure: a reappraisal. *Nephrol Dial Transplant* 1992; **7**: 379–383.
53. Franz K, Reubi F. Rate of functional deterioration in polycystic kidney disease. *Kidney Int* 1983; **23**: 526–529.
54. Fliser D, Franek E, Joest M, Stefa B, Mutschler E, Ritz E. Renal function in the elderly: Impact of hypertension and cardiac function. *Kidney Int* 1997; **51**: 1196–1204.
55. Fliser D, Zeier M, Norwack R, Ritz E. Renal function reserve in healthy elderly subjects. *J Am Soc Nephrol* 1993; **3**: 1371–1377.
56. Baylis C, Fredericks M, Wilson C, Munger K, Collins R. Renal vasodilatory response to intravenous glycine in the aging rat kidney. *Am J Kidney Dis* 1990; **15**: 244–251.
57. Emamian SA, Nielsen MB, Pedersen JF, Ytte L. Kidney dimension at sonography: Correlation with age, sex, and glomerular sclerosis. *Nephron* 1993; **58** (4): 429–436.
58. Hollenberg NK, Adams DF, Solomon HF, Rashid A, Abrams HL, Merril JP. Senescence and the renal vasculature in normal man. *Circ Res* 1974; **34**: 309–316.
59. Kaplan C, Pasternack B, Shah H, Gallo G. Age-related incidence of sclerotic glomeruli in human kidneys. *Am J Pathol* 1975; **80**: 227–234.
60. Takazakura E, Sawabu N, Handa A, Takada A, Shinoda A, Takeuchi J. Intrarenal vascular changes with age and disease. *Kidney Int* 1972; **2**: 224–230.
61. Kasiske BL. Relationship between vascular disease and age-associated changes in the human kidney. *Kidney Int* 1986; **31**: 1153–1159.
62. Wesson LG (ed.). Renal hemodynamics in physiological states. *Physiology of the Human Kidney*. Grune & Stratton, London, 1969; 96–116.
63. Davies DF, Shock NW. Age changes in glomerular filtration rate, effective plasma flow and tubular excretory capacity in adult males. *J Clin Invest* 1950; **29**: 496–507.
64. Rowe JW, Andres R, Tobin J, Norris AH, Shock NW. The effect of age on creatinine clearance in men: a cross-sectional and longitudinal study. *J Gerontol* 1976; **31**: 155–163.
65. Kaysen GA, Myers BD. The aging kidney. *Clin Geriatr Med* 1985; **1**: 207–222.
66. Lindeman RD, Tobin JD, Shock NW. Longitudinal studies on the rate of decline in renal function with age. *J Am Geriatr Soc* 1985; **33**: 278–285.
67. Feinfeld DA, Guzik H, Carvounis CP, Lynn RI, Somer B, Aronson MK, Frishman WH. Sequential changes in renal function tests in the old: results from the Bronx Longitudinal Aging Study. *J Am Geriatr Soc* 1995; **43**: 412–414.
68. Luft FC, Fineberg NS, Miller JZ, Rankin LI, Grim CE. The effects of age, race and heredity on GFR following volume expansion and contraction in normal man. *Am J Med Sci* 1980; **279**: 15–24.
69. Larsson M, Jagenburg R, Landahl S. Renal function in an elderly population: a study of S-creatinine, Cr-EDTA-clearance, C_{Cr} and maximal tubular water reabsorption. *Scand J Clin Lab Invest* 1986; **46**: 593–598.

70. Lindeman RD, Tobin JD, Shock NW. Association between blood pressure and the rate of decline in renal function with age. *Kidney Int* 1984; **26**: 861–868.
71. Feest TG, Mistry CD, Grimes DS, Mallick NP. Incidence of advanced chronic renal failure and the need for end-stage renal replacement therapy. *Br Med J* 1990; **301**: 897–900.
72. McGewon MG. Prevalence of advanced renal failure in Northern Ireland. *Br Med J* 1990; **301** (6757): 900–903.
73. Jungers P, Chaveau P, Descamps-Latscha B, Labrunie M, Giraud E, Man NK, Grünfeld JP, Jacobs C. Age and gender-related incidence of chronic renal failure in a French urban area: a prospective epidemiologic study. *Nephrol Dial Transplant* 1996; **11**: 1542–1546.
74. US Renal Data System. USRDS Annual Data Report. Incidence and prevalence of ESRD. *Am J Kidney Dis* 1998; **32** (Suppl. 1): S38–S49.
75. Berthoux F, Gellert R, Jones E, Mendel S, Valderrabano F, Briggs D, Carrera F, Cambi V, Saker L. Epidemiology and demography of treated end-stage renal failure in the elderly: from the European Renal Association (ERA-EDTA) Registry. *Nephrol Dial Transplant* 1998; **13** (Suppl. 7): 65–68.
76. Locatelli F, Marcelli D, Conte F, Limido A, Lonati F, Malberti F, Spotti D. 1983–92: Report on regular dialysis and transplantation in Lombardy. *Am J Kidney Dis* 1995; **25**: 196–205.
77. Malberti F, Conte F, Limido A, Marcelli D, Spotti D, Lonati F, Locatelli F. Ten years experience of renal replacement therapy in the elderly. *Geriatric Nephrol Urol* 1997; **7**: 1–10.
78. Simon P, Ramée MP, Autuly V, Laruelle E, Charasse C, Cam G, Ang KS. Epidemiology of primary glomerular disease in a French region. Variation according to period and age. *Kidney Int* 1994; **46**: 1192–1198.
79. Davison AM, Johnston PA. Idiopathic glomerulonephritis in the elderly. *Contrib Nephrol* 1993; **105**: 38–48.
80. Ponticelli C, Passerini P, Cresseri D. Primary glomerular diseases in the elderly. *Geriatric Nephrol Urol* 1996; **6**: 105–112.
81. Caillette A, Tabakian A, Colon S, Labeeuw M, Zech P. IgA mesangial nephropathy in over-75-year-old patients. *Contrib Nephrol* 1993; **105**: 152–156.
82. Nagai R, Cattran D, Pei Y. Steroid therapy and prognosis of focal segmental glomerulosclerosis in the elderly. *Clin Nephrol* 1994; **42**: 18–21.
83. Davison AM, Cameron JS, Keer DNS, Ogg CS, Wilkinson RW. The natural history of renal function in untreated idiopathic membranous glomerulonephritis in adults. *Clin Nephrol* 1984; **22**: 61–67.
84. Rosman JB, Langer K, Brandl M, Piers-Becht TPM, Van der Hem GK, Ter Wee PM, Donker AJM. Protein-restricted diets in chronic renal failure: a four year follow-up shows limited indications. *Kidney Int* 1989; **36** (Suppl. 27): 96–102.
85. Coggins CH, Lewis JB, Caggiula AW, Castaldo LS, Klahr S, Wang SR. Differences between women and men with chronic renal disease. *Nephrol Dial Transplant* 1998; **13**: 1430–1437.
86. West KM, Erdreich L, Stober JA. A detailed study of risk factors for retinopathy and nephropathy in diabetes. *Diabetes* 1980; **29**: 501–508.
87. Gretz N, Zeier M, Geberth S, Strauch M, Ritz E. Is gender a determinant for evolution of renal failure? A study in autosomal dominant polycystic kidney disease. *Am J Kidney Dis* 1989; **14**: 178–183.

88. Stewart JH. End-stage renal failure appears earlier in men than women with polycystic kidney disease. *Am J Kidney Dis* 1994; **24**: 181–183.
89. Tiernay WM, McDonald CJ, Luft FC. Renal disease in hypertensive adults: effect of race and type II diabetes mellitus. *Am J Kidney Dis* 1989; **13**: 485–493.
90. Hunt LP, Short CD, Mallick NP. Prognostic indicators in patients presenting with a nephrotic syndrome. *Kidney Int* 1988; **34**: 382–388.
91. Donadio JV, Torres VE, Velosa JA, Wagoner RD, Holley KE, Ikamura M, Ilstrup DM, Chu CP. Idiopathic membranous nephropathy. The natural history of untreated patients. *Kidney Int* 1988; **33**: 708–715.
92. Schieppati A, Mosconi L, Perna A, Mecca G, Bertani T, Garatinni S, Remuzzi G. Prognosis of untreated patients with idiopathic membranous nephropathy. *N Engl J Med* 1993; **329**: 85–89.
93. Ibels LS, Györy AZ. IgA nephropathy: analysis of the natural history, important factors in the progression of renal disease and review of the literature. *Med* 1994; **73**: 79–102.
94. Lopes AAS, Port FK, James SA, Agadoa L. The excess risk of treated end-stage renal disease in blacks in the United States. *J Am Soc Nephrol* 1993; **3**: 1961–1971.
95. Pugh JA, Stern MP, Haffner SM, Eifler CW, Zapata M. Excess incidence of treatment of end-stage renal disease in Mexican Americans. *Am J Epidemiol* 1988; **127**: 135–144.
96. Agodoa L, Jones C, Held P. End-stage renal disease in the USA. data from the United States Renal Data System. *Am J Nephrol* 1996; **16**: 7–16.
97. Whittle JC, Whelton PK, Seidler AJ, Klag MJ. Does racial variation in risk factors explain black-white differences in the incidence of hypertensive end-stage renal disease? *Arch Intern Med* 1991; **151**: 1359–1364.
98. Klag MJ, Whelton PK, Randall BL, Neaton JD, Brancati FL, Stamler J. End-stage renal disease in African-American and white men. *JAMA* 1997; **277**: 1293–1298.
99. Pazianas M, Eastwood JB, MacRae KD, Phillips ME. Racial origin and primary renal diagnosis in 771 patients with end-stage renal disease. *Nephrol Dial Transplant* 1991; **6**: 931–935.
100. Freedman BI, Bowden DW. The role of genetic factors in the development of end-stage renal disease. *Cur Opin Nephrol Hypertens* 1995; **4**: 230–234.
101. Ferguson R, Grim CE, Opgenorth TJ. A familial risk of chronic renal failure among blacks on dialysis? *J Clin Epidemiol* 1988; **41**: 1189–1196.
102. Freedman BI, Spray BJ, Tuttle AB, Buckalew VM Jr. The familial risk of end-stage renal disease in African Americans. *Am J Kidney Dis* 1993; **21**: 387–393.
103. Bergman S, Key BA, Kirk KA, Warnock DG, Rostand SG. Kidney disease in the first-degree relatives of African-Americans with hypertensive end stage renal disease. *Am J Kidney Dis* 1996; **27**: 341–346.
104. Freedman BI, Yu HY, Rich SS, Rothschild CB, Bowden DW. Genetic linkage analysis of growth factor loci and end-stage renal disease in African Americans. *Kidney Int* 1997; **51**: 819–825.
105. Yu H, Bowden DW, Spray BJ, Rich SS, Freedman BI. Linkage analysis between loci in the renin-angiotensin axis and end-stage renal disease in African Americans. *J Am Soc Nephrol* 1996; **7**: 2559–2564.
106. Yu H, Bowden DW, Spray BJ, Rich SS, Freedman BI. Identification of human plasma kallikrein gene polymorphisms and evaluation of their role in end-stage renal disease. *Hypertension* 1998; **31** (4): 906–911.

107. Cornoni-Hutley J, LaCroix AZ, Havlik RJ. Race and sex differentials in the impact of hypertension in the United States. The national health and nutrition examination survey I epidemiologic follow-up study. *Arch Intern Med* 1989; **149**: 780–788.
108. Cooper RS, Liao Y. Is hypertension among blacks more severe or simply more common? [Abstract]. *Circulation* 1992; **85**: 12.
109. Shulman NB, Hall WD. Renal vascular disease in African-Americans and other racial minorities. *Circulation* 1991; **83**: 1477–1479.
110. Dustan HP, Curtis JJ, Luke RG, Rostand SG. Systemic hypertension and the kidney in black patients. *Am J Cardiol* 1987; **60** (Suppl. 1): 731–771.
111. Luft FC, Miller JZ, Grim CE, Fineberg NS, Christian KC, Daugherty SA, Weinberger MH. Salt sensitivity and resistance of blood pressure. *Hypertension* 1991; **17** (Suppl. 1): 102–108.
112. Falkner B, Kushner H. Effect of chronic sodium loading on cardiovascular response in young blacks and whites. *Hypertension* 1990; **15**: 36–43.
113. Nosadini R, Semplicini A, Fioretto P, Lusiani L, Trevisan R, Donadon V, Zanette G, Nicolosi GL, Dall'Aglio V, Zanuttini D. Sodium lithium countertransport and cardiorenal abnormalities in essential hypertension. *Hypertension* 1991; **9** (Suppl. 6): S158–S159.
114. Campese V. Salt sensitivity in hypertension. *Hypertension* 1994; **23**: 531–550.
115. Summerson GH, Bell RA, Konen JC. Racial differences in the prevalence of microalbuminuria in hypertension. *Am J Kidney Dis* 1995; **26**: 577–579.
116. Bigazzi R, Bianchi S, Baldari D, Sgherri G, Baldari G, Campese VM. Microalbuminuria in salt-sensitive patients. A marker for renal and cardiovascular risk factors. *Hypertension* 1994; **23**: 195–199.
117. Muirhead EE, Pitcock JA. Histopathology of severe vascular damage in blacks. *Clin Cardiol* 1989; **12**: 58–65.
118. Dustan HP. Does keloid pathogenesis hold the key to understanding black/white differences in hypertension severity? *Hypertension* 1995; **26** (1): 858–862.
119. Walker WG, Neaton JD, Cutler JA, Neuwirth R, Cohen JD for the MRFIT Research Group. Renal function change in hypertensive members of the Multiple Risk Factor Intervention Trial. *JAMA* 1992; **268**: 3085–3091.
120. Peterson JC, Sharon A, Burkart JM, Greene T, Hebert LA, Hunsicker LG, King AJ, Klahr S, Massry SG, Seifter JL for the Modification of Diet in Renal Disease (MDRD) Study Group. Blood pressure control, proteinuria and the progression of renal disease. *Ann Intern Med* 1995; **123**: 754–762.
121. Toto RD, Mitchell HC, Smith RD, Lee HC, McIntire D, Pettinger WA. 'Strict' blood pressure control and progression of renal disease in hypertensive nephrosclerosis. *Kidney Int* 1995; **48**: 851–859.
122. Carter JS, Pugh JA, Monterrosa A. Non-insulin dependent diabetes mellitus in minorities in the United States. *Ann Intern Med* 1996; **125**: 221–236.
123. Brancati FL, Klag MJ, Whelton PK, Neaton JD, Randall BL, Ford CE. End-stage renal disease in black and white diabetic men. A prospective cohort study. *Diabetes* 1994; **43**: 26A.
124. Pugh JA, Medina RA, Cornell JC, Basu S. NIDDM is the major cause of diabetic end-stage renal disease. More evidence from a tri-ethnic community. *Diabetes* 1995; **44**: 1375–1380.
125. Gohdes D, Kaufman S, Valway S. Diabetes in American Indians: an overview. *Diabetes Care* 1993; **16** (Suppl. 1): 239.
126. McCance DR, Hanson RL, Pettitt DJ, Jacbson LT, Bennet PH, Bishop DT, Knowler

WC. Diabetic nephropathy: a risk factor for diabetes mellitus in offspring. *Diabetologia* 1995; **38** (2): 221–226.

127. Nelson RG, Bennet PH, Beck GJ, Tan M, Knowler WC, Mitch WE, Hirschman GH, Myers BD. Development and progression of renal disease in Pima Indians with non-insulin-dependent diabetes mellitus. Diabetic Renal Disease Study Group. *N Engl J Med* 1996; **335** (22): 1636–1642.
128. Pontier PJ, Patel TG. Racial differences in the prevalence and presentation of glomerular disease in adults. *Clin Nephrol* 1994; **42**: 79–84.
129. Korbet SM, Genchi RM, Borok RZ, Schwartz MM. The racial prevalence of glomerular lesions in nephrotic adults. *Am J Kidney Dis* 1996; **27**: 647–651.
130. Glicklich D, Haskell L, Senitzer D, Weiss RA. Possible genetic predisposition to idiopathic focal segmental glomerulosclerosis. *Am J Kidney Dis* 1988; **12**: 26–30.
131. Hogan SL, Nachman PH, Wilkman AS, Jennette JC, Falk RJ and the Glomerular Disease Collaborative Network. Prognostic markers in patients with antineutrophil cytoplasmic autoantibodies-associated microscopic polyangiitis and glomerulonephritis. *J Am Soc Nephrol* 1996; **7**: 23–32.
132. Quinn M, Angelico MC, Warram JH, Krowleski AS. Familial factors determine the development of diabetic nephropathy in patients with IDDM. *Diabetologia* 1996; **39**: 940–945.
133. Viberti GC, Keen H, Wiseman MJ. Raised arterial pressure in parents of proteinuric insulin dependent diabetics. *Br Med J* 1987; **295**: 515–517.
134. Krolewski AS, Canessa M, Warram JH, Laffel LM, Christlieb AR, Knowler WC, Rand LI. Predisposition to hypertension and susceptibility to renal disease in insulin-dependent diabetes mellitus. *N Engl J Med* 1988; **318**: 140–145.
135. Nelson RG, Pettitt DJ, deCourten MP, Hanson RL, Knowler WC, Bennet PH. Parental hypertension and proteinuria in Pima Indians with NIDDM. *Diabetologia* 1996; **39**: 433–438.
136. Stattin EL, Rudberg S, Dahlquist G. Hereditary risk determinants of micro- and macroalbuminuria in young IDDM patients. [Abstract]. *Diabetologia* 1996; **39**: A299.
137. Breyer JA, Bain RP, Evans JK, Nahman NS, Lewis EJ, Cooper M, McGill J, Berl T and the Microalbuminuria Collaborative Study Group. Predictors of the progression of renal insufficiency in patients with insulin-dependent diabetes and overt diabetic nephropathy. *Kidney Int* 1993; **50**: 1651–1658.
138. Schmid M, Meyers S, Wegner R, Ritz E. Increased genetic risk of hypertension in glomerulonephritis? *J Hypertens* 1990; **10**: 290–295.
139. Autuly V, Laruelle E, Benziane A, Ang KS, Cam G, Ramee M, Simon P. Increased genetic risk of hypertension in immunoglobulin A nephropathy but not in membranous nephropathy. *J Hypertens* 1991; **9**: S220–S221.
140. Del Vecchio L, Grillo P, Bernardi L, Slaviero G, Cervini P, Tarantino A, Ragni A, Roccatello D, Cusi D, Bianchi G. Hypertension and IgA nephropathy: role of clinical and familial factors in progression to renal failure. [Abstract]. *Nephrol Dial Transplant* 1997; **12** (9): A77.
141. Lei HH, Perneger TV, Klag MJ, Whelton PK, Coresh J. Familial aggregation of renal disease in a population-based case-control study. *J Am Soc Nephrol* 1998; **9** (7): 1270–1276.
142. Rees AJ. The HLA complex and susceptibility to glomerulonephritis. *Plasma Ther* 1984; **5**: 455–471.
143. Chevrier D, Giral M, Perrichot R, Latinne D, Coville P, Muller JY, Soullilou JP, Bignon

JD. Idiopathic and secondary membranous nephropathy and polymorphism at TAP1 and HLA-DMA loci. *Tissue Antigens* 1997; **50** (2): 164–169.

144. Burns AP, Fisher M, Li P, Pusey CD, Rees AJ. Molecular analysis of HLA class II genes in Goodpasture's disease. *Q J Med* 1995; **88** (2): 93–100.
145. Fisher M, Pusey CD, Vaughan RW, Rees AJ. Susceptibility to anti-glomerular basement membrane disease is strongly associated with HLA-DRB1 genes. *Kidney Int* 1997; **51** (1): 222–229.
146. Mori K, Sasazuki T, Kimura A, Ito Y. HLA-DP antigens and post-streptoccoccal acute glomerulonephritis. *Acta Paediatr* 1996; **85** (8): 916–918.
147. Rambausek MH, Waldherr R, Ritz E. Immunogenetics findings in glomerulonephritis. *Kidney Int* 1993; **43** (Suppl. 39): S3–S8.
148. Berthoux FC, Gagne A, Sabatier JC, Ducret F, Le Petit JC, Marcelin M, Mercier B, Brizard CP. HLA-Bw35 and mesangial IgA-glomerulonephritis. *N Engl J Med* 1978; **298**: 10341035.
149. Moore R. MHC gene polymorphism in primary IgA nephropathy. *Kidney Int* 1993; **43** (Suppl. 39): S9–S12.
150. Fennessy M, Hitman GA, Moore RH, Metcalfe K, Medcraft J, Sinico RA, Mustonen JT, D'Amico G. HLA-DQ gene polymorphism in primary IgA nephropathy in 3 European populations. *Kidney Int* 1996; **49** (2): 477–480.
151. Berthoux FC, Genin C, Gagne A, Le Petit JC, Sabatier JC. HLA-Bw35 antigen in mesangial IgA glomerulonephritis: a poor prognostic marker? *Proc Eur Dial Transplant Assoc* 1979; **16**: 551–555.
152. Alamartine E, Sabatier JC, Guerin C, Berliet JM, Berthoux F. Prognostic factors in mesangial IgA glomerulonephritis: an extensive study with univariate and multivariate analysis. *Am J Kidney Dis* 1991; **28** (1): 12–19.
153. Freedman BI, Spray BJ, Heise ER. HLA associations in IgA nephropathy and focal and segmental glomerulosclerosis. *Am J Kidney Dis* 1994; **23** (3): 352–357.
154. Raguenes O, Mercier B, Cledes J, Whebe B, Ferec C. HLA class II typing and idiopathic IgA nephropathy (IgAN): DQB1*0301, a possible marker of unfavourable outcome. *Tissue Antigens* 1995; **45** (4): 246–249.
155. Kam Tao Li P, Poon ASY, Kar Neng Lai. Molecular genetics of MHC class II alleles in Chinese patients with IgA nephropathy. *Kidney Int* 1994; **46**: 185–190.
156. Hiki Y, Kobayashi Y, Ookubo M, Kashiwagi N. The role of HLA-DR4 in the long-term prognosis of IgA nephropathy. *Nephron* 1990; **54** (3): 264–265.
157. Freedman BI, Spray BJ, Dunston GM, Heise ER. HLA associations in end-stage renal disease due to membranous glomerulonephritis: HLA–DR3 associations with progressive renal injury. *Am J Kidney Dis* 1994; **23** (6): 797–802.
158. Papasteriades C, Hatziyannakos D, Siakotos M, Pappas H, Tarassi K, Nikolopoulou N, Michael S, Kaninis CH, Vosnides G, Sotsiou F, Billis A. HLA antigens in microscopic polyarteritis (MP) with renal involvement. *Dis Markers* 1997; **13** (2): 117–122.
159. Welch TR, Beischel L, Balakrishnan K, Quinlan M, West CD. Major-histocompatibility-complex extended haplotypes in membranoproliferative glomerulonephritis. *N Engl J Med* 1986; **314** (23): 1476–1481.
160. Müller GA, Gebhardt M, Kmpf J, Balwin GM, Ziegenhagen D, Bohle A. Association between rapidly progressive glomerulonephritis and the properdin factor Bf-F and different HLA-D region products. *Kidney Int* 1984; **25**: 115–118.
161. Papiha SS, Rashid HU, Robets DF, Kerr DNS. A note on association of Bf and glomerulonephritis. *Clin Genetic* 1982; **22**: 67–69.

162. Mauff G, Alper CA, Dawkins R, Doxiadis G, Giles CM, Hauptmann G, Rittner C, Schneider PM. C4 nomenclature statement. *Complement Inflamm* 1990; **7**: 261.
163. Hauptmann G, Tappeiner G, Schifferli JA. Inherited deficiency of the fourth component of human complement. *Immunodef Rev* 1988; **1**: 3.
164. Schifferli JA, Steiger G, Paccaud JP, Sjöholm AG, Hauptmann J. Differences in the biological properties of the two forms of the fourth component of human complement (C4). *Clin Exp Immunol* 1986; **63**: 473.
165. Wyatt RJ, Julian BA, Woodford SY, Wang C, Roberts J, Thompson JS, Christenson MJ, McLean RH. C4A deficiency and poor prognosis in patients with IgA nephropathy. *Clin Nephrol* 1991; **36** (1): 1–5.
166. Wopenka U, Thysell H, Sjöholm AG, Truedsson L. C4 phenotypes in IgA nephropathy: disease progression associated with C4A deficiency but with C4 isotype concentration. *Clin Nephrol* 1996; **45** (3): 141–145.
167. Hubert C, Kouot AM, Corvol P, Soubrier F. Structure of the angiotensin-I-converting enzyme gene. *J Biol Chem* 1991; **266**: 15377.
168. Nakano Y, Oshima T, Hiraga H, Matsuura H, Kajiyama G, Kambe M. DD genotype of the angiotensin I-converting enzyme gene is a risk factor for early onset of essential hypertension in Japanese patients. *J Lab Clin Med* 1998; **131** (6): 502–506.
169. Cambien F, Poirier O, Lecerf L, Evans A, Cambou JP, Arveiler D, Luc G, Bard JM, Bara L, Ricard S, Tiret L, Amouyel P, Alhenc-Gelas F. Deletion polymorphism in the gene for angiotensin-converting enzyme is a potent risk factor for myocardial infarction. *Nature* 1992; **359**: 641.
170. Marian AJ, Yu Q, Workman R, Greve G, Roberts R. Angiotensin converting enzyme polymorphism in hypertrofic cardiomyopathy and sudden cardiac death. *Lancet* 1993; **342**: 1085–1086.
171. Rigat B, Hubert C, Alhenc-Gelas F, Cambien F, Corvol P, Soubrier F. An insertion/deletion polymorphism in the angiotensin I-converting enzyme gene accounting for half the variance of serum enzyme levels. *J Clin Invest* 1990; **86**: 134.
172. Yorioka T, Suehiro T, Yasuoka N, Hashimoto R, Kawada M. Polymorphism of the angiotensin converting enzyme gene and clinical aspects of IgA Nephropathy. *Clin Nephrol* 1995; **44** (2): 80–85.
173. Harden PN, Geddes C, Rowe PA, McIlroy JH, Boulton-Jones M, Rodger RS, Briggs JD, McConnel JM, Jardine AG. Polymorphism in angiotensin-converting-enzyme gene and progression of IgA nephropathy. *Lancet* 1995; **345**: 1540–1542.
174. Hunley TE, Julian BA, Phillips III JA, Summar ML, Yoshida H, Horn RG, Brown NJ, Fogo A, Ichikawa I, Kon V. Angiotensin converting enzyme gene polymorphism: potential silencer motif and impact on progression in IgA Nephropathy. *Kidney Int* 1996; **49**: 571–577.
175. Yoshida H, Mitarai T, Kawamura T, Kitajiama T, Miyazaki Y, Nagasawa R, Kawaguchi Y, Kubo H, Ichikawa I, Sakai O. Role of the deletion polymorphism of the angiotensin converting enzyme gene in the progression and therapeutic responsiveness of IgA nephropathy. *J Clin Invest* 1995; **96**: 2162–2169.
176. Schmidt S, Stier E, Hartung R, Stein G, Bahnisch J, Woodroffe A, Clarkson A, Ponticelli C, Campise MR, Mayer G, Ganten D, Ritz E. No association of converting enzyme insertion/deletion polymorphism with immunoglobulin A glomerulonephritis. *Am J Kidney Dis* 1995; **26** (5): 727–731.
177. El Deeb S, Deprèle C, Berthoux P, Cécillon S, Berthoux F. Polymorphism study in primary IgA nephritis (IgAN) of genes (ACE, AGT, AT1-R, eNOS) involved in arterial hypertension. [Abstract]. *Nephrol Dial Transplant* 1997; **12**: A47.

178. Ogura M, Yoshida H, Kawamura T, Hamaguchi A, Miyazaki Y, Mitarai T, Okada T, Eto T, Kitajima T, Sakai O. The impact of the ACE gene polymorphism on slowly progressive IgA nephropathy may be linked to the glomerular size. [Abstract]. *J Am Soc Nephrol* 1995; **6**: 398.
179. Tanaka R, Iijima K, Murakami R, Koide M, Nakamura H, Yoshikawa N. ACE gene polymorphism in childhood IgA nephropathy: associations with clinicopathologic findings. *Am J Kidney Dis* 1998; **31** (5): 774–779.
180. Frishberg Y, Becker-Cohen R, Halle D, Feigin E, Eisenstein B, Halevy R, Lotan D, Juabech I, Ish-Shalom N, Magen D, Shvil Y, Sinai-Treiman L, Drukker A. Genetic polymorphisms of the renin-angiotensin system and the outcome of focal segmental glomerulosclerosis in children. *Kidney Int* 1998; **54** (6): 1843–1849.
181. Perrichot R, Raguenes O, Mercier B, Whebe B, Lenormand JP, Ferec C, Cledes J. Genetic variation in the renin angiotensin system and membranous glomerulonephritis. [Abstract]. *J Am Soc Nephrol* 1996; **7**: 1779.
182. Marre M, Bernardet P, Gallois Y, Savagner F, Guyene TT, Hallab M, Cambien F, Passa P, Alhenc-Gelas F. Relationship between an insertion/deletion polymorphism in the angiotensin-I-converting enzyme gene polymorphism, plasma levels, and diabetic retinal and renal complications. *Diabetes* 1994; **43**: 384–388.
183. Marre M, Jeunemaitre X, Gallois Y, Rodler M, Chatellier G, Sert C, Dusselier L, Kahal Z, Chaillous L, Halimi S, Muller A, Sackmann H, Baudeuceau B, Bled F, Passa P, Alhenc-Gelas F. Contribution of genetic polymorphism in the renin-angiotensin system to the development of renal complications in insulin-dependent diabetes. Genetique de la Nephropathie Diabetique (GENEDIAB) Study Group. *J Clin Invest* 1997; **99**: 1585–1595.
184. Barnas U, Schmidt A, Illievich A, Rabensteiner D, Prager R, Mayer G. The ACE gene polymorphism in patients with diabetic nephropathy [Abstract]. *J Am Soc Nephrol* 1995; **6**: 1036.
185. Tarnow L, Cambien F, Rossing P, Nielsen FS, Hansen BV, Lecerf L, Poirier O, Danilov S, Parving HH. Lack of relationship between an insertion/deletion polymorphism in the angiotensin I-converting enzyme gene and diabetic nephropathy and proliferative nephropathy in IDDM patients. *Diabetes* 1995; **44**: 489–494.
186. Schmidt S, Schöne N, Ritz E and the Diabetic nephropathy Study Group. Association of ACE gene polymorphism and diabetic nephropathy? *Kidney Int* 1995; **47**: 1176–1181.
187. Chowdhury TA, Dronsfield MJ, Kumar S, Gough SLC, Gibson SP, Khatoon A, MacDonald F, Rowe BR, Dunger DB, Dean JD, Davies SJ, Webber J, Smith PR, Mackin P, Marshall SM, Adu D, Morris PJM, Todd JA, Barnett AH, Boulton AJM, Bain SC. Examination of two genetic polymorphisms within the renin-angiotensin system: no evidence for an association with nephropathy in IDDM. *Diabetologia* 1996; **39**: 1108–1114.
188. Doria A, Warram JH, Krolewski AS. Genetic predisposition to diabetic nephropathy: evidence for a role of the angiotensin I-converting enzyme gene. *Diabetes* 1994; **43**: 690–695.
189. Freire MB, Dijk DJ, Erman A, Boner G, Warram JK, Krolewski AS. DNA polymorphisms in the ACE gene, serum ACE activity and the risk of nephropathy in insulin-dependent diabetes mellitus. *Nephrol Dial Transplant* 1998; **13** (10): 2553–2558.
190. Marre M, Bouhanick B, Berrut G, Gallois Y, Le Jeune JJ, Chatellier G, Menard J, Alhenc-Gelas F. Renal changes on hyperglycemia and angiotensin-converting enzyme in type 1 diabetes. *Hypertension* 1999; **33** (3): 775–780.
191. Jeffers JW, Estacio R, Raynolds MV, Schrier RW. Angiotensin-converting enzyme gene

polymorphism in non-insulin dependent diabetes mellitus and its relationship with diabetic nephropathy. *Kidney Int* 1997; **52**: 473–477.

192. Grzeszczak W, Zychma MJ, Lacka B, Zukowska-Szczechowska E. Angiotensin I-converting enzyme gene polymorphisms: relationship to nephropathy in patients with non-insulin dependent diabetes mellitus. *J Am Soc Nephrol* 1998; **9**: 1664–1669.
193. Mizuiri S, Hemmi H, Inoue A, Yoshikawa H, Tanegashima M, Fushimi T, Ishigami M, Amagasaki Y, Ohara T, Shimatake H, Hasegawa A. Angiotensin-converting enzyme polymorphism and development of diabetic nephropathy in non-insulin dependent diabetes mellitus. *Nephron* 1995; **70**: 455–459.
194. Fujisawa T, Ikegami H, Shen GO, Yamamoto E, Nakagawa Y, Hamada Y, Ueda H, Rakugi H, Higaki J, Ohishi M. Angiotensin I-converting enzyme gene polymorphism is associated with myocardial infarction, but not with retinopathy or nephropathy, in NIDDM. *Diabetes Care* 1995; **18**: 983–985.
195. Kunz R, Bork JP, Fritshe L, Ringel J, Sharma AM. Association between the angiotensin-converting enzyme-insertion/deletion polymorphism and diabetic nephropathy: a methodological appraisal and systematic review. *J Am Soc Nephrol* 1998; **9** (9): 1653–1663.
196. Yoshida H, Kuriyama S, Tomonari H, Mitarai T, Hamaguchi A, Kubo H, Kawaguchi Y, Kon V, Matsuoka K, Ichikawa I, Sakai O. Angiotensin I converting enzyme gene polymorphism in non-insulin dependent diabetes mellitus. *Kidney Int* 1996; **50**: 657–664.
197. Tarnow L, Rossing P, Jacobsen P, Nielsen FS, Cambien F, Lecerf L, Poirier O, Parving HH. Progression of diabetic nephropathy and the insertion/deletion polymorphism (ACE I/D) of the angiotensin-I-converting enzyme gene. [Abstract]. *J Am Soc Nephrol* 1996; **6**: 441.
198. Van Essen GG, Rensma PL, de Zeeuw D, Sluiter WJ, Scheffer H, Apperloo AJ. Association between angiotensin-converting-enzyme gene polymorphism and failure of renoprotective therapy. *Lancet* 1996; **347**: 94–95.
199. Jacobsen P, Rossing K, Rossing P, Tarnow L, Mallet C, Poirier O, Cambien F, Parving HH. Angiotensin converting enzyme gene polymorphism and ACE inhibition in diabetic nephropathy. *Kidney Int* 1998; **53**: 1002–1006.
200. Penno G, Chaturvedi N, Talmud PJ, Cotroneo P, Manto A, Nannipieri M, Luong LA, Fuller JH. Effect of angiotensin-converting enzyme (ACE) gene polymorphism on progression of renal disease and the influence of ACE inhibition in IDDM patients: findings from the EUCLID Randomized Controlled Trial. EURODIAB Controlled Trial of Lisinopril in IDDM. *Diabetes* 1998; **47** (9): 1507–1511.
201. Missouris CG, Barley J, Jeffrey S, Carter ND, Singer DRJ, MacGregor GA. Genetic risk for renal artery stenosis: association with deletion polymorphism in angiotensin 1-converting enzyme gene. *Kidney Int* 1996; **46**: 534–537.
202. Sato H, Akai Y, Iwano M, Kurumatani N, Kurioka H, Kubo A, Yamaguchi T, Fujimoto T, Dohi K. Association of an insertion polymorphism of angiotensin-converting enzyme gene with the activity of systemic lupus erythematosus. *Lupus* 1998; **7** (8): 530–534.
203. Kario K, Kanai N, Nishiuma S, Fujii T, Saito K, Matsuo M, Shimada K. Hypertensive nephropathy and the gene for angiotensin-converting enzyme. *Arterioscler Thromb* 1997; **17** (2): 252–256.
204. Cheong HI, Park HW, Choi Y. Role of the angiotensin I converting enzyme (ACE) gene polymorphism in the development of reflux nephropathy (RNP) in children with vesico-ureteral reflux (VUR). [Abstract]. *J Am Soc Nephrol* 1996; **7**: 1383.
205. Baboolal K, Ravine D, Daniels J, Williams N, Holmans P, Coles GA, Williams JD.

Association of the angiotensin I converting enzyme gene deletion polymorphism with early onset of ESRF in PKD1 adult polycystic kidney disease. *Kidney Int* 1997; **52**: 607–613.

206. Grzeszczak W, Zukowska-Szczechowska E, Karasek D, Zychma M, Czechowska C. Role of angiotensin I converting enzyme and angiotensinogen gene polymorphisms in the development of renal failure in PKD. [Abstract]. *Nephrol Dial Transplant* 1997; **12**: A44.
207. Amoroso A, Danek G, Vatta S, Crovella S, Berrino M, Guarrera S, Fasano ME, Mazzola G, Amore A, Gianoglio B, Peruzzi L, Coppo R. Polymorphisms in angiotensin-converting enzyme gene and severity of renal disease in Henoch-Schoenlein patients. Italian Group of Renal Immunopathology. *Nephrol Dial Transplant* 1998; **13** (12): 3184–3188.
208. Zoccali C, Misefari V, Romeo G, Testa A, Spoto B, Ruggenenti P, Perna A, Matalone M, Remuzzi G. Polymorphism of the angiotensin I enzyme (ACE) gene does not predict disease progression, nor response to ACE-inhibition in non-diabetic chronic renal disease. [Abstract]. *J Am Soc Nephrol* 1997; **8**: 80A.
209. Schmidt A, Kiener HP, Barnas U, Arias I, Illievich A, Auinger M, Graninger W, Kaider A, Mayer G. Angiotensin-converting enzyme polymorphism in patients with terminal renal failure. *J Am Soc Nephrol* 1996; **7**: 314–317.
210. Burg M, Menne J, Ostendorf T, Kliem V, Floege J. Gene polymorphisms of angiotensin converting enzyme and endothelial nitric oxide synthase in patients with primary glomerulonephritis. *Clin Nephrol* 1997; **48**: 205–211.
211. Jeunemaitre X, Soubrier F, Kotelevtsev YV, Lifton RP, Williams CS, Charru A, Hunt SC, Hopkins PN, Williams RR. Molecular basis of human hypertension: Role of angiotensinogen. *Cell* 1992; **71**: 169–180.
212. Pei Y, Scholey J, Thai K, Suzuki M, Cattran D. Association of angiotensinogen gene T235 variant with progression of immunoglobulin A nephropathy in Caucasian patients. *J Clin Invest* 1997; **100** (4): 814–820.
213. Fogarty DG, Harron JC, Hughes AE, Nevin NC, Doherty CC, Maxwell AP. A molecular variant of angiotensinogen is associated with diabetic nephropathy in IDDM. *Diabetes* 1996; **45**: 1204–1208.
214. Schmidt S, Gießel R, Bergis KH, Strojek K, Grzeszczak W, Ganten D, Ritz E and the Diabetic Nephropathy Study Group. Angiotensin gene M235T polymorphism is not associated with diabetic nephropathy. *Nephrol Dial Transplant* 1996; **11**: 1755–1761.
215. Tarnow L, Cambien F, Rossing P, Nielsen FS, Hansen BV, Ricard S, Poirier O, Parving HH. Angiotensinogen gene polymorphism in IDDM patients with diabetic nephropathy. *Diabetes* 1996; **45**: 367–369.
216. Moczulski DK, Rogus JJ, Antonellis A, Warram JH, Krolewski AS. Major susceptibility locus for nephropathy in type 1 diabetes on chromosome 3q: results of novel discordant sib-pair analysis. *Diabetes* 1998; **47** (7): 1164–1169.
217. McLaughlin KJ, Jagger C, Small M, Jardine AG. Effect of angiotensinogen gene M235T variant on the development of diabetic complications in type II diabetes mellitus. *Lancet* 1995; **346**: 1160.
218. Bonnardeaux A, Davies E, Jeunemaitre X, Fery I, Charru A, Clauser E, Tiret L, Cambien F, Corvol P, Soubrier F. Angiotensin II type 1 receptor gene polymorphisms in human essential hypertension. *Hypertension* 1994; **24**: 63–69.
219. Berthoux FC, El Deeb S, Deprèle C, Cécillon S, Berthoux P, Alamartine E. Polymorphism study in primary IgA nephritis (IgAN) of genes (ACE, AGT, AT1-R, eNOS) involved in arterial hypertension. [Abstract]. *J Am Soc Nephrol* 1997; **8**: 82A.

220. Zanchi A, Moczulski D, Krolewski AS. Role of endothelial nitric oxide synthase gene (eNOS) in diabetic nephropathy (DN): Results of family studies. [Abstract]. *J Am Soc Nephrol* 1997; **8**: 121A.
221. Brown DM, Provoost AP, Daly MJ, Lander ES, Jacob HJ. Renal disease susceptibility and hypertension are under independent genetic control in the fawn-hooded rat. *Nat Genet* 1996; **12**: 44–51.
222. Yu H, Sale M, Rich SS, Spray BJ, Roh BH, Bowden DW, Freedman BI. Evaluation of markers of human chromosome 10, including the homologue of the rodent Rf-1 gene, for linkage to ESRD in black patients. *Am J Kidney Dis* 1999; **33** (2): 294–300.
223. Medcraft J, Hitman GA, Sachs JA, Whichelow CE, Raafat I, Moore RH. Autoimmune renal disease and tumor necrosis factor β gene polymorphism. *Clin Nephrol* 1993; **40**: 63–68.
224. Olmos J, A'Hern R, Heaton DA, Millward BA, Risley D, Pyke DA, Leslie RD. The significance of the concordance rate for type 1 (insulin-dependent) diabetes in identical twins. *Diabetologia* 1988; **31**: 747–750.
225. Tarnow L, Pociot F, Hansen PM, Rossing P, Nielsen FS, Hansen BV, Parving HH. Polymorphisms in the interleukin-1 gene cluster and diabetic nephropathy. [Abstract]. *J Am Soc Nephrol* 1995; **6**: 456.
226. Blakemore AI, Cox A, Gonzalez AM, Maskil JK, Hughes ME, Wilson RM, Ward JD, Duff GW. Interleukin-1 receptor antagonist allele (IL1RN*2) associated with nephropathy in diabetes mellitus. *Hum Genet* 1996; **97** (3): 369–374.
227. Yip J, Mattock MB, Morocutti A, Sethi M, Trevisan R, Viberti GC. Insulin-resistance in insulin-dependent diabetic patients with microalbuminuria. *Lancet* 1993; **342**: 883–887.
228. Groop L, Ekstrand A, Foesblom C, Widen E, Groop PH, Teppo AM, Eriksson J. Insulin-resistance, hypertension and microalbuminuria in patients with type 2 (non-insulin dependent) diabetes mellitus. *Diabetologia* 1993; **36**: 642–647.
229. Kahn CR, Saad MJA. Alterations in insulin receptor and substrate phosphorylation in hypertension and other insulin resistant states. *J Am Soc Nephrol* 1992; **3** (Suppl.1): S69–S77.
230. Krolewski AS, Doria A, Magre J, Warram JH, Housman D. Application of methods of molecular genetics to identify genes involved in the development of nephropathy in IDDM. *J Am Soc Nephrol* 1992; **3** (Suppl. 1): S9–S17.
231. Kimura H, Gejyo F, Suzuki Y, Suzuki S, Miyazaki R, Arakawa M. Polymorphisms of angiotensin converting enzyme and plasminogen activator inhibitor-1 genes in diabetes and macroangiopathy. *Kidney Int* 1998; **54** (5): 1659–1669.
232. Chase HP, Garg SK, Marshall G, Berg CL, Harris S, Jackson WE, Hamman RE. Cigarette smoking increases the risk of albuminuria among subjects with type 1 diabetes. *JAMA* 1991; **265**: 614–617.
233. Orth SR, Stockman A, Conradt C, Ritz E, Ferro M, Kreusser W, Piccoli G, Rambausek M, Roccatello D, Schafer K, Sieberth HG, Wanner C, Watschinger B, Zucchelli P. Smoking as a risk factor for endstage renal failure in men with primary renal disease. *Kidney Int* 1998; **54**: 926–931.
234. Shiiki H, Nishino T, Uyama H, Kimura T, Nishimoto K, Iwano M, Kanauchi M, Fujii Y, Dohi K. Clinical and morphological predictors of renal outcome in adult patients with focal and segmental glomerulosclerosis (FSGS). *Clin Nephrol* 1996; **46** (6): 362–368.
235. Cameron JS, Turner DR, Heaton J, Williams DG, Ogg CS, Chantler C, Haycock GB,

Hicks J. Idiopathic mesangiocapillary glomerulonephritis: comparison of types I and II in children and adults and long-term prognosis. *Am J Med* 1983; **74**: 175–192.

236. Durin S, Barbanel C, Landais P, Noel LH, Grunfeld JP. Long term course of idiopathic extramembranous glomerulonephritis. Study of predictive factors of terminal renal insufficiency in 82 untreated patients. *Nephrologie* 1990; **11** (2): 67–71.

237. Ponticelli C, Zucchelli P, Passerini P, Cesana B, Locatelli F, Pasquali S, Sasdelli M, Redaelli B, Grassi C, Pozzi C *et al.* A 10-year follow-up of a randomized study with methylprednisolone and chlorambucil in membranous nephropathy. *Kidney Int* 1995; **48** (5): 1600–1604.

238. D'Amico G, Colasanti G, Barbiano di Belgioioso G, Fellin G, Ragni A, Egidi F, Radaelli L, Fogazzi G, Ponticelli C, Minetti L. Long-term follow-up of IgA mesangial nephropathy: clinico-histological study in 374 patients. *Semin Nephrol* 1987; **4**: 355–358.

239. Donadio JV, Bergstrth EJ, Offord KP, Holley KE, Spencer DC. Clinical and histopatological associations with impaired renal function in IgA nephropathy. *Clin Nephrol* 1994; **41** (2): 65–71.

240. Ibels LS, Györy AZ, Caterson RJ, Pollock AA, Mahony JF, Waugh DA, Roger SD, Coulshed S. Primary IgA nephropathy: Natural history and factors of importance in the progression of renal impairment. *Kidney Int* 1997; **52** (Suppl. 61): S67–S70.

241. Kincaid-Smith P, Becker G. Reflux nephropathy and chronic atrophic pyelonephritis: a review. *J Infect Dis* 1978; **138** (6): 774–780.

242. Halimi JM, Ribstein J, Du Cailar G, Ennouchi JM, Mimran A. Albuminuria predicts renal function outcome after intervention in atheromatous renovascular disease. *J Hypertens* 1995; **13**: 1335–1342.

243. Iseki K, Iseki C, Ikemiya Y, Fukiyama K. Risk of developing end-stage renal diseases in cohort of mass screening. *Kidney Int* 1996; **49**: 800–805.

244. Locatelli F, Alberti D, Graziani G, Buccianti G, Redaelli B, Giangrande A. Prospective, randomised, multicentre trial of effect of protein restriction on progression of chronic renal insufficiency. Northern Italian Cooperative Study Group. *Lancet* 1991; **337** (8753): 1299–1304.

245. D'Amico G, Gentile G, Fellin G, Manna G, Cofano F. Effect of dietary protein restriction on the progression of renal failure: a prospective randomised trial. *Nephrol Dial Transplant* 1994; **9**: 1590–1594.

246. Wingen AM, Fabian-Bach C, Schaefer F, Mehls O for the European Group for Nutritional Treatment of Chronic Renal Failure in Childhood. Randomised multicentre study of a low-protein diet on the progression of chronic renal failure in children. *Lancet* 1997; **349**: 1117–1123.

247. Lewis EJ, Hunsicker LG, Raymond PB, Rohde RD for the Collaborative Study Group. The effect of angiotensin-converting-enzyme inhibition on diabetic nephropathy. *N Engl J Med* 1993; **329**: 1456–1462.

248. Praga M, Hernandez E, Montoyo C, Andres A, Ruilope LM, Rodicio JL. Long-term beneficial effects of ACE inhibition in patients with nephrotic proteinuria. *Am J Kidney Dis* 1992; **20**: 240–248.

249. Gansevoort RT, de Zeeuw D, de Jong PE. Long-term benefits of the antiproteinuric effect of ACE inhibition in non-diabetic renal disease. *Am J Kidney Dis* 1993; **2**: 202–206.

250. Apperloo AJ, de Zeeuw D, de Jong PE. Short-term antiproteinuric response to antihypertensive treatment predicts long-term GFR decline in patients with non-diabetic renal disease. *Kidney Int* 1994; **45** (Suppl. 45): S147–S178.

251. Locatelli F, Manzoni C, Marcelli D. Factors affecting progression of renal insufficiency. *Miner Electrolyte Metab* 1997; **23** (3–6): 301–305.
252. Gansevoort RT, Sluiter WJ, Hemmelder MH, de Zeeuw D, de Jong PE. Antiproteinuric effect of blood-pressure-lowering agents: a meta-analysis of comparative trials. *Nephrol Dial Transplant* 1995; **10**: 1963–1974.
253. Rossing P, Hommel E, Smidt UM, Parving HH. Reduction in albuminuria predicts a beneficial effect on diminishing the progression of human diabetic nephropathy during antihypertensive treatment. *Diabetologia* 1994; **37**: 511–516.
254. Gansevoort RT, de Zeeuw D, de Jong PE. Additive antiproteinuric effect of ACE inhibition and a low-protein diet in human renal disease. *Nephrol Dial Transplant* 1995; **10**: 497–504.
255. Gansevoort RT, de Zeeuw D, Shahinfar S, Redfield A, de Jong PE. Effects of the angiotensin II antagonist losartan in hypertensive patients with renal disease. *J Hypertens* 1994; **12** (Suppl. 2): S37–S42.
256. Rambausek MH, Rhein C, Waldherr R, Goetz R, Heidland A, Ritz E. Hypertension in chronic idiopathic glomerulonephritis: analysis of 311 biopsied patients. *Eur J Clin Invest* 1989; **19**: 176–180.
257. Kheder MA, Ben Maïz H, Abdderrhaim E, El Younsi F, Ben Moussa F, Safar ME, Ben Ayed H. Hypertension in chronic glomerulonephritis. Analysis of 359 cases. *Nephron* 1993; **63**: 140–144.
258. Oldrizzi L, Rugiu C, De Biase V, Maschio G. The place of hypertension among the risk factors for renal function in chronic renal failure. *Am J Kidney Dis* 1993; **21** (5): 119–123.
259. Kes P, Ratkovic-Gusic I. The role of arterial hypertension in progression of renal failure. *Kidney Int* 1996; **49** (Suppl. 55): S72–S74.
260. Alvestrand A, Gutierrez A, Bucht H, Bergström J. Reduction of blood pressure retards the progression of chronic renal failure in man. *Nephrol Dial Transplant* 1988; **3**: 624–632.
261. Brazy PC, Stead WW, Fitzwilliam JF. Progression of renal insufficiency: Role of blood pressure. *Kidney Int* 1989; **35**: 670–674.
262. Perry HM, Miller JP, Fornoff JR, Baty JD, Sambhi MP, Rutan G, Moskowitz DW, Carmody SE. Early predictors of 15-year end-stage renal disease in hypertensive patients. *Hypertension* 1995; **25**: 587–594.
263. Locatelli F, Marcelli D, Alberti D, Graziani G, Buccianti G, Redaelli B, Giangrande A, the Northern Italian Cooperative Study Group. Hypertension as a factor in chronic renal insufficiency progression. *High Blood Press* 1994; **3**: 175–184.
264. Rosman JB, Langer K, Brandl M, Piers-Becht TP, van der Hem GK, Ter Wee PM, Donker AJ. Protein-restricted diets in chronic renal failure: a four year follow-up shows limited indications. *Kidney Int* 1989; **27**: S96–S102.
265. Alberti D, Locatelli F, Graziani G, Buccianti G, Redaelli B, Giangrande A, Marcelli D. Hypertension and chronic renal insufficiency: the experience of the Northern Italian Cooperative Study Group. *Am J Kidney Dis* 1993; **21** (5) (Suppl. 2): 124–130.
266. Hebert LA, Kusek JW, Greene T, Agodoa LY, Jones CA, Levey AS, Breyer JA, Faubert P, Rolin HA, Wang SH and the Modification of Diet in Renal Disease Study Group. Effects of blood pressure control on progressive renal disease in blacks and whites. *Hypertension*, 1997; **30** (part I): 428–435.
267. Microalbuminuria Collaborative Study Group UK. Risk factors for development of microalbuminuria in insulin dependent diabetic patients: a cohort study. *Br Med J* 1993; **306**: 1235–1239.
268. Mathiesen ER, Ronn B, Storm B, Foght H, Deckert T. The natural course of

microalbuminuria in insulin-dependent diabetes: a 10-year prospective study. *Diabetes Med* 1995; **12**: 482–487.

269. Mogensen CE. Systemic blood pressure and glomerular leakage with particular reference to diabetes and hypertension. *J Intern Med* 1994; **235**: 297–316.
270. Kansen KW, Petersen MM, Christiansen JS, Mogensen CE. Diurnal blood pressure variations in normoalbuminuric type 1 diabetic patients. *J Intern Med* 1993; **234**: 175–180.
271. Parving HH, Smidt UM, Friisberg B, Bonnevie-Nielsen V, Andersen AR. A prospective study of glomerular filtration rate and arterial blood pressure in insulin-dependent diabetics with diabetic nephropathy. *Diabetologia* 1981; **20**: 457–461.
272. Keller CK, Bergis KH, Fliser D, Ritz E. Renal findings in patients with short term type 2 diabetes. *J Am Soc Nephrol* 1996; **7** (12): 2627–2635.
273. Pugh JA, Medina R, Ramirez M. Comparison of the course of end-stage renal disease of type 1 (insulin dependent) and type 2 (non-insulin-dependent) diabetic nephropathy. *Diabetologia* 1993; **36**: 1094–1098.
274. Biesenbach G, Janko O, Zazgornik J. Similar rate of progression in the predialysis phase in type I and type II diabetes mellitus. *Nephrol Dial Transplantat* 1994; **9**: 1097–1102.
275. Walker WG, Hermann J, Murphy RP, Patz A. Prospective study of the impact of hypertension upon kidney function in diabetes mellitus. *Nephron* 1990; **55**: 21–26.
276. Parving HH, Andersen AR, Smidt UM, Svendsen PA. Early aggressive antihypertensive treatment reduces rate of decline in kidney function in diabetic nephropathy. *Lancet* 1983; **1**: 1175–1179.
277. Wiseman M, Viberti GC, Mackintosh A, Jarret RJ, Keen H. Glycemia, arterial pressure and microalbuminuria in type 1 (insulin-dependent) diabetes. *Diabetologia* 1984; **14**: 401–405.
278. Hasslacher C, Stech W, Wahl P, Ritz E. Blood pressure and metabolic control as risk factors for nephropathy in type 1 (insulin-dependent) diabetes. *Diabetologia* 1985; **28**: 6–11.
279. Gansevoort RT, Navis GJ, Wapstra FH, de Jong PE, de Zeeuw D. Proteinuria and progression of renal disease: therapeutic implications. *Curr Opin Nephrol Hypertens* 1997; **6**: 133–140.
280. Maki DD, Ma JZ, Louis TA, Kasiske BL. Long-term effects of antihypertensive agents on proteinuria and renal function. *Arch Intern Med* 1995; **155**: 1073–1080.
281. Hansson L, Zanchetti A, Carruthers SG, Dahlof B, Elmfeldt D, Julius S, Menard J, Rahn KH, Wedel H, Westerling S. Effects of intensive blood-pressure lowering and low-dose aspirin in patients with hypertension: principal results of the Hypertension Optimal Treatment (HOT) randomised trial. HOT Study Group. *Lancet* 1998; **351** (9118): 1755–1762.
282. Weidmann P, Schneider M, Bohlen L. Therapeutic efficacy of different antihypertensive drugs in human diabetic nephropathy: an updated metanalysis. *Nephrol Dial Tranplant* 1995; **10** (Suppl. 9): 39–45.
283. Kramer HJ, Meyer-Lehnert H, Mohaupt M. Role of calcium in the progression of renal disease: experimental evidence. *Kidney Int* 1992; **41** (Suppl. 36): S2–S7.
284. Ibels LS, Alfrey AC, Huffer WE, Craswell PW, Weil R. Calcification in end-stage kidneys. *Am J Med* 1981; **71**: 33–37.
285. Gimenez LF, Solez K, Walker WG. Relation between renal calcium content and renal impairment in 246 human renal biopsies. *Kidney Int* 1987; **31**: 93–99.
286. Lau K. Nephrology forum: phosphate excess and progressive renal failure: the precipitation-calcification hypothesis. *Kidney Int* 1989; **36**: 918–937.

287. Frohling PT, Krupki F, Kokot F, Vetter K, Kaschube I, Lindenau K. What are the most important factors in the progression of renal failure? *Kidney Int* 1989; **36** (Suppl. 27): S106–S109.
288. Moorhead JF, Chan MK, El-Nahas M, Varghese Z. Lipid nephrotoxicity in chronic progressive glomerular and tubulo-interstitial disease. *Lancet* 1982; **ii** (8311): 1309–1311.
289. Grond J, Goor H, Erkelens DW, Elema JD. Glomerular sclerotic lesions in the rat. *Virchows Arch B Cell Pathol* 1986; **51**: 521–524.
290. Keane WF, Kasiske BL, O'Donnel MP. Hyperlipidemia and the progression of renal disease. *Am J Clin Nutr* 1988; **47**: 430–435.
291. El Nahas AM. Glomerulosclerosis: a form of atherosclerosis. *Nephrol* 1988; **2**: 1206–1220.
292. Keane WF, Kasiske BL, O'Donnel MP. Lipids and progressive glomerulosclerosis. A model analogous to atherosclerosis. *Am J Nephrol* 1988; **8** (4): 261–271.
293. Walker WG. Hypertension-related renal injury: a major contributor to end-stage renal disease. *Am J Kidney Dis* 1993; **22**: 164–173.
294. Krolewski AS, Warram JH, Christlieb AR. Hypercholesterolemia. A determinant of renal functional loss and deaths in IDDM patients with nephropathy. *Kidney Int* 1994; **45** (Suppl. 45): S125–S131.
295. Mänttäri M, Tiula E, Alikoski T, Manninen V. Effects of hypertension and dyslipidemia on the decline of renal function. *Hypertension* 1995; **26**: 670–675.
296. Attman PO, Samuelsson O, Alaupovic P. Lipid metabolism and renal failure. *Am J Kidney Dis* 1993; **21**: 573–592.
297. Samuelsson O, Mulec H, Knight-Gibson C, Attman PO, Kron R, Larsson R, Weiss H, Wedel H, Alaupovic P. Lipoprotein abnormalities are associated with increased rate of progression of human chronic renal insufficiency. *Nephrol Dial Transplant* 1997; **12**: 1908–1915.
298. Samuelsson O, Attman PO, Knight-Gibson C, Larsson R, Mulec H, Weiss L, Alaupovic P. Complex apolipoprotein B-containing lipoprotein particles are associated with a higher rate of progression of human chronic renal insufficiency. *J Am Soc Nephrol* 1998; **9** (8): 1482–1488.

3

Glomerulosclerosis: insights into pathogenesis and treatment

Sharon Anderson

Introduction

The progressive nature of renal disease

Loss of renal function is progressive; once the glomerular filtration rate (GFR) falls below about 25 ml/min, regardless of etiology, most patients will progress to end-stage renal disease (ESRD) [1–3]. Recent investigations have focused on the elucidation of risk factors for progression, and the mechanisms which promote the process. It has long been known that contributing factors include poorly controlled hypertension, urinary tract infection, obstruction, administration of nephrotoxic drugs, and episodes of acute renal failure. More newly validated risk factors include hyperlipidemia, cigarette smoking, poor metabolic control (in diabetes), advancing age, and genetic factors, as are detailed elsewhere in this volume.

Mechanisms of progressive renal failure

Progressive renal insufficiency results from fibrosis and sclerosis of the glomeruli, and of the tubulointerstitium. The latter mechanism is covered in detail elsewhere in this volume. The major mechanisms underlying progression of glomerular injury are listed in Table 3.1, and are discussed below.

Persistent activity of the underlying disease

The importance of controlling the underlying disease process (whether immunological, hemodynamic or metabolic) has not always been sufficiently emphasized. For example, immunotherapy of active lupus nephritis has been extensively studied and advocated, but the role of prophylactic therapy against development of this complication in patients at risk remains poorly understood. Control of the underlying immunological events in antineutrophil cytoplasmic antibody-positive vasculitides preserves renal function in a significant proportion of patients. In some diseases, such as primary glomerulonephritides, convincing data as to the efficacy

Table 3.1 Mechanisms of progressive renal injury

Persistent activity of the underlying disease
Nephrotoxic insults: drugs, contrast dye, infection, obstruction
Functional adaptations
Systemic hypertension
Glomerular capillary hypertension
Renal hypoperfusion
Proteinuria
Structural and cellular adaptations
Renal hypertrophy
Glomerular hypertrophy
Structural–functional interactions
Tubulointerstitial injury
Mediators of cellular and structural injury: peptides, cytokines, growth factors
Metabolic and dietary factors
Protein intake
Hyperlipidemia
Other factors

of specific therapy remains lacking. Hypertension is a well recognized cause of progressive renal insufficiency, particularly in certain populations, but only now are the goals and optimal regimens of antihypertensive therapy being critically evaluated (see Chapter 6). Diagnosis and therapy of renovascular hypertension remain subjects of controversy (see Chapter 9). Relatively recently, it has been shown that aggressive treatment of hyperglycemia in patients with type 1 and now type 2 diabetes slows the progression of nephropathy, but universal control remains elusive. With the aging of the population, the importance of age-associated renal disease (or susceptibility to acquired injury in the aging kidney) is becoming more apparent, but its mechanisms remain ill defined. Thus, continuing attention to this primary principle of preventing progressive renal disease is warranted.

Superimposed nephrotoxic insults

Another long recognized risk factor is the superimposition of nephrotoxic insults. Nephrotoxic drugs (in particular, non-steroidal anti-inflammatory agents and angiotensin-converting enzyme inhibitors), infection, radiocontrast dye, and partial obstruction cause little problem in normal individuals, but can accelerate loss of renal function in those already compromised by intrinsic renal disease. This problem may be particularly important in the early stages of progressive injury, when the magnitude of disease may be underestimated by the treating physician. Thus, attention to this principle also remains mandatory.

Glomerulosclerosis

Hemodynamic mechanisms

Systemic and glomerular hypertension (see also Chapter 6)

Hemodynamic mechanisms, both primary and secondary, play an important part in the initiation and perpetuation of glomerular injury. While systemic blood pressure has been quantifiable for over a century, intrarenal hemodynamic measurements have become possible only in the past few decades. The deleterious effects of systemic and glomerular hypertension are detailed in Chapters 6 and 7, but will be briefly mentioned here.

Role of systemic hypertension Hypertension is both cause and consequence of renal disease. While the incidence of ESRD solely due to hypertension is difficult to quantitate, it is believed to be the second leading cause of renal death [4]. Far greater numbers of patients suffer from chronic renal failure (CRF) due to hypertension, and to aggravation of other forms of renal disease by the added stress of inadequately controlled blood pressure. Patients with CRF [5], including diabetic nephropathy [6], exhibit not only higher blood pressure, but also loss of the usual nocturnal blood pressure decline, so that the mechanisms of hypertensive injury are more continuously operable in these high-risk patients. Once present, hypertension is associated with faster loss of renal function in patients with acquired renal disease [7,8], as well as acceleration of the more moderate loss of renal function associated with normal aging [9].

Role of glomerular capillary hypertension Studies in various experimental hypertensive renal diseases have helped to delineate mechanisms of hypertensive injury, which relate in part to the effects of elevated blood pressure on an already compromised glomerulus. When nephrons fall out due to disease, this loss of nephrons leads to adaptive functional changes in those nephrons which are least damaged. This mechanism has been most clearly shown in the rat model of subtotal nephrectomy. The initial response to loss of nephrons is structural and functional hypertrophy of the remaining nephrons. The functional adaptations have been demonstrated by micropuncture studies, which show that vascular resistance falls in the afferent and efferent arterioles, allowing an increase in the glomerular capillary plasma flow rate (Q_A). Because the decrease in afferent arteriolar resistance (R_A) is proportionately greater than that in efferent arteriolar resistance (R_E), the glomerular capillary pressure (P_{GC}) increases [10,11]. Glomerular hypertension also results from impaired afferent arteriolar autoregulation in remnant nephrons, with reduced ability to constrict in the setting of systemic hypertension [12]. Together, glomerular capillary hypertension and hyperperfusion account for the increased single nephron glomerular filtration rate (SNGFR) in the remaining nephrons.

While initially serving to sustain filtration, these adaptations in themselves may promote further nephron loss. Eventually, they are associated with progressive proteinuria, and then focal and segmental glomerulosclerosis (FSGS). The pace of remnant glomerular injury, as well as the magnitude of glomerular hemodynamic changes, correlate with the amount of renal mass excised. These observations led Brenner and colleagues to hypothesize that the compensatory increases in glomerular pressures and flows are in fact maladaptive [10,13]. As was shown by Hostetter *et al.* [10], reversal of these hemodynamic changes with dietary protein restriction leads to structural protection. Later studies established that of the glomerular hemodynamic determinants of adaptive hyperfiltration, glomerular capillary hypertension plays the key part in the eventual structural injury [11,14]. Pharmacologic or dietary regimens which control glomerular hypertension effectively limit development of proteinuria and FSGS, even when systemic hypertension is not controlled [14,15].

Accordingly, the relative roles of systemic and glomerular capillary hypertension may be clearly dissociated in studies of experimental renal disease. That glomerular rather than systemic hypertension is the critical determinant of injury in some models has been shown by demonstrating that therapeutic interventions may affect these pressures independently, and that injury correlates with levels of glomerular, rather than systemic, pressure.

Pharmacologic therapy of systemic and glomerular hypertension

Although uncontrolled hypertension is an important risk factor for acceleration of progressive renal disease, current evidence indicates that all antihypertensive regimens do not impart equivalent degrees of protection to the kidney at risk. The role of hypertension and its therapy is discussed in detail elsewhere in this volume, and will only be briefly mentioned here.

Angiotensin-converting enzyme inhibitors (ACEI) have received attention as potentially protective of the kidney at risk for progressive loss of function. Numerous studies have established their efficacy in experimental models [11,16,17]. Indeed, of the regimens tested thus far, this class of agents has proven by far the most consistently successful in slowing progression of experimental renal disease [15] These drugs exert their beneficial effects, at least in part, via hemodynamic mechanisms. Through their action to limit formation of angiotensin II (Ang II), they routinely lower efferent arteriolar resistance (R_E), and thus glomerular capillary pressure. This is a class effect, as such protection has been found with every ACEI yet studied.

Ang II potently influences many physiologic processes, and thus it is no surprise that many mechanisms have been postulated to contribute to the protective effect of blockade of Ang II production with ACEI therapy. As further detailed in Chapter 6, ACEI appear to protect by a number of mechanisms, including effects on growth, specific pro-sclerosing mediators, endothelial cell dysfunction, and others [15,18]. In further support for the role of Ang II, recent micropuncture and morphologic studies with the several non-peptide Ang II receptor AT1 antagonists confirm that Ang II receptor blockade also reproduces these hemodynamic and protective effects [17,19–22]; this too appears to be a class effect.

Surprisingly, monotherapy with diuretics has received relatively little experimental attention in terms of preventing progressive renal disease, but in general, it has not proven very effective [23–25]. Sodium restriction has been confirmed as effective in other studies [25], but diuretics alone remain understudied. Results of calcium channel blockade have been inconsistent in animal models of renal disease [15,26]. A number of studies have evaluated the efficacy of older combination regimens, usually containing a diuretic, a vasodilator, and/or a centrally acting agent. The combination of reserpine, hydralazine, and hydrochlorothiazide ('triple therapy') has been extensively studied, due to its excellent control of blood pressure, and its availability long before newer classes of drugs were developed. In some models, this regimen has provided benefit, while in others, it is ineffective, or less effective than ACE inhibition, in delaying renal injury [11,17]. Beta-blockers as monotherapy have not received intensive study in experimental models; the available evidence is not very promising [27].

Renal hypoperfusion

In some renal diseases, progressive diminution of renal blood flow, due to atherosclerotic or other forms of damage to the renal arterial supply, eventually leads to obsolescence of the underperfused glomeruli. This scenario is likely to occur as the primary lesion in some patients, and late and as a secondary event in others. Hypertension is both a consequence of interruption of renal arterial flow, and a pathogenetic mechanism for the progression of renal disease in this circumstance [28,29]. Thus, both glomerular hypoperfusion, and glomerular capillary hypertension, contribute to hypertensive injury. The former may also follow the latter when arteriolosclerosis evolves.

Chronic renal hypoxia

The role of glomerular hypertension, and its attendant mechanical stresses which induce cytokine formation and release, has been relatively well studied. Only recently has renewed attention been directed toward the other side of the hemodynamic coin: hypoperfusion, and hypoxia [30,31]. According to this hypothesis, hypoxic injury may occur after nephron loss, as a consequence of increased oxygen consumption during adaptive hypertrophy and hyperfunction [32], and decrement of oxygen delivery, resulting from peritubular capillary obliteration and expanding extracellular matrix distances [33]. Hypoxia is known to stimulate expression of a number of adverse growth factors, including PDGF [34], endothelin-1 [35], transforming growth factor (TGF)-β [36], vascular endothelial growth factor [37], and others [30,31]. Accordingly, both hyperperfusion (via mechanical stress), and hypoperfusion (via hypoxia), may lead to overexpression of the same litany of pro-sclerosing mediators. Although best described in the pathogenesis of tubulo-interstitial disease, the hypoxic theory may apply to intrarenal vascular structures as well.

Role of proteinuria

Proteinuria is another functional consequence of most forms of glomerular injury. Recently, it has been suggested that proteinuria is not only a marker, but is also a pathogenetic factor for further injury [38]. The evidence in support of this hypothesis, and mechanisms by which proteinuria might accelerate injury, are detailed in Chapter 5.

Structural and cellular adaptations

Renal and glomerular hypertrophy

Adaptations in cellular structure and function also contribute to progressive injury. Structural changes, particularly compensatory hypertrophy, comprise the earliest adaptive changes. These changes are expressed as an increase in kidney weight, due to enlargement of the glomeruli particularly in the proximal convoluted tubule mass. The true importance of hypertrophy *per se* in the pathogenesis of injury remains debatable, and the mechanisms by which growth induces injury are unclear. Nevertheless, some discussion of this venerable putative risk factor is warranted.

Renal hypertrophy

The adaptive response to loss of renal mass includes the early development of renal hypertrophy [1,3]. These changes are expressed as an increase in kidney weight, and morphologically as an increase in the cross-sectional surface area of the kidney. The increase in kidney size is due to enlargement of the glomeruli and, most prominently, the proximal convoluted tubules [39], resulting in disproportionate enlargement of the cortex in comparison to the relatively unaffected medulla.

Renal hypertrophy has long fascinated investigators in the field, leading to extensive work aimed at defining the mechanisms of compensatory enlargement. The term compensatory renal hypertrophy has generally been used to describe the aggregate changes in nephron structure and function, including both cellular hypertrophy and hyperplasia, which follow loss of renal mass. Extensive work in this area has been summarized in several reviews [40–42], and will be briefly summarized here.

Biochemical changes

The ratio of kidney protein to kidney wet weight remains constant during renal hypertrophy, though the increase in the rate of renal protein synthesis is increased as early as 3 h after uninephrectomy in the mouse [43]. Synthesis of new RNA precedes new protein synthesis [44,45]. Studies of expression of a number of genes suspected to participate in renal hypertrophy failed to demonstrate increases in either steady-state levels [46] or in transcription rates [47], suggesting that post-transcriptional mechanisms may be more important in the regulation of hypertrophy. The renal hypertrophic stimulus causes cell enlargement, and cells reaching the largest size are stimulated to divide.

Extensive work has also been directed at identification of the signals which initiate compensatory renal growth. A circulating factor has been suggested since at least 1896, when Sacerdotti [48] infused blood from bilaterally nephrectomized dogs into normal dogs, and induced renal growth in the recipients. In the 1950s, Braun Menéndez postulated the existence of a humoral renal growth factor, termed renotropin [49]. Fractions of urine, serum, and liver from uninephrectomized animals and urine and serum from humans stimulate biochemical changes, such as incorporation of radiolabeled nucleotides into DNA, in isolated renal tissue preparations, and stimulate growth in cultures of kidney-derived cells; such studies have been proposed as further evidence for the existence of renotropin [50]. Such properties do not establish that these fractions induce whole kidney growth, however, and no truly 'renotropic hormone' has been isolated.

Despite the failure to isolate a growth factor which causes selective renal hypertrophy, many mediators cause hypertrophy and/or hyperplasia of kidney cells. Factors which have been shown to promote growth, usually in cultured proximal tubule or mesangial cells, include insulin, insulin-like growth factor-1 (IGF-1), epidermal growth factor (EGF), hepatocyte growth factor (HGF), PDGF, prostaglandin E_2, and hormones including hydrocortisone, thyroxine, arginine vasopressin, and Ang II [51–56]. However, it seems likely that these factors participate in compensatory renal hypertrophy in a non-specific manner, after growth has been triggered by some unidentified, renal-specific signal. This may involve the stimulation of cyclins and the downregulation of their inhibitors. These intracellular mediators are known to regulate cellular mitosis and have been implicated in compensatory renal growth as well as other models of glomerular proliferation [57]. Once growth has been triggered, sequential production of different growth factors may be required to achieve co-ordinated growth of specific renal cell types. Moreover, factors which cause growth of kidney cells *in vitro* may not necessarily contribute importantly *in vivo* following nephron loss.

Recent studies have implicated IGF-1 in compensatory renal hypertrophy. Administration of IGF-1 increases GFR and kidney weight in intact rats, although it is not clear whether the kidneys grows disproportionally to an increase in body weight [58–61]. There is disagreement, however, concerning the time course of the increase in IGF-1 activity, and some studies have found that renal IGF-1 levels begin to increase only after compensatory hypertrophy is already detectable [58,62–64]. Whether the increased remnant kidney IGF-1 activity is associated with consistent increases in IGF-1 message and/or binding proteins is also controversial [58,63,65]. Another confounding factor is the observation that partial renal infarction increases IGF-1 activity in the adjacent renal tissue [66]. Preliminary data support a growth-promoting effect of IGF-I, as the administration of a specific IGF-I receptor antagonist blunts both compensatory and diabetic renal growth in rats [67]. Overall, the data suggest that IGF-1 participates in, but does not initiate, compensatory renal growth.

Less is known regarding the participation of other growth factors. The distal nephron produces a large amount of the precursor protein for EGF. Renal content of EGF, distribution of EGF, and receptor levels for EGF, however, all remain constant over the first few days following uninephrectomy [68–70]. Increased EGF content and reduced EGF receptor levels have been observed only after compensatory renal hypertrophy is established [70,71]. In contrast, there is a very early increase in remnant kidney HGF and HGF mRNA following uninephrectomy [71]. However, uninephrectomy and operative stress also increase HGF expression in distant organs such as the lung [72]. Thus, evidence indicates that HGF is an important morphogen for growing tubule cells, but the significance of the early increase in HGF following nephrectomy remains unclear [73].

Changes in gene expression

Availability of new techniques to assess gene expression has prompted attention to 'early response' genes, whose protein products regulate transcriptional control of large numbers of other genes. The activation of early response genes is an early step in cell proliferation and differentiation evoked by mitogens and growth factors. Thus far, studies of the expression of early response genes in the remnant kidney following uninephrectomy have not provided unequivocal information [45,46,74–77]. For example, renal activity of c-*fos* following uninephrectomy has been found to increase in some studies, but not in others [75,76]. It was recently reported that c-*fos* and c-*jun* genes and proteins may be detected following extensive renal ablation, but not uninephrectomy [79]. Increased renal activity of some early response genes induced by sham surgery and catecholamine exposure may make it hard to define the role of these genes in compensatory renal hypertrophy [77,79]. Isolation of new genes whose activities in the remnant kidney increase following nephrectomy may ultimately provide a better means to identify stimuli which trigger renal growth in this setting [80]. Some of these genes encode proteins (cyclins) known to regulate cell turnover, proliferation, and death [57]. The balance of some of these cyclins in health and disease may determine the fate of renal cells.

Other factors modulating renal growth

Though the specific stimuli for initiation and perpetuation of renal hypertrophy remain to be defined, a number of dietary, endocrine, and other factors are known to modulate the process.

Age Probably the least controversial modifier of compensatory renal hypertrophy is age. Age at nephrectomy clearly affects the magnitude of compensatory renal growth, with greater responses being seen in the younger kidneys [81–84]. The increased magnitude of compensatory renal hypertrophy in youth may reflect generally greater responsiveness of young tissue to stimuli responsible for organ growth, as similar increases have been noted in compensatory growth of other organs.

Diet Feeding a low protein diet to rats subjected to renal ablation limits remnant kidney GFR and weight, while feeding a high protein diet augments hypertrophy [85–87]. These observations suggest that the stimuli to hyperfiltration and hypertrophy associated with nephrectomy and protein feeding are additive. Restriction of other dietary components may also influence the renal hypertrophic response. As compared with values for kidney weights in nephrectomized animals receiving normal diets, kidney weights are lower in similarly nephrectomized rats ingesting diets which are restricted in sodium [23,25], phosphate [88], total calories [89], or carbohydrates [90], or high in water [91].

Hormones Manipulation of endogenous levels of various hormones has been used to examine the influence of these factors on compensatory renal hypertrophy (reviewed in [51]). While early, incompletely controlled studies concluded otherwise, the most convincing data appear to exclude an important modulating effect of pituitary ablation, thyroidectomy, adrenalectomy or congenital growth hormone (GH) deficiency. The magnitude of compensatory hypertrophy does not appear to be influenced by androgens or gender. Of interest, transgenic mice expressing excessive amounts of GH or GH-releasing factor have a predisposition to develop accelerated glomerulosclerosis [92]. Conversely, dwarf rodents or mice expressing excessive amounts of GH antagonists are resistant to glomerulosclerosis, thus suggesting a modulating role of GH in the pathogenesis of glomerulosclerosis.

Glomerular hypertrophy

The case for glomerular hypertrophy as a risk factor for glomerular sclerosis is stronger and more specific than that for enlargement of the whole kidney. Observations of an association between glomerular size and injury have led to the hypothesis that enlargement of the glomerulus is a risk factor for eventual sclerosis. Enlargement of various intraglomerular components has been noted, and linked to postulated mechanisms of injury. In the diabetic kidney, expansion of the mesangial area is prominent. In other models, enlargement includes dilatation of the glomerular capillary lumen and its radius. The combination of increased glomerular capillary luminal pressure and capillary radius are postulated to increase tension on the capillary wall (following the Laplace law), thus contributing to disruption of capillary wall integrity, and FSGS. The potential additive deleterious effects of glomerular capillary hypertension and glomerular enlargement have also prompted speculation that injury may be mediated by detrimental effects on the glomerular visceral epithelial cells [93,94]. Still another hypothesis has centered on the concept that glomerular growth promoters, released locally or circulating in response to an injurious stimulus, may possess a capacity not only to enlarge the glomerular tuft, but also to augment mesangial matrix formation and/or suppress matrix degradation processes [95].

Although contributing relatively little to the overall renal growth, the glomeruli undergo progressive enlargement [1,93,96,97]. Increased glomerular size does not necessarily parallel increased whole kidney size. Serial structure–function studies in the rat have shown that glomerular volume and SNGFR increase in parallel following uninephrectomy [98,99]. The contribution of constituent parts of the glomerulus to its expansion following nephrectomy remains controversial and incompletely characterized. Morphometric studies demonstrate an increase in the total volume occupied by cellular constituents in the remnant glomeruli of nephrectomized rats [93,96–99]. Overall, these studies indicate that the fractions of the glomerulus occupied by different structural components (mesangium, capillary lumina, endothelial and epithelial cells) remain constant as the glomerulus enlarges, at least in the early phases of adaptation. However, long-term adaptation may follow a different pattern. Schwartz and Bidani found no change in the relative volume of the mesangium and its individual components at 6 weeks after ablation [100], but subsequently found in studies of partially nephrectomized rats followed for 26 weeks (about one-fourth of the lifespan) that the mesangial volume fraction, as well as the percentage of the mesangium occupied by cells and matrix, all increase at 26 weeks [95].

It remains uncertain to what extent different glomerular cell types increase in number and in volume following renal ablation. Visceral epithelial cell number remains constant when the glomerulus grows following loss of renal mass [93,101,102]. Mesangial cell number does not appear to increase early, but may increase later, as mentioned above. The effect of glomerular hypertrophy on endothelial cell number has not been evaluated in detail, although one study found an early, non-sustained increase in proliferation of peritubular endothelial cells shortly after uninephrectomy in mice [103]. It appears that the differential responses of glomerular cells may occur in phases. Most recently, the sequential changes in glomerular cells during the first 2 weeks after partial nephrectomy in the rat were defined [104]. In that study, early epithelial cell expansion was followed later by mesangial expansion, with glomerular procollagen $\alpha 1(IV)$ mRNA levels rising only during the second (mesangial) phase of glomerular hypertrophy.

A number of investigators have noted increases in glomerular capillary length and radius, so that capillary surface area increases [95,105]. Diameters of the afferent and efferent arterioles increase as well [106]. Morphometric measurements have also been used to try to estimate the filtering capacity of the enlarged remnant glomeruli. The glomerular capillary ultrafiltration coefficient (K_f) is the product of the surface area available for filtration (S) and the hydraulic permeability of the glomerular capillary wall per unit surface area (k). It is not clear which anatomic boundary constitutes the surface corresponding to S. As estimated by measuring the glomerular capillary area in direct apposition to epithelial foot processes, S increases following nephrectomy, albeit to a slightly lesser degree than total glomerular volume [96,98]. Despite this apparent increase in the filtration surface area, most functional studies have not found an increase in K_f of remnant glomeruli following extensive renal ablation in rats [10,11,17].

As a decrease in S cannot be involved to explain the fall in K_f, it is conceivable that K is reduced. In theory, an increase in average foot process width would cause a decrease in the length of filtration slits overlying each unit area of peripheral capillary surface, and thereby could decrease k in remnant glomeruli. In fact, morphometric studies have revealed an increase in the average width of epithelial cell foot processes in rats subjected to extensive renal ablation [98]. Alternatively, it is possible that the filtering surface estimated by morphologic techniques in remnant glomeruli does not represent effective area available for filtration *in vivo*. Theoretical studies suggest that much of the glomerular capillary network is relatively underperfused in rats subjected to extensive renal ablation [107]. It is notable that no increase in S was found following uninephrectomy in rats when infusion of glomerular basement membrane (GBM) antibody was used to estimate capillary surface area *in vivo* [108]. Alternatively, it is possible that the decrease in K_f in remnant glomeruli is more functional than structural, as ACE inhibitor therapy in remnant kidney rats routinely raises K_f to supranormal levels [11,16].

In spite of a large body of evidence linking glomerular hypertrophy to sclerosis, some authors shed some doubt on such association. Striker observed that certain strains of mice (C57/Os+) carrying a mutation predisposing them to oligomeganephronia (a reduced number of large glomeruli) were resistant to ablation-induced glomerulosclerosis [109]. This contrasted with another mutated strain of mice (ROP/Os+) with similarly enlarged glomeruli who were predisposed to spontaneous and ablation-accelerated glomerulosclerosis. This led them to conclude that genetic predisposition to glomerulosclerosis affected the response of large glomeruli to injury and determined the outcome. Similarly, as discussed below, studies with antihypertensive regimens have been unable to uniformly invoke glomerular hypertrophy as a universal risk factor for sclerosis.

Modulation of glomerular hypertrophy

Recognition of the magnitude of glomerular hypertrophy following nephron loss, and observations of an association between glomerular size and injury, have led to the hypothesis that enlargement of the glomerulus is a risk factor predisposing to eventual glomerular sclerosis (discussed below). The influence of a number of dietary and pharmacologic therapies on glomerular hypertrophy has been examined [110]. Both dietary protein restriction [97,111] and dietary sodium restriction [25] limit glomerular size increases following hypertrophic stimuli. Various antihypertensive drugs have also been examined, but not without controversy. Although ACE inhibitors occasionally limit glomerular enlargement [11,112], they often do not [110,113,114]. Calcium channel blocker therapy (specifically, nifedipine) has been shown to limit glomerular enlargement somewhat more consistently [114]. Other manipulations are less well studied, although it has been reported that glomerular hypertrophy is not influenced by caloric restriction [90].

Structural–functional interactions

The various mechanisms proposed to account for remnant injury should not be regarded as mutually exclusive. Indeed, given the close apposition and functional interdependency of glomerular cell types, there are most likely extensive interactions among them. It seems likely that glomerular hypertension exerts deleterious effects on all glomerular cell constituents. Recently, innovative new techniques using a variety of *in vitro* systems have been developed to address the question of how glomerular hypertension leads to structural injury. These studies have addressed the hypothesis that increased glomerular pressures and/or plasma flow rates alter the growth and activity of glomerular component cells, inducing the elaboration or expression of cytokines and other mediators which then stimulate mesangial matrix production and promote structural injury.

Endothelial cells Hemodynamic physical forces, such as shear stress or changes in blood flow, are well recognized to influence activity of endothelial cells in extrarenal systems [115]. It seems likely that such forces exert cellular actions in the glomerulus as well. In analogy with atherosclerosis, increased P_{GC} enhances endothelial cell release of vasoactive substances (e.g. thromboxanes, endothelin), lipid deposition, and intracapillary thrombosis. For instance, growing cultured endothelial cells under conditions of increased shear stress increases the activity or expression of a variety of mediators (see ref. 115 and Chapter 6). These diverse effects of endothelial cell stimulation/injury/dysfunction may facilitate intraglomerular thrombus formation, the attraction of inflammatory cells by endothelial release of chemokines, and their adhesion and infiltration of glomerular capillaries. This may also form the basis for the prevention of progressive glomerulosclerosis through antiplatelet, anticoagulant, or anti-inflammatory strategies.

Mesangial cells Altered hemodynamics also influence activity of mesangial cells. In support of this notion, it has been postulated that expansion of the glomerular capillaries, and resultant stretching of the mesangium in response to hypertension, are forces which translate high P_{GC} into increased mesangial matrix formation [116]. Evidence for this mechanism comes from observations in microperfused rat glomeruli, in which increased hydraulic pressure was associated with increased glomerular volume [116,117] and collagen formation [118]. Additional studies have shown that in cultured mesangial cells, cyclic stretching results in enhanced synthesis of protein, collagens, laminin, fibronectin, and TGF-β; these effects are discussed in detail in Chapter 6.

Another feature of mesangial injury may be the dedifferentiation of these cells into primitive mesenchymal/myofibroblastic cells expressing α-smooth muscle actin (α-SMA) [119,120]. Such transdifferentiation of mesangial cells into myofibroblasts has been described in a wide range of experimental renal models of mesangial injury and/or proliferation. It has also been observed in mesangioproliferative glomerulonephritides in humans, where the expression of mesangial α-SMA correlated with the proliferative changes. These phenotypic changes in mesangial cells may underlie a switch in collagen synthesis by these cells to an interstitial type (I and III) of collagen. These may lead to the deposition of such collagens in scarred glomeruli precluding, in the absence of specific metalloproteinases, the breakdown of deposited collagen and leading to irreversible sclerosis. This would also be compounded by a decrease in the overall glomerular collagenolytic activity associated with experimental renal disease, thus favoring deposition rather than removal of collagen and accelerating sclerosis.

Epithelial cells The permselective defects are associated with abnormalities of epithelial cell structure, including retraction of epithelial cell foot processes and focal detachment of epithelial cells from the underlying basement membrane. Epithelial cell injury in remnant glomeruli may reflect increased capillary wall tension and the inability of highly differentiated epithelial cells to replicate as glomerular volume increases following reduced nephron number. As has been postulated by Rennke [121], distortion or damage to the filtration slit diaphragm or, in some cases, absence of the visceral epithelial cell, will produce areas of the capillary wall with a lowered resistance for convective flow. Increased local hydraulic conductivity through such areas will increase permeability to macromolecules, enhancing both proteinuria. While smaller molecules will pass through and end up in the urine, large plasma proteins are likely to be restricted from passing beyond the lamina densa, resulting in progressive upstream accumulation of plasma-derived components in the lamina rara interna. Eventually, masses of such hyaline material occlude capillary lumina, contributing to capillary collapse and FSGS [121]. Kriz [122] has also proposed that the stretching of glomerular podocytes and their detachment from the underlying GBM expose areas of denuded GBM. These areas attract parietal epithelial cells, thus facilitating the formation of capsular adhesions. These may in turn initiate segmental glomerulosclerosis through the collapse of the underlying capillaries and their hyalinosis. Furthermore, it has been observed that detachment of damaged podocytes leads to phenotypic changes, with the loss of normal characteristics and the acquisition of macrophage differentiation antigens [123].

Thus, mechanical forces engendered by the high pressure and flows promote multiple mechanisms of glomerulosclerosis. Of note, recent evidence is beginning to invoke such forces in the pathogenesis of tubulo-interstitial injury, as well. For example, subjecting proximal tubule cells to mechanical stretch has recently been shown to upregulate the mediators of oxidant injury [124].

Mediators of cellular and structural injury

An ever increasing number of hormonal mediators are postulated to play a part in the pathogenesis of tubulo-interstitial and glomerular sclerotic injury. These mediators have recently been reviewed [31,126–128], and the major factors are listed in Table 3.2 [127]. While some of those listed are primarily observed in inflammatory diseases, others have been invoked to participate in non-inflammatory progressive glomerulopathies. Prominent among these are Ang II [18,126], endothelin [128], nitric oxide [129,130], TGF-β [130–132], PDGF [133], fibroblast growth factor [133], osteopontin [134], and others. Each of these, in turn, has been linked to a number of injury pathways. For example, Ang II may promote injury by causing systemic and glomerular hypertension; increasing macromolecular flux into the mesangium; stimulating growth and proto-oncogenes; increasing proteinuria; promoting interstitial fibrosis; and stimulating the production and/or release of other injurious mediators, including endothelin, TGF-β, PDGF, ammonia, fibronectin, and others [126]. For some of these, such as Ang II, specific blockers have been shown to ameliorate injury; for others, such blockers are under development but not yet available for widespread study. However, while evidence for a pathogenetic role of several of these is quite strong, the complexity of disease processes has made it difficult to ascribe more than contributory activity to any one cytokine. As was recently reviewed by Johnson [127], problems with interpretation of cytokine blocking studies are multiple. Blockade may be ineffective due to compensatory mechanisms; contrasting or opposing effects in different cell types or diseases; heterogeneity of responses under different circumstances; or problems with incomplete blockade. These problems notwithstanding, it seems likely that anti-cytokine thera-

Table 3.2 Major cytokines/growth factors in renal injury

Proinflammatory molecules:
Complement activation products (C5a, C5b-9)
Proinflammatory cytokines (IL-1, TNF-α, γ-interferon, MIF)
Chemokines (MCP-1, IL-8, MiP-2, etc.)
Osteopontin
Tissue factor
Vasoactive substances:
Vasoconstrictors: angiotensin II, endothelin-1, thromboxanes
Vasodilators: nitric oxide, prostaglandins
Growth factor/matrix promoting substances
Proliferative: PDGF, bFGF, IGF-1
Matrix-stimulating: TGF-β, cTGF
Extracellular matrix/proteases:
Type IV collagen
Matrix metalloproteinases (MMP-2, MMP-9)
SPARC
Decorin
Thrombospondin 1

Reproduced from Ref. 133 with permission. Abbreviations: IL, interleukin; TNF, tumor necrosis fator; MIF, macrophage inhibitory factor; MCP, monocyte chemoattractant protein; MiP-2, macrophage inhibitory peptide-2; PDGF, platelet-derived growth factor; bFGF, basic fibroblast growth factor; IGF, insulin-like growth factor; TGF, transforming growth factor; cTGF, connective tissue growth factor; MMP, metalloproteinase; SPARC, secreted protein, acidic and rich in cysteine.

pies will be a prominent part of our therapeutic armamentarium in the decades to come.

A better understanding of the mediators involved in the pathogenesis of glomerulosclerosis has suggested a wide range of pharmacological interventions. These have included the inhibition of the release of systemic hormones such as GH with octreotide, the blockade of autacoids such as Ang II, endothelin, and nitric oxide, as well as the inhibition of cytokines and growth factors. Preliminary observations have suggested a potential therapeutic efficacy of antagonists of inflammatory chemokines and cytokines such as interleukin (IL)-1 and tumor necrosis factor-α as well as of growth factors such as PDGF and TGF-β in the prevention of experimental glomerulosclerosis. Furthermore, recent evidence also points to a therapeutic role for anti-inflammatory cytokines such as IL-4 and IL-10 in experimental glomerulonephritis [135]. Accordingly, the processes and mediators which eventuate in glomerulosclerosis are being elucidated by a variety of physiological, biochemical, morphometric, and molecular biologic techniques. A useful schematic integrating these pathways has recently been published by Terzi *et al.*, and is shown in Fig. 3.1 [30].

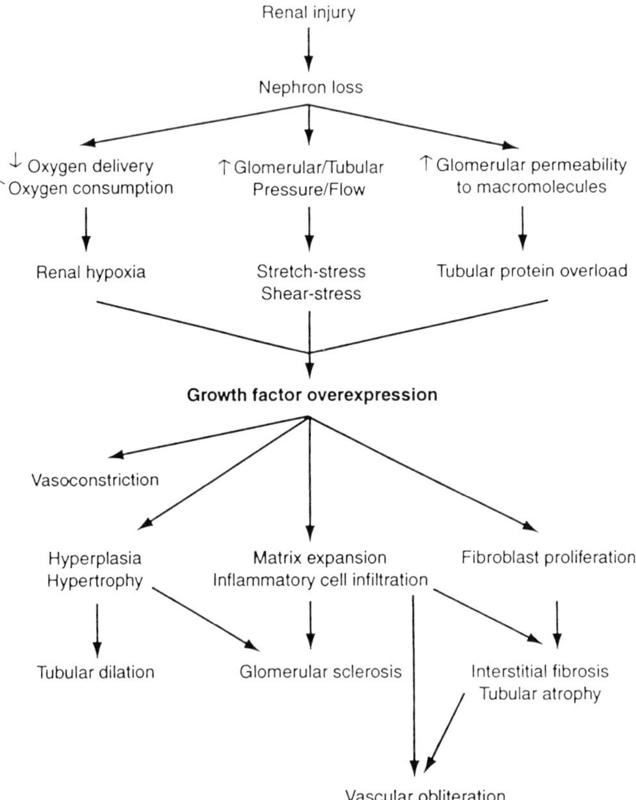

Fig. 3.1 Hypothetical schema of pathways that link nephron reduction to the development of renal lesions via hemodynamic forces and growth factor overexpression. Reproduced from ref. 30 with permission.

Other factors in progressive renal disease

Metabolic and dietary factors

Protein intake

Dietary interventions have been attractive to investigators and clinicians for over half a century. Most prominent is dietary protein restriction, which was initially used to ameliorate uremic symptoms, and later proposed to slow the progression of renal disease. Although almost uniformly effective in animal models, dietary protein restriction has remained a controversial issue clinically. The well known Modification of Diet in Renal Disease trial did not show an unequivocal benefit, although studies in some of the subgroups have shown a beneficial effect [136]. Mechanisms by which protein restriction protects the kidney include attenuation of hemodynamic adaptations, limitation of renal and glomerular growth, beneficial effects on serum lipids, effects on renal metabolism and reduction of oxygen consumption, reduction of oxidant stress, effects on T-cell function, and suppression of Ang II and TGF-β, among others [137].

Hyperlipidemia and glomerular lipid deposition

In experimental animals and humans, glomerular deposits of lipids have been described in the course of nephropathies. It has been suggested that glomerular deposition of circulating lipids contributes to progressive glomerular injury in renal disease [138]. This area of research has received intensive attention in recent years, and has been summarized in several recent reviews [138–140]. In numerous animal models of progressive renal disease, feeding a high cholesterol diet accelerates injury, whereas hypolipidemic therapy slows progression (reviewed in [139]). Mechanisms of lipid-induced injury include a proliferative response of mesangial cells to low-density lipoprotein (LDL) [141,142]; synergistic interactions among LDL, endothelin, PDGF, and IGF-1 [141]; aggravation of glomerular macrophage influx, and stimulation of monocyte chemoattractant protein (MCP-1) [143]; effects on mesangial type IV collagen synthesis [141]; and increased TGF-β expression by infiltrating macrophages [144]. Also, recent data suggest that exposure of mesangial cells in culture to oxidized LDL induces apoptosis [145].

Hypolipidemic therapy with lovastatin has been shown to influence mesangial cell metabolism, by inhibiting serum-induced proliferation [146], inhibiting PDGF-induced mesangial cell mitogenesis [147], and inhibiting MCP-1 and IL-6 mRNA expression and protein secretion [148]. As in atherosclerosis, hyperlipidemia may act synergistically with other risk factors, such as hypertension, in promoting glomerular injury [149].

Other nutrients

Phosphate intake has been proposed to promote injury, and in experimental models, limitation of phosphate intake is protective. Phosphorus restriction may protect remnant nephrons by lowering circulating lipid levels, reducing tubule energy consumption, altering remnant glomerular hemodynamic function, or reducing glomerular volume [137]. Although not well studied, increasing water intake has also been shown to ameliorate experimental sclerosis [91]. Total caloric restriction has long been noted to modify progression of renal disease [89], particularly that associated with aging [150].

Summary

This brief overview has highlighted some of the mechanisms which, acting together, drive the progression from an initial (even transient) insult, to extensive glomerular and tubulo-interstitial sclerosis, and finally leading to ESRD. Intensive, ongoing research using innovative models and techniques is anticipated to refine further our understanding of these processes, and to lead to new clinical strategies for slowing the progression of renal disease.

Key references

Anderson S, Meyer TW. Pathophysiology and nephron adaptation in chronic renal failure. In: Schrier RW, Gottschalk CW (eds), *Diseases of the Kidney*. New York: Little Brown 1997: 2555–2579.

Anderson S, Rennke HG, Brenner BM. Therapeutic advantage of converting enzyme inhibitors in arresting progressive renal disease associated with systemic hypertension in the rat. *J Clin Invest* 1986; **77**: 1993–2000.

Fine LG, Orphanides C, Norman JT. Progressive renal disease: the chronic hypoxia hypothesis. *Kidney Int* 1998; **53** (Suppl. 65): S74–S78.

Hostetter TH, Meyer TW, Rennke HG, Brenner BM. Chronic effects of dietary protein on renal structure and function in the rat with intact and reduced renal mass. *Kidney Int* 1986; **30**: 509–517.

Rennke HG, Anderson S, Brenner BM. Structural and functional correlations in the progression of renal disease. In: Tisher CC, Brenner BM (eds), *Renal Pathology*. Philadelphia: JB Lippincott, 1994: pp. 116–142.

References

1. Rennke HG, Anderson S, Brenner BM. Structural and functional correlations in the progression of renal disease. In: Tisher CC, Brenner BM (eds), *Renal Pathology*. Philadelphia: JB Lippincott, 1994: pp. 116–142.
2. Brunskill N, Klahr S. Mechanisms of progressive renal failure. In: El Nahas AM, Mallick NP, Anderson S (eds), *Prevention of Progressive Chronic Renal Failure*. Oxford: Oxford University Press, 1993: 1–61.
3. Anderson S, Meyer TW. Pathophysiology and nephron adaptation in chronic renal failure. In: Schrier RW, Gottschalk CW (eds), *Diseases of the Kidney*. New York: Little Brown 1997: 2555–2579.
4. Agodoa L, Jones C, Held P. End-stage renal disease in the USA. Data from the United States Renal Data System. *Am J Nephrol* 1996; **16**: 7–16.
5. Portaluppi F, Montanari L, Massari M, Di Chiara V, Capanna M. Loss of nocturnal decline of blood pressure in hypertension due to chronic renal failure. *Am J Hypertension* 1991; **4**: 20–26.
6. Weigman TB, Herron KG, Chonko AM, Macdougall ML, Moore WV. Recognition of hypertension and abnormal blood pressure burden with ambulatory blood pressure recordings in type I diabetes mellitus. *Diabetes* 1990; **39**: 1556–1560.
7. Brazy PC, Stead WW, Fitzwilliam JF. Progression of renal insufficiency: role of blood pressure. *Kidney Int* 1989; **35**: 670–674.
8. Klag MJ, Whelton PK, Randall BL, Neaton JD, Brancati FL, Ford E, Shulman NB, Stamler J. Blood pressure and end-stage renal disease in men. *N Engl J Med* 1996; **334**: 13–18.
9. Lindeman RD, Tobin JD, Shock NW. Association between blood pressure and the rate of decline in renal function with age. *Kidney Int* 1984; **26**: 861–868.
10. Hostetter TH, Olson JL, Rennke HG, Venkatachalam MA, Brenner BM. Hyperfiltration in remnant nephrons: a potentially adverse response to renal ablation. *Am J Physiol* 1981; **241**: F85–F93.
11. Anderson S, Rennke HG, Brenner BM. Therapeutic advantage of converting enzyme inhibitors in arresting progressive renal disease associated with systemic hypertension in the rat. *J Clin Invest* 1986; **77**: 1993–2000.

12. Bidani AK, Schwartz MM, Lewis EJ. Renal autoregulation and vulnerability to hypertensive injury in remnant kidneys. *Am J Physiol* 1987; **252**: F1003–F1010.
13. Brenner BM, Meyer TW, Hostetter TH. Dietary protein intake and the progressive nature of kidney disease. *N Engl J Med* 1982; **307**: 652–660.
14. Anderson S, Brenner BM. The role of nephron mass and of intraglomerular pressure in initiation and progression of experimental hypertensive-renal disorders. In: Laragh JH, Brenner BM (eds), *Hypertension: Pathophysiology, Diagnosis and Management*. New York: Raven Press, 1995: 1553–1568.
15. Anderson S. Pharmacologic interventions in experimental animals. In: El Nahas AM, Mallick NP, Anderson S (eds), *Prevention of Progressive Chronic Renal Failure*. Oxford: Oxford University Press 1993: 173–209.
16. Zatz R, Dunn BR, Meyer TW, Anderson S, Rennke HG, Brenner BM. Prevention of diabetic glomerulopathy by pharmacological amelioration of glomerular capillary hypertension. *J Clin Invest* 1986; **77**: 1925–1930.
17. Lafayette RA, Mayer G, Park SK, Meyer TW. Angiotensin II receptor blockade limits glomerular injury in rats with reduced renal mass. *J Clin Invest* 1992; **90**: 766–771.
18. Wolf G, Ziyadeh FN. The role of angiotensin II in diabetic nephropathy: emphasis on nonhemodynamic mechanisms. *Am J Kidney Dis* 1997; **29**: 153–163.
19. Anderson S, Jung FF, Ingelfinger JR. Renin-angiotensin system in diabetic rats: functional, immunohistochemical, and molecular biologic correlations. *Am J Physiol* 1993; **265**: F477–F486.
20. Ziai F, Ots M, Provoost AP, Troy JL, Rennke HG, Brenner BM, Mackenzie HS. The angiotensin receptor antagonist, irbesartan, reduces renal injury in experimental chronic renal failure. *Kidney Int* 1996; **50** (Suppl. 57): S132–S136.
21. Remuzzi A, Perico N, Amuchastegui CS, Malanchini B, Mazerska M, Battaglia C, Bertani C, Remuzzi G. Short- and long-term effect of angiotensin II receptor blockade in rats with experimental diabetes. *J Am Soc Nephrol* 1993; **4**: 40–49.
22. Shihab FS, Bennett WM, Tanner AM, Andoh TF. Angiotensin II blockade decreases TGF-β1 and matrix proteins in cyclosporine nephropathy. *Kidney Int* 1997; **52**: 660–673.
23. Benstein JA, Feiner HD, Parker M, Dworkin LD. Superiority of salt restriction over diuretics in reducing renal hypertrophy and injury in uninephrectomized SHR. *Am J Physiol* 1990; **258**: F1675–F1681.
24. Ercole LB, Inserra F, Romano LA, Ferder L. Failure of renal protection by chronic administration of thiazide. *J Am Soc Nephrol* 1996; **7**: 1731 (Abstr.).
25. Daniels BS, Hostetter TH. Adverse effects of growth in the glomerular microcirculation. *Am J Physiol* 1990; **258**: F1409–F1416.
26. Bakris GL. Renal effects of calcium antagonists in diabetes mellitus. An overview of studies in animal models and humans. *Am J Hypertension* 1991; **4**: 487S–493S.
27. Zoja C, Perico N, Bergamelli A, Pasini M, Morigi M, Dadan J, Belloni A, Bertani T, Remuzzi G. Ticlodipine prevents renal disease progression in rats with reduced renal mass. *Kidney Int* 1990; **37**: 934–942.
28. Jacobson HR. Ischemic renal disease: an overlooked clinical entity? *Kidney Int* 1998; **34**: 729–743.
29. Breyer JA, Jacobson HR. Ischemic nephropathy. *Curr Opinion Nephrol Hypertension* 1993; **2**: 216–224.
30. Terzi F, Burtin M, Friedlander G. Early molecular mechanisms in the progression of renal failure: role of growth factors and protooncogenes. *Kidney Int* 1998; **53** (Suppl. 65): S68–S73.

31. Fine LG, Orphanides C, Norman JT. Progressive renal disease: the chronic hypoxia hypothesis. *Kidney Int* 1998; **53** (Suppl. 65): S74–S78.
32. Harris DC, Chan L, Schrier RW. Remnant kidney hypermetabolism and progression of chronic renal failure. *Am J Physiol* 1988; **254**: F267–F276.
33. Bohle A, Gise H, Mackensen HS, Stark JB. The obliteration of the postglomerular capillaries and its influence upon the function of both glomeruli and tubuli. Functional interpretation of morphologic findings. *Klin Wochenschr* 1981; **59**: 1043–1051.
34. Kourembanas S, Hannan RL, Faller DV. Oxygen tension regulates the expression of the platelet-derived growth factor-B chain gene in human endothelial cells. *J Clin Invest* 1990; **86**: 670–674.
35. Ong ACAC, Jowett TP, Firth JD, Burton s Karet FE, Fine LG. An endothelin-1 mediated autocrine growth loop involved in human renal tubular regeneration. *Kidney Int* 1995; **48**: 390–401.
36. Orphanides C, Fine LG, Norman JT. Hypoxia stimulates proximal tubular cell matrix production via a TGF-β1-independent mehanism. *Kidney Int* 1997; **52**: 637–647.
37. Schweiki D, Itin A, Soffer D, Keshet E. Vascular endothelial growth factor induced by hypoxia may mediate hypoxia-initiated angiogenesis. *Nature* 1992; **359**: 843–845.
38. Remuzzi G, Bertani T. Is glomerulosclerosis a consequence of altered glomerular permeability to macromolecules? *Kidney Int* 1990; **38**: 384–394.
39. Hayslett JP, Kashgarian M, Epstein FH. Functional correlates of compensatory renal hypertrophy. *J Clin Invest* 1968; **47**: 774–799.
40. Wesson LG. Compensatory growth and other growth responses of the kidney. *Nephron* 1989; **51**: 149–184.
41. Norman JT, Fine LG. Renal growth and hypertrophy. In: Massry SG, Glassock RJ (eds), *Textbook of Nephrology*. Baltimore: Williams & Wilkins, 1995: 146–158.
42. Fine LG, Norman J. Cellular events in renal hypertrophy. *Annu Rev Physiol* 1989; **51**: 19–32.
43. Johnson HA, Roman JMV. Compensatory renal enlargement. Hypertrophy versus hyperplasia. *Am J Pathol* 1966; **49**: 1–13.
44. Ouellette AJ. Messenger RNA regulation during compensatory renal growth. *Kidney Int* 1983; **23**: 575–580.
45. Ouellette AJ, Moonka R, Zelenetz AD, Malt RA. Regulation of ribosome synthesis during compensatory renal hypertrophy in mice. *Am J Physiol* 1987; **253**: C506–C513.
46. Norman JT, Bohman RE, Fischmann G, Bowen JW, McDonough A, Slamon D, Fine LG. Patterns of mRNA expression during early cell growth differ in kidney epithelial cells destined to undergo compensatory hypertrophy versus regenerative hyperplasia. *Proc Natl Acad Sci USA* 1988; **85**: 6768–6772.
47. Norman JT. Regulation of gene expression in renal compensatory growth. *Am J Kidney Dis* 1991; **17**: 638–640.
48. Sacerdotti C. Über die compensatorische hypertrophie der nieren. *Virch Arch Pathol Anat* 1896; **146**: 267–297.
49. Braun Menéndez E. Hypertension and relation between kidney and body weight. *Stanford Med Bull* 1952; **10**: 65–72.
50. Preuss HG. Does renotropin have a role in the pathogenesis of hypertension? *Am J Hypertension* 1989; **2**: 65–71.
51. Fine LG. Cellular events in renal hypertrophy. *Annu Rev Physiol* 1989; **51**: 19–32.
52. Igawa T, Kanetake H, Saitoh Y, Ichihara A, Tomita Y, Nakamura T. Hepatocyte growth factor is a potent mitogen for cultured rabbit renal tubular epithelial cells. *Biochem Biophys Res Commun* 1991; **174**: 831–838.

53. Fine LG, Hammerman MR, Abboud HE. Evolving role of growth factors in the renal response to acute and chronic disease. *J Am Soc Nephrol* 1992; **2**: 1163–1170.
54. Mendley SR, Toback FG. Cell proliferation in the end-stage kidney. *Am J Kidney Dis* 1990; **16**: 80–84.
55. Kujubu DA, Fine LG. Polypeptide growth factors and their relation to renal disease. *Am J Kidney Dis* 1989; **14**: 61–73.
56. Patt LM, Houck JC. Role of polypeptide growth factors in normal and abnormal growth. *Kidney Int* 1983; **23**: 603–610.
57. Shankland SJ. Cell-cycle control and renal disease. *Kidney Int* 1997; **52**: 294–308.
58. Lajara R, Rotwein P, Bortz JD, Hansen VA, Sadow JL, Betts CR, Rogers SA, Hammerman MR. Dual regulation of insulin-like growth factor I expression during renal hypertrophy. *Am J Physiol* 1989; **257**: F252–F261.
59. Miller SB, Hansen VA, Hammerman MR. Effects of growth hormone and IGF-I on renal function in rats with normal and reduced renal mass. *Am J Physiol* 1990; **259**: F747–F757.
60. Quaife CJ, Mathews LS, Pinkert CA, Hammer RE, Brinster RL, Palmiter RD. Histopathology associated with elevated levels of growth hormone and insulin-like growth factor I in transgenic mice. *Endocrinol* 1989; **124**: 40–48.
61. Mehls O, Irzynjec T, Ritz E, Eden S, Kovàcs KG, Floege J, Mall G. Effects of rhGH and rhIGF-1 on renal growth and morphology. *Kidney Int* 1993; **44**: 1251–1258.
62. Stiles AD, Sosenko IR, Dercole AJ, Smith BT. Relation of kidney tissue somatomedin-C/insulin-like growth factor I to postnephrectomy renal growth in the rat. *Endocrinology* 1985; **117**: 2397–2401.
63. Fagin JA, Melmed S. Relative increase in insulin-like growth factor I messenger ribonucleic acid levels in compensatory renal hypertrophy. *Endocrinology* 1987; **120**: 718–724.
64. Flyvbjerg A, Ussing O, Næraa R, Ingerslev J, Ørskov H. Kidney tissue somatomedin C and initial renal growth in diabetic and uninephrectomized rats. *Diabetologia* 1988; **31**: 310–314.
65. Hise MK, Lahn JS, Shao ZM, Mantzouris NM, Fontana JA. Insulin-like growth factor-I receptor and binding proteins in rat kidney after nephron loss. *J Am Soc Nephrol* 1993; **4**: 62–68.
66. Rogers SA, Miller SB, Hammerman MR. Enhanced renal IGF-I expression following partial kidney infarction. *Am J Physiol* 1993; **264**: F963–F967.
67. Hickling HM, El Eter F, Haylor J, Hardisty C, El Nahas MA. IGF type 1 receptor antagonist (JB3) inhibits kidney growth in diabetic and Unx rats. *J Am Soc Nephrol* 1997; **8**: 638A (Abstr.).
68. Behrens MT, Corbin AL, Hise MK. Epidermal growth factor receptor regulation in rat kidney: two models of renal growth. *Am J Physiol* 1989; **257**: F1059–F1064.
69. Sack EM, Arruda JA. Epidermal growth factor binding to cortical basolateral membranes in compensatory renal hypertrophy. *Regulatory Peptides* 1991; **33**: 339–348.
70. Miller SB, Rogers SA, Estes CE, Hammerman MR. Increased distal nephron EGF content and altered distribution of peptide in compensatory renal hypertrophy. *Am J Physiol* 1992; **262**: F1032–F1038.
71. Nagaike M, Hirao S, Tajima H, Noji S, Taniguchi S, Matsumoto K, Nakamura T. Renotropic functions of hepatocyte growth factor in renal regeneration after unilateral nephrectomy. *J Biol Chem* 1991; **266**: 22781–22784.
72. Yanagita K, Nagaike M, Ishibashi H, Matsumoto K, Nakamura T. Lung may have an endocrine function producing hepatocyte growth factor in response to injury of distal organs. *Biochem Biophys Res Commun* 1992; **182**: 802–809.

73. Montesano R, Matsumoto K, Nakamura T, Orci L. Identification of a fibroblast-derived epithelial morphogen as hepatocyte growth factor. *Cell* 1991; **67**: 901–908.
74. Beer DG, Zweifel KA, Simpson DP, Pitot HC. Specific gene expression during compensatory renal hypertrophy in the rat. *J Cell Physiol* 1987; **131**: 29–35.
75. Sawczuk IS, Olsson CA, Hoke G, Buttyan R. Immediate induction of c-fos and c-myc transcripts following unilateral nephrectomy. *Nephron* 1990; **55**: 193–195.
76. Nakamura T, Ebihara I, Tomino Y, Koide H, Kikuchi K, Koiso K. Gene expression of growth-related proteins and ECM constituents in response to unilateral nephrectomy. *Am J Physiol* 1992; **262**: F389–F396.
77. Kujubu DA, Norman JT, Herschman HR, Fine LG. Primary response gene expression in renal hypertrophy and hyperplasia: evidence for different growth initiation processes. *Am J Physiol* 1991; **260**: F823–F827.
78. Terzi F, Ticozzi C, Burtin M, Motel V, Beaufils H, Laouari D, Assael BM, Kleinknecht C. Subtotal but not unilateral nephrectomy induces hyperplasia and protooncogene expression. *Am J Physiol* 1995; **268**: F793–F801.
79. Rosenberg ME, Hostetter TH. Effect of angiotensin II and norepinephrine on early growth response genes in the rat kidney. *Kidney Int* 1993; **43**: 601–609.
80. Kojima R, Troy J, Brenner BM, Gullans SR. Identification and characterization of novel genes induced by uninephrectomy. *J Am Soc Nephrol* 1993; **4**: 774 (Abstract).
81. Hayslett JP. Effect of age on compensatory renal growth. *Kidney Int* 1983; **23**: 599–602.
82. Galla JH, Klein-Robbenhaar T, Hayslett JP. Influence of age on the compensatory response in growth and function to unilateral nephrectomy. *Yale J Biol Med* 1974; **47**: 218–226.
83. MacKay EM, Mackay LL, Addis T. The degree of compensatory renal hypertrophy following unilateral nephrectomy. *I Influence Age J Exp Med* 1932; **56**: 225–232.
84. O'Donnell MP, Kasiske BL, Raij L, Keane WF. Age is a determinant of the glomerular morphologic and functional responses to chronic nephron loss. *J Lab Clin Med* 1985; **106**: 308–313.
85. Hostetter TH, Meyer TW, Rennke HG, Brenner BM. Chronic effects of dietary protein on renal structure and function in the rat with intact and reduced renal mass. *Kidney Int* 1986; **30**: 509–517.
86. Kenner CH, Evan AP, Blomgren P, Aronoff GR, Luft FC. Effect of protein intake on renal function and structure in partially nephrectomized rats. *Kidney Int* 1985; **27**: 739–750.
87. Kaysen GA, Rosenthal C, Hutchison FN. GFR increases before renal mass or ODC activity increase in rats fed high protein diets. *Kidney Int* 1989; **36**: 441–446.
88. Klahr S, Buerkert J, Purkerson ML. Role of dietary factors in the progression of chronic renal disease. *Kidney Int* 1983; **24**: 579–587.
89. Kobayashi S, Venkatachalam MA. Differential effects of caloric restriction on glomeruli and tubules of the remnant kidney. *Kidney Int* 1992; **42**: 710–717.
90. Kleinknecht C, Laouari D, Hinglais N, Habib R, Dodu C, Lacour B, Broyer M. Role of amount and nature of carbohydrates in the course of experimental renal failure. *Kidney Int* 1986; **30**: 687–693.
91. Bouby N, Bachmann S, Bichet D, Bankir L. Effect of water intake on the progression of chronic renal failure in the 5/6 nephrectomized rat. *Am J Physiol* 1990; **258**: F973–F979.
92. Chen NY, Chen WY, Kopchick JJ. Liver and kidney growth hormone receptors are regulated differently in diabetic GH and GH antagonist transgenic mice. *Endocrinology* 1997; **138**: 851–854.

93. Fries JWU, Sandstrom DJ, Meyer TW, Rennke HG. Glomerular hypertrophy and epithelial cell injury modulate progressive glomerulosclerosis in the rat. *Lab Invest* 1989; **60**: 205–218.
94. Schwartz MM, Evans J, Bidani AK. The mesangium in the long-term remnant kidney model. *J Lab Clin Med* 1994; **124**: 644–651.
95. Fogo A, Ichikawa I. Evidence for the central role of glomerular growth promoters in the development of sclerosis. *Semin Nephrol* 1989; **9**: 329–342.
96. Olivetti G, Anversa P, Rigamonti W, Vitali-Mazza L, Loud AV. Morphometry of the renal corpuscle during normal postnatal growth and compensatory hypertrophy. A light microscope study. *J Cell Biol* 1977; **75**: 573–585.
97. Dworkin LD, Hostetter TH, Rennke HG, Brenner BM. Hemodynamic basis for glomerular injury in rats with desoxycorticosterone-salt hypertension. *J Clin Invest* 1984; **73**: 1448–1461.
98. Shea SM, Raskova J, Morrison AB. A stereologic study of glomerular hypertrophy in the subtotally nephrectomized rat. *Am J Pathol* 1978; **90**: 201–210.
99. Olivetti G, Anversa P, Melissari M, Loud AV. Morphometry of the renal corpuscle during postnatal growth and compensatory hypertrophy. *Kidney Int* 1980; **17**: 438–454.
100. Schwartz MM, Bidani AK. Mesangial structure and function in the remnant kidney. *Kidney Int* 1991; **40**: 226–237.
101. Nagata M, Kriz W. Glomerular damage after uninephrectomy in young rats. I. Hypertrophy and distortion of capillary architecture. *Kidney Int* 1992; **42**: 136–147, 160.
102. Nagata M, Schärer K, Kriz W. Glomerular damage after uninephrectomy in young rats. II. Mechanical stress on podocytes as a pathway to sclerosis. *Kidney Int* 1992; **42**: 148–160.
103. Kanda S, Hisamatsu H, Igawa T, Eguchi J, Taide M, Sakai H, Kanetake H, Saito Y, Yoshitake Y, Nishikawa K. Peritubular endothelial cell proliferation in mice during compensatory renal growth after unilateral nephrectomy. *Am J Physiol* 1993; **265**: F712–F716.
104. Lee GSL, Nast CC, Peng SC, Artishevsky A, Ihn-G, Guillermo R, Levin PS, Glassock RJ, LaPage J, Adler SG. Differential response of glomerular epithelial and mesangial cells after subtotal nephrectomy. *Kidney Int* 1998; **52**: 1389–1398.
105. Bidani AK, Mitchell KD, Schwartz MM, Navar LG, Lewis EJ. Absence of glomerular injury or nephron loss in a normotensive rat remnant kidney model. *Kidney Int* 1990; **38**: 28–38.
106 Kimura K, Tojo A, Hirata Y, Matsuoka H, Sugimoto T. Morphometric analysis of renal arterioles in subtotally nephrectomized rats. *J Lab Clin Med* 1993; **22**: 273–283.
107. Shea SM, Raskova J. Glomerular hemodynamics and vascular structure in uremia: a network analysis of glomerular path lengths and maximal blood transit times computed for a microvascular model reconstructed from serial ultrathin sections. *Microvascular Res* 1984; **28**: 37–50.
108. Knutson DW, Chieu F, Bennett CM, Glassock RJ. Estimation of relative glomerular capillary surface area in normal and hypertrophic rat kidneys. *Kidney Int* 1978; **14**: 437–443.
109. Striker LJ. Nephron reduction in man—lessons from the OS mouse. *Nephrol Dial Transplant* 1998; **13**: 543–545.
110. Lafferty HM, Brenner BM. Are glomerular hypertension and 'hypertrophy' independent risk factors for progression of renal disease? *Semin Nephrol* 1990; **10**: 294–304.
111. Miller PL, Scholey JW, Rennke HG, Meyer TW. Glomerular hypertrophy aggravates epithelial cell injury in nephrotic rats. *J Clin Invest* 1990; **85**: 1119–1126.

112. Yoshida Y, Kawamura T, Ikoma M, Fogo A, Ichikawa I. Effects of antihypertensive drugs on glomerular morphology. *Kidney Int* 1989; **36**: 626–635.
113. Scholey JW, Miller PL, Rennke HG, Meyer TW. Effect of converting enzyme inhibition on the course of adriamycin-induced nephropathy. *Kidney Int* 1989; **36**: 816–822.
114. Dworkin LD, Levin RI, Benstein JA, Parker M, Ullian ME, Kim Y, Feiner HD. Effect of nifedipine and enalapril on glomerular injury in rats with desoxycorticosterone-salt hypertension. *Am J Physiol* 1990; **259**: F598–F604.
115. Griendling KK, Alexander RW. Endothelial control of the cardiovascular system: recent advances. *FASEB J* 1996; **10**: 283–292.
116. Riser BL, Cortes P, Zhao X, Bernstein J, Dumler F, Narins RG. Intraglomerular pressure and mesangial stretching stimulate extracellular matrix formation in the rat. *J Clin Invest* 1992; **90**: 1932–1943.
117. Cortes P, Zhao X, Riser BL, Narins RG. Regulation of glomerular volume in normal and partially nephrectomized rats. *Am J Physiol* 1996; **270**: F356–F370.
118. Cortes P, Zhao X, Riser BL, Narins RG. Role of glomerular mechanical strain in the pathogenesis of diabetic nephropathy. *Kidney Int* 1997; **51**: 57–68.
119. Johnson RJ, Iida H, Alpers CE, Majesky MW, Schwartz SM, Pritzi P, Gordon K, Gown AM. Expression of smooth muscle cell phenotype by rat mesangial cells in immune complex nephritis. Alpha-smooth muscle actin is a marker of mesangial cell proliferation. *J Clin Invest* 1991; **87**: 847–858.
120. El Nahas AM, Muchaneta-Kubara EC, Zhang GZ, Adam A, Goumenos D. Phenotypic modulation of renal cells during experimental and clinical renal scarring. *Kidney Int* 1996; **49** (Suppl. 54): S23–S27.
121. Rennke HG. How does glomerular epithelial cell injury contribute to progressive glomerular damage? *Kidney Int* 1994; **45** (Suppl. 45): S58–S63.
122. Kriz W. Progressive renal failure—inability of podocytes to replicate and the consequences for glomerulosclerosis. *Nephrol Dial Transplant* 1996; **11**: 1738–1742.
123. Bariety J, Nochy D, Mandet C, Jacquot C, Glotz D, Meyrier A. Podocytes undergo phenotypic changes and express macrophagic-associated markers in idiopathic collapsing glomerulopathy. *Kidney Int* 1998; **53**: 918–925.
124. Ricardo SD, Ding G, Eufemio M, Diamond JR. Antioxidant expression in experimental hydronephrosis: role of mechanical stretch and growth factors. *Am J Physiol* 1997; **272**: F789–F798.
125. Ong ACM, Fine LG. Tubular-derived growth factors and cytokines in the pathogenesis of tubulointerstitial fibrosis: implications for human renal disease progression. *Am J Kidney Dis* 1994; **23**: 205–209.
126. Egido J. Vasoactive hormones and renal sclerosis. *Kidney Int* 1996; **49**: 578–597.
127. Johnson RJ. Cytokines, growth factors, and renal injury: Where do we go now? *Kidney Int* 1997; **52** (Suppl. 63): S2–S6.
128. Perico N, Remuzzi G. Role of endothelin in glomerular injury. *Kidney Int* 1993; **43** (Suppl. 39): S76–S80.
129. Raij L, Baylis C. Glomerular actions of nitric oxide. *Kidney Int* 1995; **48**: 20–32.
130. Ketteler M, Border WA, Noble NA. Cytokines and l-arginine in renal injury and repair. *Am J Physiol* 1994; **267**: F197–F207.
131. Border WA, Noble NA. Transforming growth factor-β in tissue fibrosis. *N Engl J Med* 1994; **331**: 1286–1292.
132. Border WA, Noble NA, Ketteler M. TGF-β: a cytokine mediator of glomerulosclerosis and a target for therapeutic intervention. *Kidney Int* 1995; **47** (Suppl. 49): S59–S61.

133. Johnson RJ. The glomerular response to injury: progression or resolution? *Kidney Int* 1994; **45**: 1769–1782.
134. Giachelli CM, Pichler R, Lombardi D, Denhardt DT, Alpers CE, Schwartz SM, Johnson RJ. Osteopontin expression in angiotensin II-induced interstitial nephritis. *Kidney Int* 1994; **45**: 515–524.
135. Ring GH, Lakkis FG. T lymphocyte-derived cytokines in experimental glomerulonephritis: testing the Th1/Th2 hypothesis. *Nephrol Dial Transplant* 1998; **13**: 1101–1103.
136. Levey AS, Adler S, Caggiula AW, England BK, Greene T, Hunsicker LG, Kusek JW, Rogers NL, Teschan P. Effect of dietary protein restriction on the progression of advanced renal disease in the Modification of Diet in Renal Disease Study. *Am J Kidney Dis* 1996; **27**: 652–663.
137. Modi KS, O'Donnell MP, Keane WF. Dietary interventions for progressive renal disease in experimental animal models. In: El NahasAM, Mallick NP, Anderson S (eds), *Prevention of Progressive Chronic Renal Failure*. Oxford: Oxford University Press, 1993: 117–172.
138. Keane WF. Lipids and the kidney. *Kidney Int* 1994; **46**: 910–920.
139. Walli AK, Gröne E, Miller B, Gröne H-J, Thiery J, Seidel D. Role of lipoproteins in progressive renal disease. *Am J Hypertension* 1993; **1993** (6): 358S–366S.
140. Schlondorff D. Cellular mechanisms of lipid injury in the glomerulus. *Am J Kidney Dis* 1993; **22**: 72–82.
141. Gröne EF, Abboud HE, Höhne M, Walli AK, Gröne H-J, Stüker D, Robenek H, Wieland E, Seidel D. Actions of lipoproteins in cultured human mesangial cells: modulation by mitogenic vasoconstrictors. *Am J Physiol* 1992; **263**: F686–F696.
142. Keane WF, O'Donnell MP, Kasiske BL, Kim Y. Oxidative modification of low density lipoproteins by mesangial cells. *J Am Soc Nephrol* 1993; **4**: 187–194.
143. Rovin BH, Tan LC. LDL stimulates mesangial fibronectin production and chemoattractant expression. *Kidney Int* 1993; **43**: 218–225.
144. Ding GH, Pesek-Diamond I, Diamond JR. Cholesterol, macrophages, and gene expression of TGF-β1 and fibronectin during nephrosis. *Am J Physiol* 1993; **264**: F577–F584.
145. Sharma P, Reddy K, Franki N, Sanwal V, Sankaran R, Ahuja TS, Gibbons N, Mattana J, Singhal PC. Native and oxidized low density lipoproteins modulate mesangial cell apoptosis. *Kidney Int* 1996; **50**: 1604–1611.
146. O'Donnell MP, Kasiske BL, Kim Y, Atluru D, Keane WF. Lovastatin inhibits proliferation of rat mesangial cells. *J Clin Invest* 1993; **91**: 83–87.
147. O'Donnell MP, Kasiske BL, Kim Y, Atluru D, Keane WF. Platelet-derived growth factor stimulation of mesangial cell DNA synthesis is dependent on the isoprenoid farnesyl. *J Am Soc Nephrol* 1993; **4**: 473 (Abstr.).
148. Guijarro C, O'Donnell MP, Kasiske BL, Kim Y, Atluru D, Keane WF. Differential effects of lovastatin on human mesangial cell mRNA for cytokines involved in proliferation and matrix turnover. *J Am Soc Nephrol* 1993; **4**: 770 (Abstr.).
149. Mulec H, Johnsen SA, Wiklund O, Björck S. Cholesterol: a renal risk factor in diabetic nephropathy? *Am J Kidney Dis* 1993; **22**: 196–201.
150. Van Liew JB, David FB, Davis PJ, Noble B, Bernardis LL. Calorie restriction decreases microalbuminuria associated with aging in barrier-raised Fischer 344 rats. *Am J Physiol* 1992; **263**: F554–F561.

4

Experimental insights into the mechanisms of tubulo-interstitial scarring

Stephanie M. Jernigan and Allison A. Eddy

Overview

The relationship of chronic tubulo-interstitial disease to the decline in renal function and long-term prognosis was first highlighted in the landmark structure–function studies by Risdon *et al.* [1] and Schainuck *et al.* [2]. Investigators today continue to reaffirm the importance of chronic damage to tubules and the surrounding interstitial space to renal failure progression [3,4] and to search for the mechanisms involved in the development of glomerular and tubulo-interstitial fibrosis. It is likely that the pathogenesis is similar in each compartment of the kidney but not identical. In addition, pathways involved in interstitial fibrosis overlap with the normal repair process in tissues and may be reversible at some level. In this chapter current concepts of the pathogenesis of renal interstitial fibrosis will be reviewed. A schematic overview of these pathways is summarized in Fig. 4.1. Several theories have been proposed as initiating events in the pathogenesis of interstitial scarring (Table 4.1).

The effect of interstitial scarring on the tubulo-interstitial cells is critical. Local and systemic cytokines and vasoactive substances stimulate cellular participants. Resident kidney cells as well as migrating and transformed cells contribute to increased extracellular matrix (ECM) production. Ultimately, the tubules and peritubular capillaries disappear. Tubular loss likely explains the close relationship between interstitial fibrosis and declining renal function. In some cases relatively intact glomeruli may persist, leading to the appearance of 'atubular glomeruli', a histological feature of progressive renal disease that was first highlighted by Marcussen [5]. As illustrated in Fig. 4.2, detailed studies of renal structure have confirmed that as the interstitial area increases due to matrix protein accumulation, the area occupied by tubules declines. In fact, the tubules may be considered one of the primary victims of interstitial fibrosis. It is now time for studies to address the important question of why tubules die. Ischemia due to loss of peritubular capillaries and to the constriction of efferent arterioles is likely to be important [6–8]. Whether the mechanism of tubular death is due to necrosis or apoptosis is currently unknown, although speculation suggests that apoptosis predominates [9]. Figure 4.3 illustrates numerous apoptotic tubular cells in an experimental model of interstitial fibrosis

Table 4.1 Pathogenesis of tubulo-interstitial fibrosis: the theories

Ammoniogenesis increased [215]
Ischemia [7,157,216]
Lipiduria [210,217]
Proteinuria [218,219]
Chemoattractants [67–69,220]
Complement [74,75]
Cytokines [172,221]
Lysosomal enzymes [222]
Transferrin/iron [223–225]
Tubular obstruction [226]
T-cell-mediated immune response [227–230]
Tubular hypermetabolism [231,232]
Tubulo-interstitial crystalline deposits [233–235]

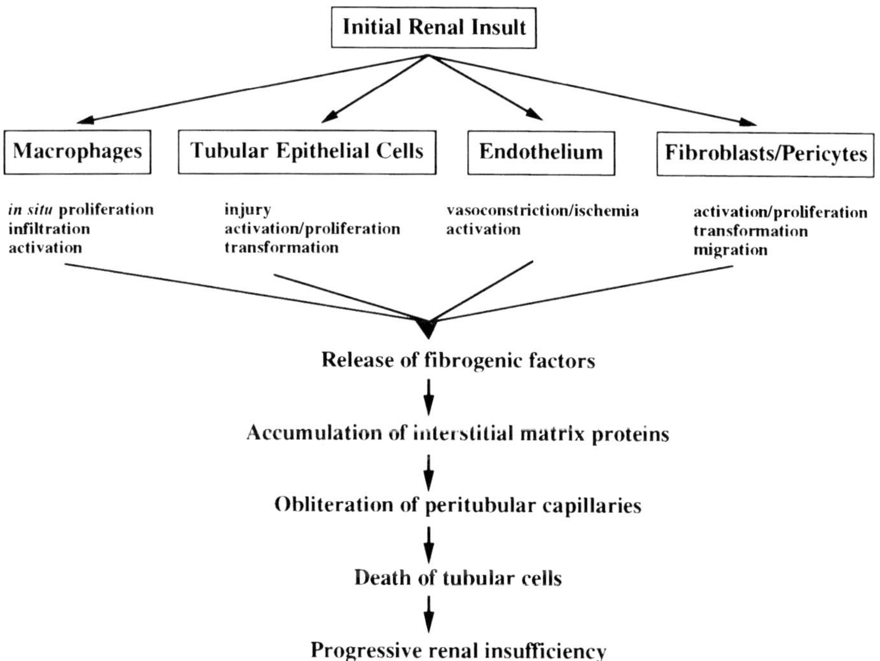

Fig. 4.1 Overview of the key participants in the pathogenesis of tubulo-interstitial fibrosis.

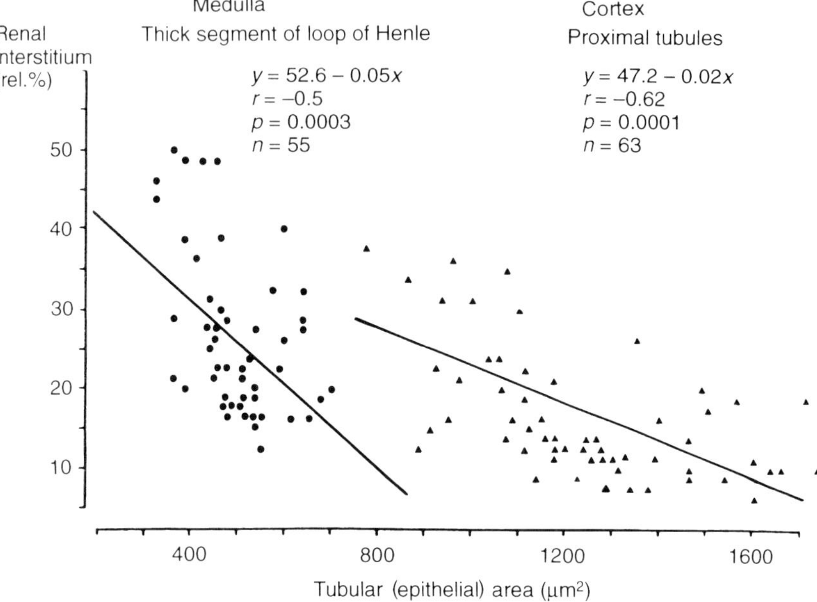

Fig. 4.2 Relationship of the epithelial area of the proximal tubules and the thick ascending limb of the loop of Henle to the relative interstitial area in the cortex and outer stripe of the outer medulla in human renal diseases. (From Mackensen-Haen S, Bohle A, Christensen M, Wehrmann M, Kendziorra H, Korot F. The consequences for renal function of widening of the interstitium and changes in the tubular epithelium of the cortex and outer medulla in various renal diseases. *Clin Nephrol* 1992; **37**: 70–72. Copyright permission of DUSTRI-VERLAG.)

due to cyclosporine nephrotoxicity. Inadequate matrix degradation also appears to play a part in interstitial matrix accumulation. As the functioning unit of the kidney is replaced by interstitial scar tissue, renal function declines and kidney failure is the final outcome.

Composition of interstitial scar

Interstitial fibrosis is the excess accumulation of matrix proteins in the renal interstitium. The composition of this matrix is quite complex (Table 4.2) and is made up of both normal interstitial proteins (collagens I, III, V, VII, XV) and proteins normally restricted to other structures such as the TBM (collagen IV, laminin) (Fig. 4.4). It is not clear that each component of the interstitial scar has a detrimental effect on renal structure. Some components may actually attenuate damage, as suggested by the observation that glomerular injury is more severe in mice that are genetically deficient in tenascin [10]. Qualitative changes in the molecular composition of the normal interstitial matrix also characterize interstitial

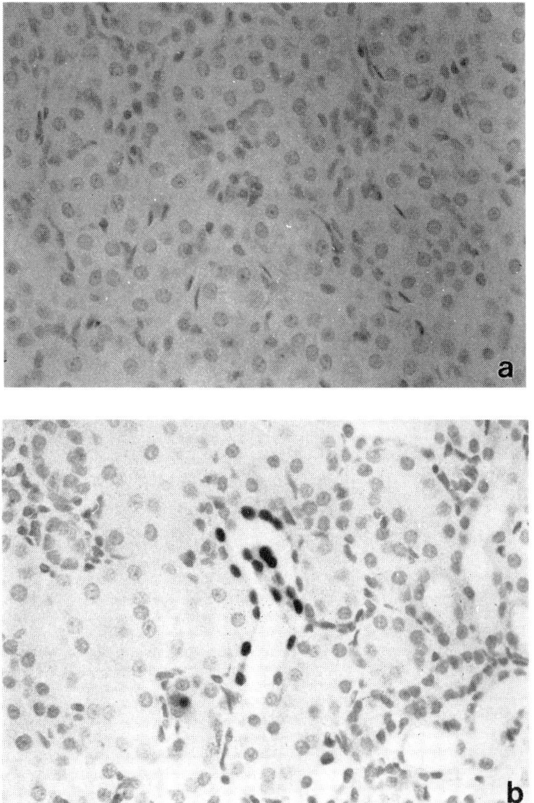

Fig. 4.3 Apoptotic tubular epithelial cells. Using the TUNEL (terminal deoxynucleotidyl transferase-mediated dUTP nick end-labeling) method, apoptotic tubular epithelial cells are difficult to find in normal rat kidneys (a). In contrast, several apoptotic cells (black nuclear bodies) are seen along the wall and within the lumen of renal tubules is a rat with cyclosporine-induced interstitial fibrosis (b). (Photo: Dr Susan Thomas, University of Washington.)

fibrogenesis. Take, for example, the adhesive glycoprotein fibronectin. Fibronectin is often the first protein on the scene in the formation of a 'scar.' It is thought to form a scaffold for further matrix deposition as well as acting as a fibroblast chemoattractant [11]. In experimental models of anti-glomerular basement membrane (anti-GBM) nephritis, anti-tubular basement membrane (anti-TBM) nephritis [12], chronic graft versus host disease and chronic serum sickness [13], the splicing pattern of fibronectin is different from the pattern found in normal kidneys. Studies by Viedt and associates [14] also found that human tubular epithelial cells cultured in the presence of transforming growth factor (TGF)-β1 synthesized increased quantities of fibronectin but most of this newly synthesized protein was of the alternatively spliced variant. Although the biological significance of this alteration is currently unknown, the variant fibronectin may have distinct functions. All of the

Table 4.2 Matrix proteins that accumulate in the interstitium during renal fibrosis

Interstitial matrix proteins
Collagens I, III, V, VII, XV
Fibronectin
Tenascin
Basement membrane proteins
Collagen IV
Laminin
Extracellular proteoglycans*
Large chondroitin sulfate proteoglycans (aggrecan, versican)
Small proteoglycans (decorin, fibromodulin, biglycan)
Basement membrane proteoglycans (heparan sulfate proteoglycan, perlecan)
Polysaccharides and glycoproteins*
Hyaluronan
Thrombospondin
Secreted protein, acidic, and rich in cysteine (SPARC)

* Studies on the accumulation of extracellular proteoglycans, polysaccharides, and glycoproteins are in their infancy. Modified from Eddy AA: Molecular insights into renal interstitial fibrosis. *J Am Soc Nephrol* 1996; 7: 2495–2508. Copyright permission from Williams and Wilkins.

cells that are thought to participate in the interstitial fibrogenic response may express matrix receptors, particularly the integrins, but their part in progressive renal injury has received little attention to date. A recent study in human renal biopsies reports increased expression of the α_5 integrin chain by interstitial cells and increased expression of the α_v integrin chains by tubular cells in damaged kidneys [15]. Both of these chains bind fibronectin and may play a part in its assembly into an insoluble matrix.

Understanding the significance of the accumulation of proteoglycans, polysaccharides, and glycoproteins in the renal interstitium is in the early stages of investigation [16] and the role of these molecules in fibrosis remains unclear. Hyaluronan [17], decorin [18], thrombospondin [19], and SPARC (secreted protein, acidic, and rich in cysteine) [20,21] have been shown to accumulate in the interstitium during progressive renal disease. These molecules may regulate the function of cells and cytokines within the tubulo-interstitium [22]. SPARC may even be antifibrogenic due to antiproliferative properties and to its ability to inhibit some growth factors [23]. Hyaluronan is found in large quantities in healing fetal wounds and may play a part in the prevention of scarring that typifies healed fetal injuries [24]. Whether hyaluronan plays a similar protective part in the renal interstitium is unknown. Other proteoglycans may serve as a reservoir for fibrogenic growth factors such as basic fibroblast growth factor (bFGF) and TGF-β. Sequestered at these sites and functionally inactivated, these growth factors may be released by proteases to propagate fibrosis [22]. Thrombospondin is known to activate latent TGF-β1 *in vitro* [25,26], an effect that might facilitate interstitial scarring.

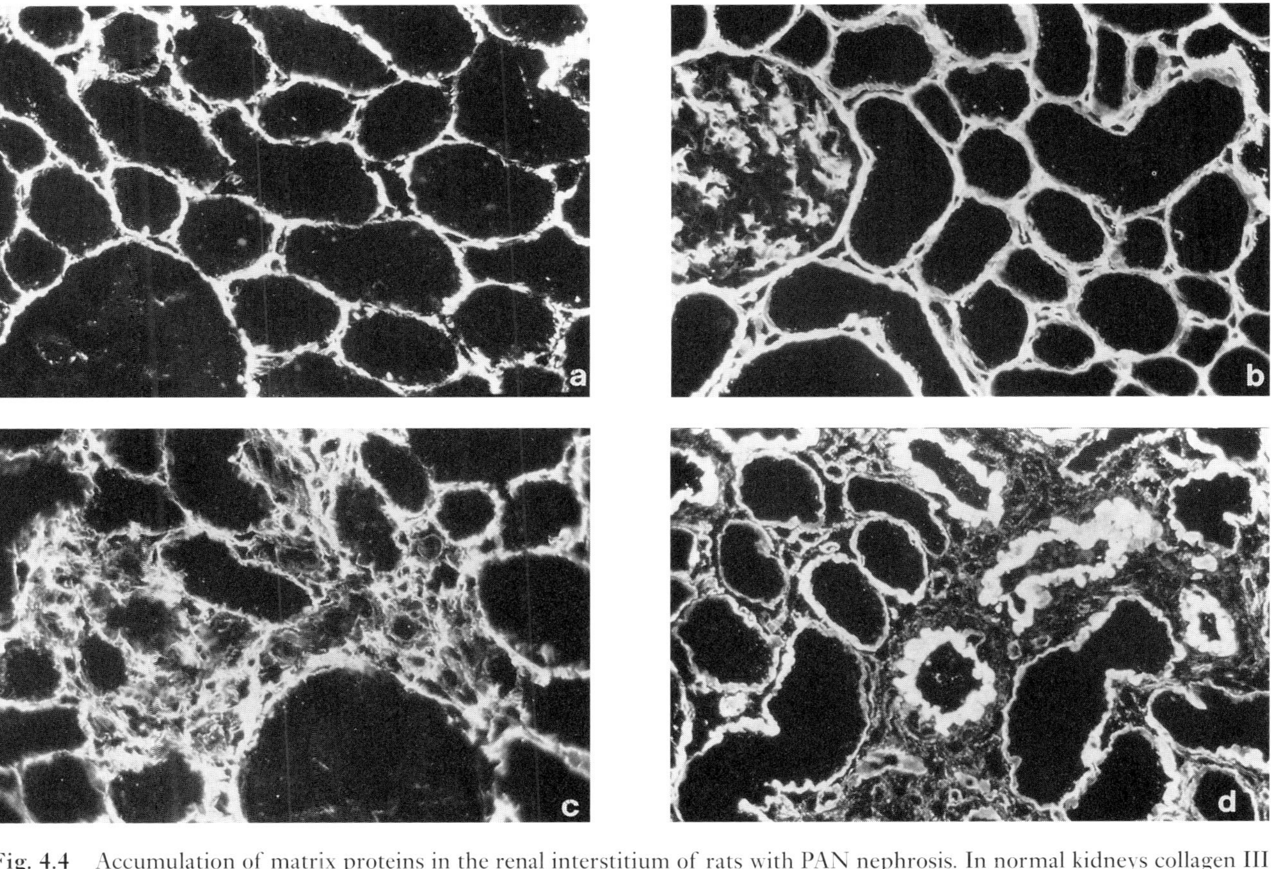

Fig. 4.4 Accumulation of matrix proteins in the renal interstitium of rats with PAN nephrosis. In normal kidneys collagen III is found in small quantities through the interstitium (a) and collagen IV is limited to tubular and glomerular basement membranes (b). After 13 weeks of proteinuria, rats develop severe interstitial fibrosis. Interstitial deposits of collagen III are greatly increased (c). Collagen IV not only accumulates along the thickened tubular basement membranes but it appears *de novo* in the interstitium (d).

The various matrix proteins that are secreted into the interstitium become assembled into a complex three-dimensional scaffold. Although the enzymes that are involved in the reorganization of interstitial matrix proteins into the 'scar' are unknown, cross-linking of polypeptide chains is clearly important. Not only does this reorganization provide greater structural stability, but as a consequence the matrix becomes more resistant to degradation by proteases. Two enzymes that mediate cross-linking of polypeptide chains have been studied in the kidney. In association with an increase in the kidney content of collagen cross-links, lysyl oxidase expression was found to be increased in rats with adriamycin-induced interstitial fibrosis [27]. Renal transglutaminase activity increases in association with rising renal levels of ε-(γ-glutamyl) lysine cross-links during interstitial fibrosis in the rat remnant kidney model [28]. Prior to these important post-translational changes in the interstitial matrix, interstitial fibrosis may even be reversible as reported in rats with focal interstitial fibrosis due to acute and reversible PAN-induced nephrosis [29].

Cells involved in interstitial fibrosis

Tubular epithelial cells

Tubuloepithelial cells line the tubules of the kidney and normally produce the matrix proteins that comprise the basement membrane. The relative contribution of tubular cells to the pool of matrix proteins that accumulate in the renal interstitium during renal fibrosis is unknown. Tubuloepithelial cells have been shown to overproduce collagen IV in experimental models of diabetes [30] and there is evidence that tubular epithelial cells behave differently after exposure to fibrogenic cytokines. For example, Creely *et al.* [31] demonstrated an eightfold increase in collagen I production after rat epithelial cells were exposed to TGF-β1 while collagen IV production remained unchanged. TGF-β1 stimulates increased fibronectin and proteoglycan synthesis by rabbit proximal tubular cells [32]. Nadasdy *et al.* [33] identified cells within the interstitium of end-stage human kidneys that expressed epithelial markers specific for the distal nephron suggesting that migration of tubuloepithelial cells may also occur.

In more recent reports, Strutz *et al.* [34] have introduced evidence that tubular epithelial cells may transdifferentiate, a process of phenotypic change into mesenchymal cells, specifically fibroblasts. This hypothesis followed the cloning and characterization of a fibroblast-specific protein (FSP1) in mice [35]. In normal renal interstitium, a small population of interstitial cells express this marker. In models of chronic renal inflammation and fibrosis, interstitial staining for FSP1 dramatically increases. *In vitro* as well as *in vivo* studies have demonstrated that selected tubular epithelial cells start expressing FSP1 *de novo* suggesting the onset of transdifferentiation. The stimuli for tubular cell transdifferentiation remain unclear but alterations in the ECM milieu and exposure to growth factors such as TGF-β1 are considered candidates. Further work with FSP1 as well as the identification of additional markers specific for fibroblasts are needed to understand the extent of tubular epithelial cell transdifferentiation and its contribution to renal fibrosis.

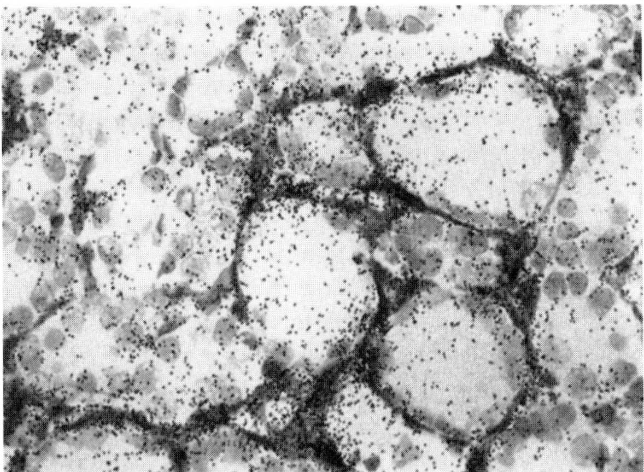

Fig. 4.5 Interstitial myofibroblasts produce increased quantities of collagen III in rats with PAN nephrosis. *In situ* hybridization with a ^{33}P anti-sense procollagen α1(III) riboprobe shows a large number of transcripts (black grains) associated with cells that express α-SMA (black-stained cells). (From Tang WW, Van GY, Qi M. Myofibroblast and α_1(III) collagen expression in experimental tubulo-interstitial nephritis. *Kidney Int* 1997; **51**: 926–931. Copyright permission of Blackwell Science Inc.)

Fibroblasts

To determine the cellular origin of the matrix proteins that accumulate in the interstitium of diseased kidneys, most studies have concentrated on the identification of the cells that produce 'normal' interstitial proteins such as collagens I and III and fibronectin. In rat models of puromycin aminonucleoside (PAN) or adriamycin-induced renal fibrosis, increased renal mRNA levels and rates of matrix synthesis support the view that increased production of these proteins contribute to the fibrogenic process [29,36,37]. In a rabbit model of anti-GBM nephritis, renal collagen I mRNA levels on day 7 predicted the severity of interstitial fibrosis at day 30 [38]. *In situ* hybridization studies to identify the matrix-producing cells have highlighted interstitial cells [29,39,40]; cells of the fibroblast lineage appear most important (Fig. 4.5). Owing to the lack of specific cellular markers it has not yet been possible to determine the origin and specific role of fibroblasts during the active phase of interstitial fibrosis.

The number of 'classical' interstitial fibroblasts increases during renal fibrosis but the extent of the increase appears to be relatively modest. In a rat model of PAN nephrosis [36], interstitial fibroblasts were counted after immunostaining with ST3, a monoclonal antibody raised against rat bone-marrow fibroblasts which reacts with a subset of interstitial fibroblasts. A gradual increase in ST3 positive fibroblasts was observed over a 13-week period, reaching a maximum fourfold increase. Recent work with FSP1 also documents a relatively small increase in FSP-1-positive interstitial fibroblasts [35]. It remains unclear whether fibroblast proliferation *per se* is an essential component of the fibrogenic process.

In contrast, behavioral and phenotypic changes in the renal fibroblast cell population appear to be critical components in the cascade of events that leads to interstitial fibrosis. Experimental evidence comes from both *in vitro* and *in vivo* observations. Renal fibroblasts have functional differences depending on their external milieu. For example, cultured fibroblasts spontaneously synthesize different collagens depending on their site of origin (e.g. dermal versus kidney fibroblasts; kidney fibroblasts from normal versus fibrotic kidneys) [41]. Studies by Rodemann [42] and Müller [43] have shown that fibroblasts derived from fibrotic human kidneys synthesize more total collagen than those from normal kidneys. In addition, the site of origin also determines the response of cultured fibroblasts to mitogens. For example, Lonnemann *et al.* [44] found that fibroblasts derived from a fibrotic environment proliferated in response to interleukin (IL)-1β while proliferation of fibroblasts from normal kidneys was inhibited by IL-1β.

In addition to these 'behavioral' changes, resident fibroblasts have a unique phenotypic plasticity that appears to be important in renal fibrosis. In particular, the appearance of a large number of interstitial myofibroblasts characterizes most progressive renal diseases [45–51]. These myofibroblasts are identified as interstitial cells that express the myocyte protein alpha smooth muscle actin (α-SMA). In the normal kidney α-SMA-positive cells are restricted to arterioles and rare interstitial cells. The origin of these myofibroblasts that appear in the interstitium is not completely clear. It may be that resident fibroblasts are able to assume a myofibroblastic phenotype, possibly representing a state of activation. TGF-β1 [52] and platelet-derived growth factor B (PDGF-B) [53] can stimulate transformation of fibroblasts to myofibroblasts. The second possibility is that these myofibroblasts have their origin in the perivascular regions of the kidney and that they migrate into the interstitium during the fibrogenic process. In a model of anti-GBM nephritis, Wiggins and associates [54] showed that the earliest increase in mRNA transcripts for procollagen α1(I) occurred in the perivascular cells. Studies by Ronnov-Jessen *et al.* [55] in a human breast cancer model suggest that myofibroblasts come from venules and that the migration of these cells from the perivascular areas into the interstitium compromises vascular support and leads to capillary obliteration (a common finding in progressive renal interstitial fibrosis as well). Whether transdifferentiated tubular cells are a potential source of myofibroblasts remains to be proven. The importance of the interstitial myofibroblast population is highlighted by *in situ* hybridization studies that indicate these cells as the main site of interstitial collagen synthesis during interstitial fibrosis (Fig. 4.5). Early studies in human renal biopsies obtained from patients with crescentic nephritis [45], IgA nephropathy [46], and membranous nephropathy [56] suggest that the presence of interstitial myofibroblasts is predictive of progressive renal disease.

Monocytes/macrophages

Interstitial macrophages are potential players in renal fibrosis. Macrophages may be an important source of fibrosis-promoting growth factors, vasoactive molecules, and even matrix proteins [57]. In kidneys with progressive renal disease an interstitial infiltrate of macrophages is routinely present and experimental manipulations to prevent the influx of monocytes into the interstitium have been shown to attenuate interstitial fibrosis [58–63]. Circulating monocytes migrate into the interstitium of kidneys when inflammation is present. The chemotactic factors and adhesion molecules that are involved in interstitial monocyte recruitment remain to be determined. Several candidates have been identified but it has been very difficult to design a method to block a single monocyte chemoattractant or adhesion molecule and prevent the interstitial influx of monocytes, likely due to the great genetic redundancy in potential mechanisms of monocyte recruitment to sites of inflammation. Monocyte chemoattractant protein-1 (MCP-1) and activated complement components may be exceptions, although current data are conflicting. Increased tubular production of MCP-1 has been reported in several animal and human models of progressive renal disease [64–66]. MCP-1 is a small 14–23 kDa protein that can be detected in the urine [67,68]. Urinary MCP-1 levels have been reported to correlate with the severity of interstitial fibrosis in patients with IgA nephropathy [69]. In a recent study [70] administration of an MCP-1 neutralizing antibody was reported to reduce significantly the number of interstitial macrophages on day 6 in rats with PAN nephrosis; however, treatment with the same antibody failed to attenuate interstitial inflammation in another study that examined the kidneys on day 7 [71].

Proximal tubular cells may play an important role in the complement pathway. Tubular cells can be stimulated to synthesize complement components C_3 and C_4 [72,73] and they may activate complement proteins via the alternative pathway [74]. The appearance of complement proteins along tubular brush border membranes may be observed in proteinuric renal diseases associated with interstitial inflammation. In the past it was thought that these complement deposits represented proteins that had been filtered from the plasma and that they did not play a part in monocyte recruitment occurring beyond the basolateral membrane. However, two recent studies using complement depletion with cobra venom factor or complement inhibition with the soluble complement receptor type I provide evidence that the complement cascade does participate in interstitial monocyte recruitment in rats with PAN nephrosis [75] and mesangial proliferative glomerulonephritis [76].

To date most of the studies that have been designed to determine mechanisms of interstitial monocyte recruitment have been based on experimental models of primary glomerular disease. Figure 4.6 summarizes the pathways that have been implicated. It is also important to consider that the number of interstitial monocytes may increase by *in situ* proliferation as illustrated in rats with anti-GBM nephritis [77].

Fibrogenic signals

Several cytokines, growth factors and vasoactive molecules are known to promote fibrosis *in vitro* (Table 4.3) [78–80]. The relative contribution of each of these molecules to interstitial fibrosis is currently unclear. To date, most of the investigations have focused on three of these: TGF-β1, angiotensin II (ANG II) and endothelin-1 (ET-1).

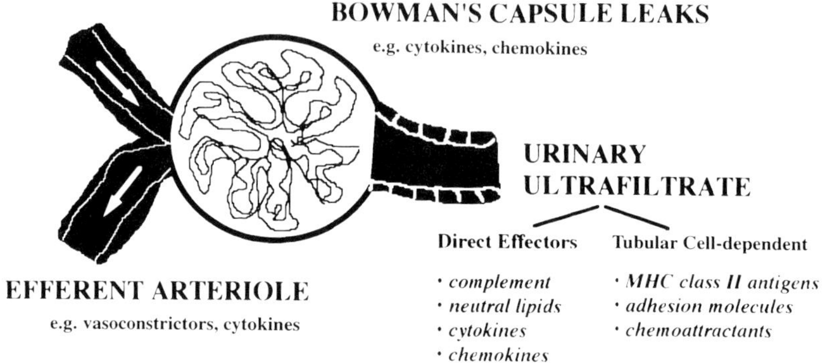

Fig. 4.6 Potential pathways of mediation of interstitial monocyte recruitment in primary glomerular diseases.

Table 4.3 Fibrogenic molecules

Cytokines	Interleukin-1α, interleukin-1β, tumor necrosis factor α
Growth factors:	Connective tissue growth factor, basic fibroblast growth factor, platelet-derived growth factor, transforming growth factor-α, transforming growth factor-β
Vasoactive molecules	Angiotensin II
	Endothelin-1

Transforming growth factor-β1

TGF-β1 is currently considered to be the premier fibrogenic cytokine and it is the most extensively studied growth factor with respect to renal interstitial fibrosis. Active TGF-β1 elicits a variety of responses that may play a part in fibrosis. Its actions include stimulated synthesis of matrix proteins as well as decreased matrix degradation [81–83]. The net effect of TGF-β1 is to mediate the accumulation of matrix proteins and ultimately to cause 'scar' formation if the activity of TGF-β1 is left unchecked. TGF-β1 activity is regulated at several steps that are summarized in Fig. 4.7: synthesis; activation; receptor binding; sequestration in ECM and elimination from the circulation.

TGF-β1 is a homodimeric peptide with three distinct isoforms in mammals. It is released as a latent, biologically inactive, peptide containing the N-terminal sequence latency associated peptide (LAP). Activation must occur prior to receptor binding. This occurs by cleavage of the active TGF-β1 peptide from LAP [25,84]. Activation *in vitro* can be accomplished by acidic pH, thrombospondin, insulin-like growth factor-II/mannose-6-phosphate receptor, transglutaminase, and proteolytic cleavage

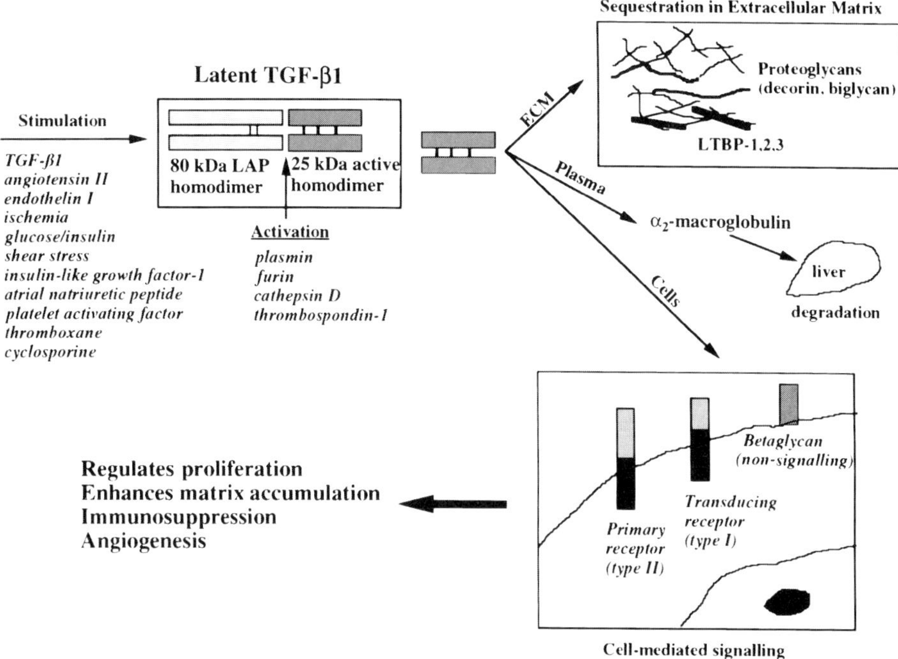

Fig. 4.7 Pathways involved in regulating the synthesis and bioactivity of TGF-β1. Abbreviations: LAP, latency-associated peptide; ECM, extracellular matrix; LTBP, latent TGF-β binding protein.

by plasmin, cathepsin D, furin, and glycosidases [25,26,84,85]. How TGF-β1 is activated *in vivo* remains unclear. This activation step may prove to be a major step in the regulation of TGF-β1 effects.

There are many other steps within the TGF-β1 pathway where TGF-β1 bioactivity can be increased or decreased. TGF-β1 secreted into the plasma is found almost exclusively bound to α_2 macroglobulin (a fact that makes plasma measurements of TGF-β1 difficult) [26]. In addition, TGF-β1 belongs to a group of molecules referred to as 'crinopectins' [86]. This term refers to molecules that are secreted by cells but maintained in a latent form after secretion through binding to pericellular structures. In the case of TGF-β1 these structures include small proteoglycans such as decorin [26,83,87,88], betaglycan [26,89], biglycan [87,83], fibromodulin [87], endoglin [90], and fucoidan [26,91]. These molecules may play a part in keeping active TGF-β1 where it is needed [26]. There is little information on the accumulation of TGF-β1-binding glycoproteins during interstitial fibrosis. Decorin increases in the interstitium of rats with obstructive uropathy [18]. Endoglin (which also forms part of the TGF-β1 receptor complex) has been reported to be increased in the interstitium of human kidneys in association with areas of chronic damage [92].

TGF-β1 receptors are ubiquitously expressed [93]. Little is known about changes in their expression in renal disease. Tamaki *et al.* [37] reported progressive increases in renal mRNA levels for receptors II and III in the model of adriamycin nephrosis. TGF-β1 type II receptors are upregulated in the renal cortex of diabetic rats [94]. The soluble form of the TGF-β1 type II receptor is a potent inhibitor of TGF-β1 [95]. This observation may be used to advantage experimentally but whether soluble forms of the receptor are formed *in vivo* is unknown. Another protein complex, latent TGF-β1-binding protein (LTBP), may also alter the bioavailability of TGF-β1. LTBP has features in common with the ECM and therefore may play a part in targeting TGF-β1 to the interstitium [26]. Three LTBP are now known to exist. Although not detected in normal rat kidneys [96], LTBP is found in the interstitium of rats with adriamycin nephrosis [97]. Finally, the LAP cleaved during TGF-β1 activation, has the ability to non-covalently re-associate with mature TGF-β1, an interaction that results in TGF-β1 inactivation [25,93]. Administration of recombinant LAP has been an effective way to block TGF-β1 in TGF-β1 overexpressing mice [98].

Increased production of TGF-β1 has been reported in essentially every animal and human model of progressive renal disease investigated to date (Table 4.4). TGF-β1 transgenic mice with high plasma levels of active TGF-β1 develop chronic tubulo-interstitial disease after the onset of glomerulosclerosis [99,100]. More recently a transgenic mouse has been generated in which the TGF-β1 transgene is under the control of the phosphoenolpyruvate carboxykinase promotor [101]. In these mice overexpression of TGF-β1 by tubular cells is associated with interstitial fibrosis (Fig. 4.8). In the context of renal allograft fibrosis, it is noteworthy that cyclosporine A can stimulate TGF-β1 transcription [102].

During the course of interstitial fibrosis TGF-β1 may be synthesized by several cell types [21,63,103]. Tubular epithelial cells appear to be an important source in some renal diseases [104,105]. In rats with acute PAN nephrosis [63] TGF-β1 mRNA levels in proximal tubular cells were increased to twice the control levels. By *in situ* hybridization, tubular cells were found to be an important site of TGF-β1 transcription in rats with interstitial fibrosis due to overload proteinuria [106]. Several studies have reported increased tubular immunostaining for TGF-β1 in kidneys with chronic interstitial damage. Fibroblasts [21] and myofibroblasts [103] are also an important source of TGF-β1. In a rat model of five-sixths nephrectomy, α-SMA-positive myofibroblasts were shown to express TGF-β1 protein [107]. In the chronic model of Thy-1 nephritis [103], interstitial myofibroblasts were identified as the primary source of TGF-β1 production. Finally, interstitial macrophages may also be an important source of TGF-β1. In studies of rats with PAN nephrosis, a reduction in the number of interstitial macrophages induced by dietary protein restriction prevented the increase in renal TGF-β1 mRNA levels and the rise in total kidney collagen [63].

Little is known about the *in vivo* stimulation of TGF-β1 synthesis although several agonists are proposed (Fig. 4.7). It is also important to remember that TGF-β1 is auto-induced, that is, TGF-β1 stimulates cells at the site of tissue injury to increase its own production [108]. This auto-induction has the potential to establish a vicious cycle of TGF-β1-dependent responses.

Table 4.4 Increased transforming growth factor (TGF)-β expression in renal interstitial fibrosis

Renal disease	References
Human studies	
Diabetic nephropathy	[236]
Glomerulonephritis, chronic	[237]
HIV nephropathy	[238,239]
IgA nephropathy	[240]
Renal allograft rejection, chronic	[241,242,243]
Animal studies	
Acute tubular necrosis	[105,244]
Adriamycin nephropathy	[37,97]
Anti-glomerular basement membrane nephritis	[245]
Anti-Thy-1 nephritis, chronic	[103]
Cyclosporine nephrotoxicity	[21,246]
Diabetic nephropathy	[94,236]
Diet-induced hypercholesterolemia	[210]
FK506 nephrotoxicity	[247]
Heymann nephritis	[248]
HIV nephropathy	[249]
Immune complex nephritis	[121]
Murine lupus nephritis	[250]
Obese Zucker rats	[251]
Obstructive uropathy	[65,104,136]
Polycystic kidney disease	[252]
Protein-overload proteinuria	[106]
Puromycin aminonucleoside nephrosis	[29,36,63]
Remnant kidney	[139,253]
TGF-β1-overproducing mice	[99,100,101]

Modified from Eddy AA: Molecular insights into renal interstitial fibrosis. *J Am Soc Nephrol* 1996; 7: 2495–2508. Copyright permission from Williams and Wilkins.

Despite the tight association between TGF-β1 production and interstitial fibrosis, definitive proof that TGF-β1 causes interstitial fibrosis is still lacking. This is because there are currently no effective strategies to inhibit TGF-β1 chronically. In a model of acute transient injury to the glomerulus induced in rats with anti-Thy-1 antiserum, Border and colleagues have inhibited TGF-β1 with neutralizing antiserum [109] or the neutralizing proteoglycan decorin [110,111]. Although the degree of glomerulosclerosis was reduced in the first week of renal injury, prolonged inhibition of TGF-β1 to study progressive interstitial fibrosis remains to be done. Short-term neutralization of TGF-β1 has also been shown to attenuate matrix gene expression in experimental diabetes [112]. Major problems arise with prolonged systemic depletion of TGF-β1 [113,114]. For example, TGF-β1 knockout mice die within weeks of weaning due cardiopulmonary inflammation, highlighting the

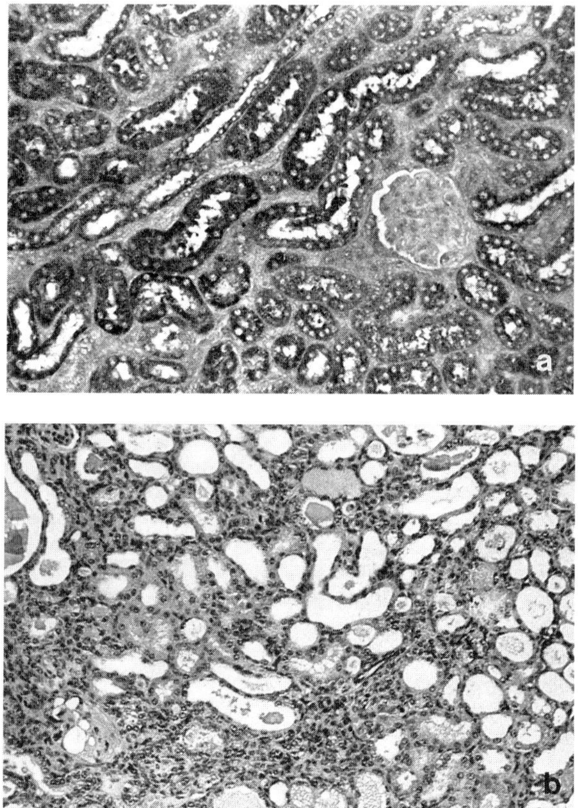

Fig. 4.8 Interstitial fibrosis in TGF-β overexpressing mice. Using regulatory sequences of the rat phosphoenolpyruvate carboxykinase gene to induce the production of active human TGF-β1 in the renal tubules of transgenic mice, significant renal interstitial fibrosis developed. Increased staining for PAI-1 indicates the presence of biologically active TGF-β1 in the tubules of the transgenic mice (a). Staining with Masson's trichrome identifies areas of interstitial inflammation and fibrosis surrounding proximal tubules (b). (From Clouthier DE, Comerford SA, Hammer RE. Hepatic fibrosis, glomerulosclerosis, and a lipodystrophy-like syndrome in PEPCK-TGF-β1 transgenic mice. *J Clin Invest* 1997; **100**: 2697–2713. Copyright permission of the American Society of Clinical Investigation).

important role of TGF-β1 in regulating immune responses. The challenge ahead of us is to develop strategies to target TGF-β1 inhibitors to the kidney to avoid these important systemic effects.

Angiotensin II

Emerging as an important *in vivo* stimulus for TGF-β1 production is ANG II. Wolfe and associates [115] first reported that ANG II stimulates TGF-β1 production by renal tubular cells. Angiotensin has been noted to upregulate TGF-β1 in fibroblasts as well [116]. ANG II inhibitors and ANG II type I receptor antagonists have been shown to decrease renal TGF-β1 levels and attenuate renal fibrosis in several animal models [117–124]. It is important to note that, although ANG may upregulate TGF-β1 expression, its presence is not essential. In mice with a homozygous null mutation in the angiotensinogen gene, histologic evidence of mild interstitial fibrosis is present within 3 weeks of postnatal age [125]. Renal disease in these mice is accompanied by an increase in expression of TGF-β1. Concurrent upregulation of PDGF observed in these mice might be responsible for the increase in TGF-β1.

In addition to its function as a TGF-β1 agonist, ANG II may have other fibrosis-promoting effects. ANG II has long been known as an important part of the autocrine system that regulates blood pressure, maintains intravascular volume and regulates renal perfusion. There is now evidence that proximal tubular cells not only express mRNA for renin, angiotensinogen, and angiotensin-converting enzyme (ACE) but that they also posses all the necessary substrates and enzymes to generate, bind, and inactivate ANG II [126,127]. This has led to the investigation of ANG II as part of a local paracrine system and a growth factor within the kidney. There is evidence that the hypertrophic response of glomeruli may be pathogenetically linked to glomerulosclerosis. Although this hypothesis has been controversial, if proven true, there is reason to speculate that the cellular events that contribute to tubular cell hypertrophy may also contribute to the development of progressive renal disease [128]. The relationship between tubular hypertrophy and progressive tubulo-interstitial disease has not yet been systematically evaluated.

Our knowledge of ANG II as a growth factor comes largely from studies in vascular smooth muscle cells, although there is growing evidence that it is a hypertrophogenic cytokine for renal tubular cells as well [127,129]. ANG II has the ability to promote hyperplasia or hypertrophy of smooth muscle cells and mesangial cells *in vitro*. TGF-β1 appears to mediate these responses, at least in part [130,131]. In contrast, the effect of ANG II on proximal tubule cells appears to be limited to hypertrophy [132]. This occurs in a dose-dependent manner and is accompanied by increases in *de novo* protein synthesis, total protein content, and cellular enlargement. ANG II stimulates proximal tubular cells to increase transcription and synthesis of collagen IV but not collagen I. As collagen IV is an integral basement membrane protein this may simply be an appropriate response to cell enlargement [127]. After *in vitro* exposure to ANG II renal interstitial fibroblasts also undergo hyperplasia in a time- and dose-dependent manner [116]. This response is associated with increases in mRNA levels for fibronectin and collagen I and increased production of soluble fibronectin.

There are two ANG II receptors, AT1 and AT2. AT1 appears to mediate the classic actions of ANG II and is more abundant in human tissue [130]. In the kidney, immunohistochemical localization of rat AT1 revealed its presence in the proximal tubule, mesangial cells, and small arteries and arterioles [133]. The receptors are expressed on both the apical and basolateral membranes of the proximal tubule [127]. Hypertrophy of cultured proximal tubule cells induced by ANG II is mediated by the AT1 receptor [134]; blockade of this receptor eliminates the hypertrophic response. AT2 may counterbalance AT1 and have antifibrogenic actions [130].

The most compelling evidence that ANG II plays a part in interstitial fibrosis comes from studies of ANG II inhibition and antagonism. For many years the beneficial effects of ACE inhibition were thought to be mediated by its effects on glomerular hemodynamics. In a study of five-sixths nephrectomized rats given ANG II receptor antagonists, ACE inhibitors or other classes of antihypertensives, only rats in the angiotensin blockade groups had significantly reduced transcapillary pressure, proteinuria, and glomerulosclerosis [135]. However, in recent years it has become evident that ANG II inhibition has additional beneficial effects due to its' ability to block the proliferative and fibrogenic effects of ANG II. Results from studies in rats with obstructive nephropathy are particularly convincing. In this model both ACE inhibitors and ANG II receptor antagonists have been shown to decrease interstitial fibrosis as compared with untreated animals or animals treated with other classes of antihypertensive drugs [117,119,136,137]. Additional findings in the angiotensin blockade groups have included significantly decreased TGF-β1 levels, decreased collagen IV mRNA levels, and preservation of the renal interstitial architecture. Even delaying treatment with enalapril for several days after the onset of ureteral obstruction slows the progression of interstitial fibrosis in rats with obstructive nephropathy [136]. In uninephrectomized spontaneously hypertensive rats, ACE inhibitors and AT1 receptor antagonists were also shown to attenuate the accumulation of matrix proteins, even when treatment was delayed for 16 weeks [138].

ACE inhibition has been shown to decrease fibrosis and TGF-β1 levels in several other animal models including chronic aminonucleoside nephrosis [122], rat remnant kidney [123,139], aging mice [124], deoxycorticosterone acetate (DOCA)-salt hypertension [140], spontaneously hypertensive rats [141], cyclosporine nephropathy [142], and chronic immune complex nephritis [121]. Together these studies support an important part for ANG II in the progression of renal fibrosis and upregulated renal expression of TGF-β1 as an integral part of this process.

Endothelin-1

ET-1, a potent vasoconstrictor, is gaining support as a contributor to renal fibrosis. First identified in 1988 by Yanagisawa [143], there are actually three endothelin isoforms. ET-1 is the primary endothelin found in the kidney. Small amounts of ET-3 are also found [144]. In the kidney, endothelin is produced by proximal and distal tubules, cortical and medullary collecting ducts [145], endothelial cells [143], fibroblasts [146,147], and macrophages [148]. Increased expression of ET-1 has been reported in the rat remnant kidney model where it was mainly produced by tubular cells [149]. Macrophages also secrete abundant ET-1 in response to inflammation [148]. Neutrophils do not secrete ET-1, but can convert latent prepro ET-1 to the biologically active peptide [130]. Prepro ET-1 mRNA levels in cultured endothelial and mesangial cells increase following exposure to several agents including TGF-β1 [150], PDGF [130], thrombin [150], shear stress [151], tumor necrosis factor (TNF)-α [152], thromboxane A_2 [150], and cyclosporine [153]. Proximal tubular cells exposed to increased concentrations of proteins such as albumin, immunoglobulin G, or transferrin may respond with an increase in ET-1 production [154]. The release of ET-1 was primarily basolateral in these latter studies suggesting a possible link between proteinuria and interstitial injury that is ET-1 mediated. ANG II also stimulates prepro-ET-1 expression in cultured endothelial cells [155]. There are two known receptors for ET-1. Growth effects of ET-1 appear to be mediated by ET_A receptor while the ET_B receptor mediates vasoconstriction [130]. The expression of ET-1 can also be auto-induced via the ET_B receptor [156].

ET-1 has several effects that may contribute to interstitial fibrosis. As a potent vasoconstrictor, ET-1 may induce interstitial ischemia and subsequent fibrogenic responses. *In vitro* studies by Orphanides and Norman [157] have shown that tubular cells exposed to an hypoxic environment respond with an increase in matrix protein synthesis and a decrease in net metalloproteinase (MMP) activity (Fig. 4.9). Hypoxia also induces intercellular adhesion molecule-1 expression by renal tubular cells [158]. In addition, ET-1 may have fibrosis-promoting effects by directly stimulating the synthesis of matrix proteins [159,160], stimulating tubular cell proliferation [161], and decreasing collagenase activity [160], or indirectly by upregulating TGF-β1 expression [130]. The relative importance of these direct and indirect effects in ET-1-mediated fibrosis remains to be determined.

Two lines of experimental evidence support the hypothesis that ET-1 may be an important mediator of renal fibrosis *in vivo*. First, ET-1 antagonists and/or ET-1 receptor blockers preserve renal function and decrease histologic injury in experimental models of chronic cyclosporine nephrotoxicity [162], murine lupus nephritis [163] and five-sixths nephrectomy [164]. Second, is the observation that transgenic mice that overexpress the human ET-1 gene develop tubular cysts, interstitial fibrosis, and a progressive decline in renal function, all in the absence of systemic hypertension [165] (Fig. 4.10).

Other fibrogenic mediators

Very little is currently known about the role of other cytokines with fibrogenic potential in the pathogenesis of renal interstitial fibrosis. These include bFGF, IL-1, TNF-α, TGF-α, and PDGF (Table 4.3). PDGF likely participates in interstitial fibrosis due to its ability to transform fibroblasts to myofibroblasts and through an indirect mechanism mediated by its mitogenic action on renal cells. Treatment of rats with recombinant PDGF-BB leads to tubulo-interstitial cell proliferation, appearance of myofibroblasts and macrophages in the interstitium and ultimately interstitial fibrosis [53]. This effect of PDGF was probably not mediated via TGF-β1 as TGF-β1 mRNA levels were not increased in the treated rats. In a rat model of five-sixths nephrectomy and progressive interstitial fibrosis [47], increased expression of PDGF B-chain and the PDGF receptor B subunit in tubules and interstitial cells has been reported. In regions of tubulo-interstitial injury induced by ANG II infusion, PDGF B-chain expression is increased [48]. Increased interstitial expression of the β receptor for PDGF has been observed in diseased human kidneys [166,167]. Unfortunately, it has not been possible to determine the role of PDGF

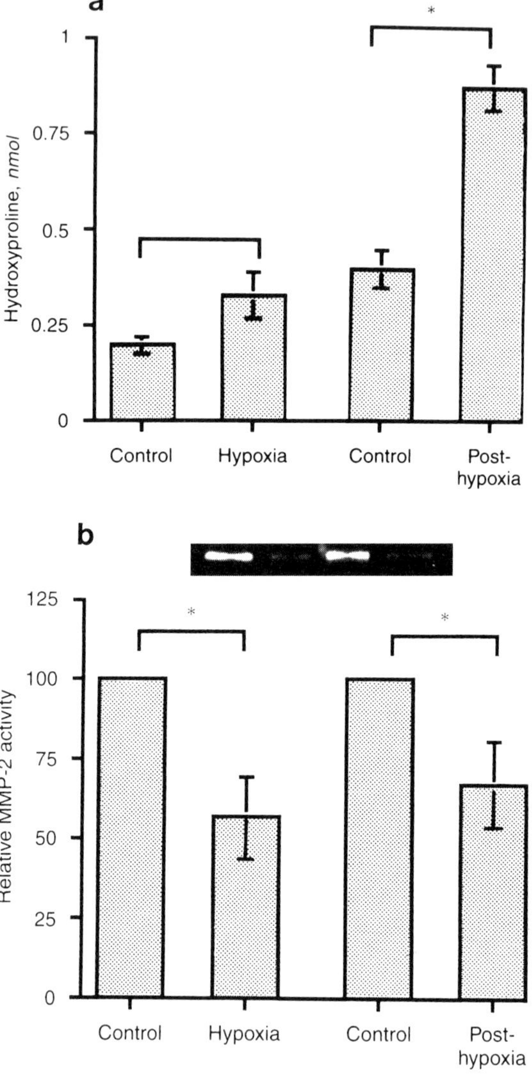

Fig. 4.9 Hypoxia induces a fibrogenic response in renal tubules. Human proximal tubular cells cultured in 1% oxygen respond with a significant increase in the quantity of collagen (measured as hydroxyproline) synthesized in the immediate post-hypoxic period (a). During both the 24h period of hypoxia and the 24h after hypoxia, the 72kDa gelatinase (MMP-2) activity detected by substrate gel zymography of culture supernatants was significantly less than the MMP-2 activity of tubular cells cultured in 21% oxygen (b). (From Orphanides C, Fine LG, Norman JT: Hypoxia stimulates proximal tubular cell matrix production via a TGF-β1-independent mechanism. *Kidney Int* 1997; **52**: 637–647. Copyright permission of Blackwell Science Inc.).

by investigating renal disease models in mice that are genetically deficient in this growth factor. The PDGF-B null phenotype is embryonically lethal [168]. The mice have an absence of mesangial cells and glomerular capillary tufts. The PDGF-A knockout animals either die *in utero* or within a few weeks of birth due to pulmonary emphysema associated with a deficiency of alveolar myofibroblasts [169].

IL-1 is a cytokine that is increased in several models of experimental and human glomerulonephritis. IL-1 is a pro-inflammatory protein that stimulates fibroblast proliferation and possibly matrix production [78,79,170]. IL-1 positive interstitial cells are seen in patients with primary glomerular disease and declining renal function. In IgA nephropathy [171] the number of IL-1-positive cells has been shown to correlate with the extent of interstitial damage. This same study in IgA nephropathy patients also found a significant positive correlation between a more complete cytokine profile (IL-1, IL-6, IL-8, TNF-α) and the extent of tubulo-interstitial damage. Administration of a soluble recombinant IL-1 receptor antagonist to rats with crescentic glomerulonephritis prevented tubular atrophy and interstitial fibrosis [172,173]. Although encouraging, this finding may be an indirect consequence of a decrease in the acute renal injury and the inflammatory response mediated by IL-1.

There is some evidence to suggest that bFGF plays a part in the pathogenesis of renal interstitial fibrosis. Production of bFGF by interstitial cells has been observed in biopsy specimens from patients with chronic renal disease [174]. After a nephrotoxic insult, increased bFGF expression has been reported in interstitial and tubular cells [175]. In a model of HIV-associated nephropathy [176], bFGF and its receptor co-localize to areas of interstitial matrix accumulation. Finally, in a recent report by Phillips *et al.* [177], bFGF was shown to stimulate the release of preformed latent TGF-β1 from renal proximal tubular cells. It did not stimulate TGF-β1 gene transcription or translation. In what appears to be a positive feedback loop, TGF-β1 then induces the proximal tubular cells to increase bFGF mRNA followed by a time-dependent increase in bFGF production. These investigators propose that this feedback loop may play a part in the progressive nature of renal fibrosis *in vivo*. Hepatocyte growth factor (HGF) is a mitogen for tubular cells. Increased tubular production of HGF has been reported in human kidney biopsies in areas of tubular damage [178].

Nitric oxide (NO) is a gaseous free radical with numerous biologic effects. There is some evidence that nitric oxide may attenuate renal interstitial fibrosis as shown by the beneficial effect of L-arginine (an NO precursor) in rats with obstructive nephropathy [179]. This beneficial effect may be an indirect one as a consequence of the decreased influx of monocytes into the interstitium. NO is known to inhibit leukocyte adhesion to endothelial cells. However, NO may also decrease matrix protein synthesis more directly via a mechanism that appears to be TGF-β1 independent.

Alterations in matrix turnover

In addition to the abundance of data confirming that renal fibrosis results from increased ECM production, there is also an expanding body of evidence that ECM

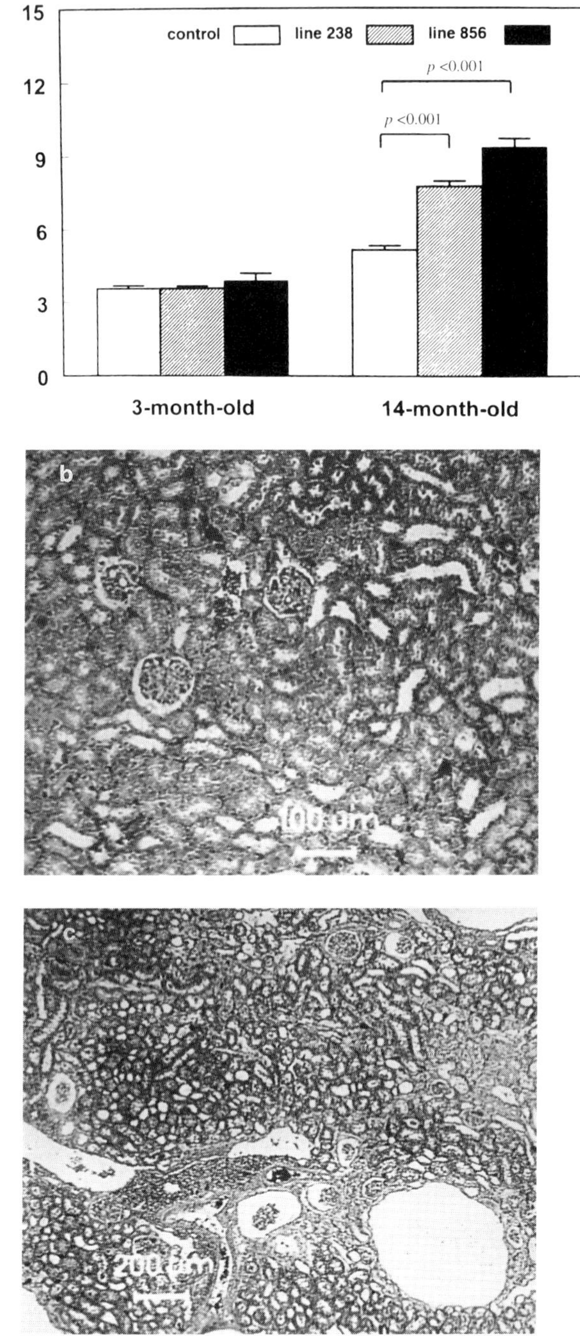
a
Interstitial fibrosis in ET-1 tg Mice
Fibrotic area (% of total area)
15
12
9
6
3
0
control
line 238
line 856
p <0.001
p <0.001
3-month-old
14-month-old
b
100 µm
c
200 µm

degradation is also impaired during the active phase of renal interstitial fibrosis. The importance of alterations in the degradation pathway were first appreciated by González-Avila and co-workers [180]. In experimental models of interstitial fibrosis induced by ligation of a renal vein or ureter, these investigators failed to document an increase in the rate of collagen synthesis. In contrast, impressive reductions in renal collagenolytic activity were seen. Evidence of active intrarenal matrix degradation pathways also comes from studies that suggest that the early stages of 'scar' formation may be reversible. For example, in studies of rats with PAN nephrosis [29], the early foci of interstitial fibrosis seen at 3 weeks disappear again by 6 weeks. Transient accumulation of fibronectin has also been reported in rats with acute tubular necrosis [181].

There are four families of connective tissue proteases (Table 4.5). Of these, the MMP and the serine proteases of the plasmin cascade have been the most extensively studied with respect to their part in renal fibrosis. The remaining two classes, the aspartic and cysteine proteinases, consist primarily of lysosomal cathepsins.

The MMP are a large family of zinc- and calcium-dependent enzymes [182] (Fig. 4.11). They are secreted as zymogens and then activated by proteolytic cleavage. Based on their substrate specificity, the extracellular MMP are subclassified into three groups—the interstitial collagenases, gelatinases, and stromelysins. Collectively, they can degrade all major components of the ECM [183,184]. *In vitro* studies have shown that tubular cells as well as fibroblasts and macrophages are a source of MMP [185]. The specific enzymes expressed depend in part on the matrix composition of the substrate upon which they are cultured. Available data suggest that

Table 4.5 Major classes of matrix protein protease

Class	Enzymes	pH activity range
Aspartic proteinases	Cathepsin D	3–5
Cysteine proteinases	Cathepsins B, L, H	3–8
Serine proteinases	Plasmin, thrombin, tPA, uPA, elastase, cathepsin G, granzymes	6–9
Metalloproteinases	Stromelysin, collagenase, gelatinase	6–9

Fig. 4.10 Interstitial fibrosis develops in transgenic mice that overexpress human endothelin-1 (ET-1) in the absence of systemic hypertension (a). In contrast with the renal histology of normal wild-type mice (b), the kidneys of the ET-1 overexpressing mice are characterized by significant peritubular fibrosis and by the presence of several cysts at 14 months of age (c). (From Hocher B, Thöne-Reineke C, Rohmeiss P, Schmager F, Slowinski T, Burst V, Siegmund F, Quertermous T, Bauer C, Neumayer H-H, Schleuning W-D, Theuring F. Endothelin-1 transgenic mice develop glomerulosclerosis, interstitial fibrosis, and renal cysts but not hypertension. *J Clin Invest* 1997; **99**: 1380–1389. Copyright permission of the American Society of Clinical Investigation).

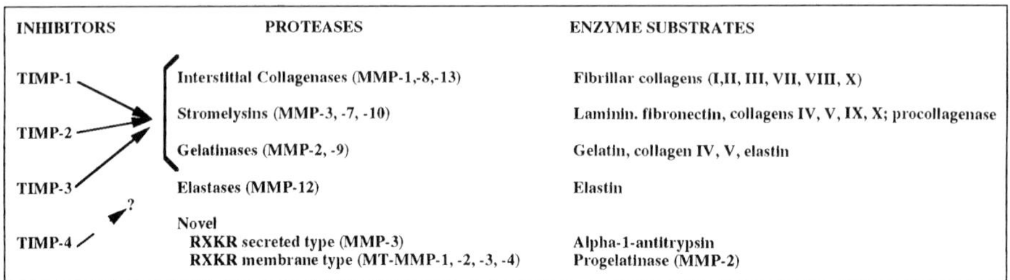

Fig. 4.11 Members of the metalloproteinase family of matrix-degrading proteases and their inhibitors. Abbreviations: TIMP, tissue inhibitor of metalloproteinases; MMP, metalloproteinase; MT, membrane-type; RXKR, a furin enzyme recognition site Arg-X-Lys-Arg. (Modified from Eddy AA. Molecular insights into renal interstitial fibrosis. *J Am Soc Nephrol* 1996; 7: 2495–2508. Copyright permission from Williams and Wilkins).

tubular cells mainly synthesize gelatinase A and B, fibroblasts, predominantly gelatinase A, and both produce interstitial collagenase [186]. Tubular epithelial cells may secrete MMP both apically and basolaterally [187]. While it is thought that basolateral secretion is involved in basement membrane turnover, the role of apical activity remains unclear.

There are currently four described tissue inhibitors of MMP: TIMP-1, -2, -3, and -4. These enzyme inhibitors may neutralize several members of this family by non-covalent binding to the active enzyme and in some cases to the proenzyme as well. TIMP-1 and -2 are soluble while TIMP-3 may be insoluble and can be found bound to ECM [182]. TIMP-4, first described in 1996 [188] remains unstudied in renal fibrosis. Low levels of TIMP-4 mRNA transcripts are found in normal kidneys.

TIMP-1 inhibits all of the latent pro-MMP, is the most extensively studied in renal interstitial fibrosis, and is emerging as a likely contributor to the fibrogenic process. TIMP-1 is not detected by immunostaining in normal rat kidneys but appears in the interstitium during renal fibrosis. By *in situ* hybridization in the protein-overload model of fibrosis, TIMP-1 transcripts localized to both interstitial cells and tubular epithelial cell [189]. TIMP-1 was detected in tubular and interstitial cells in kidney biopsies obtained from patients with diabetic nephropathy [190]. TIMP-1 mRNA levels correlated with the extent of tubulo-interstitial damage in that study. Renal mRNA levels for TIMP-1 are elevated in essentially all experimental models of interstitial fibrosis studied (Table 4.6). Proof that upregulated expression of TIMP-1 plays an acute part in the pathogenesis of renal interstitial fibrosis is not yet available. It is noteworthy however, that renal metalloproteinase mRNA levels fail to increase during the period of increased matrix protein synthesis and upregulated TIMP-1 expression. These findings predict that while matrix protein production is amplified in response to renal injury, the renal MMPs that would normally counterbalance and regulate this response are inactivated, an effect that should facilitate the interstitial fibrogenic response. Recently, Heidland *et al.*

Table 4.6 Increased TIMP-1 expression in models of interstitial fibrosis

Model/disease	Relative mRNA level	References
Anti-tubular basement membrane nephritis	11×	[254]
Cyclosporine nephropathy	ND	[255]
Diabetic nephropathy	1.4×	[256]
Heymann nephritis	3.3×	[248]
Hypercholesterolemia	2.7×	[210]
Murine lupus nephritis	15×	[257]
Obese Zucker rats	ND	[251]
Obstructive uropathy	14–30×	[136,258,259]
Polycystic kidney disease	9×	[260]
Protein-overload proteinuria	2.3×	[106]
Puromycin aminonucleoside nephrosis	11×	[29,36]

* mRNA level relative to control kidneys.
ND, not done.

[191] have reported that treatment with a protease cocktail (phlogenzyme) for 6–7 weeks has decreased fibrosis in the rat remnant kidney model and the Goldblatt hypertension model. TIMP-1 may have other biologic roles that could be relevant to the fibrogenic response such as growth-modulating activities and inhibition of angiogenesis [182]. What stimulates TIMP-1 expression *in vivo* in the kidney remains unclear. Several TIMP-1 agonists have been identified using *in vitro* studies including cytokines (IL-1, IL-6, IL-10), growth factors (epidermal growth factor, PDGF, TGF-α, TGF-β1, TNF-α), oncostatin M, endotoxin, thrombin, glucose, and hypoxia [182].

In contrast to TIMP-1, relatively little is known about changes in TIMP-2, -3, and -4 during interstitial fibrosis. In rodents, TIMP-2 and -3 transcripts are relatively abundant in normal kidneys. TIMP-2 expression is thought to be largely constitutive [192]. TIMP-3 expression is subject to cell cycle regulation [193] and the protein has an affinity for ECM [194].

Whether downregulation of MMP themselves plays a part in the pathogenesis of interstitial fibrosis is unknown. Decreased glomerular metalloproteinase and cysteine protease activity have been reported in models of glomerulosclerosis observed in obese Zucker rats [195], aging rat kidneys [196,197], Goldblatt hypertension [198], and the remnant kidney [199]. Macrophage biosynthesis of MMPs is suppressed by interferon-γ, IL-4, and IL-10 [200]. ANG II inhibits the activity of collagenases and gelatinases in proximal tubular cells. TGF-β1 usually decreases the activity of collagenases and cathepsins in fibroblasts, and mesangial and tubular cells [201], although increased expression has occasionally been reported [202].

It has recently been appreciated that MMP may have pro-inflammatory effects. Using anti-MMP-2 ribozymes, Turck *et al.* [203] reported significant changes in cultured glomerular mesangial cells. When MMP-2 secretion was inhibited, the mesangial cells reverted from an 'active' phenotype of proliferation and matrix synthesis to a 'quiescent' phenotype. Transfected mesangial cells expressing stromelysin show increased proliferation rates [204] while infusion of active gelatinase A into the renal artery also increases mesangial cell proliferation [205]. MMPs have other effects that could theoretically accentuate fibrosis. Matrilysin (MMP-7) activates plasminogen and pro-urokinase [206]. In humans with idiopathic dilated cardiomyopathy, cardiac fibrosis was associated with a net increase in cardiac collagenase and gelatinase activity [207]. These investigators suggested that an increase in cardiac metalloproteinase activity in the presence of increased collagen synthesis is actually harmful due to the ability of the MMP to degrade collagen fibrils into poorly cross-linked, immature, and unstable fibrils with damaging consequences. Norman and co-workers [187] also found increased gelatinase and stromelysin activity at the early phase of autosomal dominant polycystic kidney disease. Thus, until MMP activity is blocked *in vivo*, it remains unknown whether metalloproteinase activity is a beneficial response in the face of increased collagen synthesis or whether it has detrimental effects.

The second matrix degradation pathway that appears to be important in renal interstitial fibrosis is the plasmin-dependent pathway (Fig. 4.12). Although historically known best for its part in the coagulation cascade, there is growing evidence that this group of enzymes also plays a part in such diverse processes as cell migration, tissue remodeling, wound healing, morphogenesis, tumor development and metastasis, and angiogenesis. Plasmin not only converts latent procollagenases to active collagenases but it may also directly degrade some matrix proteins such as fibronectin, laminin, entactin, tenascin-C, and proteoglycan core protein. Plasminogen is present in relatively high concentrations in the plasma, although 40% of

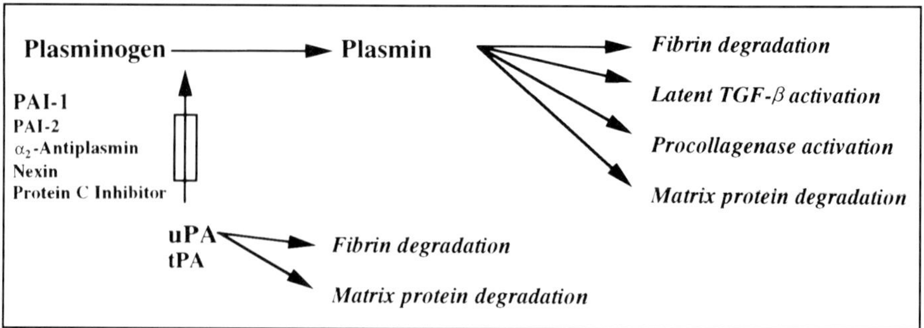

Fig. 4.12 Members of the plasmin-dependent cascade that may play a part in renal interstitial fibrosis. Abbreviations: PAI, plasminogen activator inhibitor; uPA, urokinase-type plasminogen activator; tPA, tissue-type plasminogen activator. (Modified from Eddy AA. Molecular insights into renal interstitial fibrosis. *J Am Soc Nephrol* 1996; 7: 2495–2508. Copyright permission from Williams and Wilkins).

circulating plasminogen migrates to extravascular sites [208]. The majority of plasminogen is synthesized in the liver but plasminogen mRNA has been detected in the kidney [209]. Plasminogen is proteolytically cleaved to plasmin by both tissue-type plasminogen activator (tPA) and urokinase-type plasminogen activator (uPA). Thus far, significant expression of tPA by the tubulo-interstitial compartment of the kidney has not been reported. In contrast, uPA is normally produced in significant quantities by proximal and distal tubular epithelial cells and large quantities of uPA are present in normal urine. The pattern of tubular uPA production during the course of interstitial fibrosis has not been studied in any detail. In one study in the rat model of diet-induced hypercholesterolemia, renal uPA mRNA levels were significantly reduced throughout the 12-week study period as focal interstitial fibrosis developed [210].

The activity of the plasmin-dependent cascade can be blocked by four protease inhibitors (Fig. 4.12). The one of greatest interest in the context of renal fibrosis is plasminogen activator inhibitor-1 (PAI-1), the major inhibitor *in vivo*. Relatively little is currently known about the role of the plasminogen activator/plasmin pathway in renal interstitial fibrosis, although increased expression of PAI-1 has been detected in several experimental models (Table 4.7). In a murine model of lupus nephritis, PAI-1 levels in renal tissue were found to correlate with the severity of the disease and by *in situ* hybridization PAI-1 transcripts localized not only to glomerular cells but to tubular epithelial cells and interstitial inflammatory mononuclear cells [211]. In rats with radiation-induced nephropathy, ANG II blockade has been reported to normalize renal PAI-1 mRNA levels (compared with a ninefold increase in the untreated animals at 12 weeks) in association with an attenuation in glomerular and interstitial fibrosis [212].

Despite this circumstantial evidence, definitive proof that depressed intrarenal plasmin activity facilitates interstitial fibrosis is lacking. Noteworthy is the fact that plasmin is also known to activate TGF-β1 *in vitro* [213]. If plasmin mediates a similar effect *in vivo*, the argument could be made that increased intrarenal plasmin

Table 4.7 Increased PAI-1 expression in association with interstitial fibrosis

Model/disease	Relative mRNA level	References
Anti-tubular basement membrane nephritis	12×	[254]
Cyclosporine nephropathy	ND	[246,261]
Endotoxemia	ND	[262]
FK506 nephrotoxicity	5–10×	[247]
Hypercholesterolemia	1.3×	[210]
Murine lupus nephritis	ND	[263]
Protein-overload proteinuria	2.1×	[106]
Puromycin aminonucleoside nephrosis	2.0×	[264]
Radiation nephropathy	9×	[212]
Renal allograft rejection	ND	[241,265,266]

activity would aggravate rather than attenuate fibrosis. However, recent studies based on an experimental model of pulmonary fibrosis found that enhanced plasmin activity attenuates pulmonary fibrosis [214]. These studies, in the model of bleomycin-induced lung fibrosis, reported significantly worse fibrosis in mice that genetically overexpressed PAI-1 and significantly less fibrosis in mice that were genetically deficient in PAI-1. Whether the same outcome will be true in renal interstitial fibrosis remains to be determined.

The relevance of progressive tubulo-interstitial fibrosis to the progression of renal diseases stems from the close correlations between the severity of these histological changes and renal function [1–4]. However, the precise mechanisms linking tubulo-interstitial fibrosis and progressive renal insufficiency remain speculative. For instance, it has been postulated that these changes lead to the strangulation of renal vessels precipitating ischemia, hypoxia, and further renal functional decline [157,267]. It has also been suggested that interstitial fibrosis would reduce the diameter of postglomerular capillaries thus exacerbating glomerular hypertension and the ensuing glomerulosclerosis [7]. Narrowing of afferent arterioles would also lead to glomerular ischemia and obsolescence.

In summary, it is an exciting time for scientists and clinicians interested in advancing our understanding of the pathogenesis and treatment options for chronic renal disease. For many patients with renal disease, definitive treatment is not currently available. For others, a narrow window of opportunity has been missed and they first come to medical attention after progressive renal insufficiency is inevitable. Returning to the schematic overview presented in Fig. 4.1 as a reference point, we are now in a position to focus in on the primary mediators of interstitial fibrosis with the goal of developing new therapeutic strategies to alter the natural history of this relentless course in our patients.

Acknowledgements

The authors acknowledge the assistance of Jennifer Samson with referencing and formatting of the manuscript. For our own work that is cited we would like to acknowledge research grant support from the Kidney Foundation of Canada; the Medical Research Council of Canada; Baxter Healthcare Inc.; The Hospital for Sick Children Research Institute, University of Toronto; and the Children's Hospital and Regional Medical Center, University of Washington.

Key references

Clouthier D, Comerford S, Hammer R. Hepatic fibrosis, glomerulosclerosis, and lipodystrophy-like syndrome in PEPCK-TGF-β1 transgenic mice. *J Clin Invest* 1997; **100**: 2697–2713.

Egido J. Vasoactive hormones and renal sclerosis. *Kidney Int* 1996; **49**: 578–597.

Eitzman D, McCoy R, Zheng X, *et al.* Bleomycin-induced pulmonary fibrosis in transgenic mice that either lack or overexpress the murine plasminogen activator inhibitor-1 gene. *J Clin Invest* 1996; **97**: 232–237.

González-Avila G, Vadillo-Ortega F, Pérez-Tamayo R. Experimental diffuse interstitial renal fibrosis. A biochemical approach. *Lab Invest* 1988; **59**: 245–252.

Hocher B, Thone-Reineke C, Rohmeiss P, *et al.* Endothelin-1 transgenic mice develop glomerulosclerosis, interstitial fibrosis, and renal cysts but not hypertension. *J Clin Invest* 1997; **99**: 1380–1389.

Ruoslahti E, Yamaguchi Y. Proteoglycans as modulators of growth factor activities. *Cell* 1991; **64**: 867–869.

Wolf G, Mueller E, Stahl R, Ziyadeh F. Angiotensin II-induced hypertrophy of cultured murine proximal tubular cells is mediated by endogenous transforming growth factor-β. *J Clin Invest* 1993; **92**: 1366–1372.

References

1. Risdon RA, Sloper JC, de Vardener HE. Relationship between renal function and histologic changes found in renal-biopsy specimens from patients with persistent glomerulonephritis. *Lancet* 1968; **ii**: 363–366.
2. Schainuck LI, Stricker GE, Cutler RE, Benditt EP. Structural-functional correlations in renal disease. Part II Correlations. *Hum Pathol* 1970; **1**: 631–641.
3. Kim KH, Kim Y, Gubler MC, *et al.* Structural-functioning relationships in Alport syndrome. *J Am Soc Nephrol* 1995; **5**: 1659–1668.
4. Mackensen-Haen S, Bohle A, Christensen J, Wehrmann M, Kendziorra H, Korot E. The consequences for renal function of widening of the interstitium and changes in the tubular epithelium of the renal cortex and outer medulla in various renal diseases. *Clin Nephrol* 1992; **37**: 70–77.
5. Marcussen N. Biology of disease. Atubular glomeruli and the structural basis for chronic renal failure. *Lab Invest* 1992; **66**: 265–284.
6. Ljungquist A. The intrarenal arterial pattern in the normal and diseases human kidney. *Acta Med Scand* 1963; **174**: 5–34.
7. Bohle A, Gise HV, Mackensen-Haen S, Start-Jacob B. The obliteration of the postglomerular capillaries and its influence upon the function of both glomeruli and tubuli. *Klin Wochenschr* 1981; **59**: 1043–1051.
8. Serón D, Alexopoulos E, Raftery MJ, Hartley B, Cameron JS. Number of interstitial capillary cross sections assessed by monoclonal antibodies: Relation to interstitial damage. *Nephrol Dial Transplant* 1990; **5**: 889–893.
9. Lieberthal W, Levine JS. Mechanisms of apoptosis and its potential role in renal tubular epithelial cell injury. *Am J Physiol* 1996; **271**: F477–F488.
10. Nakao N, Yoshiki A, Hiraiwa N, Kusakabe M. Tenascin is an important matrix protein during the healing process of murine mesangial proliferative glomerulonephritis. *J Am Soc Nephrol* 1995; **6**: 903.
11. Gharaee-Kermani M, Wiggins R, Wolber F, Goyal M, Phan SH. Fibronectin is the major fibroblast chemoattractant in rabbit anti-glomerular basement membrane disease. *Am J Pathol* 1996; **148**: 961–967.
12. Tang WW, Feng L, Xia Y, Peters J, Wilson CB. Expression of embryonic (E) fibronectins (FN) due to alternative splicing after immune renal injury. *J Am Soc Nephrol* 1993; **4**: 667.
13. Bergijk EC, Baelde JJ, Kootstra CJ, De Heer E, Killen PD, Bruijn JA. Cloning of the mouse fibronectin V-region and variation of its splicing pattern in experimental immue complex glomerulonephritis. *J Pathol* 1996; **178**: 462–468.

14. Viedt C, Büuger A, Hänsch GM. Fibronectin synthesis in tubular epithelial cells: Up-regulation of the EDA splice variant by transforming growth factor β. *Kidney Int* 1995; **48**: 1810–1817.
15. Roy-Chaudhury P, Hillis G, McDonald S, Simpson JG, Power DA. Importance of the tubulointerstitium in human glomerulonephritis. II. Distribution of integrin chains beta 1, alpha 1–6 and alpha V. *Kidney Int* 1997; **52**: 103–110.
16. Davies M, Kastner S, Thomas GJ. Proteoglycans: Their possible role in renal fibrosis. *Kidney Int* 1996; **49**: S55–S60.
17. Hällgren R, Gerdin B, Tufveson G. Hyaluronic acid accumulation and redistribution in rejecting rat kidney graft. Relationship to the transplantation edema. *J Exp Med* 1990; **171**: 2063–2076.
18. Diamond J, Levinson M, Kreisberg R, Ricardo SD. Increased expression of decorin in experimental hydronephrosis. *Kidney Int* 1997; **51**: 1133–1139.
19. Hugo C, Shankland SJ, Pichler R, Couser WG, Johnson RJ. Thrombospondin 1 precedes and predicts the development of tubulointerstitial fibrosis in glomerular disease in the rat. *Kidney Int* 1998; **53**: 302–311.
20. Wu LL, Cox A, Roe CJ, Dziadek M, Cooper ME, Gilbert RE. Secreted protein acidic and rich in cysteine expression after subtotal nephrectomy and blockade of the renin-angiotensin system. *J Am Soc Nephrol* 1997; **8**: 1373–1382.
21. Pichler RH, Franceschini N, Young BA, *et al.* Pathogenesis of cyclosporine nephropathy. Roles of angiotensin II and osteopontin. *J Am Soc Nephrol* 1995; **6**: 1186–1196.
22. Ruoslahti E, Yamaguchi Y. Proteoglycans as modulators of growth factor activities. *Cell* 1991; **64**: 867–869.
23. Pichler RH, Bassuk JA, Hugo C, *et al.* SPARC is expressed by mesangial cells in experimental mesangial proliferative nephritis and inhibits platelet-derived-growth-factor-mediated mesangial cell proliferation in vitro. *Am J Pathol* 1996; **48**: 1153–1167.
24. West DC, Shaw DM, Lorenz P, Adzick NS, Longaker MT. Fibrotic healing of adult and late gestation fetal wounds correlates with increased hyaluronidase activity and removal of hyaluronan. *Int J Biochem Cell Biol* 1997; **29**: 201–210.
25. Bottinger EP, Letterio JJ, Roberts AB. Biology of TGF-beta in knockout and transgenic mouse models. *Kidney Int* 1997; **51**: 1355–1360.
26. Munger JS, Harpel JG, Gleizes PE, Mazzieri R, Nunes I, Rifkin DB. Latent transforming growth factor-β: structural features and mechanisms of activation. *Kidney Int* 1997; **51**: 1376–1382.
27. DiDonato A, Ghiggeri GM, DiDuca M, *et al.* Lysyl oxidase expression and collagen cross-linking during chronic adriamycin nephropathy. *Nephron* 1997; **76**: 192–200.
28. Johnson TS, Griffin M, Thomas GL, *et al.* The role of transglutaminase in the rat subtotal nephrectomy model of renal fibrosis. *J Clin Invest* 1997; **99**: 2950–2959.
29. Jones CL, Buch S, Post M, McCulloch L, Liu E, Eddy AA. Renal extracellular matrix accumulation in acute puromycin aminonucleoside nephrosis in rats. *Am J Pathol* 1992; **141**: 1381–1396.
30. Ceol M, Nerlich A, Baggio B, *et al.* Increased glomerular α1 (IV) collagen expression and deposition in long-term diabetic rats is prevented by chronic glycosaminoglycan treatment. *Lab Invest* 1996; **74**: 484–495.
31. Creely JJ, DiMari SJ, Howe AM, Haralson MA. Effects of transforming growth factor-β on collagen synthesis by normal rat kidney epithelial cells. *Am J Pathol* 1992; **140**: 45–55.
32. Humes HD, Nakamura T, Cieslinski DA, Miller D, Emmons RV, Border WA. Role of

proteoglycans and cytoskeleton in the effects of TGF-beta 1 on renal proximal tubule cells. *Kidney Int* 1993; **43**: 575–584.
33. Nadasdy T, Laszik Z, Blick KE, Johnson DL, Silva FG. Tubular atrophy in the end-stage kidney: a lectin and immunohistochemical study. *Hum Pathol* 1994; **25**: 22–28.
34. Strutz F, Müller GA, Neilson EG. Transdifferentiation: a new angle on renal fibrosis. *Exp Nephrol* 1996; **4**: 267–270.
35. Strutz F, Okada H, Lo CW, *et al.* Identification and characterization of a fibroblast marker: FSP1. *J Cell Biol* 1995; **130**: 393–405.
36. Jones CL, Buch S, Post M, McCulloch L, Liu E, Eddy AA. The pathogenesis of interstitial fibrosis in chronic purine aminonucleoside nephrosis. *Kidney Int* 1991; **40**: 1020–1031.
37. Tamaki K, Okuda S, Ando T, Iwamoto T, Nakayama M, Fujishima M. TGF-β1 in glomerulosclerosis and interstitial fibrosis of adriamycin nephropathy. *Kidney Int* 1994; **45**: 525–536.
38. Lee S-K, Goyal M, de Miguel M, *et al.* Renal biopsy collagen I mRNA predicts scarring in rabbit anti-GBM disease: comparison with conventional measures. *Kidney Int* 1997; **52**: 1000–1015.
39. Tang WWGY, Qi M. Myofibroblast and α_1 (III) collagen expression in experimental tubulointerstitial nephritis. *Kidney Int* 1997; **51**: 926–931.
40. Sharma AK, Mauer SM, Kim Y, Michael AF. Interstitial fibrosis in obstructive nephropathy. *Kidney Int* 1993; **44**: 774–788.
41. Alvarez RJ, Sun MJ, Haverty TP, Iozzo RV, Myers JC, Neilson EG. Biosynthetic and proliferative characteristics of tubulointerstitial fibroblasts probed with paracrine cytokines. *Kidney Int* 1992; **41**: 14–23.
42. Rodemann HP, Müller GA. Characterization of human renal fibroblasts in health and disease: II. In vitro growth, differentiation, and collagen synthesis of fibroblasts from kidneys with interstitial fibrosis. *Am J Kidney Dis* 1991; **17**: 684–686.
43. Müller GA, Rodemann HP. Characterization of human renal fibroblasts in health and disease: I. Immunophenotyping of cultured tubular epithelial cells and fibroblasts derived from kidneys with histologically proven interstitial fibrosis. *Am J Kidney Dis* 1991; **17**: 680–683.
44. Lonnemann G, Shapiro L, Engler-Blum G, Muller GA, Koch KM, Dinarello CA. Cytokines in human renal interstitial fibrosis. I. Interleukin-1 is a paracrine growth factor for cultured fibrosis-derived kidney fibroblasts. *Kidney Int* 1995; **47**: 837–844.
45. Alpers CE, Hudkins KL, Floege J, Johnson RJ. Human renal cortical interstitial cells with some features of smooth muscle cells participate in tubulointerstitial and crescentic glomerular injury. *J Am Soc Nephrol* 1994; **5**: 201–210.
46. Goumenos DS, Brown CB, Shortland J, El Nahas AM. Myofibroblasts, predictors of progression of mesangial IgA nephropathy? *Nephrol Dial Transplant* 1994; **9**: 1418–1425.
47. Kliem V, Johnson RJ, Alpers CE, *et al.* Mechanisms involved in the pathogenesis of tubulointerstitial fibrosis in 5/6-nephrectomized rats. *Kidney Int* 1996; **49**: 666–678.
48. Johnson RJ, Alpers CE, Yoshimura A, *et al.* Renal injury from angiotensin II-mediated hypertension. *Hypertension* 1992; **19**: 464–474.
49. Eng E, Veniant M, Floege J, *et al.* Renal proliferative and phenotypic changes in rats with two-kidney, one-clip Goldblatt hypertension. *Am J Hypertension* 1994; **7**: 177–185.
50. Diamond JR, Goor H, Ding G, Engelmyer E. Myofibroblasts in experimental hydronephrosis. *Am J Pathol* 1995; **146**: 121–129.

51. Zhang G, Moorhead PJ, El Nahas AM. Myofibroblasts and the progression of experimental glomerulonephritis. *Exp Nephrol* 1995; **3**: 308–318.
52. Desmoulière A, Geinoz A, Gabbiani F, Gabbiani G. Transforming growth factor-β1 induces α-smooth muscle actin expression in granulation tissue myofibroblasts and in quiescent and growing cultured fibroblasts. *J Cell Biol* 1993; **122**: 103–111.
53. Tang WW, Ulich TR, Lacey DL, *et al.* Platelet-derived growth factor-BB induces renal tubulointerstitial myofibroblast formation and tubulointerstitial fibrosis. *Am J Pathol* 1996; **148**: 1169–1180.
54. Wiggins R, Goyal M, Merritt S, Killen PD. Vascular adventitial cell expression of collagen I messenger ribonucleic acid in anti-glomerular basement membrane antibody-induced crescentic nephritis in the rabbit. A cellular source for interstitial collagen synthesis in inflammatory renal disease. *Lab Invest* 1993; **68**: 557–565.
55. Ronnov-Jessen L, Petersen OW, Koteliansky VE, Bissell MJ. The origin of the myfibroblasts in breast cancer. Recapitulation of tumor environment in culture unravels diversity and implicates converted fibroblasts and recruited smooth muscle cells. *J Clin Invest* 1995; **95**: 859–873.
56. Roberts ISD, Burrows C, Shanks JH, Venning M, McWilliam LJ. Intersitial myofibroblasts: predictors of progression in membranous nephropathy. *J Clin Pathol* 1997; **50**: 123–127.
57. Nathan CF. Secretory products of macrophages. *J Clin Invest* 1987; **79**: 319–326.
58. Diamond JR, Pesek-Diamond I. Sublethal X-irradiation during acute puromycin nephrosis prevents late renal injury: role of macrophages. *Am J Physiol* 1991; **260**: F779–F786.
59. Harris KPG, Lefkowith JB, Klahr S, Schreiner GF. Essential fatty acid deficiency ameliorates acute renal dysfunction in the rat after the administration of the aminonucleoside of puromycin. *J Clin Invest* 1990; **86**: 1115–1123.
60. Saito T, Atkins RC. Contribution of mononuclear leukocytes to the progression of experimental focal glomerular sclerosis. *Kidney Int* 1990; **37**: 1076–1083.
61. Nakamura T, Ebihara I, Fukui M, Tomino Y, Koide H. Effects of methylprednisolone on glomerular and medullary mRNA levels for extracellular matrices in puromycin aminonucleoside nephrosis. *Kidney Int* 1991; **40**: 874–881.
62. Gattone VHII, Cowley BD Jr, Barash BD, *et al.* Methylprednisolone retards the progression of inherited polycystic kidney disease in rodents. *Am J Kidney Dis* 1995; **25**: 302–313.
63. Eddy AA. Protein restriction reduces transforming growth factor-β and interstitial fibrosis in nephrotic syndrome. *Am J Physiol* 1994; **266**: F884–F893.
64. Zoja C, Liu X-H, Donadelli R, *et al.* Renal expression of monocyte chemoattractant protein-1 in lupus autoimmune mice. *J Am Soc Nephrol* 1997; **8**: 720–729.
65. Diamond JR, Kees-Folts D, Ding G, Frye JE, Restrepo NC. Macrophages, monocyte chemoattractant peptide-1, and TGF-β1 in experimental hydronephrosis. *Am J Physiol* 1994; **226**: F926–F933.
66. Prodjosudjadi W, van Gerritsma JSJ, Es LA, Daha MR, Bruijn JA. Monocyte chemoattractant protein-1 in normal and diseased human kidneys: an immunohistochemical analysis. *Clin Nephrol* 1995; **44**: 148–155.
67. Noris M, Bernasconi S, Casiraghi F, *et al.* Monocyte chemoattractant protein-1 is excreted in excessive amounts in the urine of patients with lupus nephritis. *Lab Invest* 1995; **73**: 804–809.
68. Rovin BH, Doe N, Tan LC. Monocyte chemoattractant protein-1 levels in patients with glomerular disease. *Am J Kidney Dis* 1996; **27**: 640–646.

69. Grandaliano G, Gesualdo L, Ranieri E, *et al.* Monocyte chemotactic peptide-1 expression in acute and chronic human nephritides: a pathogenic role in interstitial monocytes recruitment. *J Am Soc Nephrol* 1996; **7**: 906–913.
70. Tang WW, Qi M, Van Warren JS, GY. Chemokine expression in experimental tubulointerstitial nephritis. *J Immunol* 1997; **159**: 870–876.
71. Eddy AA, Warren JS. Expression and function of monocyte chemoattractant protein-1 in experimental nephrotic syndrome. *Clin Immunol Immunopathol* 1996; **78**: 140–151.
72. Welch TR, Beischel LS, Witte DP. Differential expression of complement C3 and C4 in the human kidney. *J Clin Invest* 1993; **92**: 1451–1458.
73. Witte DP, Welch TR, Beischel LS. Detection and cellular localization of human C4 gene expression in the renal tubular epithelial cells and other extrahepatic epithelial sources. *Am J Pathol* 1991; **139**: 717–724.
74. Camussi G, Rotunno M, Segoloni G, Brentjens JR, Andres GA. *In vitro* alternative pathway activation of complement by the brush border of proximal tubules of normal rat kidney. *J Immunol* 1982; **128**: 1659–1663.
75. Nomura A, Morita Y, Maruyama S, *et al.* Role of complement in acute tubulointerstitial injury of rats with aminonucleoside nephrosis. *Am J Pathol* 1997; **151**: 539–547.
76. Morita Y, Nomura A, Yuzawa Y, *et al.* The role of complement in the pathogenesis of tubulointerstitial lesions in rat mesangial proliferative glomerulonephritis. *J Am Soc Nephrol* 1997; **8**: 1363–1372.
77. Lan HY, Nikokic-Paterson DJ, Mu W, Atkins RC. Local macrophage proliferation in the progression of glomerular and tubulointerstitial injury in rat anti-GBM glomerulonephritis. *Kidney Int* 1995; **48**: 753–760.
78. Kovacs EJ. Fibrogenic cytokines: the role of immune mediators in the development of scar tissue. *Immunol Today* 1991; **12**: 17–23.
79. Kovacs EJ, DiPietro LA. Fibrogenic cytokines and connective tissue production. *FASEB J* 1994; **8**: 854–861.
80. Korfhagen TR, Swantz RJ, Wert SE, *et al.* Respiratory epithelial cell expression of human transforming growth factor-α induces lung fibrosis in transgenic mice. *J Clin Invest* 1994; **93**: 1691–1699.
81. Border WA, Noble NA. Transforming growth factor β in tissue fibrosis. *N Engl J Med* 1994; **331**: 1286–1292.
82. Sharma K, Ziyadeh FN. The emerging role of transforming growth factor-β in kidney diseases. *Am J Physiol* 1994; **266**: F829–F842.
83. Border WA, Noble NA. TGF-β in kidney fibrosis: a target for gene therapy. *Kidney Int* 1997; **51**: 1388–1396.
84. Ketteler M, Noble NA, Border WA. Transforming growth factor-β and angiotensin II. the missing link from glomerular hyperfiltration to glomerulosclerosis. *Annu Rev Physiol* 1995; **57**: 279–295.
85. Dubois CM, Laprise M-H, Blanchette F, Gentry LE, Leduc R. Processing of transforming growth factor β1 precursor by human furin convertase. *J Biol Chem* 1995; ••: 10618–10624.
86. Feige JJ, Baird A. Crinopexy: extracellular regulation of growth factor action. *Kidney Int* 1995; **47**: S15–S18.
87. Hildebrand A, Romaris M, Rasmussen LM, *et al.* Interaction of the small interstitial proteoglycans biglycan, decorin and fibromodulin with transforming growth factor beta. *Biochem J* 1994; **302**: 527–534.
88. Yamaguchi Y, Mann DM, Ruoslahti E. Negative regulation of transforming growth factor-beta by the proteoglycan decorin. *Nature* 1990; **346**: 281–284.

89. Lopez-Casillas F, Cheifetz S, Doody J, Andres JL, Lane WS, Massagué J. Structure and expression of the membrane proteolycan betaglycan, a component of the TGF-beta receptor system. *Cell* 1991; **67**: 785–795.
90. Yamashita H, Ichijo H, Grimsby S, Móren A, ten-Dijke P, Miyazono K. Endoglin forms a heteromeric complex with the signaling receptors for transforming growth factor-beta. *J Biol Chem* 1994; **269**: 1995–2001.
91. McCaffrey TA, Falcone DJ, Vincente D, Du B, Consigli S, Borth W. Protection of transforming growth factor-beta 1 activity by heparin and fucoidan. *J Cell Physiol* 1994; **159**: 51–59.
92. Roy-Chaudhury P, Simpson JG, Power DA. Endoglin, a transforming growth factor-beta-binding protein, is upregulated in chronic progressive renal disease. *Exp Nephrol* 1997; **5**: 55–60.
93. Miyazono K, Ichijo H, Heldin CH. Transforming growth factor-β: latent forms, binding proteins and receptors. *Growth Factors* 1993; **8**: 11–22.
94. Ziyadeh FN, Han DC. Involvement of transforming growth factor-β and its receptors in the pathogenesis of diabetic nephropathy. *Kidney Int* 1997; **52** (Suppl. 60): S7–S11.
95. Yamamoto H, Ueno H, Ooshima A, Takeshita A. Adenovirus-mediated transfer of a truncated transforming growth factor-β (TGF-β) type II receptor completely and specifically abolishes diverse signaling by TGF-β in vascular wall cells in primary culture. *J Biol Chem* 1996; **271**: 16253–16259.
96. Ando T, Okuda S, Tamaki K, Yoshitomi K, Fujishima M. Localization of transforming growth factor-β and latent transforming growth factor-β binding protein in rat kidney. *Kidney Int* 1995; **47**: 733–739.
97. Tamaki K, Okuda S, Miyazono K, Nakayama M, Fujishima M. Matrix-associated latent TGF-β with latent TGF-β binding protein in the progressive process in adriamycin-induced nephropathy. *Lab Invest* 1995; **73**: 81–89.
98. Bottinger EP, Factor VM, Tsang ML, *et al.* The recombinant proregion of transforming growth factor β1 (latency-associated peptide) inhibits active transforming growth factor β1 in transgenic mice. *Proc Natl Acad Sci USA* 1996; **93**: 5877–5882.
99. Sanderson N, Factor V, Nagy P, *et al.* Hepatic expression of mature transforming growth factor β1 in transgenic mice results in multiple tissue lesions. *Proc Natl Acad Sci USA* 1995; **92**: 2572–2576.
100. Kopp JB, Factor VM, Mozes M, *et al.* Transgenic mice with increased plasma levels of TGF-β1 develop progressive renal disease. *Lab Invest* 1996; **74**: 991–1003.
101. Clouthier DE, Comerford SA, Hammer RE. Hepatic fibrosis, glomerulosclerosis, and lipodystrophy-like syndrome in PEPCK-TGF-β1 transgenic mice. *J Clin Invest* 1997; **100**: 2697–2713.
102. Pankewycz OG, Miao L, Isaacs R, *et al.* Increased renal tubular expression of transforming growth factor beta in human allografts correlates with cyclosporine toxicity. *Kidney Int* 1996; **50**: 1634–1640.
103. Yamamoto T, Noble NA, Miller DE, Border WA. Sustained expression of TGF-β1 underlies development of progressive kidney fibrosis. *Kidney Int* 1994; **45**: 916–927.
104. Wright EJ, McCaffrey TA, Robertson AP, Vaughan ED Jr, Felsen D. Chronic unilateral ureteral obstruction is associated with intersitial fibrosis and tubular expression of transforming growth factor-β. *Lab Invest* 1996; **74**: 528–537.
105. Basile DP, Rovak JM, Martin DR, Hammerman MR. Increased transforming growth factor-β1 expression in regenerating rat renal tubules following ischemic injury. *Am J Physiol* 1996; **270**: F500–F509.
106. Eddy AA, Giachelli CM. Renal expression of genes that promote interstitial inflamma-

tion and fibrosis in rats with protein-overload proteinuria. *Kidney Int* 1995; **47**: 1546–1557.

107. Muchaneta-Kubara EC, El Nahas AM. Myofibroblast phenotypes expression in experimental renal scarring. *Nephrol Dial Transplant* 1997; **12**: 904–915.
108. Van Obberghen-Schilling E, Roche NS, Flanders KC, Sporn MB, Roberts AB. Transforming growth factor β1 positively regulates its own expression in normal and transformed cells. *J Biol Chem* 1988; **263**: 7741–7746.
109. Border WA, Okuda S, Languino LR, Sporn MB, Ruoslahti E. Suppression of experimental glomerulonephritis by antiserum against transforming growth factor β1. *Nature* 1990; **346**: 371–374.
110. Border WA, Noble NA, Yamamoto T, *et al.* Natural inhibitor of transforming growth factor-β protects against scarring in experimental kidney disease. *Nature* 1992; **360**: 361–364.
111. Isaka Y, Brees DK, Ikegaya K, *et al.* Gene therapy by skeletal muscle expression of decorin prevents fibrotic disease in rat kidney. *Nature Med* 1996; **2**: 418–423.
112. Sharma K, Jin Y, Guo J, Ziyadeh FN. Neutralization of TGF-β by anti-TGF-β antibody attenuates kidney hypertrophy and the enhanced extracellular matrix gene expression in STZ-induced diabetic mice. *Diabetes* 1996; **45**: 522–530.
113. Boivin GP, Molina JR, Ormsby I, Stemmermann G, Doetschman T. Gastric lesions in transforming growth factor β-1 heterozygous mice. *Lab Invest* 1996; **74**: 513–518.
114. Kulkarni AB, Ward JM, Yaswen L, *et al.* Transforming growth factor-β1 null mice. An animal model for inflammatory disorders. *Am J Pathol* 1995; **146**: 264–275.
115. Wolf G, Mueller E, Stahl RAK, Ziyadeh FN. Angiotensin II-induced hypertrophy of cultured murine proximal tubular cells is mediated by endogenous transforming growth factor-β. *J Clin Invest* 1993; **92**: 1366–1372.
116. Ruiz-Ortega M, Egido J. Angiotensin II modulates cell growth-related events and synthesis of matrix proteins in renal interstitial fibroblasts. *Kidney Int* 1997; **52**: 1497–1510.
117. Pimentel JL Jr, Sundell CL, Wang S, Kopp JB, Montero A, Martínez-Maldonado M. Role of angiotensin II in the expression and regulation of transforming growth factor-β in obstructive nephropathy. *Kidney Int* 1995; **48**: 1233–1246.
118. Kaneto H, Morrissey J, Klahr S. Increased expression of TGF-β1 mRNA in the obstructed kidney of rats with unilateral ureteral ligation. *Kidney Int* 1993; **44**: 313–321.
119. Ishidoya S, Morrissey J, McCracken R, Reyes A, Klahr S. Angiotensin II receptor antagonist ameliorates renal tubulointerstitial fibrosis caused by unilateral ureteral obstruction. *Kidney Int* 1995; **47**: 1285–1294.
120. Burdmann EA, Andoh TF, Nast CC, *et al.* Prevention of experimental cyclosporin-induced interstitial fibrosis by losartan and enalapril. *Am J Physiol* 1995; **269**: F491–F499.
121. Ruiz-Ortega M, González S, Serón D. *et al.* ACE inhibition reduces proteinuria, glomerular lesions and extracellular matrix production in a normotensive rat model of immune complex nephritis. *Kidney Int* 1995; **48**: 1778–1791.
122. Diamond JR, Anderson S. Irreversible tubulointerstitial damage associated with chronic aminonucleoside nephrosis. Amelioration by angiotensin I converting enzyme inhibition. *Am J Pathol* 1990; **137**: 1323–1332.
123. Norman JT, Gallego C, Bridgeman DA. Enalapril ameliorates interstitial fibrosis in the remnant kidney of the rat. *J Am Soc Nephrol* 1992; **3**: 746.
124. Inserra F, Romano LA, de Cavanagh EMV, Ercole L, Ferder LF, Gomez RA. Renal interstitial sclerosis in aging: effects of enalapril and nifedipine. *J Am Soc Nephrol* 1996; **7**: 676–680.

125. Niimura F, Labosky PA, Kakuchi J, *et al.* Gene targeting in mice reveals a requirement for angiotensin in the development and maintenance of kidney morphology and growth factor regulation. *J Clin Invest* 1995; **96**: 2947–2954.
126. Harris RC, Cheng HF. The intrarenal renin-angiotensin system: a paracrine system for the local control of renal function separate from the systemic axis. *Exp Nephrol* 1996; **4** (Suppl. 1): 2–7.
127. Wolf G, Neilson EG. Angiotensin II as a hypertrophogenic cytokine for proximal tubular cells. *Kidney Int* 1993; **43** (Suppl. 39): S100–S107.
128. Wolf G, Ziyadeh FN. Renal tubular hypertrophy induced angiotensin II. *Semin Nephrol* 1997; **17**: 448–454.
129. Wolf G, Neilson EG. Angiotensin II as a renal growth factor. *J Am Soc Nephrol* 1993; **3**: 1531–1540.
130. Egido J. Vasoactive hormones and renal sclerosis. *Kidney Int* 1996; **49**: 578–597.
131. Gibbons GH, Pratt RE, Dzau VJ. Vascular smooth muscle cell hypertrophy vs. hyperplasia. Autocrine transforming cell growth factor-beta 1 expression determines growth response to angiotensin II. *J Clin Invest* 1992; **90**: 456–461.
132. Wolf G, Neilson EG. Angiotensin II induces cellular hypertrophy in cultured murine proximal tubular cells. *Am J Physiol* 1990; **259**: F768–F777.
133. Paxton WG, Runge M, Horaist C, Cohen C, Alexander RW, Bernstein KE. Immunohistochemical localization of rat angiotensin II AT1 receptor. *Am J Physiol* 1993; **264**: F989–F995.
134. Wolf G, Zahner G, Mondorf U, Schoeppe W, Stahl RA. Angiotensin II stimulates cellular hypertrophy of LLC-PK1 cells through the AT1 receptor. *Nephrol Dial Transplant* 1993; **8**: 128–133.
135. Lafayette RA, Mayer G, Park SK, Meyer TW. Angiotensin II receptor blockade limits glomerular injury in rats with reduced renal mass. *J Clin Invest* 1992; **90**: 766–771.
136. Ishidoya S, Morrisey J, McCracken R, Klahr S. Delayed treatment with enalapril halts tubulointerstitial fibrosis in rats with obstructive nephropathy. *Kidney Int* 1996; **49**: 1110–1119.
137. Klahr S, Ishidoya S, Morrissey J. Role of angiotensin II in the tubulointerstitial fibrosis of obstructive nephropathy. *Am J Kidney Dis* 1995; **26**: 141–146.
138. Geiger H, Fierlbeck W, Mai M, *et al.* Effects of early and late antihypertensive treatment on extracellular matrix proteins and mononuclear cells in uninephrectomized SHR. *Kidney Int* 1997; **51**: 750–761.
139. Junaid A, Hostetter TH, Rosenberg ME. Interaction of angiotensin II and TGF-β1 in the rat remnant kidney. *J Am Soc Nephrol* 1997; **8**: 1732–1738.
140. Kim S, Ohta K, Hamaguchi A, *et al.* Role of angiotensin II in renal injury of deoxycorticosterone acetate-salt hypertensive rats. *Hypertension* 1994; **24**: 195–204.
141. Ohta K, Kim S, Hamaguchi A, *et al.* Role of angiotensin II in extracellular matrix and transforming growth factor-β1 expression in hypertensive rats. *Eur J Pharmacol* 1994; **269**: 115–119.
142. Shihab FS, Bennett WM, Tanner AM, Andoh TF. Angiotensin II blockade decreases TGF-β1 and matrix proteins in cyclosporine nephropathy. *Kidney Int* 1997; **52**: 660–673.
143. Yanagisawa M, Kurihara H, Kimura S, *et al.* A novel potent vasoconstrictor peptide produced by vascular endothelial cells. *Nature* 1988; **332**: 411–415.
144. Kohan DE. Endothelins in the kidney: physiology and pathophysiology. *Am J Kidney Dis* 1993; **22**: 493–510.

145. Fine LG, Norman JT, Ong A. Cell-cell cross-talk in the pathogenesis of renal interstitial fibrosis. Kidney Int, 1995; **47**: S48–S50.
146. Kawaguchi Y, Suzuki K, Hara M, *et al.* Increased endothelin-1 production in fibroblasts derived from patients with systemic sclerosis. *Ann Rheum Dis* 1994; **53**: 506–510.
147. Fujisaki H, Ito H, Hirata Y, *et al.* Natriuretic peptides inhibit angiotensin II-induced proliferation of rat cardiac fibroblasts by blocking endothelin-1 gene expression. *J Clin Invest* 1995; **96**: 1059–1065.
148. Ehrenreich H, Anderson RW, Fox C, *et al.* Endothelins, peptides with potent vasoactive properties, are produced by human macrophages. *J Exp Med* 1990; **172**: 1741–1748.
149. Bruzzi I, Corna D, Zoja C, *et al.* Time course and localization of endothelin-1 gene expression in a model of renal disease progression. *Am J Pathol* 1997; **151**: 1241–1247.
150. Zoja C, Orisio S, Perico N, *et al.* Constitutive expression of endothelin gene in cultured human mesangial cells and its modulation by transforming growth factor-β, thrombin, and a thromboxane A_2 analogue. *Lab Invest* 1991; **64**: 16–20.
151. Morita T, Kurihara H, Maemura K, Yoshizumi M, Yazaki Y. Disruption of cytoskeletal structures mediates shear stress-induced endothelin-1 gene expression in cultured porcine aortic endothelial cells. *J Clin Invest* 1993; **92**: 1706–1712.
152. Kohan DE. Production of endothelin-1 by rat mesangial cells: regulation by tumor necrosis factor. *J Lab Clin Med* 1992; **119**: 477–484.
153. Bunchman TE, Brookshire CA. Cyclosporine-induced synthesis of endothelin by cultured human endothelial cells. *J Clin Invest* 1991; **88**: 310–314.
154. Zoja C, Morigi M, Figliuzzi M, *et al.* Proximal tubular cell synthesis and secretion of endothelin-1 on challenge with albumin and other proteins. *Am J Kidney Dis* 1995; **26**: 934–941.
155. Chua BH, Chua CC, Diglio CA, Siu BB. Regulation of endothelin-1 mRNA by angiotensin II in rat heart endothelial cells. *Biochim Biophys Acta* 1993; **1178**: 201–206.
156. Iwasaki S, Homma T, Matsuda Y, Kon V. Endothelin receptor subtype B mediates autoinduction of endothelin-1 in rat mesangial cells. *J Biol Chem* 1995; **270**: 6997–7003.
157. Orphanides C, Fine LF, Norman JT. Hypoxia stimulates proximal tubular cell matrix production via a TGF-β1-independent mechanism. *Kidney Int* 1997; **52**: 637–647.
158 Combe C, Burton CJ, Dufourcq P, *et al.* Hypoxia induces intracellular adhesion molecule-1 on cultured human tubular cells. *Kidney Int* 1997; **51**: 1703–1709.
159. Gómez-Garre D, Largo R, Liu X-H *et al.* An orally active ET_A/ET_B receptor antagonist ameliorates proteinuria and glomerular lesions in rats with proliferative nephritis. *Kidney Int* 1996; **50**: 962–972.
160. Guarda E, Katwa LC, Myers PR, Tyagi SC, Weber KT. Effects of endothelins on collagen turnover in cardiac fibroblasts. *Cardiovasc Res* 1993; **27**: 2130–2134.
161. Ong ACM, Jowett TP, Firth JD, Burton S, Karet FE, Fine LG. An endothelin-1 mediated autocrine growth loop involved in human renal tubular regeneration. *Kidney Int* 1995; **48**: 390–401.
162. Kon V, Hunley TE, Fogo A. Combined antagonism of endothelin A/B receptors links endothelin to vasoconstriction whereas angiotensin II effects fibrosis. Studies in chronic cyclosporine nephrotoxicity in rats. *Transplantation* 1995; **60**: 89–95.
163. Nakamura T, Ebihara I, Tomino Y, Koide H. Effect of a specific endothelin A receptor antagonist on murine lupus nephritis. *Kidney Int* 1995; **47**: 481–489.
164. Benigni A, Zoja C, Corna D, *et al.* Blocking both type A and B endothelin receptors in

the kidney attenuates renal injury and prolongs survival in rats with remnant kidney. *Am J Kidney Dis* 1996; **27**: 416–423.

165. Hocher B, Thone-Reineke C, Rohmeiss P, *et al.* Endothelin-1 transgenic mice develop glomerulosclerosis, interstitial fibrosis, and renal cysts but not hypertension. *J Clin Invest* 1997; **99**: 1380–1389.
166. Fellström B, Klareskog L, Heldin CH, *et al.* Platelet-derived growth factor receptors in the kidney—Upregulated expression in inflammation. *Kidney Int* 1989; **36**: 1099–1102.
167. Gesualdo L, Di Paolo S, Milani S, *et al.* Expression of platelet-derived growth factor receptors in normal and diseased human kidney. *J Clin Invest* 1994; **94**: 50–58.
168. Levéen P, Pekny M, Gebre-Medhin S, Swolin B, Larsson E, Betsholtz C. Mice deficient for PDGF B show renal, cardiovascular, and hematological abnormalities. *Genes Dev* 1994; **8**: 1875–1887.
169. Bostrom H, Willetts K, Pekny M, *et al.* PDGF-A signaling is a critical event in lung alveolar myofibroblast development and alveogenesis. *Cell* 1996; **85**: 863–873.
170. Nikolic-Paterson DJ, Main IW, Tesch GH, Lan HY, Atkins RC. Interleukin-1 in renal fibrosis. *Kidney Int* 1996; **49**: S88–S90.
171. Yoshioka K, Takemura T, Murakami K, *et al.* *In situ* expression of cytokines in IgA nephritis. *Kidney Int* 1993; **44**: 825–833.
172. Lan HY, Nikolic-Paterson DJ, Zarama M, Vannice JL, Atkins RC. Suppression of experimental crescentic glomerulonephritis by the interleukin-1 receptor antagonist. *Kidney Int* 1993; **43**: 479–485.
173. Lan HY, Nikolic-Paterson DJ, Wu W, Vannice JL, Atkins RC. Interleukin-1 receptor antagonist halts the progression of established crescentic glomerulonephritis in the rat. *Kidney Int* 1995; **47**: 1303–1309.
174. Morita H, Shinzato T, David G, *et al.* Basic fibroblast growth factor-binding domain of heparan sulfate in the human glomerulosclerosis and renal tubulointerstitial fibrosis. *Lab Invest* 1994; **71**: 528–535.
175. Ichimura T, Maier JAM, Maciag T, Zhang G, Stevens JL. FGF-1 in normal and regenerating kidney: expression in mononuclear, interstitial, and regenerating epithelial cells. *Am J Physiol* 1995; **269**: F653–F662.
176. Ray PE, Bruggeman LA, Weeks BS, *et al.* bFGF and its low affinity receptors in the pathogenesis of HIV-associated nephropathy in transgenic mice. *Kidney Int* 1994; **46**: 759–772.
177. Phillips AO, Steadman R, Morrisey K, Williams JD. Polarity of stimulation and secretion of transforming growth factor-β1 by cultured proximal tubular cells. *Am J Pathol* 1997; **150**: 1101–1111.
178. Taniguchi Y, Yorioka N, Yamashita K, *et al.* Hepatocyte growth factor localization in primary glomerulonephritis and drug-induced interstitial nephritis. *Nephron* 1996; **73**: 357–358.
179. Morrissey JJ, Ishidoya S, McCracken R, Klahr S. Nitric oxide generation ameliorates the tubulointerstitial fibrosis of obstructive nephropathy. *J Am Soc Nephrol* 1996; **7**: 2202–2212.
180. González-Avila G, Vadillo-Ortega F, Pérez-Tamayo R. Experimental diffuse interstitial renal fibrosis. A biochemical approach. *Lab Invest* 1988; **59**: 245–252.
181. Walker PD. Alterations in renal tubular extracellular matrix components after ischemia-reperfusion injury to the kidney. *Lab Invest* 1994; **70**: 339–346.
182. Gomez DE, Alonso DF, Yoshiji H, Thorgeirsson UP. Tissue inhibitors of metalloproteinases: structure, regulation and biological functions. *Eur J Cell Biol* 1997; **74**: 111–122.

183. Birkedal-Hansen H, Moore WGI, Bodden MK, *et al.* Matrix metalloproteinases: a review. *Crit Rev Oral Biol Med* 1993; **4**: 197–250.
184. Stetler-Stevenson WG. Dynamics of matrix turnover during pathologic remodeling of the extracellular matrix. *Am J Pathol* 1996; **148**: 1345–1350.
185. Lewis MP, Fine LG, Norman JT. Pexicrine effects of basement membrane components on paracrine signaling by renal tubular cells. *Kidney Int* 1996; **49**: 48–58.
186. Norman JT, Gatti L, Wilson PD, Lewis M. Matrix metalloproteinases and tissue inhibitor of matrix metalloproteinases expression by tubular epithelia and interstitial fibroblasts in the normal kidney and in fibrosis. *Exp Nephrol* 1995; **3**: 88–89.
187. Norman JT, Lewis MP. Matrix metalloproteinases (MMPs) in renal fibrosis. *Kidney Int* 1996; **49**: S61–S63.
188. Greene J, Wang M, Lui YE, Raymond LA, Rosen C, Shi YE. Molecular cloning and characterization of human tissue inhibitor of metalloproteinase 4. *J Biol Chem* 1996; **271**: 30375–30380.
189. Eddy AA. Expression of genes that promote renal interstitial fibrosis in rats with proteinuria. *Kidney Int* 1996; **49**: S49–S54.
190. Suzuki D, Miyazaki M, Jinde K, *et al. In situ* hybridization studies of matrix metalloproteinase-3, tissue inhibitor of metalloproteinase-1 and type IV collagen in diabetic nephropathy. *Kidney Int* 1997; **52**: 111–119.
191. Heidland A, Sebekova K, Paczek L, Teschner M, Dämmrich J, Gaciong Z. Renal fibrosis: role of impaired proteolysis and potential therapeutic strategies. *Kidney Int* 1997; **52**: S32–S35.
192. Stetler-Stevenson WG, Brown PD, Onisto M, Levy AT, Liotta LA. Tissue inhibitor of metalloproteinases-2 (TIMP-2) mRNA expression in tumor cell lines and human tumor tissues. *J Biol Chem* 1990; **265**: 13933–13938.
193. Wick M, Bürger C, Brüsselbach S, Lucibello FC, Müller R. A novel member of human tissue inhibitor of metalloproteinases (TIMP) gene family is regulated during G_1 progression, mitogenic stimulation, differentiation, and senescence. *J Biol Chem* 1994; **269**: 18953–18960.
194. Anand-Apte B, Bao L, Smith R, *et al.* A review of tissue inhibitor of metalloproteinases-3 (TIMP-3) and experimental analysis of its effect on primary tumor growth. *Biochem Cell Biol* 1996; **74**: 853–862.
195. Teschner M, Paczek L, Schaefer RM, Heidland A. Obese Zucker rat: potential role of intraglomerular proteolytic enzymes in the development of glomerulosclerosis. *Res Exp Med* 1991; **191**: 129–135.
196. Reckelhoff JF, Baylis C. Glomerular metalloprotease activity in the aging rat kidney: inverse correlation with injury. *J Am Soc Nephrol* 1993; **3**: 1835–1838.
197. Schaefer L, Teschner M, Ling H, Oldakowska U, Heidland A, Schaefer RM. The aging rat kidney displays low glomerular and tubular proteinase activities. *Am J Kidney Dis* 1994; **24**: 499–504.
198. Paczek L, Teschner M, Schaefer RM, Kovar J, Romen W, Heidland A. Proteinase activity in isolated glomeruli of Goldblatt hypertensive rats. *Clin Exp Hypertens A* 1991; **13**: 339–356.
199. Schaefer L, Meier K, Hafner C, Teschner M, Heidland A, Schaefer RM. Protein restriction influences glomerular matrix turnover and tubular hypertrophy by modulation of renal proteinase activities. *Miner Electrolyte Metab* 1996; **22**: 162–167.
200. Lacraz S, Nicod LP, Chicheportiche R, Welgus H, Dayer JM. IL-10 inhibits metalloproteinase and stimulates TIMP-1 production in human mononuclear phagocytes. *J Clin Invest* 1995; **96**: 2304–2310.

201. Edwards DR, Murphy G, Reynolds JJ, *et al.* Transforming growth factor beta modulates the expression of collagenase and metalloproteinase inhibitor. *EMBO J* 1987; **6**: 1899–1904.
202. Marti HP, Lee L, Kashgarian M, Lovett DH. Transforming growth factor-beta 1 stimulates glomerular mesangial cell synthesis of the 72-kd type IV collagenase. *Am J Pathol* 1994; **144**: 82–94.
203. Turck J, Pollock AS, Lee LK, Marti HP, Lovett DH. Matrix metalloproteinase 2 (gelatinase A) regulates glomerular mesangial cell proliferation and differentiation. *J Biol Chem* 1996; **271**: 15074–15083.
204. Kitamura M, Shirasawa T, Maruyama N. Gene transfer of metalloproteinase transin induces aberrant behavior of cultured mesangial cells. *Kidney Int* 1994; **45**: 1580–1586.
205. Turck J, Pollock AS, Lovett DH. Gelatinase A is a glomerular mesangial cell growth and differentiation factor. *Kidney Int* 1997; **51**: 1397–1400.
206. Marcotte PA, Kozan IM, Dorwin SA, Ryan JM. The matrix metalloproteinase pump-1 catalyzes formation of low molecular weight (Pro) urokinase in cultures of normal human kidney cells. *J Biol Chem* 1992; **267**: 13803–13806.
207. Gunja-Smith Z, Morales AR, Romanelli R, Woessner JF Jr. Remodeling of human myocardial collagen in idiopathic dilated cardiomyopathy. *Am J Pathol* 1996; **148**: 1639–1648.
208. Romer J, Bugge TH, Pyke C, *et al.* Impaired wound healing in mice with a disrupted plasminogen gene. *Nature Med* 1996; **2**: 287–292.
209. Meroni G, Buraggi G, Mantovani R, Taramelli R. Motifs resembling hepatocyte nuclear factor 1 and activator protein 3 mediate the tissue specificity of the human plasminogen gene. *Eur J Biochem* 1996; **236**: 373–382.
210. Eddy AA. Interstitial inflammation and fibrosis in rats with diet-induced hypercholesterolemia. *Kidney Int* 1996; **50**: 1139–1149.
211. Keeton M, Ahn C, Eguchi Y, Burlingame R, Loskutoff DJ. Expression of type 1 plasminogen activator inhibitor in renal tissue in murine lupus nephritis. *Kidney Int* 1995; **47**: 148–157.
212. Oikawa T, Freeman M, Lo W, Vaughan DE, Fogo A. Modulation of plasminogen activator inhibitor-1 *in vivo*: a new mechanism for the anti-fibrotic effect of renin-angiotensin inhibition. *Kidney Int* 1997; **51**: 164–172.
213. Lyons RM, Gentry LE, Purchio AF, Moses HL. Mechanism of activation of latent recombinant transforming growth factor beta 1 by plasmin. *J Cell Biol* 1990; **110**: 1361–1367.
214. Eitzman DT, McCoy RD, Zheng X, *et al.* Bleomycin-induced pulmonary fibrosis in transgenic mice that either lack or overexpress the murine plasminogen activator inhibitor-1 gene. *J Clin Invest* 1996; **97**: 232–237.
215. Nath KA, Hostetter MK, Hostetter TH. Pathophysiology of chronic tubulointerstitial disease in rats: Interactions of dietary acid load, ammonia and complement component C3. *J Clin Invest* 1985; **76**: 667–675.
216. Fine LG, Ong ACM, Norman JT. Mechanisms of tubulo-interstitial injury in progressive renal diseases. *Eur J Clin Invest* 1993; **23**: 259–265.
217. Moorhead JF, Chan MK, El-Nahas M, Varghese Z. Lipid nephrotoxicity in chronic progressive glomerular and tubulo-interstitial disease. *Lancet* 1982; **2**: 1309–1311.
218. Bertani T, Cutillo F, Zoja C, Broggini M, Remuzzi G. Tubulo-interstitial lesions mediate renal damage in adriamycin glomerulopathy. *Kidney Int* 1986; **30**: 488–496.
219. Eddy AA, McCulloch L, Liu E, Adams J. A relationship between proteinuria and acute

tubulointerstitial disease in rats with experimental nephrotic syndrome. *Am J Pathol* 1991; **138**: 1111–1123.

220. Kees-Folts D, Sadow JL, Schreiner GF. Tubular catabolism of albumin is associated with the release of an inflammatory lipid. *Kidney Int* 1994; **45**: 1697–1709.
221. Hirschberg R. Bioactivity of glomerular ultrafiltrate during heavy proteinuria may contribute to renal tubulo-interstitial lesions. *J Clin Invest* 1996; **98**: 116–124.
222. Maack T, Park CH, Camargo MJF. Renal filtration, transport, and metabolism of proteins, In: Seldin DW, Giebisch G (eds), *The Kidney: Physiology and Pathophysiology*. Raven Press, New York, 1985: 1773–1803.
223. Alfrey AC, Foment DH, Hammond WS. Role of iron in tubulo-interstitial injury in nephrotoxic serum nephritis. *Kidney Int* 1989; **36**: 753–759.
224. Nankivell BJ, Tay Y-C, Boadle RA, Harris DCH. Dietary protein alters tubular iron accumulation after partial nephrectomy. *Kidney Int* 1994; **45**: 1006–1013.
225. Chen L, Boadle RA, Harris DCH. Toxicity of holotransferrin but not albumin in proximal tubule cells in primary culture. *J Am Soc Nephrol* 1998; **9**: 77–84.
226. Kumar S, Muchmore A. Tamm-Horsfall protein–uromodulin (1950–90). *Kidney Int* 1990; **37**: 1395–1401.
227. Neilson EG, Jimenez SA, Phillips SM. Cell-mediated immunity in interstitial nephritis. III. T Lymphocyte-mediated fibroblast proliferation and collagen synthesis: an immune mechanism for renal fibrogenesis. *J Immunol* 1980; **125**: 1708–1714.
228. Kelly CJ, Roth DA, Meyers CM. Immune recognition and response to the renal interstitium. *Kidney Int* 1991; **39**: 518–530.
229. Rubin-Kelley VE, Jevnikar AM. Antigen presentation by renal tubular epithelial cells. *J Am Soc Nephrol* 1991; **2**: 13–26.
230. Weiss RA, Madaio MP, Tomaszewski JE, Kelly CJ. T cells reactive to an inducible heat shock protein induce disease in toxin-induced interstitial nephritis. *J Exp Med* 1994; **180**: 2239–2250.
231. Schrier RW, Harris DCH, Chan L, Shapiro JI, Caramelo C. Tubular hypermetabolism as a factor in the progression of chronic renal failure. *Am J Kidney Dis* 1988; **3**: 243–249.
232. Schrier RW, Shapiro JI, Chan L, Harris DCH. Increased nephron oxygen consumption: potential role in progression of chronic renal disease. *Am J Kidney Dis* 1994; **23**: 176–182.
233. Maschio G, Oldrizzi L, Tessitore N, *et al.* Effects of dietary protein and phosphorus restriction on the progression of early renal failure. *Kidney Int* 1982; **22**: 371–376.
234. Barsotti G, Giannoni A, Morelli E, *et al.* The decline of renal function slowed by very low phosphorus intake in chronic renal patients following a low nitrogen diet. *Clin Nephrol* 1984; **21**: 54–59.
235. Lau K. Phosphate excess and progressive renal failure: the precipitation-calcification hypothesis (clinical conference). *Kidney Int* 1989; **36**: 918–937.
236. Yamamoto T, Nakamura T, Noble NA, Ruoslahti E, Border WA. Expression of transforming growth factor β is elevated in human and experimental diabetic nephropathy. *Proc Natl Acad Sci USA* 1993; **90**: 1814–1818.
237. Yamamoto T, Noble NA, Cohen AH, *et al.* Expression of transforming growth factor-β isoforms in human glomerular diseases. *Kidney Int* 1996; **49**: 461–469.
238. Yamamoto T, Noble NA, Miller DE, Gold LI, Hishida A, Nagase M, Cohen AH, Border WA. Increased levels of transforming growth factor-beta in HIV-associated nephropathy. *Kidney Int* 1999; **55**: 579–592.
239. Bódi I, Kimmel PL, Abraham AA, Svetkey LP, Klotman PE, Kopp JB. Renal TGF-beta in HIV-associated kidney diseases. *Kidney Int* 1997; **51**: 1568–1577.

240. Niemir ZI, Stein H, Noronha IL, *et al.* PDGF and TGF-β contribute to the natural course of human IgA glomerulonephritis. *Kidney Int* 1995; **48**: 1530–1541.
241. Shihab FS, Yamamoto T, Nast CC, *et al.* Transforming growth factor-beta and matrix protein expression in acute and chronic rejection of human renal allografts. *J Am Soc Nephrol* 1995; **6**: 286–294.
242. Sharma VK, Bologa RM, Xu GP, *et al.* Intragraft TGF-β1 mRNA. a correlate of interstitial fibrosis and chronic allograft nephropathy. *Kidney Int* 1996; **49**: 1297–1303.
243. Gaciong Z, Koziak Religa P, *et al.* Increased expression of growth factors during chronic rejection of human kidney allograft. *Transplant Proc* 1995; **27**: 928–929.
244. Goes N, Urmson J, Ramassar V, Halloran PF. Ischemic acute tubular necrosis induces an extensive local cytokine response. Evidence for induction of interferon-gamma, transforming growth factor-beta 1, granulocyte-macrophage colony-stimulating factor, interleukin-2, and interleukin-10. *Transplantation* 1995; **59**: 565–572.
245. Coimbra T, Wiggins R, Noh JW, Merritt S, Phan SH. Transforming growth factor-β production in anti-glomerular basement membrane disease in the rabbit. *Am J Pathol* 1991; **138**: 223–234.
246. Shihab FS, Andoh TF, Tanner AM, *et al.* Role of transforming growth factor-β1 in experimental chronic cyclosporine nephropathy. *Kidney Int* 1996; **49**: 1141–1151.
247. Shihab FS, Bennett WM, Tanner AM, Andoh TF. Mechanism of fibrosis in experimental tacrolimus nephrotoxicity. *Transplantation* 1997; **64**: 1829–1837.
248. Eddy AA, Li Z, Liu E, McCulloch L. Macrophages may mediate interstitial fibrosis via the release of transforming growth factor β1 in passive Heymann nephritis. *J Am Soc Nephrol* 1991; **2**: 573.
249. Kopp JB, McCune BK, Notkins AL, Sporn MB, Klotman PE. Increased expression of transforming growth factor β in HIV-transgenic mouse kidney. *J Am Soc Nephrol* 1991; **3**: 600 (Abstr.).
250. Nakamura T, Ebihara I, Nagaoka I, Osada S, Tomino Y, Koide H. Effect of methylprednisolone on transforming growth factor-beta, insulin-like growth factor-I, and basic fibroblast growth factor gene expression in the kidneys of NZB/W F1 mice. *Renal Physiol Biochem* 1993; **16**: 105–116.
251. Lavaud S, Heudes D, Bariéty J, Chevalier J. Mediators involved in the pathogenesis of interstitial fibrosis in the obese Zucker rat model. *J Am Soc Nephrol* 1997; **8**: 520 (Abstr.).
252. Nakamura T, Ebihara I, Nagaoka I, *et al.* Growth factor gene expression in kidney of murine polycystic kidney disease. *J Am Soc Nephrol* 1993; **3**: 1378–1386.
253. Coimbra TM, Carvalho J, Fattori A, Da Silva CG, Lachat JJ. Transforming growth factor-beta production during the development of renal fibrosis in rats with subtotal renal ablation. *Int J Exp Pathol* 1996; **77**: 167–173.
254. Tang WW, Feng L, Xia Y, Wilson CB. Extracellular matrix accumulation in immune-mediated tubulointerstitial injury. *Kidney Int* 1994; **45**: 1077–1084.
255. Duymelinck C, Deng JT, Dauwe SE, De Broe ME, Verpooten GA. Inhibition of the matrix metalloproteinase system in a rat model of chronic cyclosporine nephropathy. *Kidney Int* 1998; **54**: 804–818.
256. Wu K, Setty S, Mauer SM, *et al.* Altered kidney matrix gene expression in early stages of experimental disease. *Acta Anat* 1997; **158**: 155–165.
257. Nakamura T, Ebihara I, Osada S, *et al.* Gene expression of metalloproteinases and their inhibitor in renal tissue of New Zealand black/white F1 mice. *Clin Sci* 1993; **85**: 295–301.
258. Sharma AK, Mauer SM, Kim Y, Michael AF. Altered expression of matrix metallo-

proteinase-2, TIMP, and TIMP-2 in obstructive nephropathy. *J Lab Clin Med* 1995; **125**: 754–761.

259. Engelmyer E, Goor H, Edwards DR, Diamond JR. Differential mRNA expression of renal cortical tissue inhibitor of metalloproteinase-1-2, and -3 in experimental hydronephrosis. *J Am Soc Nephrol* 1995; **5**: 1675–1683.
260. Schaefer L, Han X, Gretz N, *et al.* Tubular gelatinase A (MMP-2) and its tissue inhibitors in polycystic kidney disease in the Han:SPRD Rat. *Kidney Int* 1996; **49**: 75–81.
261. Duymelinck C, Dauwe SE, Nouwen EJ, DeBroe ME, Verpooten GA. Cholesterol feeding accentuates the cyclosporin-induced elevation of renal plasminogen activator inhibitor type I. *Kidney Int* 1997; **51**: 1818–1830.
262. Moll S, Schifferli JA, Huarte J, Lemoine R, Vassalli J-D, Sappino A-P. LPS induces major changes in the extracellular proteolytic balance in the murine kidney. *Kidney Int* 1994; **45**: 500–508.
263. Keeton M, Eguchi Y, Sawdey M, Ahn C, Loskutoff DJ. Cellular localization of type 1 plasminogen activator inhibitor messenger RNA and protein in murine renal tissue. *Am J Pathol* 1993; **142**: 59–70.
264. Eddy AA. Expression of genes that promote renal interstitial fibrosis in rats with proteinuria. *Kidney Int* 1996; **54**: S49–S54.
265. Wang Y, Pratt JR, Hartley B, Evans B, Zhang L, Sacks SH. Expression of tissue type plasminogen activator and type 1 plasminogen activator inhibitor, and persistent fibrin deposition in chronic renal allograft failure. *Kidney Int* 1997; **52**: 371–377.
266. Shihab FS, Tanner AM, Shao Y, Weffer MI. Expression of TGF-beta 1 and matrix proteins is elevated in rats with chronic rejection. *Kidney Int* 1996; **50**: 1904–1913.
267. Fine LG, Orphanides C, Norman JT. Progressive renal disease: the chronic hypoxia hypothesis. *Kidney Int* 1998; **53** (Suppl. 65): S74–S78.

5

Proteinuria: implications for progression and management

Kevin P. G. Harris

Introduction

It is a well established observation from both human and animal studies of renal disease, that once a degree of renal damage has occurred then the progression of kidney failure is inexorable, even if the original injurious process has resolved [1]. Such observations have led to the hypothesis that following renal damage of any aetiology a maladaptive response occurs in the remaining nephrons which results in their eventual destruction by a common pathogenic mechanism. In support of this, the histological appearance of the kidney in end-stage renal disease is similar whatever the initial cause of the renal injury; within the glomerulus there are localised areas of cellular proliferation, deposition of excess extracellular matrix (ECM) and there is collapse of the glomerular capillary. Within the interstitium there is tubular cell atrophy, a mononuclear cell infiltrate, fibroblast proliferation, and ECM deposition. These events lead to the replacement of the functioning renal tissue by scar tissue, and affects both the glomeruli and the tubulo-interstitium, culminating in glomerulosclerosis and tubulo-interstitial fibrosis, respectively. This process which is more accurately defined as 'nephrosclerosis' causes the subsequent development of chronic renal failure (CRF).

A variety of potential 'maladaptive responses' have been identified including hemodynamic abnormalities [2,3], lipid abnormalities [4], and renal growth [5]. However, it is likely that the process is multifactorial [6]. There has also been considerable controversy regarding the relative importance of glomerular and interstitial pathology as it has been shown that even in primary glomerular disease there is a better correlation of renal function with markers of interstitial disease than with markers of glomerular pathology [7,8].

The development of proteinuria in which large amounts of medium and high molecular weight proteins are found in the urine is a characteristic finding in most progressive renal diseases. Proteinuria has traditionally been viewed as merely a 'marker' of renal disease—the more severe the renal disease the greater the degree of proteinuria. However, over recent years a hypothesis has developed suggesting that that proteinuria may itself be an independent determinant of the progression of renal disease, i.e. a cause of, rather than merely the consequence of progressive renal

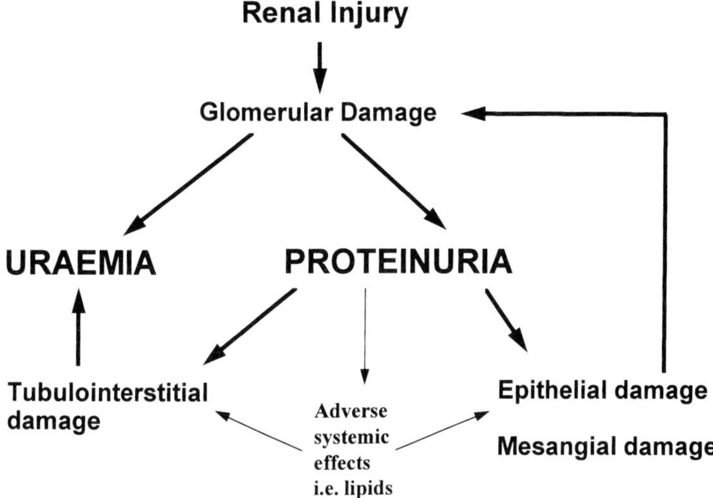

Fig. 5.1 Proteinuria as a cause of renal damage. Rather than being a consequence of renal damage proteinuria may cause further renal damage in its own right. Proteinuria may promote both glomerular and tubulo-interstitial injury.

damage (Fig. 5.1). This is an attractive hypothesis as it not only provides a mechanism by which progressive renal scarring may occur independently of the initial renal insult but also a means by which glomerular disease may ultimately result in interstitial scarring. Under normal circumstances only low molecular weight macromolecules gain access to the urinary space, larger molecules being excluded by an intact glomerular barrier. In glomerular disease, the barrier is disrupted and much larger serum proteins including albumin, gain access to both the mesangium and tubular fluid. Hence the potential exists for one or more of these abnormally filtered proteins to interact adversely with the mesangium and or the cells lining the tubular space promoting further glomerular and interstitial damage.

The evidence supporting the hypothesis that the development of proteinuria is of direct pathophysiological importance to the progression of renal disease, together with the therapeutic implications will be reviewed in the this chapter. However, it should be noted that in addition to a direct toxic effect of proteinuria, renal toxicity could be the result of changes that occur secondary to the development of proteinuria. Lipid and lipoprotein abnormalities (which are commonly found in proteinuric states) have been most extensively studied in this regard; this work is beyond the scope of this chapter but has been reviewed elsewhere [9,10].

Proteinuria: implications from experimental models of renal disease

Proteinuria is a universal finding in all experimental models of progressive CRF. The most extensively studied model is that of the 'remnant kidney' in the rat in which following a surgical reduction in renal mass, the animals develop proteinuria, hypertension, and progressive renal failure with histological evidence of glomerulosclerosis and tubulo-interstitial fibrosis [11]. These changes are essentially similar to those found in human CRF and observations made in this model have formed the basis of the majority of the hypotheses on the aetiology of progressive renal scarring. In this model, all manoeuvres which protect the animal against the development of progressive renal impairment are associated with a reduction in the severity of the proteinuria. For example in many studies the beneficial effects of antihypertensive agents on the evolution of the renal disease are associated with a reduction in the magnitude of the proteinuria. The use of angiotensin-converting enzyme (ACE) inhibitors and more recently angiotensin II receptor antagonists have been shown to have a more dramatic beneficial effect on the evolution of renal disease in this model than other antihypertensive agents. Theoretical considerations and experimental observations would suggest that these agents should be particularly effective in reducing the severity of proteinuria. It is of note that in one study ACE inhibitors reduced the level of proteinuria in the 'remnant kidney' rats to values comparable with controls, an effect that could not be reproduced by an alternative antihypertensive regimen. In parallel the degree of structural damage in the glomeruli and the tubulo-interstitium was reduced to a much greater degree in animals treated with ACE inhibitors than with the alternative regimen [12]. Similarly, dietary manipulation studies have demonstrated that feeding the animals with low protein diets or diets composed of soya rather than casein significantly reduces the amount of proteinuria and abrogates the development of renal failure [13,14]. Thus in this model the degree of proteinuria, the degree of structural damage, and the degree of renal impairment are all closely correlated.

Similar observations in a wide variety of different experimental renal diseases generally support the hypothesis that the severity of proteinuria correlates with structural changes within the kidney; for example, a recent meta-analysis of experimental models has shown a strong positive correlation between urinary protein excretion and glomerulosclerosis [15]. While such observations provide support to the hypothesis that proteinuria may be directly toxic to the kidney they cannot prove a cause and effect relationship.

Evidence in support of proteinuria having a direct renal toxic effect comes from observations made in two other animal models of proteinuria, namely puromycin aminonucleoside (PAN) nephrosis and protein overload nephropathy. These models are characterized by the development of heavy proteinuria which is accompanied by marked changes within the tubulo-interstitium. Following a single dose of PAN the animals develop nephrotic range proteinuria as a result of the direct toxicity of PAN to glomerular epithelial cells. The proteinuria worsens up to 14 days, associated with renal impairment and then returns to normal. Closely related to the time course for proteinuria there is an influx into the interstitium of chronic inflammatory cells including macrophages and lymphocytes [16]. There is a clear relationship between the degree of the proteinuria and the severity of the interstitial infiltrate and both are reduced by dietary protein restriction [17]. As the proteinuria develops there is a significant increase in renal mRNA for the chemokine monocyte chemoattractant protein 1 (MCP-1) [18], although neutralizing antibodies to MCP-1 do not attenuate macrophage recruitment. This model is also characterized by foci of tubulo-interstitial fibrosis and mRNA levels for genes encoding ECM proteins, tissue inhibitors of metalloproteinases and transforming growth factor β1 are all increased in association with the development of proteinuria and the interstitial infiltrate. The institution of dietary protein restriction to reduce proteinuria reverses these effects [17].

Proteinuria can also be induced in rats by intraperitoneal injection of large amounts (5 g/day) of bovine serum albumin (BSA) (protein overload nephropathy). The animals develop heavy proteinuria with no evidence of immune complex deposition in the glomeruli or the interstitium, nor is there evidence of circulating anti-BSA antibodies. Ultrastructural examination of the glomeruli in this model indicates widespread foot process effacement, although the cause of this is unknown [19]. As the proteinuria increases there is an influx of chronic inflammatory cells into the interstitium and an accumulation of ECM proteins [20,21]. The aetiology of the interstitial infiltrate is complex but there is a significant increase in renal mRNA for the chemotactic substances MCP-1 and osteopontin in association with the development of the proteinuria [21]. In this model there is also evidence of changes in tubular cell turnover with increases in both proliferation and apoptosis [22]. As this is a non-immune model of heavy proteinuria without significant renal impairment, in the absence of any other explanation it has been proposed that the changes that occur within the kidney are a result of the proteinuria that develops. The proteinuria could be directly toxic to the tubular epithelial cells altering their phenotype. Alternatively, the recruitment of macrophages and lymphocytes into the interstitium [20], could provide a mechanism for the increased matrix protein synthesis and altered matrix degradation and remodelling [21] (see section on mechanisms of toxicity of proteinuria). Recent studies have suggested that the severity of tubulo-interstitial damage that develops in this model is dependent on the fatty acid composition of the albumin that is injected, with the degree of macrophage infiltration and tubular apoptosis being significantly less in rats injected with albumin devoid of fatty acids compared with those given fatty acid replete albumin [22]. This was despite both groups having comparable degrees of proteinuria and suggests that it may not be the albumin protein *per se* that is damaging to the kidney but the uptake and metabolism of albumin-associated fatty acids.

In some studies the correlation between the development of heavy proteinuria and renal scarring has been more difficult to demonstrate. For example in Adriamycin nephrosis and Heymann nephritis there is heavy proteinuria but little renal structural damage in the short term [23]. However, it is now clear from longer-term studies using these models that protracted proteinuria is associated with glomerular and tubulo-interstitial injury and that manoeuvres which reduce the severity of the proteinuria reduce the renal structural damage and preserve renal function [24–26].

Proteinuria: implications from human renal diseases

Clinical observations made over the past few decades have clearly demonstrated a strong correlation between the rate of progression of CRF and the quantity of

Table 5.1 Human renal diseases in which the presence and or severity of proteinuria has been associated with a faster rate of progression and a poor renal outcome

Nephrotic syndrome
Membranous
Focal segmental glomerular sclerosis
Mesangiocapillary glomerulonephritis
Glomerulonephritis
IgA nephropathy
Acute endocapillary glomerulonephritis
Lupus nephritis
Others
Diabetic nephropathy
Reflux nephropathy
Chronic transplant glomerulopathy

proteinuria in a number of very different renal diseases (see Table 5.1). Such observations would lend support but do not prove that proteinuria may have a causal role in the development of progressive renal failure. Perhaps the best studied renal disease in this regard is diabetic nephropathy in which the development of proteinuria is known to predict the subsequent progression of the nephropathy (see chapter 7). The adverse prognostic significance of proteinuria has also been demonstrated for a variety of different primary renal diseases. For example in 40 consecutive patients with focal and segmental glomerulosclerosis followed from 6 to 16 years, those presenting with nephrotic syndrome had a worse prognosis than those presenting with less proteinuria [27]. Similar observations have been made in mesangiocapillary glomerulonephritis type I, where the presence and persistence of nephrotic syndrome predicted renal failure [28] and in patients with idiopathic membranous nephropathy, where 41% of patients presenting with nephrotic syndrome (followed for a mean of 54.8 months) developed progressive renal failure, compared with none of those presenting with less than nephrotic range proteinuria [29]. Similarly a recent study of patients with idiopathic membranous glomerulonephritis determined that the highest sustained six-month period of proteinuria was an important predictor of progression to CRF [30]. In addition a study of nearly 300 patients with IgA nephropathy demonstrated that proteinuria of more than 1 g/day was an independent variable associated with poor renal prognosis [31]. In transplanted kidneys the development of proteinuria correlates with the development of chronic rejection [32]. Indeed, review of renal outcome in a variety of different primary renal diseases would suggest that the renal outcome is better predicted by the magnitude of proteinuria than by the underlying renal diagnosis [33].

Further studies have also been able to demonstrate a more direct correlation between the magnitude of the proteinuria and the subsequent decline in renal function, with patients with more severe proteinuria having a faster rate of progression. A study from the UK demonstrated a significant correlation between the degree of proteinuria and the rate of decline in renal function for three different renal diseases (proliferative, membranoproliferative and membranous glomerulonephritis) [34] and data from the Medical Research Council (UK) glomerulonephritis registry demonstrated that the magnitude of the proteinuria initially was predictive of subsequent plasma creatinine over a mean 52-month follow-up period. Furthermore, a retrospective analysis of patients with CRF in Sweden indicated that an increasing magnitude of proteinuria was an adverse prognostic factor for progression irrespective of the aetiology of the renal disease [35]. Such data support the view that excessive glomerular protein filtration may play an important aetiological role in the development of subsequent renal injury.

The predictive value of the severity of proteinuria on the rate of progression of CRF has recently been confirmed in several large prospective studies of progressive CRF, including studies in the USA (the Modification of Diet in Renal Disease study) [36] and Europe (the Ramipril Efficacy in Nephropathy study) [37]. In these studies the degree of proteinuria clearly predicted the rate of progression of the renal disease. Those patients with lesser degrees of proteinuria has a slower rate of progression than those with greater degrees of proteinuria. Using the Cox proportional hazard regression model to identify only those factors which are significantly associated with renal survival, the degree of proteinuria has been shown to be an even more important prognostic factor for renal death than hypertension. Furthermore, the cumulative renal survival of patients whose proteinuria decreased during the trial follow-up was better than those of patients without changes [38]. Others have confirmed that proteinuria is the best independent predictor of the progression of CRF and have speculated that hypertension may contribute to the acceleration of disease progression by enhancing the traffic of macromolecules through the damaged glomerular barrier.

Thus the rate of progression of CRF in a variety of very different primary renal pathologies is predicted by the severity of proteinuria suggesting a potential pathogenic link between proteinuria and the development of renal scarring.

Which particular component of the proteinuric urine is responsible for its nephrotoxic effect is little understood. A recent study examining sodium dodecyl sulphate–polyacrylamide gel electrophoresis patterns has identified that the presence of low molecular weight ('tubular') proteins in the urine of humans with progressive glomerulonephritis has a predictive value for renal outcome in focal and segmental glomerulosclerosis and membranous glomerulonephritis. This pattern of proteinuria may also be of predictive value for responsiveness to therapy [39]. However, such observations may merely reflect the toxic potential of glomerular proteinuria to the tubulo-interstitium rather than suggest a pathogenic role for low molecular weight proteins in the development of renal scarring.

Histological evaluation of renal biopsies from patients with proteinuria have demonstrated a marked interstitial infiltrate of monocytes/macrophages [40,41]; the presence of such biologically active cells within the interstitium provides further evidence for tubulo-interstitial damage in response to proteinuria and provides a mechanism whereby interstitial fibrosis may be initiated as monocytes/macrophages are potent sources of proinflammatory and profibrotic cytokines.

One of the major potential flaws in the arguments in favour of proteinuria having a pathogenic role in the progression of renal scarring is the absence of chronic renal damage found in patients with minimal change glomerulonephritis [42]. This condition is characterized by very large amounts of protein, predominantly albumin leaking through the glomerulus and appearing in the urine and yet renal scarring and renal failure are rare. This discrepancy may be explained by the limited duration of the proteinuria in minimal change disease, which is usually readily sensitive to steroids in contrast to progressive renal diseases in which the proteinuria is prolonged. Increased excretion of the tubular protein *N*-acetyl-β-glucosaminidase (NAG) has been shown in minimal change nephrotic syndrome [43] indicating a degree of tubular damage. The NAG excretion returns to normal when proteinuria decreases during remission of the disease. In addition a tubulo-interstitial infiltrate of macrophages/monocytes is observed in renal biopsies taken when the patients have heavy proteinuria [41]. Therefore, in minimal change disease the tubular injury is either of insufficient degree to result in long-term changes or it is of insufficient duration. An alternative explanation to this paradox may be provided by the observation that the effect of albumin on tubular cell function *in vitro* is dependent on the fatty acid composition of the albumin (discussed on pages 162–163). Significantly, urinary albumin in minimal change disease has a markedly lower fatty acid content compared with that from adult nephrotic patients [44] and could therefore have a lower potential for initiating injury.

Intervention studies: implications for therapy in human proteinuric renal disease

If it is accepted that proteinuria is of pathogenic importance to the progression of CRF, the prospect exists that strategies aimed at decreasing the level of proteinuria (or modifying it qualitatively) could have a significant impact on the evolution of CRF. Such strategies could prevent or at least delay the need for initiation of renal replacement therapy. Evidence is now accumulating that this is the case.

Control of blood pressure

It is now well established that the control of hypertension delays the decline in renal function in both diabetic [45] and non-diabetic renal [46] diseases. In the majority of studies control of hypertension (achieved with a variety of different therapies) is associated with a reduction in proteinuria. and retardation of the progression of CRF irrespective of the aetiology. However, it is difficult to define the respective roles of lowering blood pressure and reducing proteinuria on progression, although it is of note that the magnitude of the initial reduction in proteinuria brought about by the control of hypertension has been shown to correlate with the beneficial effect of the therapy in slowing the long-term decline in renal function [37,47].

Angiotensin-converting enzyme inhibition

In recent years the use of ACE inhibitors have been shown to be of particular benefit in slowing the progression of diabetic [48] and non-diabetic [37,49,50] proteinuric renal diseases. The use of ACE inhibitors is generally associated with a larger reduction in the degree of proteinuria that other classes of anti-hypertensive agent, especially the dihydropyridine calcium channel blockers which have been reported to have untoward effects on the level of proteinuria in some studies (reviewed in [51]). Thus, although calcium channel blockers are effective antihypertensive agents and may have renoprotective actions in their own right (independent of any antiproteinuric effect), they should not necessarily be considered as first-line therapy in proteinuric renal diseases where other agents (especially ACE inhibitors) have been shown to be more effective in delaying progression.

The significance of proteinuria to the progression of renal disease has recently been further supported by several studies demonstrating that a reduction in proteinuria accomplished with the use of an ACE inhibitor is associated with a slowing of the rate of progression of renal failure. The short-term antiproteinuric effect of ACE inhibition has been shown to predict the long-term renal outcome [52]. Furthermore, Praga *et al.* demonstrated that the beneficial effect of ACE inhibition on progression was only observed in those patients in whom the drug brought about a reduction in the level of proteinuria [53]. In addition, a recent study using the ACE inhibitor Ramipril in patients with proteinuric non-diabetic nephropathy demonstrated the percentage reduction in proteinuria achieved by the ACE inhibitor was significantly inversely correlated with the decline in glomerular filtration rate and predicted the reduction in risk of progressive renal failure [37].

Although ACE inhibitors appear to have clear advantages in both reducing proteinuria and delaying progression, not all patients will respond favourably and in some there will be unacceptable side-effects, including hyperkalemia and acute renal failure, especially if renal artery stenosis is present. Thus it would be useful to be able to predict those patients who would benefit from the use of ACE inhibition. It has been suggested that the renoprotective effect of ACE inhibitors might be predicted by the renin response to a frusemide challenge [54]. Recent studies have examined the role of ACE gene polymorphism on the progression of renal diseases. The majority of studies have demonstrated that the deletion polymorphism (especially the homozygote DD) is a risk factor for the accelerated loss of renal function [55]. However, conflicting results exist on the predictive value of ACE gene polymorphism on the antiproteinuric and renoprotective effects of ACE inhibition. A Japanese study in patients with IgA nephropathy showed that homozygote DD genotype predicted the therapeutic effect of ACE inhibition on proteinuria (and therefore potentially on progression) [56], while a European study has associated the DD genotype with a reduction in the beneficial effects of ACE inhibition [55]. In a recent study of insulin-dependent diabetics those with the II genotype were particularly likely to benefit from the renoprotective effects of ACE inhibition [57].

Other therapies

The effects of dietary protein restriction on delaying progression of renal disease in humans continue to be much debated. Animal studies clearly demonstrate a benefit which is associated with a reduction in proteinuria. Studies in humans are less clear-cut [36], but a correlation between the effect of diet on the decline in renal function and the reduction in proteinuria has previously been reported [58].

Similar uncertainty also exists on any potential benefits on progression of treating the hyperlipidemia commonly found in proteinuric renal diseases. While such interventions have been shown to have a beneficial effect on the evolution of a variety of different experimental renal diseases [10], to date there are no studies clearly demonstrating a therapeutic benefit of lipid lowering strategies on the progression of human renal disease.

Potential mechanisms for the toxicity of proteinuria

The majority of the evidence that proteinuria is a determinant of progression of renal failure remains circumstantial and is predominantly based on correlations and/or responses to therapy such as ACE inhibition. As already discussed such evidence is open to interpretation because *in vivo* it is difficult to dissect cause from effect. However, in the past few years several lines of investigation have provided plausible potential mechanisms to explain how proteinuria might lead to progressive renal injury [59–61]. In addition, there is now a large body of evidence mostly from *in vitro* studies supportive of a potential nephrotoxic potential for proteinuria.

Any pathological processes leading to injury to the glomerulus will cause damage to the glomerular basement membrane which is the principal structure responsible for the permeability properties of the glomerulus. As a result of damage to this barrier circulating proteins will gain access to both the mesangial area and glomerular ultrafiltrate, two areas from which such proteins would normally be excluded by an intact glomerular basement membrane. Mesangial toxicity may result from mesangial overload with abnormally filtered macromolecules and tubulo-interstitial disease could result from induction of proximal tubular cell dysfunction as a result of abnormal amounts and/or types of protein being presented to the proximal tubular brush border. Experimental evidence suggests that either or both of these processes could occur. Such observations could thus provide a mechanism whereby proteinuria promotes progressive renal scarring affecting both the mesangium and tubulo-interstitial compartments of the kidney; these changes are the histological hallmark of end-stage kidney in both experimental studies and human renal disease.

Glomerular toxicity of proteinuria

In proteinuric renal diseases of diverse aetiologies which progress to CRF, the glomerular histological changes are characterised by reactive proliferation of mesangial cells, the infiltration of activated macrophages and the deposition of ECM within the mesangium and glomerular basement membrane leading to focal and segmental glomerular hyalinosis and sclerosis. In proteinuric states there is increased mesangial trafficking of macromolecules. Segmental accumulation of serum proteins including immunoglobulin M, complement, fibrinogen, and lipoproteins is found in the glomerular mesangium in a variety of animal models of progressive renal failure [23]. Furthermore, following uninephrectomy intravenously administered colloidal carbon localizes in those glomerular areas where sclerosis subsequently develops [62]. The pathological consequences of such changes have been most extensively studied in two rat models of the nephrotic syndrome, namely PAN nephrosis and Adriamycin nephrosis [23], but similar changes are also found in the histologic lesions of the rat remnant kidney model of CRF [63]. Such experimental observations have led to the hypothesis that mesangial accumulation of these macromolecules with subsequent 'mesangial overload' may produce mesangial cell injury, mesangial cell proliferation, increased production of mesangial matrix, and hence glomerulosclerosis.

The exact mechanisms whereby mesangial overload might lead to glomerulosclerosis remain uncertain. However, the close similarities between the histological changes of glomerulosclerosis and atherosclerosis [64] has raised the possibility that the mesangial deposition of lipids and lipoproteins may be of pathogenic importance. Using immunohistochemical techniques the apolipoprotein B of low-density lipoprotein (LDL) and very low-density lipoprotein (VLDL) and apolipoprotein (a) of lipoprotein (a) have been found in glomeruli in proteinuric states [65,66]. The ability of lipoproteins to modulate mesangial cell biology appears to be receptor mediated. Receptors for both LDL and VLDL are found on human mesangial cells [67] and these lipoproteins can stimulate mesangial cell proliferation [68]. *In vitro* studies have demonstrated that the interaction of LDL with its receptor on human mesangial cells stimulates the production of the oncogenes, c-*fos* and c-*jun* [67] and hence causes cell proliferation and hypertrophy [68]. In addition LDL promotes the production of the ECM protein fibronectin by mesangial cells and induces the production of chemokines (MCP-1) [69], and platelet-derived growth factors (PDGF) [67]. Thus LDL promotes a series of cellular events in mesangial cells which may propagate glomerulosclerosis, including the recruitment of macrophages which play a pivotal role in the transition from glomerular injury to glomerular sclerosis [70].

Once within the mesangium LDL may undergo oxidation either by macrophages or mesangial cells themselves to form oxidized LDL. LDL modified in this way can be taken up by the scavenger receptors of macrophages resulting in macrophage activation and further promotion of the sclerotic response. In addition, oxidized LDL is known to be more cytotoxic to mesangial cells than LDL itself [71] and may therefore promote the transition from the hypercellular response seen within an acutely injured glomerulus to the hypocelluar and fibrotic response characteristic of the sclerotic glomerulus.

Tubulo-interstitial toxicity proteinuria

It has been known for many years that in chronic renal disease the histological changes within the tubulo-interstitial compartment of the kidney closely predict the level of renal function. A number of investigators have demonstrated that there is a close inverse correlation between various aspects of interstitial pathology and renal function while the correlation between glomerular disease and renal function is generally poor [8,72]. More recently, Howie *et al.* [73], using an immunohistochemical stain for proximal tubular brush border has shown that loss of brush border is correlated with loss of renal function, measured by the reciprocal of serum creatinine, indicating that changes in tubular cell function may be of importance in this process.

Unlike glomerular pathology it is not immediately obvious why interstitial pathology should result in a decrease in renal function, although a variety of mechanisms have been proposed. As the predominant cell within this part of the kidney is the tubular cell, it is reasonable to propose that it may be responsible for orchestrating the tubulo-interstitial inflammatory response.

The mechanism of tubulo-interstitial damage in diseases of glomerular origin has been much debated; however, the development of proteinuria, which is an inevitable consequence of glomerular disease, has the potential to produce marked effects on tubular cell function and the cell biology of the tubulo-interstitium. Potential mechanisms whereby proteinuria may induce tubulo-interstitial damage are summarized in Fig. 5.2.

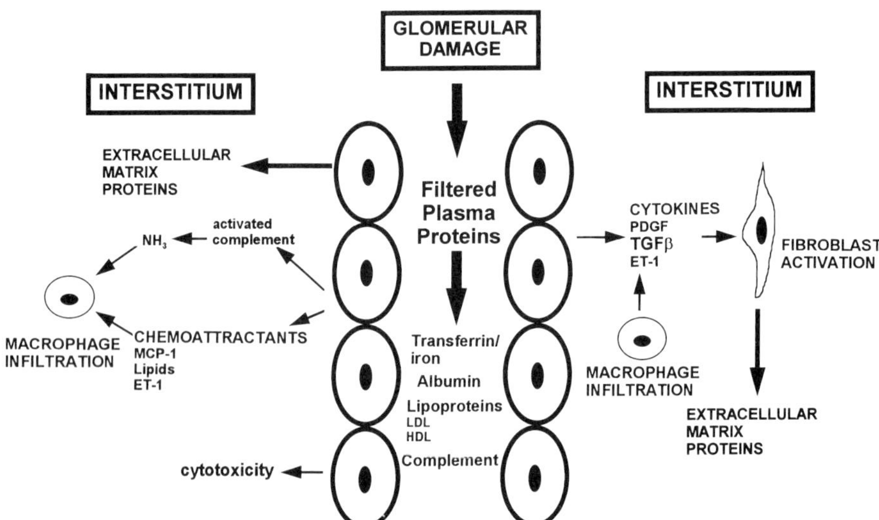

Fig. 5.2 The mechanisms by which filtered proteins may cause interstitial inflammation and scarring. Following glomerular damage proteins appear in the tubular lumen where they can be taken up by the tubular epithelium. This potentially alters the cell biology of the tubular epithelial cells, resulting in the release into the interstitium of proinflammatory cytokines, chemoattractants, and ECM proteins. Macrophage infiltration occurs with further release of cytokines and recruitment and stimulation fibroblasts. The subsequent increase in ECM results in interstitial scarring.

Uptake of proteins by tubular cells

Experimental work in the 1930s identified that proteins filtered by the glomerulus are taken up by the proximal convoluted tubule [74]. Since that time, the use of electron microscopy has identified that proteins are taken up by an apical endocytic pathway which is comprised of clathrin-coated endocytic invaginations, endocytic vesicles and vacuoles, dense apical tubules, and lysosomes [75–77]. The endocytic invaginations bud to form small endocytic vesicles or larger endocytic vacuoles [77] which then fuse with lysosomes containing enzymes for the digestion of proteins [78,79]. Proteins absorbed and transported to lysosomes are rapidly digested to amino acids [80,81]. The dense apical tubules are connected to endocytic vacuoles and form a mechanism by which membrane from vacuoles is recycled to the apical plasma membrane [82].

Investigation of albumin reabsorption in the isolated perfused proximal tubule [83] and of dextran and lysozyme reabsorption in renal cortical slices [84] has shown that protein is largely taken up by an adsorptive process with only a small contribution (2%) from non-specific fluid phase reabsorption. There is less information on the protein processing of proximal tubular cells in culture in which tubular cell ultrastructure, particularly the microvilli are less well maintained. However, in the immortalized opossum proximal tubular cell line (OK) it has been shown that uptake of albumin occurs via specific receptor-mediated endocytosis as well as by non-specific fluid phase uptake. The specific mechanism exceeds the non-specific by more than 10-fold [85]. Further studies have provided evidence for the involvement of a glycoprotein(s) in the binding of albumin to proximal tubular cells and have suggested that the receptors may be members of the family of scavenger receptors [86]. In addition, it has been shown that PI3-kinase regulates an early step in the receptor-mediated endocytosis of albumin by kidney proximal tubular cells [87] and that the uptake of albumin by its specific receptors on the cell surface is G-Protein linked [88].

Mechanisms of tubular toxicity of proteinuria

Direct toxicity It is known that higher molecular weight proteins when filtered by a damaged glomerulus are reabsorbed and metabolized by the proximal tubule which would then be vulnerable to any adverse effects that these proteins may produce. Adverse effects of proteinuria could result from either the quantity of protein in the tubular fluid or from the effects of a particular biologically active protein (or associated molecule) which is not normally found in the urine.

A variety of proteins have been demonstrated to be directly toxic to tubular epithelial cells [89]. In proteinuric states so called tubular proteins appear in the urine suggesting that there is toxic damage to the tubular epithelium. Tubular absorption of lysozyme is a high-capacity, low-affinity process and the presence of lysozyme in the final urine is a good indicator of failure of tubular reabsorption [90]. The urinary excretion of lysozyme has been shown to correlate closely with the degree of albumin excretion in passive Heymann nephritis and lysozymuria is decreased by treatments which lower albuminuria such as low protein diets or ACE inhibitors [91]. It is, however, possible that competition for protein reabsorption could result in increased urinary lysozyme in the absence of tubular damage which makes interpreting lysozymuria as a marker of tubular damage in the presence of proteinuria difficult. NAG is produced by tubular cells and released into the urine when they are injured. It is a more specific marker of tubular damage as NAG is a large protein (>125 kDa) and is only present in the serum in very low concentrations so its presence in the urine cannot be accounted for by filtration through the glomerular barrier [92]. An increase in NAG excretion has been demonstrated in patients with the nephrotic syndrome [93] and a strong correlation between the degree of proteinuria and urinary NAG excretion exists in children with a variety of glomerular disorders [43].

There is therefore evidence of direct injury to tubular cells in the presence of proteinuria, although the mechanism for this is unknown. One possible explanation is that the sheer quantity of protein required to be reabsorbed by proximal tubular cells results in injury to them as it is known that the increased trafficking of protein across the proximal tubular cell as a consequence of proteinuria results in increased lysosomal enzyme activity [94]. The leakage of lysosomal enzymes into the cytoplasm of the tubular cell and the consequent cell injury would then stimulate inflammation and scarring [83,95].

In addition to having a direct toxic effect on the tubular epithelium, increasing evidence suggests that proteins may directly modulate tubular cell function altering both their growth characteristics and their phenotypic expression of cytokines and matrix proteins.

Alteration in tubular cell growth Cell growth may represent a maladaptive response which contributes to the progression of renal failure [96]. It occurs in many renal diseases associated with proteinuria. Albumin is able to induce proliferation of OK cells in culture [97]. Furthermore, urine from nephrotic rats has been shown to induce proliferation of OK cells to a greater extent than albumin alone [98] and this effect occurs at a concentration of protein that micropuncture studies suggest may be present in proximal tubular fluid.

Proliferation of tubular cells is seen in models of proteinuria such as protein overload nephropathy. However, in this model there is a concomitant and greater degree of apoptosis of cells within the tubulo-interstitium [22]. Such observation suggest a mechanism whereby proteinuria may lead to tubular atrophy which is a characteristic feature of CRF.

Alteration in tubular cell biology An increasing body of evidence has demonstrated that proximal tubular cells have the necessary armoury to take part in an inflammatory and scarring response including the ability to secrete matrix proteins and a variety of proinflammatory and profibrotic cytokines such as PDGF and transforming growth factor-β and chemokines such as MCP-1. This is not surprising given their origin as mesenchymal cells [99].

Cultured human cortical epithelial cells will produce MCP-1 on exposure to a variety of cytokines [100,101]. Tubular cells have also been shown to produce a number of other potentially pro-inflammatory cytokines. Tubular cells grown from human kidney biopsies express mRNA for interleukin-6, granulocyte macrophage-colony stimulating factor and PDGF-B with greater amounts of mRNA for these cytokines being found in tubular cells derived from diseased kidneys in comparison to those from normal kidneys [102]. Supernatants from tubular cells in culture are also able to stimulate fibroblasts to produce the ECM protein, fibronectin [103], and again the effect is greatest using media produced by tubular cells derived from diseased kidneys. In addition, the production by tubular cells of a chemoattractant with properties similar to a non-polar lipid has been described (see below).

Using a polarized cell culture system, our laboratory has examined the effects of the addition of protein to the apical surface of human proximal tubular cells in order to mimic *in vitro* the effects of proteinuria. These experiments demonstrated that tubular cells could directly contribute to the fibrogenic process within the tubulo-interstitium by secreting PDGF and the matrix protein fibronectin predominantly into the basolateral compartment [104]. Furthermore, exposure of the apical surface of these cells to 1.0 mg/ml of serum proteins (a concentration which could be found in tubular fluid in nephrotic states) resulted in a significant increase in basolateral release of PDGF and fibronectin. The active component of serum was localized to a fraction of molecular weight 40–100 kDa. This size would readily be filtered by a damaged but not a normal glomerulus. The nature of the stimulating protein and the mechanisms of its effect are under current investigation.

The production of endothelin-1 by proximal tubular cells has also been implicated in the pathogenesis of progressive tubulo-interstitial injury [105]. Basolateral release of endothelin-1 could promote the recruitment of macrophages into the interstitium and result in interstitial fibroblast proliferation and ECM synthesis [106]. Endothelin-1 is produced by proximal tubular cells in culture [107] and in experimental models of proteinuric renal disease its production appears to be related to the severity of the proteinuria [24,25].

Ammoniagenesis Ammonia generation within the kidney may play a part in the development of progressive interstitial disease (reviewed in [108]). The development of proteinuria would result in increased intrarenal ammonia production as a result of the catabolism of the increased amount of reabsorbed proteins. In support of this the level of urinary ammonia correlates well with the level of proteinuria in patients with glomerulonephritis [109]. Ammonia is known to activate complement by the alternative pathway [108] and once activated complement has a number of proinflammatory effects including chemoattraction by C5a and cell lysis by C5b-9 [110]. C5b-9 in sublytic concentrations has also been shown to release cytokines and also to stimulate collagen synthesis in glomerular epithelial cells [111]. Thus an increase in ammonia production secondary to increased tubular catabolism of proteins from proteinuria could result in the activation of complement and consequent inflammation and scarring within the kidney. It is therefore of note that correction of acidosis in patients with CRF and proteinuria using oral sodium bicarbonate, reduces proximal renal tubular peptide catabolism and ammoniagenesis, and results in a lesser degree of tubular damage as assessed by surrogate markers [112].

Exacerbation of hypoxia by proteinuria In tubular cells which are already stressed by hypoxia the additional energy required to reabsorb and digest large amounts of proteins could result in hypoxic damage to those cells. In models of renal ischemia in rats produced by clamping of the renal artery for a fixed time or by induction of hemorrhagic shock, injection of myoglobin, ribonuclease, or lysozyme has been shown to worsen the development of acute tubular necrosis [113]. This study suggests that when tubular cells have to reabsorb low molecular weight proteins experimental ischaemic injury is exacerbated. Furthermore, in the hemorrhagic shock model it has been shown that there is a greater depletion of adenine nucleotides in the presence of the low molecular weight proteins which could be the result of the extra work required in reabsorption of these proteins [114]. There is no reason to suppose that the reabsorption of high molecular weight proteins requires any less energy than reabsorption of low molecular weight proteins. Oxygen tension in the kidney is known to be less than systemic arterial oxygen tension [115] and hence tubular cells are vulnerable to relatively small changes in oxygen requirement and delivery. In glomerular disease this vulnerability could be amplified by damage to the postglomerular capillaries induced by the transmission of glomerular hypertension, causing a further decrease in oxygen delivery [116]. In support of this studies of human biopsy specimens have demonstrated loss of postglomerular capillaries [117]. Once scarring has started the increased distance between tubular cells and peritubular capillaries would further exacerbate any ischaemic effect.

Effects of specific proteins

Whether the potential adverse effects of proteinuria are attributable to an individual protein or the molecules it carries or due to the combined effects of the many proteins filtered by a damaged glomerulus remains unknown.

Albumin *In vitro* work has provided conflicting evidence as to the potential pathogenic role for albuminuria in promoting tubulo-interstitial injury. Purified human albumin at pathologically relevant concentrations was unable to reproduce the stimulation of the basolateral secretion of ECM seen with the addition of serum proteins to the apical surface of human proximal tubular cells [104]. However, in another study using materials derived from different species BSA at a concentration of 0.5 mg/ml increased mRNA for MCP-1 in rat proximal tubular cells. To demonstrate an increase in the production of MCP-1 protein a much larger concentrations of BSA (10 mg/ml) was required and a similar effect was also seen with transferrin, suggesting it may not be an effect specific to albumin [118]. BSA has also been shown to increase the production of endothelin-1 by rabbit proximal tubular cells in culture, predominantly in a basolateral direction [107]. However, this effect was also not specific to albumin but was also seen with immunoglobulin and transferrin The relevance of these findings to those likely to be found *in vivo* in humans is less clear.

The biological activity of albumin could alternatively be the result of a molecule carried by the protein (and potentially removed during purification) rather than the protein *per se*. Albumin is one of the body's major lipoproteins carrying a variety of different fatty acids. This has led to the hypothesis that it is the metabolism of fatty acids carried on albumin rather than the protein which initiates tubulo-interstitial injury [119]. In support of this hypothesis, studies using OK cells have demonstrated that the ability of albumin to modulate cell growth and proliferation is dependent on the fatty acid content of the albumin with oleate albumin but not palmitate albumin causing cell proliferation [97].

Further evidence supporting a role of albumin in stimulating the development of interstitial inflammation through the molecules it carries has been provided by the observation that rat proximal tubules in short-term culture will produce a powerful chemoattractant for monocytes/macrophages if exposed to BSA [120]. Further investigation of this chemoattractant has shown that it is a lipid and that its production by tubular cells is dependent on the fatty acid content of the albumin to which they were exposed, with lipid-free BSA having no effect. It has also been shown that this lipid chemoattractant is present in the urine of rats with protein overload proteinuria [121]. Such observations could provide an explanation for the differential effects on tubulo-interstitial pathology of the administration of fatty acid replete and deplete albumin in this model [22].

Two lines of evidence argue against the hypothesis that albumin *per se* is the pathogenic protein in this process. These are minimal change glomerulonephritis (discussed previously) and the analbuminaemic rat. The analbuminaemic rat is genetically unable to manufacture albumin and hence serum albumin is essentially undetectable. Thus when these animals develop renal disease such as PAN nephrosis [122] or following partial nephrectomy [123] the levels of proteinuria are much lower than in normal animals and albuminuria is absent; nevertheless, these animals go on to progressive renal failure with the same histological changes as control animals. Although the quantity of proteinuria is less than the controls the animals still have high molecular weight proteinuria suggesting that the absolute quantity of proteinuria is not as significant as the types of protein that it contains.

Lipoproteins Abnormalities of lipid metabolism result from the development of proteinuria and may play a part in the progression of renal disease [4,10]. Both high-density lipoprotein (HDL) and LDL appear in nephrotic urine in significant quantities [124] and as previously discussed albumin which comprises the majority of the filtered load also contains high-affinity fatty acid binding sites and is also an important lipoprotein [125]. Lipid laden tubular cells have been found in nephrotic urine [126] and lipid droplets have been demonstrated in tubular cells in renal biopsies from nephrotic patients indicating that tubular cells interact with lipoproteins [127]. Both apolipoprotein A and B have been found in tubular cells in patients with the nephrotic syndrome [128]. Human proximal tubular cells in culture are able to take up both HDL and LDL [129] and oxidized LDL or minimally modified LDL can cause cell injury and detachment of cells from culture plates. Tubular cells themselves may possess LDL oxidizing ability and it is postulated that transferrinuria accompanying lipoproteinuria could provide a source of iron to catalyse the oxidative process [129]. Human tubular cells exposed to HDL have been shown to increase production of endothelin-1 [130]. Endothelin-1 in turn may modify the renal microcirculation [131], have effects on fibroblasts [132], and act as a monocyte chemoattractant [133]. Hence, through these effects HDL could influence tubulo-interstitial inflammation and scarring.

Transferrin Transferrin, which has a molecular weight only slightly greater than albumin, is filtered in glomerular disease and urinary transferrin has been proposed as a mediator of tubulo-interstitial injury [134]. As fluid passes down the tubule it becomes increasingly acidic. Under these conditions transferrin will release the iron that it carries [135]. Free Fe^{2+} ions are known to be cytotoxic and could therefore injure tubular cells. It has been demonstrated that exposure of tubular cells in culture to transferrin-iron but not transferrin or albumin increases lactate dehydrogenase release and cytosolic lipid peroxide malondialdehyde. This suggests that reabsorption of transferrin-iron results in the release of reactive iron in the proximal tubular cell causing peroxidative injury.

A pathogenic role for iron in progressive renal injury is provided by the demonstration that in rats with nephrotoxic serum nephritis there is a correlation with the quantity of iron excreted in the urine and the degree of tubulo-interstitial injury [136]. A marked increase in the urinary excretion of iron has been noted in patients with diabetic nephropathy and may be of pathogenic importance in the progressive renal injury seen in this disease [137]. There is, however, some evidence that urinary iron is protective in renal ischemia [135] so the effects of iron are complex.

Cell culture studies in which proximal tubular cells are exposed to transferrin have produced conflicting results. An upregulation of mRNA for MCP-1 in rat proximal tubular cells exposed to bovine transferrin has been shown [118]. These studies used high concentrations of transferrin (1–8 mg/ml) where as other studies using partially iron saturated transferrin at a lower concentrations (which may more closely mimic the pathophysiological concentrations likely to be found *in vivo*) had no effect on tubular cell production of matrix proteins [104].

Complement The activation of complement by ammonia is a mechanism by which proteinuria could influence interstitial inflammation and scarring. Increased glomerular permeability may allow circulating complement components to filter into the tubular fluid. Alternatively, complement components can be synthesized *de novo* by tubular epithelial cells [138]. Recent studies have demonstrated that tubular cell synthesis of complement is upregulated when the cells are exposed to serum proteins of a molecular weight range likely to be filtered in glomerular disease (S. H. Sacks, personal communication). Thus proteinuria may activate the complement cascade and provide a potential mechanism for cell damage. In support of this the C5b-9 membrane attack complex has been found in the urine in membranous nephropathy [139], diabetic nephropathy [140], and focal segmental glomerular sclerosis [140]. In membranous nephropathy, this is thought to represent leakage of C5b-9 from active glomerular disease. However, in the other conditions no glomerular deposition of the complex has been detected suggesting a tubular origin. The proximal tubular brush border can activate complement via the alternative pathway [141] and hence urinary C5b-9 may represent activation of filtered complement components by the tubular brush border.

Bence Jones protein Low molecular weight light chains if produced in excess will be freely filtered by the glomerulus and appear in the urine in the presence of an otherwise normal kidney. The presence of Bence Jones proteinuria is associated with the development of renal failure in some patients [142], although why some patients with Bence Jones proteinuria develop renal disease while others do not is unknown [89]. Several alterations in tubular function on exposure to light chains have been described. *In vivo* proximal tubular dysfunction occurs in the presence of urinary light chains, as evidenced by the development of 'tubular-type' proteinuria [143]. Transport of ammonium and glucose is inhibited [144] as is the sodium potassium ATPase of rat cortical tubules [145]. Sodium-dependent alanine and glucose uptake of brush border membrane vesicles from proximal tubular cells are also inhibited by urinary light chains [146]. Thus in the presence of a normal kidney some types of Bence Jones proteinuria have significant effects on tubular cell functions and are known to cause renal failure, although the relevance of such observations to the development of progressive renal scarring seen in glomerular disease is doubtful.

Filtered growth factors Growth factors are carried in the circulation bound to high-molecular weight binding proteins and as are such are normally excluded from or present only in low concentrations in the glomerular ultrafiltrate. With development of proteinuria the binding proteins and their associated growth factors will be found in the tubular fluid where they will be able to interact with receptors on proximal tubular cells. For example it has been shown that insulin-like growth factor (IGF)-I in conjunction with IGF-binding protein-2 is found in biologically significant concentrations in the urine of nephrotic rats. Proximal tubular fluid from nephrotic but not control rats autophosphorylates IGF-I receptors, increases the ^{3}H-thymidine incorporation, and promotes the secretion of collagen types I and IV in cultured proximal tubular cells. These effects are partially neutralized by IGF-I receptor antibodies [147].

Conclusions

The current evidence that proteinuria is a determinant of progression of renal failure depends predominantly on correlations between the severity of proteinuria and clinical outcomes. Such correlations cannot exclude the possibility that proteinuria is merely a marker of bad glomerular disease and bad glomerular disease progresses more rapidly. There are, however, an increasing number of intervention strategies which lend support to the hypothesis that proteinuria is damaging to the kidney. In addition, plausible hypotheses have been formulated to explain how proteinuria might influence progression of renal disease and these are now supported by *in vitro* experimental evidence.

It is beyond dispute that proteinuria is associated with a bad prognosis and therefore it is logical that therapeutic strategies aimed at non-specifically reducing proteinuria, such as tight blood pressure control, ACE inhibition, and possibly low protein diets should be employed if at all possible; indeed such strategies have generally been shown to have a beneficial effect on the rate of progression of CRF in humans. Further understanding of how subtle differences in the quality of proteinuria may affect the propagation of renal scarring holds the prospect of developing more specific therapies in the future.

Key references

Burton C, Harris KPG. The role of proteinuria in the progression of chronic renal failure. *American Journal of Kidney Diseases* 1996; **27**: 765–775.

Ledingham JGG. Tubular toxicity of filtered proteins. *American Journal of Nephrology* 1990; **10**: 52–57.

Locatelli F, Marcelli D, Comelli M, *et al.* Proteinuria and blood pressure as causal components of progression to end-stage renal failure. *Nephrology Dialysis Transplantation* 1996; **11**: 461–467.

Perna A, Remuzzi G. Abnormal permeability to proteins and glomerular lesions: A meta-analysis of experimental and human studies. *American Journal of Kidney Diseases* 1996; **27**: 34–41.

Remuzzi G, Bertani T. Is glomerulosclerosis a consequence of altered glomerular permeability to macromolecules? *Kidney International* 1990; **38**: 384–394.

References

1. Walser M. Progression of chronic renal failure in man. *Kidney International* 1990; **37**: 1195–1210.
2. Hostetter TH, Olson JL, Rennke HG, *et al.* Hyperfiltration in remnant nephrons: a potentially adverse response to renal ablation. *American Journal of Physiology* 1981; **10**: F85–F93.
3. Brenner BM. Hemodynamically mediated glomerular injury and the progressive nature of kidney disease. *Kidney International* 1983; **23**: 647–655.
4. Moorhead JF, Chan MK, El-Nahas M, Varghese Z. Lipid nephrotoxicity in chronic progressive glomerular and tubulo-interstitial disease. *Lancet* 1982; **2**: 1309–1311.
5. Fogo A, Ichikawa I. Evidence for a pathogenic linkage between glomerular hypertrophy and sclerosis. *American Journal of Kidney Disease* 1991; **17**: 666–669.
6. Klahr S, Schreiner G, Ichikawa I. The progression of renal disease. *New England Journal of Medicine* 1988; **318**: 1657–1666.
7. Risdon R, Sloper J, de Wardener H. Relationship between renal function and histological changes found in renal-biopsy specimens from patients with persistent glomerular nephritis. *Lancet* 1966; **ii**: 363–366.
8. Schainuck L, Striker G, Cutler R, Benditt E. Structural-functional correlations in renal disease. Part II. the correlations. *Human Pathology* 1970: 631–641.
9. Schmitz P, Kasiske B, Mp OD, Keane W. Lipids and progressive renal injury. *Seminars Nephrology* 1989; **9**: 354–369.
10. Grone E, Walli A, Grone J, Miller B, Seidel D. The role of lipids in nephrosclerosis and glomerulosclerosis. *Atherosclerosis* 1994; **107**: 1–13.

11. Chanutin A, Ferris E. Experimental renal insufficiency produced by partial nephrectomy. *Archives of Internal Medicine* 1932; **49**: 767–787.
12. Anderson S, Rennke H, Brenner B. Therapeutic advantage of converting enzyme inhibitors in arresting progressive renal disease associated with systemic hypertension in the rat. *Journal of Clinical Investigations* 1986; **77**: 1993–2000.
13. El Nahas AM, Paraskevakou H, Zoob S, Rees A, Evans D. Effect of dietary protein restriction on the development of renal failure after subtotal nephrectomy in rats. *Clinical Science* 1983; **65**: 399–406.
14. Williams AJ, Baker F, Walls J. Effect of varying quantity and quality of dietary protein intake in experimental renal disease in rats. *Nephron* 1987; **46**: 83–90.
15. Perna A, Remuzzi G. Abnormal permeability to proteins and glomerular lesions: a meta-analysis of experimental and human studies. *American Journal of Kidney Disease* 1996; **27**: 34–41.
16. Eddy AA, McCulloch L, Liu E, Adams J. A relationship between proteinuria and acute tubulointerstitial disease in rats with experimental nephrotic syndrome. *American Journal of Pathology* 1991; **138**: 1111–1123.
17. Eddy AA. Protein restriction reduces transforming growth factor-beta and interstitial fibrosis in nephrotic syndrome. *American Journal of Physiology* 1994; **266**: F884–F893.
18. Eddy A, Warren J. Expression and function of monocyte chemoattractant protein 1 in puromycin aminonucleoside nephrosis. *Journal of the American Society of Nephrology* 1993; **4**: 600A.
19. Andrews P. A scanning and transmission electron microscopic comparison of puromycin aminonucleoside induced nephritis to hyperalbuminemia induced proteinuria with emphasis on podocyte pedicel loss. *Laboratory and Investigations* 1977; **36**: 183–197.
20. Eddy AA. Interstitial nephritis induced by protein-overload proteinuria. *American Journal of Pathology* 1989; **135**: 719–733.
21. Eddy AA, Giachelli CM, McCulloch L, Liu E. Renal expression of genes that promote interstitial inflammation and fibrosis in rats with protein-overload proteinuria. *Kidney International* 1995; **47**: 1546–1557.
22. Thomas M, Brunskill N, Pringle H, Harris K, Walls J. Macrophage infiltrate and tubular apoptosis in protein overload proteinuria. *Journal of the American Society of Nephrology* 1997; **8**: 631A.
23. Grond J, Weening JJ, Elema JD. Glomerular sclerosis in nephrotic rats. Comparison of the long-term effects of adriamycin and aminonucleoside. *Laboratory Investigations* 1984; **51**: 277–285.
24. Zoja C, Corna D, Bruzzi I, *et al.* Passive Heymann nephritis: evidence that angiotensin-converting enzyme inhibition reduces proteinuria and retards renal structural injury. *Experimental Nephrology* 1996; **4**: 213–221.
25. Zoja C, Liu XH, Abbate M, *et al.* Angiotensin II blockade limits tubular protein over-reabsorption and the consequent upregulation of endothelin 1 gene in experimental membranous nephropathy. *Experimental Nephrology* 1998; **6**: 121–131.
26. Jovanovic D, Dimitrijevic J, Varagic J, Jovovic D, Starcevic A, Djukanovic L. Effects of captopril on morphologic changes in kidney of spontaneously hypertensive rats with adriamycin nephropathy. *Renal Failure* 1998; **20**: 451–458.
27. Cameron J, Turner D, Ogg C, Chantler C, Williams D. The long term prognosis of patients with focal segmental glomerulosclerosis. *Clinical Nephrology* 1978; **10**: 213–218.
28. Cameron J, Turner D, Heaton J *et al.* Idiopathic mesangiocapillary glomerulonephritis.

Comparison of types I and II in children and adults and long term prognosis. *American Journal of Medicine* 1983; **74**: 175–192.

29. Erwin D, Donadio D, KEH. The clinical course of idiopathic membranous nephropathy. *Mayo Clinic Proceedings* 1973; **48**: 697–712.
30. Cattran DC, Pei Y, Greenwood CM, Ponticelli C, Passerini P, Honkanen E. Validation of a predictive model of idiopathic membranous nephropathy: its clinical and research implications. *Kidney International* 1997; **51**: 901–907.
31. D'Amico G, Minetti L, Ponticelli C, *et al.* Prognostic indicators in idiopathic IgA mesangial nephropathy. *Quaterly Journal of Medicine* 1986; **228**: 363–378.
32. Massy Z, Guijarro C, Wiederkehr M, Ma J, Kasiske B. Chronic renal allograft rejection: Immunologic and nonimmunologic risk factors. *Kidney International* 1996; **49**: 518–524.
33. Cattran D. Predicting outcome in the idiopathic glomerulopathies. *Journal of Nephrology* 1998; **11**: 57–60.
34. Williams P, Fass G, Bone J. Renal pathology and proteinuria determine progression in untreated mild/moderate chronic renal failure. *Quarterly Journal of Medicine* 1988; **67**: 343–354.
35. Stenvinkel P, Alvestrand A, Bergström J. Factors influencing progression in patients with chronic renal failure. *Journal of Internal Medicine* 1989; **226**: 183–188.
36. Klahr S, Levey AS, Beck GJ, *et al.* The effects of dietary protein restriction and blood-pressure control on the progression of chronic renal disease. *New England Journal of Medicine* 1994; **330**: 877–884.
37. The GISEN Group. Randomised placebo-controlled trial of effect of ramipril on decline in glomerular filtration rate and risk of terminal renal failure in proteinuric, non-diabetic nephropathy. *Lancet* 1997; **349**: 1857–1863.
38. Locatelli F, Marcelli D, Comelli M, *et al.* Proteinuria and blood pressure as causal components of progression to end-stage renal failure. *Nephrology, Dialysis, and Transplantation* 1996; **11**: 461–467.
39. Bazzi C, Petrini C, Rizza V, Arrigo G, Beltrame A, D'Amico G. Characterization of proteinuria in primary glomerulonephritides. SDS-PAGE patterns: Clinical significance and prognostic value of low molecular weight ('tubular') proteins. *American Journal of Kidney Disease* 1997; **29**: 27–35.
40. Boucher A, Droz D, Adafer E, Noel L. Characterisation of mononuclear cell subsets in renal cellular interstitial infiltrates. *Kidney International* 1986; **29**: 1043–1049.
41. Furness PN, Rogers-Wheatley L, Harris KP. Semiautomatic quantitation of macrophages in human renal biopsy specimens in proteinuric states. *Journal of Clinical Pathology* 1997; **50**: 118–122.
42. Mak S, Short C, Mallick N. Long term outcome of adult-onset minimal-change disease. *Nephrology, Dialysis, and Transplantation* 1996; **11**: 2192–2201.
43. Kunin C, Chesney R, Craig W, England A, DeAngelis C. Enzymuria as a marker of renal injury and disease: Studies of N-acetyl-β-glucosaminidase in the general population and in patients with renal disease. *Pediatrics* 1978; **62**: 751–760.
44. Ghiggeri G, Ginevri F, Candiano G, *et al.* Characterization of cationic albumin in minimal change nephropathy. *Kidney International* 1987; **32**: 547–553.
45. Mogensen C. Long-term antihypertensive treatment inhibiting progression of diabetic nephropathy. *British Medicine Journal* 1982; **285**: 685–688.
46. Alvestrand A, Gutierrez A, Bucht H, Bergström J. Reduction of blood pressure retards the progression of chronic renal failure in man. *Nephrology, Dialysis, and Transplantation* 1988; **35**: 624–631.

47. Apperloo A, De Zeeuw D, De Jong P. Short-term anti-proteinuric response to anti-hypertensive treatment predicts long-term GFR decline in patients with non-diabetic renal disease. *Kidney International* 1994; **45** (Suppl): S174–S178.
48. Lewis E, Hunsicker L, Bain R, Rhode R. The effect of angiotensin-converting enzyme inhibition on diabetic nephropathy. *New England Journal of Medicine* 1993; **329**: 1456–1462.
49. Ihle BU, Whitworth JA, Shahinfar S, Cnaan A, Kincaid-Smith PS, Becker GJ. Angiotensin-converting enzyme inhibition in nondiabetic progressive renal insufficiency: a controlled double-blind trial. *American Journal of Kidney Disease* 1996; **27**: 489–495.
50. Kamper AL, Strandgaard S, Leyssac PP. Late outcome of a controlled trial of enalapril treatment in progressive chronic renal failure. Hard end-points and influence of proteinuria. *Nephrology, Dialysis, and Transplantation* 1995; **10**: 1182–1188.
51. Kloke H, Branten A, Huysmans F, Wetzels J. Antihypertensive treatment of patients with proteinuric renal diseases: Risks or benefits of calcium channel blockers? *Kidney International* 1998; **53**: 1559–1573.
52. Wapstra FH, Navis G, De Jong PE, De Zeeuw D. Prognostic value of the short-term antiproteinuric response to ACE inhibition for prediction of GFR decline in patients with nondiabetic renal disease. *Experimental Nephrology* 1996; **4**: 47–52.
53. Praga M, Hernandez E, Montoyo C, Andres A, Ruilope LM, Rodicio JL. Long-term beneficial effects of angiotensin-converting enzyme inhibition in patients with nephrotic proteinuria. *American Journal of Kidney Disease* 1992; **20**: 240–248.
54. Fuji Y, Kishimoto T, Dohi K. Response to the furosemide test may predict the effects of delapril on renal function in patients with chronic renal insufficiency. *Journal of Nara Medicine Association* 1997; **48**: 293–299.
55. Van Essen G, Rensma P, De Zeeuw D, *et al.* Association between angiotensin-converting-enzyme gene polymorphism and failure of renoprotective therapy. *Lancet* 1996; **347**: 94–95.
56. Yoshida H, Mitarai T, Kawamura T, *et al.* Role of the deletion polymorphism of the angiotensin converting enzyme gene in the progression and therapeutic responsiveness of IgA nephropathy. *Journal of Clinical Investigations* 1995; **96**: 2162–2169.
57. Jacobsen P, Rossing K, Rossing P, *et al.* Angiotensin converting enzyme gene polymorphism and ACE inhibition in diabetic nephropathy. *Kidney International* 1998; **53**: 1002–1006.
58. El Nahas A, Masters-Thomas A, Brady S, *et al.* Selective effect of low protein diets in chronic renal diseases. *British Medicine Journal* 1984; **289**: 1337–1341.
59. Remuzzi G, Bertani T. Is glomerulosclerosis a consequence of altered glomerular permeability to macromolecules? *Kidney International* 1990; **38**: 384–394.
60. Bruzzi I, Benigni A, Remuzzi G. Role ofcreased glomerular protein traffic in the progression of renal failure. *Kidney International*1997; **51** (Suppl.): S29–S31.
61. Burton C, Harris KPG. The role of proteinuria in the progression of chronic renal failure. *American Journal of Kidney Disease* 1996; **27**: 765–775.
62. Grond J, Schilthuis MS, Koudstaal J, Elema JD. Mesangial function and glomerular sclerosis in rats after unilateral nephrectomy. *Kidney International* 1982; **22**: 338–343.
63. Purkerson M, Hoffsten P, Klahr S. Pathogenesis of the glomerulopathy associated with renal infarction in rats. *Journal of Clinical Investigations* 1988; **9**: 407–417.
64. Diamond J, Karnovsky M. Focal and segmental glomerulosclerosis: analogies to atherosclerosis. *Kidney International* 1988; **33**: 917–924.

65. Lee HS, Lee JS, Koh HI, Ko KW. Intraglomerular lipid deposition in routine biopsies. *Clinical Nephrology* 1991; **36**: 67–75.
66. Sato H, Suzuki S, Ueno M, *et al.* Localization of apolipoprotein (a) and B-100 in various renal diseases. *Kidney International* 1993; **43**: 430–435.
67. Grone EF, Abboud HE, Hohne M, *et al.* Actions of lipoproteins in cultured human mesangial cells: Modulation by mitogenic vasoconstrictors. *American Journal of Physiology* 1992; **263**: F686–F696.
68. Wheeler DC, Persaud JW, Fernando R, Sweny P, Varghese Z, Moorhead JF. Effects of low-density lipoproteins on mesangial cell growth and viability in vitro. *Nephrology Dialysis Transplantation* 1990; **5**: 185–191.
69. Rovin BH, Tan LC. LDL stimulates mesangial fibronectin production and chemoattractant expression. *Kidney International* 1993; **43**: 218–225.
70. Van Goor H, Ding G, Kees-Folts D, Grond J, Schreiner GF, Diamond JR. Macrophages and renal disease. *Laboratory and Investigations* 1994; **71**: 456–464.
71. Wheeler DC, Chana RS, Topley N, Petersen MM, Davies M, Williams JD. Oxidation of low density lipoprotein by mesangial cells may promote glomerular injury. *Kidney International* 1994; **45**: 1628–1636.
72. Risdon R, Sloper J, de Wardener H. Relationship between renal function and histological changes found in renal biopsy specimens from patients with persistent glomerular nephritis. *Lancet* 1968; **ii**: 363–366.
73. Howie A, Gunson B, Sparke J. Morphometric correlates of renal excretory function. *Journal of Pathology* 1990; **160**: 245–253.
74. Gerard P, Cordier R. Question ofterpretation of granular formations found in cells of convoluted tubule of kidney in vertebrates. *Bulletin of the Academy of Royal Society of Medicine Belgique* 1934; **14**: 160–185.
75. Lin C, Garbern J, Wu J. Light and electron microscopic immunocytochemical localisation of clathrin in rat cerebellum and kidney. *Journal of Histochemistry and Cytochemistry* 1992; **30**: 853–863.
76. Rodman J, Kerjaschki D, Merisko E, Farquhar M. Presence of an extensive clathrin coat on the apical plasmalemma of the rat kidney proximal tubule cell. *Journal of Cell Biology* 1984; **98**: 1630–1636.
77. Christensen E, Nielson S. Structural and functional features of protein handling in the kidney proximal tubule. *Seminars in Nephrology* 1991; **11**: 414–439.
78. Straus W. Isolation and biochemical properties of droplets from the cells of rat kidney. *Journal of Biological Chemistry* 1954; **207**: 745–755.
79. Straus W. Concentration of acid phosphatase, ribonuclease, desoxyribonucleases, b glucuronidase and cathepsin in droplets isolated from the kidney cells of normal rats. *Journal of Biophysics Biochemistry and Cytology* 1956; **2**: 513–521.
80. Davidson S. Protein absorption by renal cells II. Very rapid lysosomal digestion of exogenous ribonuclease in vitro. *Journal of Cell Biology* 1973; **59**: 213–222.
81. Hjelle J, Peterson D. Subcellular sites ofsulin hydrolysis in renal proximal tubules. *American Journal of Physiology* 1984; **246**: F409–416.
82. Maunsbach A. Cellular mechanisms of tubular protein transport. In: Thurau K (ed.), *International Review of Physiology Kidney and Urinary Physiology*. Baltimore: University Park Press, 1976: 145–167.
83. Park CH, Maack T. Albumin absorption and catabolism by isolated perfused proximal convoluted tubules of the rabbit. *Journal of Clinical Investigations* 1984; **73**: 767–777.
84. Christensen E, Maunsbach A. Effects of dextran on lysosomal ultrastructure and protein digestion in renal proximal tubule. *Kidney International* 1979; **16**: 301–311.

85. Schwegler J, Heppleman B, Mildenberger S, Silbernagl S. Receptor mediated endocytosis of albumin in cultured opossum kidney cells: a model for proximal tubular protein reabsorption. *Pflügers Archives* 1991; **418**: 383–392.
86. Brunskill NJ, Nahorski S, Walls J. Characteristics of albumin binding to opossum kidney cells and identification of potential receptors. *Pflügers Archives of European Journal of Physiology* 1997; **433**: 497–504.
87. Brunskill NJ, Stuart J, Tobin AB, Walls J, Nahorski S. Receptor-mediated endocytosis of albumin by kidney proximal tubule cells is regulated by phosphatidylinositide 3-kinase. *Journal of Clinical Investigations* 1998; **101**: 2140–2150.
88. Brunskill NJ, Cockcroft N, Nahorski S, Walls J. Albumin endocytosis is regulated by heterotrimeric GTP-binding protein Galpha (i–3) in opossum kidney cells. *American Journal of Physiology* 1996; **271**: F356–F364.
89. Ledingham JGG. Tubular toxicity of filtered proteins. *American Journal of Nephrology* 1990; **10**: 52–57.
90. Sumpio BE, Maack T. Kinetics, competition, and selectivity of tubular absorption of proteins. *American Journal of Physiology* 1982; **12**: F379–F392.
91. Agarwal A, Nath KA. Effect of proteinuria on renal interstitium: Effect of products of nitrogen metabolism. *American Journal of Nephrology* 1993; **13**: 376–384.
92. Guder WG, Hofmann W. Markers for the diagnosis and monitoring of renal tubular lesions. *Clin Nephrol* 1992; **38**: Suppl 1 S3–S7.
93. Kind PRN. *N*-acetyl-beta-(D)-glucosaminidase in urine of patients with renal disease, and after renal transplants and surgery. *Clinical Chim Acta* 1982; **119**: 89–97.
94. Olbricht CJ, Cannon JK, Garg LC, Tisher CC. Activities of cathepsins B and L in isolated nephron segments from proteinuric and nonproteinuric rats. *American Journal of Physiology* 1986; **250**: F1055–F1066.
95. Maack T, Mackensie D, Kinter W. Intracellular pathways of renal reabsorption of lysozyme. *American Journal of Physiology* 1971; **221**: 1609–1616.
96. Wolf G, Neilson EG. Molecular mechanisms of tubulointerstitial hypertrophy and hyperplasia. *Kidney International* 1991; **39**: 401–420.
97. Thomas ME, Schreiner GP. Contribution of proteinuria to progressive renal injury: Consequences of tubular uptake of fatty acid bearing albumin. *American Journal of Nephrology* 1993; **13**: 385–398.
98. Burton CJ, Bevington A, Harris KPG, Walls J. Growth of proximal tubular cells in the presence of albumin and proteinuric urine. *Experimental Nephrology* 1994; **2**: 345–350.
99. Kuncio GS, Neilson EG, Haverty T. Mechanisms of tubulointerstitial fibrosis. *Kidney International* 1991; **39**: 550–556.
100. Schmouder RL, Strieter RM, Kunkel SL. Interferon-gamma regulation of human renal cortical epithelial cell-derived monocyte chemotactic peptide. *Kidney International* 1993; **44**: 43–49.
101. Prodjosudjadi W, Gerritsma JSJ, Klar-Mohamad N, *et al.* Production and cytokine-mediated regulation of monocyte chemoattractant protein-1 by human proximal tubular epithelial cells. *Kidney International* 1995; **48**: 1477–1486.
102. Frank J, Engler-Blum G, Rodemann H, Muller G. Human renal cells as a cytokine source: PDGF-B, GM-CSF IL-6 mRNA expression *in vitro*. *Experimental Nephrology* 1992; **1**: 26–35.
103. Frank J, Engler-Blum G, Rodemann H, Muller G. Proinflammatory cytokines induce GM-CSF and enhance IL-6 transcription in renal fibroblasts. *Journal of the American Society of Nephrology* 1992; **3**: 588A.

104. Burton CJ, Combe C, Walls J, Harris KPG. Fibronectin production by human tubular cells: The effect of apical protein. *Kidney International* 1996; **50**: 760–767.
105. Remuzzi G, Benigni A. Progression of proteinuric diabetic and nondiabetic renal diseases: a possible role for renal endothelin. *Kidney International* 1997; **58** (Suppl): S66–S68.
106. Benigni A, Remuzzi G. Glomerular protein trafficking and progression of renal disease to terminal uremia. *Seminars in Nephrology* 1996; **16**: 151–159.
107. Zoja C, Morigi M, Figliuzzi M, *et al.* Proximal tubular cell synthesis and secretion of endothelin-1 on challenge with albumin and other proteins. *American Journal of Kidney Disease* 1995; **26**: 934–941.
108. Clark E, Nath K, Hostetter M, Hostetter M. Role of ammonia in progressive interstitial nephritis. *American Journal of Kidney Disease* 1991; **17**: 15–19.
109. Rustom R, Maltby P, Grime JS, *et al.* Tubular peptide hypermetabolism and urinary ammonia in chronic renal failure in man: a maladaptive response? *Nephron* 1998; **79**: 306–311.
110. Koski C, Ramm L, Hammer C, Mayer M, Skin M. Cytolysis of nucleated cells by complement: Cell death displays multi-hit characteristics. *Proceedings of the National Academy of Science, USA* 1983; **80**: 3816–3820.
111. Torbohm I, Schönermark M, Wingen A, Berger B, Rother K, Hänsch G. C5b-8 and C5b-9 modulate the collagen release of human glomerular epithelial cells. *Kidney International* 1990; **37**: 1098–1104.
112. Rustom R, Grime JS, Costigan M, *et al.* Oral sodium bicarbonate reduces proximal renal tubular peptide catabolism, ammoniogenesis, and tubular damage in renal patients. *Renal Failure* 1998; **20**: 371–382.
113. Zarger R, Teubner E, Adler S. Low molecular weight proteinuria exacerbates experimental ischaemic renal injury. *Laboratory Investigations* 1987; **56**: 180–188.
114. Zager R. Myoglobin depletes renal adenine nucleotide pools in the presence and absence of shock. *Kidney International* 1991; **39**: 111–119.
115. Brezis M, Rosen S, Silva P, Epstein F. Renal ischemia: a new perspective. *Kidney International* 1984; **26**: 375–383.
116. Fine L, Ong A, Norman J. Mechanisms of tubulo-interstitial injury in progressive renal diseases. *European Journal of Clinical Investigations* 1993; **23**: 259–265.
117. Bohle A, Gise H, Mackensen-Haen S, Stark-Jacob B. The obliteration of the postglomerular capillaries and its influence upon the function of both glomeruli and tubuli. *Klinische Wochenschrift* 1981; **59**: 1043–1051.
118. Wang Y, Chen J, Chen L, Tay YC, Rangan GK, Harris DCH. Induction of monocyte chemoattractant protein-1 in proximal tubule cells by urinary protein. *Journal of the American Society of Nephrology* 1997; **8**: 1537–1545.
119. Schreiner G. Renal toxicity of albumin and other lipoproteins. *Current Opinion in Nephrological Hypertension* 1995; **4**: 369–373.
120. Kees-Folts D, Schreiner G. A lipid chemotactic factor associated with proteinuria and interstitial nephritis induced by protein overload. *Journal of the American Society of Nephrology* 1991; **2**: 548A.
121. Kees-Folts D, Diamond J. Relationship between hyperlipidemia, lipid mediators and progressive glomerulosclerosis in the nephrotic syndrome. *American Journal of Nephrology* 1993; **13**: 365–375.
122. Okuda S, Oochi N, Wakisaka M, *et al.* Albuminuria is not an aggravating factor in experimental focal glomerulosclerosis and hyalinosis. *Journal of Laboratory and Clinical Medicine* 1992; **119**: 245–253.

123. Fujihara C, Limongi D, Falzone R, Graudenz M, Zatz R. Pathogenesis of glomerular sclerosis in subtotally nephrectomised analbuminemic rats. *American Journal of Physiology* 1991; **261**: F256–F264.
124. Shore V, Forte T, Licht H, Lewis S. Serum and urinary lipoproteins in the human nephrotic syndrome: evidence for renal catabolism of lipoproteins. *Metabolism* 1982; **31**: 258–268.
125. Spector A. Plasma albumin as a lipoproteins. In: Scanu A, Spector A (eds). *Biochemistry and Biology of Plasma Lipoproteins, Vol 2: the Biochemistry of Disease*. New York: Marcel Dekker, 1986: 247–279.
126. Olson J. The nephrotic syndrome. In: Heptinstall R (ed.). *Pathology of the Kidney*. Boston: Brown and Co, 1992: 779–870.
127. Neverov N, Ivanov A, Severgina E, Kolonduck N, Srinivas K, Tareyeva I. Cytoplasmic lipid inclusions and low-density lipoprotein depositions in renal biopsies of nephrotic patients. *Nephrological, Dialysis and Transplantation* 1991; **10**: 776A.
128. Kashyap M, Ooi B, Hynd R, Gluek C, Pollak V, Robinson K. Sequestration and excretion of high density and low density lipoproteins by the kidney in human nephrotic syndrome. *Artery* 1979; **6**: 108–121.
129. Ong ACM, Moorhead JF. Tubular lipidosis: Epiphenomenon or pathogenetic lesion in human renal disease? *Kidney International* 1994; **45**: 753–762.
130. Ong ACM, Jowett T, Moorhead JF, Owen J. Human high density lipoproteins stimulate endothelin-1 release by cultured human renal proximal tubular cells. *Kidney International* 1994; **46**: 1315–1321.
131. Kon V, Yoshioka T, Fogo A, Ichikawa I. Glomerular actions of endothelin in vivo. *Journal of Clinical Investigations* 1989; **83**: 1762–1767.
132. Ong ACM, Jowett T, Firth J, Burton S, Kitamura M, Fine LG. A new paracrine loop implicated in human tubulo-interstitial disease: Tubular-derived endothelins modulate renal interstitial fibroblast function. *Journal of the American Society of Nephrology* 1993; **4**: 473A.
133. Achmad T, Rao G. Chemotaxis of human blood monocytes towards endothelin-1 and the influence of calcium channel blockers. *Biochemistry and Biophysics Research Communications* 1992; **189**: 994–1000.
134. Alfrey A. Role of iron and oxygen radicals in the progression of chronic renal failure. *American Journal of Kidney Disease* 1994; **23**: 183–187.
135. Zager R, Schimpf B, Bredi C, Gmur D. Inorganic iron effects on in vitro hypoxic proximal tubular cell injury. *Journal of Clinical Investigations* 1993; **91**: 702–708.
136. Alfrey A, Froment D, Hammond W. A role of iron in tubulointerstitial injury in nephrotoxic serum nephritis. *Kidney International* 1989; **36**: 753–759.
137. Howard R, Buddington B, Alfrey A. Urinary albumin excretion, transferrin and iron excretion in diabetic patients. *Kidney International* 1991; **40**: 923–926.
138. Song D, Zhou W, Sheerin SH, Sacks SH. Compartmental localization of complement component transcripts in the normal human kidney. *Nephron* 1998; **78**: 15–22.
139. Schulze M, Donadio J, Pruchno C, *et al.* Elevated urinary excretion of the C5b-9 complex in membranous nephropathy. *Kidney International* 1991; **40**: 533–538.
140. Ogradowski J, Herbert L, Sedmak K, Cosio F, Tamerius J, Kolb W. Measurement of C5b-9 in urine in patients with the nephrotic syndrome. *Kidney International* 1991; **40**: 1141–1147.
141. Camussi G, Tetta C, Mazzuccco G, Vercellone A. The brush border of proximal tubules of normal human kidney activates the alternative pathway of the complement system in vitro. *Annals of the New York Academy of Science* 1983; **420**: 321–324.

142. DeFronzo R, Cooke C, Wright J, Humphrey R. Renal function in patients with multiple myeloma. *Medicine (Baltimore)* 1978; **57**: 151–166.
143. Cooper E, Forbes M, Crockson R, Maclennan I. Proximal renal tubular function in myelomatosis: Observations in the fourth medical research council trial. *Journal of Clinical Pathology* 1984; **37**: 852–858.
144. Preuss H, Weiss F, Iammarino R, Hammack W, Murdaugh H. Effects on rat kidney slice function in vitro of proteins from the urines of patients with myelomatosis and nephrosis. *Clinical Science and Molecular Medicine* 1974; **46**: 283–294.
145. McGeogh J, Falconer-Smith J, Ledingham J, Ross B. Inhibition of active-transport sodium-potassium ATP-ase by myeloma protein. *Lancet* 1978; **ii**: 17–18.
146. Batuman V, Sastrasinh M, Sastrasinh S. Light chain effects on alanine and glucose uptake by renal brush border membranes. *Kidney International* 1986; **30**: 662–665.
147. Hirschberg R. Bioactivity of glomerular ultrafiltrate during heavy proteinuria may contribute to renal tubulo-interstitial lesions: evidence for a role for insulin-like growth factor I. *Journal of Clinical Investigations* 1996; **98**: 116–124.

6

Hypertension in renal parenchymal disease: role in progression

Lance D. Dworkin and Mathew R. Weir

Introduction

Hypertension is both a cause and consequence of chronic renal disease. After diabetic nephropathy, systemic hypertension is the second most common factor identified as causing end-stage renal disease (ERSD) and accounts for approximately one-fourth of all patients currently receiving dialysis in the United States. Even in those individuals in whom hypertension is not the primary cause of renal disease, elevations in systemic blood pressure may accelerate the rate at which kidney function is lost. This is particularly true for patients with glomerular disease and clinically evident proteinuria. Numerous studies in experimental animals and in humans suggest that antihypertensive drugs can slow the rate at which glomerular filtration rate (GFR) declines in chronic renal disease. Drugs that inhibit the renin–angiotensin system may be particularly effective in retarding renal disease progression.

Evidence suggests that hypertension damages the kidney by several mechanisms. Because autoregulation of glomerular pressure is impaired in chronic renal disease, elevated blood pressure is transmitted to the glomerular capillaries causing glomerular hypertension. Increased glomerular capillary hydraulic pressure leads to increased protein filtration and endothelial damage, causing release of cytokines and other soluble mediators that promote the replacement of normal kidney by fibrous tissue. An important factor contributing to progressive loss of kidney function in chronic renal disease is activation of the renin–angiotensin system, which not only tends to raise blood pressure but also to promote cellular proliferation, inflammation, and matrix accumulation.

This chapter will review experimental data that form the basis for our current understanding of the association between hypertension and chronic renal disease. The pathogenesis of increased blood pressure in chronic renal disease, the mechanisms by which systemic hypertension promotes progressive kidney failure, and the impact of antihypertensive agents on experimental kidney damage will be considered. Relevant clinical studies examining the relationship between elevation in systemic blood pressure and the development and progression of chronic renal disease will be considered. The effects of antihypertensive agents on the progression of non-diabetic chronic disease in humans as well as specific recommendations for the treatment of hypertension in chronic renal disease will be discussed. The impact of hypertension and its therapy on diabetic renal disease will not be considered in this chapter but are presented in Chapter 7.

Hypertension as a result of chronic renal disease

Hypertension is common in renal parenchymal disease and its prevalence increases as the GFR declines [1]. The prevalence of hypertension also varies with the renal diagnosis. Patients with glomerular diseases such as diabetic nephropathy or primary or secondary forms of glomerulonephritis, vascular diseases such as progressive systemic sclerosis, or polycystic kidney disease are more commonly affected than those with minimal change or membranous glomerulopathy or chronic tubulo-interstitial disease [1]. As recently reviewed [2], a number of factors have been implicated in the genesis of hypertension in chronic renal disease, including salt and water retention leading to extracellular fluid volume expansion as well as abnormal activity of vasoconstrictor pathways including the renin–angiotensin and sympathetic nervous system.

Lumping all diagnoses together, underlying renal disease is the most common cause of secondary hypertension in the general population, accounting for 2.5–5% of all cases of systemic hypertension [3]. Data from the 1991–1994 National Health and Nutrition Examination Survey (NHANES III) suggested that there were over 28 million individuals with hypertension in the United States in 1994 [4]. Therefore, it follows that between 700 000 and 1 400 000 Americans have hypertension secondary to intrinsic renal disease. Nevertheless, because essential hypertension is also a common cause of kidney disease (see below), it may be difficult in individual patients to determine whether hypertension is a consequence of renal disease. Therefore, the existence of an underlying renal disease may remain unrecognized in many hypertensive individuals, particularly prior to the development of significant impairment in renal function.

Hypertension as a risk factor for chronic renal disease

The incidence of ESRD in the United States has been progressively increasing for more than a decade attaining a rate of 253 cases per million population in 1995. As a result, in 1993, more than 257 000 people were being treated for ESRD under the Medicare program [5]. Because these data do not include patients with ESRD who are not covered by Medicare or those that develop ESRD but do not receive dialysis for more than several months, the numbers underestimate the true incidence and prevalence of ESRD in the United States. Shown in Fig. 6.1, hypertension is the second most common attributed cause of ESRD. Not shown, the risk of developing ESRD as a consequence of hypertension varies markedly according to race and is sixfold greater among black as compared with white Americans [5]. Native Americans are also at increased risk of developing hypertension associated ESRD [5]. Although the explanation for the excess risk of hypertensive renal disease in these

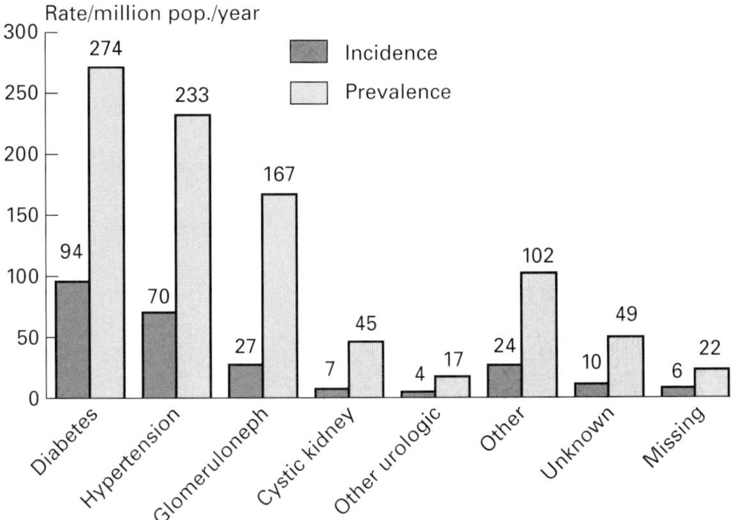

Fig. 6.1 Total treated ESRD incidence and prevalence by primary diagnoses, 1993–95. Rates by diagnoses adjusted for age, sex, and race. The category of hypertension in this classification includes diseases that affect the renal arteries such as main renal artery stenosis and occlusion and cholesterol emboli. However, renal artery disease and cholesterol emboli are very rarely invoked as the primary cause of ESRD and, therefore, the category of hypertension is presumed to be predominately composed of ESRD attributed to hypertensive nephrosclerosis. Source: USRDS, 1997 Annual Report, NIH internet site.

populations is uncertain, evidence suggests that it does not result solely from socioeconomic factors and/or from differences in access to care [6].

Epidemiological data provide additional support for the link between hypertension and ESRD. Klag and coworkers [7] examined the rate of developing ESRD as a function of systolic or diastolic blood pressure in 332 544 men ages 35–57 that were screened for inclusion in the Multiple Risk Factor Intervention Trial (MRFIT) study. They found a strong, positive correlation between hypertension and risk of ESRD. Shown in Fig. 6.2, the risk was greatest in individuals with severe hypertension (22-fold excess in individuals with blood pressure ≥210/120 mmHg as compared with those with an optimal pressure of <120/80). However, the presence of even stage 1 hypertension (140–159/90–99 mmHg) tripled the risk of developing ESRD, suggesting that hypertensive kidney damage may be a continuous function of systemic blood pressure with injury even occurring in the large subset of individuals with relatively mild hypertension. Furthermore, because the prevalence in the population of a high normal blood pressure and stage I hypertension is much greater than that of stage II and II hypertension, most hypertension-related ESRD will develop in milder hypertensives. It follows that hypertensive renal disease can only be prevented if all hypertensive patients are diagnosed and treated.

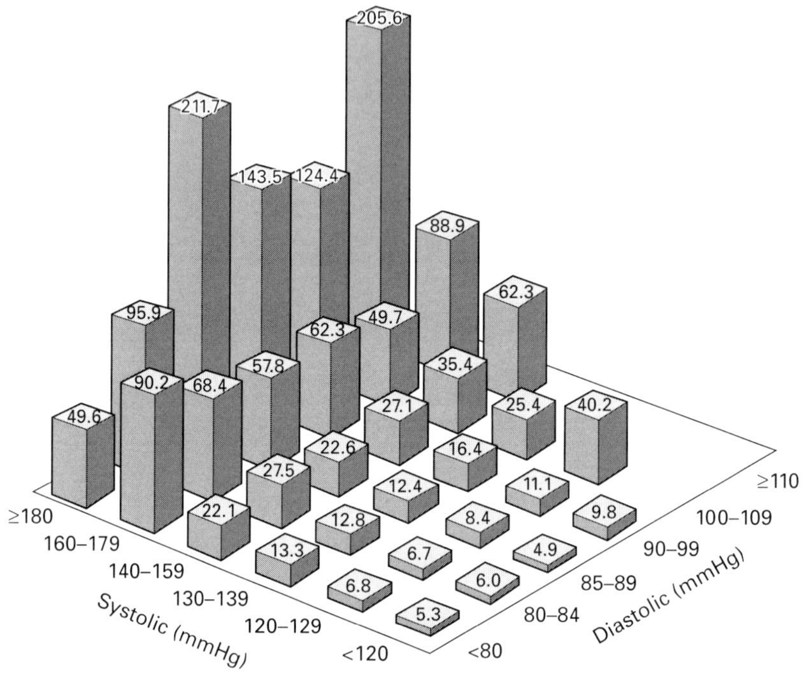

Fig. 6.2 Age-adjusted rate of end-stage renal disease due to any cause per 100 000 patient years according to systolic and diastolic blood pressure in over 300 000 men screened for the MRFIT study. The risk of developing end-stage renal disease rises with increasing systolic and/or diastolic blood pressure. Source: reference 7.

Interestingly, in the data of Klag *et al.* [7] elevation in systolic pressure was an even stronger predictor of ESRD than increased diastolic pressure. This issue may be particularly relevant to older individuals, that have an increased risk of developing both isolated systolic hypertension and ESRD [8]. Nevertheless, most clinical trials of have focused on changes in mean arterial pressure (MAP) rather than systolic blood pressure. Because they have the same MAP of 92 mmHg, patients with blood pressures of 125/75 and 156/60 are treated as similar in this type of analysis. In fact, the data displayed in Fig. 6.2 suggests this assumption is invalid. As yet, the relative impact of lowering systolic versus diastolic hypertension on progression of renal disease has not been systematically evaluated.

Undoubtedly, included in the group of patients in whom ESRD is attributed to hypertension are individuals with primary renal diseases of diverse etiologies. A subset of these patients lose kidney function as a result of processes that can be directly linked to systemic hypertension such as atherosclerotic occlusive disease of the main renal arteries, atheroembolic disease, or hypertensive nephrosclerosis. Other individuals have an underlying primary renal disease, such as chronic interstitial nephritis, that is unrecognized prior to the onset of moderate renal insufficiency and secondary hypertension. At present, the exact prevalence of these diagnoses among the many individuals with ESRD attributed to hypertension is unknown.

Even in individuals in whom the initial renal injury is caused by another process, elevation in systemic pressure accelerates the rate at which kidney function is lost [9]. Therefore, adequacy of blood pressure control is a major determinant of renal outcome in the vast majority of patients with chronic renal disease. This is particularly true for patients with glomerular diseases such as diabetic nephropathy or chronic glomerulonephritis [1]. Whether or not systemic hypertension also contributes to loss of kidney function in patients with tubulo-interstitial or polycystic kidney disease is less certain [10,11]. Nevertheless, recent clinical data suggest that reducing systemic blood pressure to the normal range is important in preventing progressive kidney failure in all individuals with chronic renal disease that excrete more than 1 g of protein per day [10,11].

Hypertension: role in progression of chronic renal disease

Glomerular pressure correlates with glomerular injury

Following a partial loss of kidney function, secondary processes develop that contribute to progression of chronic renal disease. Among these are a decrease in resistance in the preglomerular, afferent arteriole which, when associated with systemic hypertension, leads to increases in glomerular capillary hydraulic pressure (P_{GC}), renal plasma flow, and GFR. Based upon studies in animals with hypertension and renal disease in which P_{GC} has been reduced by alterations in protein intake [12–15] or by administration of antihypertensive agents [16–23], glomerular capillary hypertension has been identified as the hemodynamic alteration most closely associated with the development of glomerular sclerosis and progressive kidney failure. The direct relationship between glomerular pressure and injury is illustrated in Fig. 6.3, which displays the values for the absolute of reduction in P_{GC} achieved and the percent reduction in glomerular injury in observed in five separate studies in which rats with several forms of renal disease were treated with a similar combination of antihypertensive agents including hydralazine, reserpine, and a thiazide diuretic, so-called triple therapy [18–22]. As shown, significant protection was only observed when glomerular pressure fell by more than 6 mmHg. These and other similar studies demonstrate that one major mechanism by which antihypertensive agents prevent kidney damage is by reducing P_{GC}. However, the relationship between systemic blood pressure and glomerular capillary hydraulic pressure is complex and this has major implications for the treatment of patients with hypertension and renal disease.

Control of glomerular capillary hydraulic pressure

The vascular anatomy of the glomerulus is unusual in that the glomerular capillaries are arranged in series between two resistance vessels, the afferent and efferent arterioles (Fig. 6.4). These arterioles respond independently to vasoactive stimuli,

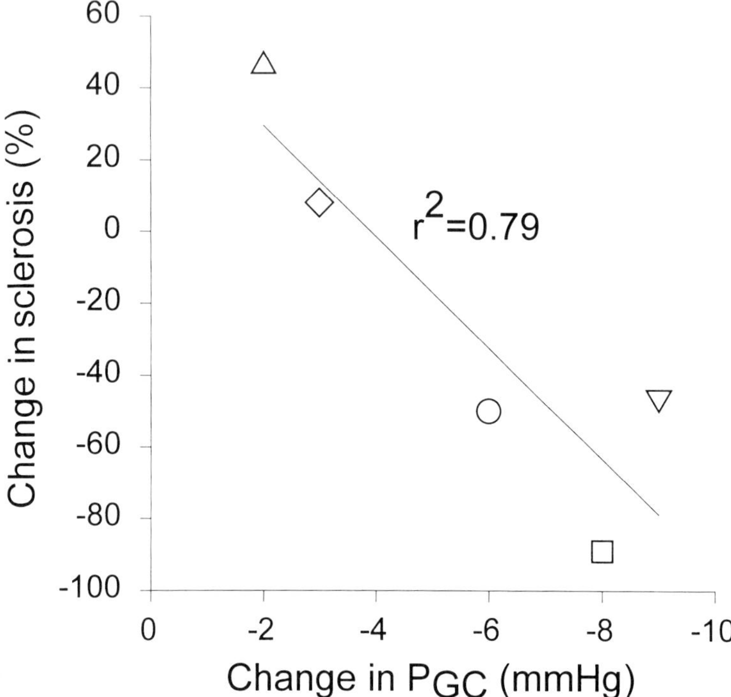

Fig. 6.3 Relationship between the absolute changes in glomerular capillary pressure (P_{GC}) and the percent of sclerotic glomeruli in five studies in which triple antihypertensive therapy was given to rats with various types of renal disease. There is a significant correlation between the magnitude of the decline in P_{GC} produced by therapy and degree of reduction in glomerular injury that was observed. Circle = UNX SHR uninephrectomized spontaneously hypertensive rat, square = REM-HD remnant kidney given high-dose triple therapy, upward pointing triangle = DOC-SALT desoxycorticosterone-salt induced hypertension, downward pointing triangle = NSN nephrotoxic serum nephritis, diamond = REM-LD remnant kidney rat given low dose triple therapy. Solid line indicates linear regression. Data adapted from references 18–22.

allowing divergent adjustment of afferent (R_A) and efferent (R_E) arteriolar resistance in response to changes in renal perfusion pressure [24]. Physiologically, glomerular capillary pressure is determined by three factors: MAP and the relative values of R_A and R_E. The predicted effects of selective changes in MAP, R_A, and R_E on glomerular pressure are summarized in Table 6.1. In general, increases or decreases in MAP are predicted to cause parallel changes in P_{GC}. Changes in R_A have inverse effects; an increase in preglomerular resistance causes a greater pressure drop across the afferent arteriole and a reduction in P_{GC}. In contrast, glomerular pressure is not reduced and may even increase in response to a rise in R_E because the high downstream resistance sustains glomerular pressure even as plasma flow rate declines. Under normal conditions, the afferent and efferent arterioles respond instantly to

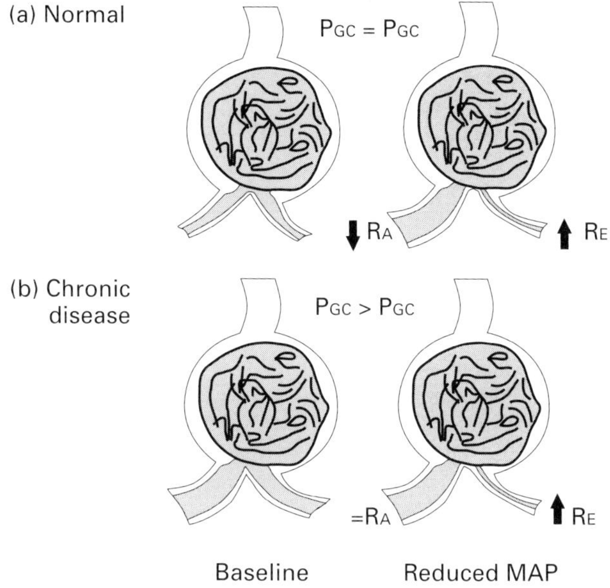

Fig. 6.4 Baseline status and changes in afferent and efferent resistance and glomerular capillary pressure in response to a reduction in MAP in (a) a glomerulus from a normal kidney and (b) a glomerulus from a chronically diseased kidney. Under normal conditions, in response to a reduction in MAP, afferent resistance (R_A) declines and efferent resistance (R_E) increases maintaining glomerular capillary pressure (P_{GC}) constant. In chronic renal disease, afferent and efferent arterioles are relatively dilated at baseline with reduced resistance. The capacity to reduce R_A is limited so that P_{GC} tends to decline with reductions in MAP.

changes in systemic blood pressure so that glomerular capillary pressure remains relatively constant over a wide range of perfusion pressures (Fig. 6.4). However, this property of the renal circulation, termed autoregulation of glomerular pressure, may be impaired in the setting of chronic renal disease or by administration of certain antihypertensive agents that dilate the afferent arteriole (see below). In this setting, glomerular pressure may vary more directly with changes in systemic blood pressure; however, the magnitude of this effect is often difficult to predict (Fig. 6.5). On the other hand, it has been suggested that the efferent arteriole is more sensitive to the vasoconstrictor effect of angiotensin II than is the afferent arteriole. Therefore, administration of drugs that block the renin–angiotensin system may be more likely to cause declines in R_E and glomerular pressure.

Antihypertensive agents, systemic and glomerular pressure, and glomerular injury

In fact, the exact relationship between systemic and glomerular pressure in animals treated with antihypertensive agents has not been systematically examined. However,

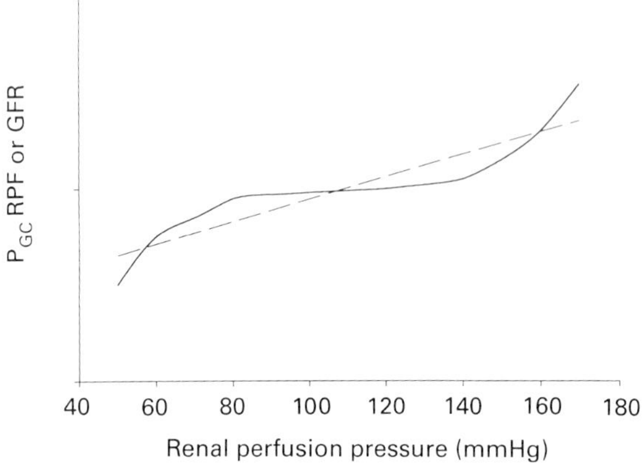

Fig. 6.5 Hypothetical renal autoregulation in normal (solid line) and diseased (dashed line) kidneys. Under normal conditions, glomerular pressure (P_{GC}), renal plasma flow (RPF), and glomerular filtration rate (GFR) remain relatively constant of a wide range of perfusion pressures. In contrast, in chronic renal disease, P_{GC}, RPF, and GFR vary more directly with changes in perfusion pressure.

Table 6.1 Effect of selective changes in mean arterial pressure, afferent, and efferent resistance on glomerular pressure

Change in determinant	Predicted change in P_{GC}
Mean arterial pressure	
⇧	⇧
⇩	⇩
Afferent resistance	
⇧	⇩
⇩	⇧
Efferent resistance	
⇧	⇧
⇩	⇩

Under normal conditions, the afferent and efferent arterioles respond to changes in perfusion pressure so that P_{GC} remains relatively constant over values for MAP from about 70 to 140 mmHg.

some insight can be gained by examining multiple studies in which a similar antihypertensive regimen was administered and these parameters measured. Figure 6.6 shows data from the same five studies utilized in Fig. 6.3, in which rats with various types of renal disease were given triple therapy [18–22]. As can be seen, although triple therapy produced significant declines in MAP in every case, no

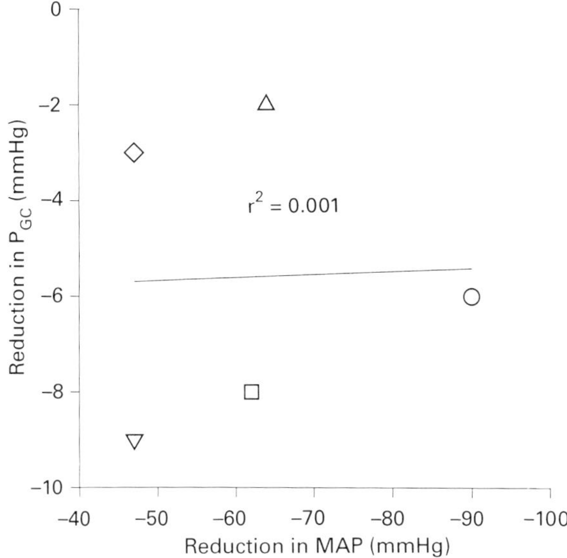

Fig. 6.6 Relationship between the percent reductions in MAP and the absolute reduction in P_{GC} in five studies of triple therapy in experimental chronic renal disease. There was no correlation between the drug-induced decline in MAP and change in P_{GC} in these studies. Symbols and abbreviations are as defined in the legend to Fig. 6.1. Data adapted from references 18–22.

real correlation exists between the absolute reductions in MAP and P_{GC} that were achieved. Similarly and shown in Fig. 6.7, because glomerular injury is a function of glomerular rather than systemic blood pressure, there was also no correlation between the changes in MAP and glomerular injury in these studies. These data suggest that, even when the response to a single type of drug therapy is examined, the magnitude of reduction in the systemic blood pressure may be a poor indicator of changes in glomerular pressure or the risk of injury in animals with hypertension and renal disease. This lack of correlation probably results from the fact that baseline afferent and efferent arteriolar resistance and, therefore, drug-induced changes in R_A, R_E, and P_{GC} vary greatly among the various models of renal disease. However, similar variability in R_A and R_E and in the effect of antihypertensive therapy on P_{GC} is likely to occur in human renal disease. In addition, blood pressure may be highly variable in chronic renal disease and its true magnitude not adequately assessed by intermittent office measurements [25,26]. In individual cases, these factors make it difficult to predict from standard office measurements of systemic blood pressure whether a particular therapy will slow the rate of progression of renal disease.

On the other hand, when increasing doses of specific drugs were administered to animals with a single type of renal disease a more predictable response was observed. In general, the greater the decline in systemic blood pressure, the more likely it is

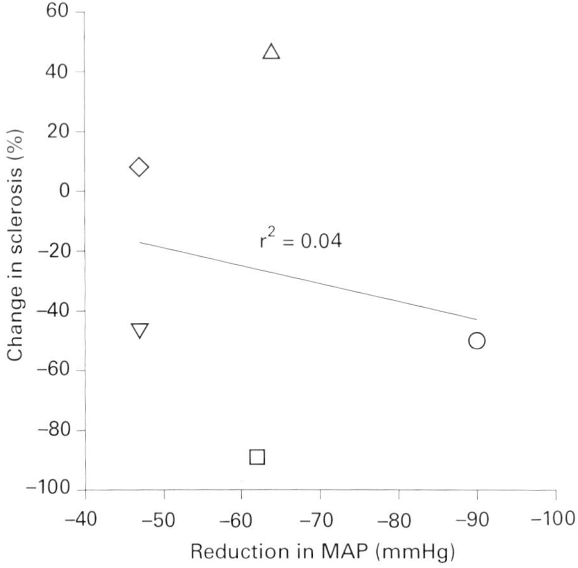

Fig. 6.7 Relationship between the percent reduction in MAP and glomerular sclerosis in five studies of triple therapy in experimental chronic renal disease. There was no significant correlation. Symbols are as defined in the legend to Fig. 6.1. Data adapted from references 18–22.

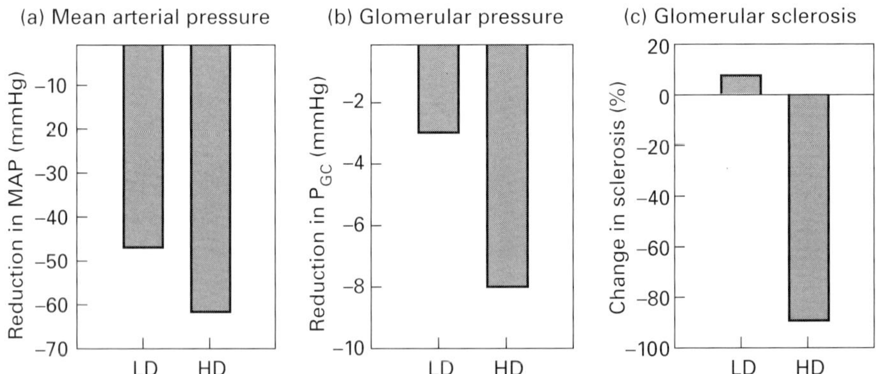

Fig. 6.8 The effects of low dose versus high triple therapy (hydralazine, thiazide, reserpine) on MAP, glomerular capillary pressure, and glomerular sclerosis in rats with remnant kidneys. Data adapted from references 21 and 22.

that a marked reduction in P_{GC} and injury will result This phenomena is illustrated by Fig. 6.8 which shows the effects of low-dose versus high-dose of triple therapy on systemic and glomerular pressure and glomerular injury in remnant kidney rats [21,22]. As shown, although low-dose triple therapy only reduced systemic blood pressure, administration of a higher dose led to an additional 15 mmHg reduction in MAP and a significant decline in glomerular pressure and injury. These data suggest that the greater the decline in systemic pressure, the more likely it is that glomerular hypertension and injury will also be averted.

A similar relationship whereby only the most marked declines in systemic pressure are associated with reduced glomerular pressure and renal protection is observed in animals treated with calcium channel blockers. This relationship is suggested by Fig. 6.9, which summarizes the results of three separate studies ([27,28]; unpublished observations) that examined the effects of different dihydropyridine calcium antagonists on glomerular hemodynamics and injury in a single model, the uninephrectomized spontaneously hypertensive rat. Although the maximally tolerated dose of drug was administered in each case, the effects on systemic blood pressure were somewhat variable. As can be seen, glomerular pressure and injury varied directly with systemic pressure with the greatest declined in P_{GC} and glomerular protection observed in the group that experienced the largest decline in MAP. Consistent with these data, Reams and coworkers [29] reported that administration of a high but not a low dose of the calcium channel blocker manidipine reduced systemic blood pressure and glomerular injury in UNX SHR.

Further insight into the relationship between systemic pressure and glomerular injury as well as the impact of antihypertensive therapy on these parameters has been provided by Griffen and coworkers [26,30]. These authors suggested that the poor performance of the systemic blood pressure response as a predictor of renal outcomes in the intervention studies cited above resulted from the fact that blood pressure is highly variable in these models and was measured only infrequently. Using

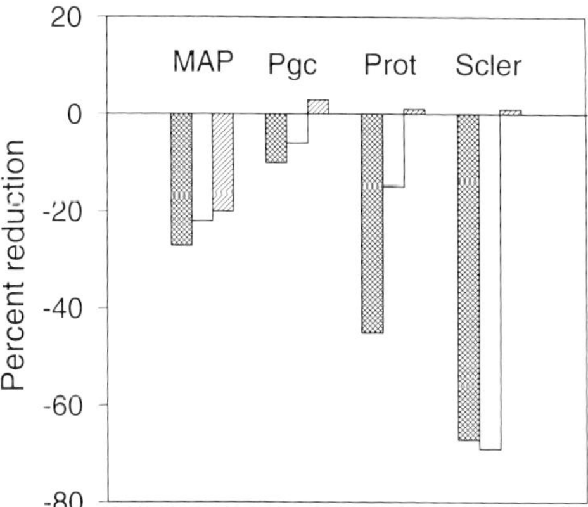

Fig. 6.9 The percent changes in MAP, glomerular pressure, proteinuria (Prot), and glomerular sclerosis (Scler) in three studies in which a calcium channel blocker was administered to UNX-SHR. Injury was only reduced when P_{GC} declined, and this was dependent on the percent reduction in MAP. cross hatched bars = rats treated nifedipine, open bars = rats treated with felodipine, diagonal hatched bars = rats treated with amlodipine. Data adapted from references 16 and 17 and unpublished observations.

radiotelemetric monitoring to assess continuously, and presumably more accurately, time-averaged systemic blood pressure, these authors found a strong correlation between blood pressure and glomerular injury in rats with remnant kidneys [26]. Shown in Fig. 6.10, in these studies, antihypertensive agents prevented glomerular injury in direct proportion to the magnitude of decline in blood pressure that was achieved in individual animals. Based on studies demonstrating that autoregulation of renal blood flow is impaired in rats with chronic renal failure [31], they proposed that autoregulation of glomerular pressure was defective as well and that P_{GC} varied directly with changes in perfusion pressure. In addition to this general observation, various classes of antihypertensive agents were found to have different effects on autoregulatory ability in remnant kidneys. Thus, autoregulation was partially impaired in control and angiotensin-converting enzyme (ACE) inhibitor treated rats, but was completely abolished by administration of a calcium channel blocker [30]. In this latter group, the slope of the relationship between blood pressure and renal injury was steep indicating that there was marked dependency of renal protection on the magnitude of blood pressure lowering in calcium channel blocker treated animals. It is important to recognize that, except for triple therapy, Griffen and colleagues did not investigate the effects of varying doses of antihypertensive drugs on pressure and injury. Rather all rats received similar doses of particular drugs, that resulted by chance in variable degrees of blood pressure lowering and protection in individual animals. In fact, when the effects of increasing doses of triple therapy were examined, these authors were unable to demonstrate improved outcomes with higher doses [26]. Therefore, while lower average blood pressures were convincingly associated with less injury, these data do not establish that higher doses of specific, antihypertensive agents will improve outcomes in the setting of hypertension and chronic renal disease.

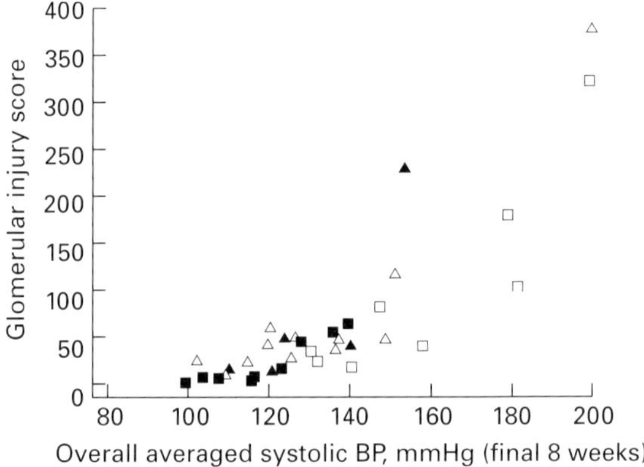

Fig. 6.10 Correlation of glomerular injury score with overall averaged systolic blood pressure. Rats received either no treatment (open squares), enalapril (closed squares), triple therapy (open triangles), or high-dose triple therapy (closed triangles). $r = 0.84$. Reproduced from reference 26.

Links between systemic and glomerular hypertension and progressive kidney damage

A theoretical construct linking systemic and glomerular hypertension to the progression of chronic renal disease is presented in Fig. 6.11. According to this hypothesis, the adverse effects of increases in glomerular pressure primarily result from increases in protein filtration and from capillary wall damage, both causing release of various cytokines and growth factors, activation of the processes of inflammation and abnormal matrix production, matrix degradation, and apoptosis in kidney cells. Alterations in these cellular functions promote the accumulation of matrix and the premature demise of renal glomerular and tubular cells leading eventually to the replacement of normal kidney by fibrous tissue. Also important in this process is

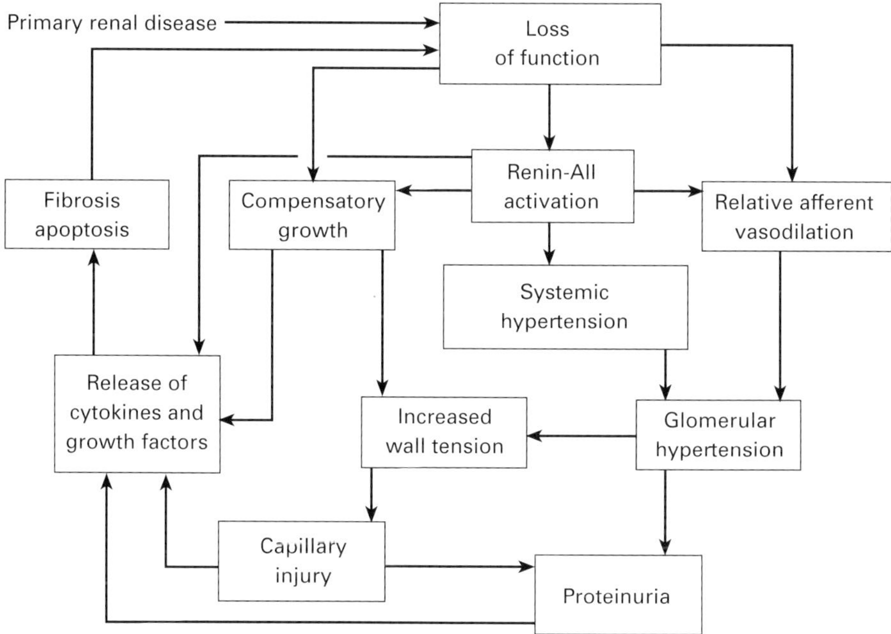

Fig. 6.11 Theoretical construct identifying various factors involved in the progression of chronic renal disease and emphasizing the importance of systemic hypertension in this process. Following a partial loss of kidney function, a number of adaptations occur including stimulation of compensatory growth and afferent vasodilation leading to an increase in function in surviving nephrons. Relative activation of the renin–angiotensin system is also common in renal disease and contributes to the development of systemic hypertension. The combination of systemic hypertension and afferent vasodilatation leads to an increase in glomerular pressure and capillary wall tension. Protein filtration is increased as a result of altered hemodynamics and also of capillary injury and these abnormalities promote production and release of numerous cytokines and growth factors that promote apoptosis and progressive fibrosis.

activation of the renin–angiotensin–aldosterone system which not only tends to increase systemic and glomerular blood pressure but also directly impairs the glomerular capillary wall barrier to macromolecule filtration and stimulates the release of factors that promote cell growth and matrix accumulation. The remainder of this chapter will examine the individual components of this pathophysiologic sequence in greater detail.

Proteinuria as a mechanism of renal injury

A considerable body of data supports the hypothesis that increased filtration of macromolecules promotes glomerular and tubulo-interstitial injury. In numerous clinical studies of various types of glomerular disease, it has generally been observed that patients with greater amounts of proteinuria have a worse renal prognosis. For example, increasing proteinuria was a predictor of more rapid loss of kidney function in both the Modification of Diet in Renal Disease (MDRD) Study [10] and in the more recent Ramipril Efficacy in Nephropathy (REIN) trial [32]. The latter study examined the effects of administration of an ACE inhibitor on the rate of loss of kidney function in patients with non-diabetic renal disease. The study included patients with creatinine clearances from 20 to 70 ml/min per 1.73 m^2 and 24-h urinary protein excretion rates of at least 1 g. The subjects were further divided into two groups with initial protein excretion rates of less than or greater than or equal to 3 g/24 h. Subsequent determinations of GFR revealed a more rapid rate of decline in GFR in patients with more than 3 g of proteinuria. Furthermore, in the patients that did not receive the ACE inhibitor, the greater the baseline protein excretion rate, the more rapid was the rate of decline in GFR. Of note, the correlation between protein excretion rate and GFR decline was less consistent in the ACE inhibitor treated group, suggesting that not all of the beneficial actions of these drugs are mediated by reductions protein excretion rate. The complex interaction between the renin–angiotensin system and various factors that contribute to progression of chronic renal disease is discussed in detail below.

A number of mechanisms have been proposed to explain the adverse effects of macromolecule filtration on kidney function. Filtered proteins cause phenotypic changes in glomerular mesangial and tubular epithelial cells that may have pathogenic significance. In proximal tubular cells, protein loading overwhelms organelles leading to lysosomal rupture and release of toxic enzymes into the renal interstitium [33]. Proteins also induce expression of chemokines in renal epithelial cells, including monocyte chemoattractant protein-1 (MCP-1) [34] and osteopontin [35]. These substances attract monocytes thereby promoting interstitial inflammation. Endothelin production by cultured proximal tubular cells is also enhanced by exposure to proteins [36]. Of note, an increase in local renal endothelin synthesis has been observed in several models of progressive kidney failure, including the remnant kidney [37] and passive Heyman nephritis [38], and administration of an endothelin receptor antagonist ameliorates injury in these models [38,39].

As recently reviewed [40], mesangial deposition of lipoproteins and albumin is also common in glomerular diseases [41,42] and these substances have adverse effects on glomerular cells. Mesangial cells express receptors for both low-density (LDL) and very low-density lipoproteins (VLDL) [43] and binding of these lipoproteins induces multiple phenotypic changes that may promote glomerular sclerosis. For example, binding of LDL and/or VLDL increases expression of transcription factors c-*fos* and c-*jun* as well as platelet-derived growth factor (PDGF) and these changes may contribute to mesangial cell proliferation, hypertrophy, and matrix production [43–45]. Chemokine release is also induced favoring migration of macrophages into the glomerular tuft [46]. Macrophages further contribute to injury by releasing reactive oxygen species that oxidize LDL producing modified lipoproteins that are directly toxic to mesangial cells [47,48].

Increased capillary wall tension promotes capillary injury

One-of the most obvious adaptations to a partial loss of renal function is compensatory kidney growth leading to hyperplasia and hypertrophy of surviving nephron structures. As recently reviewed [49], a large body of evidence suggests that abnormal growth also contributes to progressive kidney damage. For example, maneuvers that reduce renal growth but not glomerular pressure, including dietary salt restriction [50–52] and administration of certain antihypertensive drugs [53,54] also lessen glomerular injury. Consistently, ureteral diversion, which leads to an increase in glomerular pressure but not glomerular size is not associated with marked glomerular injury [55]. On the other hand, hypertrophy without hypertension also produces only a mild degree of injury [56]. Taken together, these data suggest that injury is most severe when glomerular hypertension and hypertrophy coexist. One-factor that has been suggested to explain the synergistic effects of glomerular growth and hypertension in promoting injury is an increase in glomerular capillary wall tension. As summarized in Fig. 6.12, this hypothesis proposes that the hydraulic stress

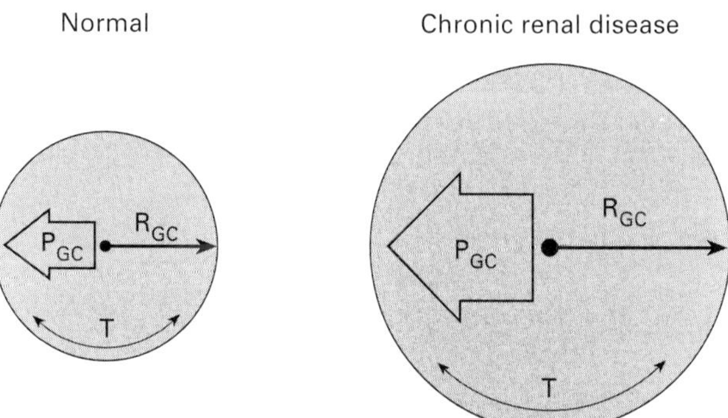

Fig. 6.12 The wall tension hypothesis. According to the LaPlace equation, wall tension in a blood vessel is equal to the product of the transcapillary hydraulic pressure and the radius of the vessel. In chronic renal disease, glomerular capillary wall tension rises because of increases in both glomerular capillary pressure (P_{GC}) and radius (R_{GC}).

experienced by glomerular capillaries is a function of the tension within the capillary wall. According to the LaPlace equation, wall tension in a tubular structure like a glomerular capillary is determined by the product of the transmural hydraulic pressure gradient and the radius of the tube. Therefore, in a hypertensive and hypertrophied glomerular capillary, wall tension will increase because both glomerular pressure and glomerular capillary radius rise.

Morphologic confirmation that glomerular capillary dilatation actually occurs in experimental chronic renal disease has come from the precise anatomical investigations of Kriz and coworkers. These investigators observed focal areas of capillary enlargement in glomeruli from remnant kidneys [57] as well as in a genetic model of progressive glomerular sclerosis [58] (see Fig. 6.13). Localized increases in capillary radius and, therefore, wall tension may help to explain the focal nature of glomerular injury in the initial stages of many chronic renal diseases. Increased capillary wall tension may have several adverse consequences including damage to glomerular endothelial cells and activation mesangial cells [59,60] leading to a release of soluble mediators of inflammation and fibrosis. In addition, because glomerular epithelial cells have a relatively limited ability to proliferate, capillary dilation results in gaps in epithelial integrity with resultant alterations in the filtration of macromolecules and water [61,62]. As discussed above, evidence suggests that increased transglomerular passage of proteins and other large molecules promotes glomerular and interstitial fibrosis.

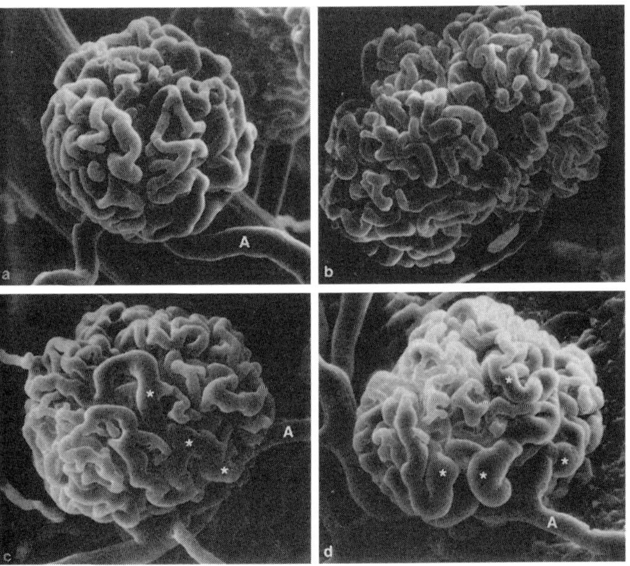

Fig. 6.13 Scanning electron micrographs of vascular casts of glomerular capillaries from normal rats (A,B) and rats with remnant kidneys (C,D). The remnant glomeruli display focal areas of capillary dilatation (indicated by the stars). From reference 57.

Phenotypic changes in endothelial and mesangial cells in response to mechanical stress

Regardless of whether increased wall tension is the major determinant of hydraulic stress to the glomerular capillary wall, mechanical trauma induces phenotypic changes in vascular endothelial and glomerular mesangial cells that tend to promote glomerular sclerosis. In endothelial cells, mechanical stress induces expression of multiple transcription factors including AP-1 [63] as well as growth factors PDGF and basic fibroblast growth factor [64]. PDGF released by stressed epithelial cells in conjunction with that released from platelets adhering to damaged capillary loops in hypertensive glomeruli may promote mesangial cell proliferation and progressive glomerular sclerosis. Endothelial cells subjected to mechanical stretch also increase production and release of endothelin-1 (ET-1) [65]. As discussed above, increased local production of endothelin has been implicated in the progression of experimental renal disease. Finally, studies suggest that mechanical stress stimulates endothelial production of chemokines [66] and alters expression of adhesion molecules [67] in a manner that may promote migration of inflammatory cells into the renal parenchyma.

The effects of increased pressure and mechanical stretch have also been studied in mesangial cells. Yasuda and coworkers [68], subjected cultured mesangial cells to cyclic stretch and examined the regulation of extracellular matrix (ECM) turnover. Stretching mesangial cells induced the expression of multiple matrix genes including types I, III, and IV collagen, fibronectin, and laminin in a time- and force-dependent fashion. A reduction in matrix degradation was also evident, probably mediated by a decrease in the production of a specific metalloproteinase. These alterations are similar to those observed in cells exposed to transforming growth factor (TGF)-β and expression of this cytokine was increased in stretched cells. However, many of the observed changes occurred after only 12 or 24 h of stretch, whereas the increase in TGF-β production was maximal at 48 h. The authors concluded that hydraulic stress induced changes in mesangial cell function that might promote progression to ESRD that were both dependent and independent of TGF-β production. Of note, this same group reported that stretching also induces expression of immediate early genes [69] and, therefore, may promote cell proliferation as well as matrix accumulation by these cells.

It should be noted that, although Akai *et al.* [69] observed fibrosis promoting changes in mesangial cells in response to cyclic stretch, the cells they studied were not actually exposed to increased hydraulic pressure, as would occur in a hypertensive glomerulus. To examine the effects of increased pressure *per se* on mesangial cell function, Mattana and Singhal [70] grew cells in a sealed chamber under normal (40–50 mmHg) or increased (50–60 mmHg) barometric pressure. Consistent with the findings in cells exposed to stretch, prolonged exposure to high barometric pressure stimulated mesangial cell growth and matrix production. Higher than normal pressure also inhibited metalloproteinase activity and degradation of type IV collagen [71]. All of these observations are consistent with the hypothetical construct presented in Fig. 6.11, in which increased glomerular pressure activates multiple cellular pathways tending to promote glomerular sclerosis.

Role of the renin–angiotensin–aldosterone system in renal disease progression

Hemodynamically mediated effects

As suggested in Fig. 6.11, activation of the renin–angiotensin system is a key event promoting progression of chronic renal disease by both hemodynamically and non-hemodynamically mediated mechanisms. Discussed above, renin and angiotensin levels are either elevated or, at least not appropriately suppressed for the degree of blood pressure elevation and volume overload that are characteristic of chronic renal disease and this contributes to the increase in systemic blood pressure in this setting [2]. The importance of systemic hypertension in the genesis of glomerular hypertension and, therefore, injury in chronic renal disease has been examined by comparing renal structure and function in models in which renal mass is reduced by resection [72] or infarction. The increases in renal size, renal blood flow, and GFR produced by these maneuvers are similar, however, because the degree of activation of the renin–angiotensin system may be greater following renal infarction [73], systemic and glomerular hypertension and glomerular injury are also largely limited to this group. The importance of systemic hypertension in the progression of chronic renal disease is also supported by studies that compared the effects of renal mass reduction on systemic and glomerular pressure and glomerular injury in different strains of rat. Typically, subtotal renal ablation by infarction in rats produces a syndrome of systemic and glomerular hypertension, proteinuria, and progressive glomerular sclerosis [74]. However, in Wistar–Kyoto rats (the normotensive controls for spontaneously hypertensive rats) systemic hypertension does not develop following five-sixths nephrectomy and glomerular hypertension and injury are also not observed in this strain [75]. Thus, one critical mechanism by which activation of the renin–angiotensin system promotes glomerular hypertension and injury in chronic renal disease is by contributing to the development of systemic hypertension.

In addition to its action to increase systemic vascular resistance and MAP, angiotensin II has direct effects of the renal microcirculation that tend to increase glomerular capillary hydraulic pressure. Thus, although both pre- and post-glomerular vessels constrict in response to angiotensin II, on balance, the glomerular microcirculatory response to angiotensin II is characterized by a proportionally greater increase efferent as opposed to afferent arteriolar resistance [76]. As summarized above (see Table 6.1) because the efferent arterioles are downstream from the glomerular capillaries, relative efferent vasoconstriction tends to cause glomerular capillary pressure to rise, particularly in the presence of systemic hypertension. That this phenomena is relevant to the progression of renal disease is suggested by studies in which various antihypertensive agents were given to rats with chronic renal disease and their effects on glomerular hemodynamics assessed. Drugs that block the renin–angiotensin system are more likely than other agents to cause reductions in efferent arteriolar resistance and, therefore, declines in glomerular pressure and injury [21,73,77].

Cellular pathways

The process of renal disease progression involves multiple phenotypic changes within various kidney cells. Important alterations in cell function that contribute to the progression of chronic renal disease include proliferation of glomerular mesangial cells and interstitial fibroblasts, stimulation of apoptosis leading to the demise of normal kidney cells, increased matrix production and decreased degradation contributing to the replacement of normal by fibrous tissue. Central to these alterations is an increase in the production of multiple cytokines and growth factors by cells within the glomeruli and tubulo-interstitial regions of damaged kidneys. Many of these pathways are also regulated, at least in part, by components of the renin–angiotensin system.

Renal growth

A considerable body of data supports the hypothesis that angiotensin II is a renotropic factor [78]. Within the glomerulus, angiotensin II stimulates proliferation [79] and/or hypertrophy [80] of mesangial cells. The type of response may depend upon whether or not the cells are in an activated state as determined by factors such as mechanical stretch [81]. Evidence suggests that the proliferative response to angiotensin II is mediated via AT type 1 (AT1) receptors and, therefore, should be blocked by both ACE inhibitors and commercially available angiotensin receptor antagonists. At least some of the growth responses to angiotensin II may be secondarily mediated, as angiotensin II induces synthesis of several mitogens including PDGF [78] and TGF-β [82]. Angiotensin II induced expression of immediate early genes, that signal entry into the G_0–G_1 phase of the cell cycle from which mitosis is possible, in mesangial cells has also been reported by some [78], but not all investigators [83].

Proximal tubule cells contain mRNA [84,85] for all of the components of the renin–angiotensin system including AT1 [86] and AT2 [87] receptors. Angiotensin II has a number of effects on proximal tubular cells including stimulation of Na^+/H^- exchange and ammoniagenesis [78]. By itself, angiotensin II primarily induces hypertrophy of tubular cells [88]; however, proliferative responses to other growth factors may be enhanced in the presence of angiotensin II [89]. As in mesangial cells, angiotensin II also induces immediate-early genes in tubular epithelial cells [88]. However, despite these dramatic effects on cell growth *in vitro*, the importance of angiotensin II as a renal growth factor *in vivo* is still uncertain. For example, chronic infusion of angiotensin II does not induce marked renal hypertrophy of hyperplasia in normal rats [90] and blockade of the renin–angiotensin system has inconsistent effects of renal growth in animals with reduced renal mass [21,91].

Matrix production and degradation

The renin–angiotensin system participates in the regulation of matrix production and degradation both directly, and indirectly by affecting the production of other fibrogenic cytokines. At the level of the glomerulus, angiotensin II induces production of ECM proteins such as thrombospondin [92] and collagen [79] in mesangial cells. Transfection of glomeruli *in vivo* with the renin and angiotensinogen genes induced type I and type III collagen expression and expansion of the ECM [93]. In part, this may result from angiotensin II mediated induction of TGF-β. Sustained, abnormal production of TGF-β alters both the production and degradation of ECM [94] and has been associated with the development of glomerular sclerosis in several models of renal disease [95]. Lee *et al.* [96] reported that enhanced glomerular TGF-β gene expression in remnant kidneys was localized to glomerular endothelial cells where angiotensinogen mRNA levels were also increased. Of note, all of these abnormalities including increased matrix gene expression could be blocked by administration of an angiotensin II receptor antagonist. They proposed that activation of the tissue renin–angiotensin system promoted glomerular sclerosis via a TGF-β mediated process. A similar pathophysiologic sequence has been proposed to explain the development of tubulo-interstitial nephritis following unilateral ureteral obstruction in rats [97]. Gene expression of TGF-β, type IV collagen and a tissue inhibitor of metalloproteinase (TIMP)-1 is enhanced in the kidneys of these rats and administration of an ACE inhibitor reduces mRNA levels for these compounds as well as morphologic evidence of interstitial fibrosis.

In addition to its effects of mesangial and renal tubular cells, activation of the renin–angiotensin system may promote progression of chronic renal disease by activating renal interstitial fibroblasts. Proliferation and increased production of cytokines and matrix proteins [98] by these cells is considered to be a major factor leading to interstitial fibrosis. Interstitial fibroblasts [99] in culture express the AT1 receptor and binding of angiotensin II to this receptor induces expression of the early activating gene c-*fos* and cell proliferation. Angiotensin II also induces interstitial fibroblasts to increase production of TGF-β as well as matrix components fibronectin and type I collagen. Activation of interstitial fibroblasts by angiotensin II also induces endogenous angiotensinogen gene expression, forming a positive feedback loop promoting progressive interstitial fibrosis.

Accumulation of ECM may result from increased synthesis and/or decreased degradation of component proteins. In fact, activation of degradative pathways has the potential not only to prevent but even to reverse glomerular fibrosis [100]. ECM degradation is a highly regulated process and the renin–angiotensin system participates in this regulation [101]. Matrix proteins are degraded by several different families of proteinases including the metalloproteinases. Summarized in Fig. 6.14, activation of the renin–angiotensin system inhibits metalloproteinase activity by at least two mechanisms. First, by both type 1 receptor dependent and independent pathways, angiotensin II induces plasminogen activator inhibitor (PAI) [102,103]. PAI inhibits matrix degradation by reducing the action of plasminogen activators that convert plasminogen to plasmin. Plasmin, in turn, converts latent to active

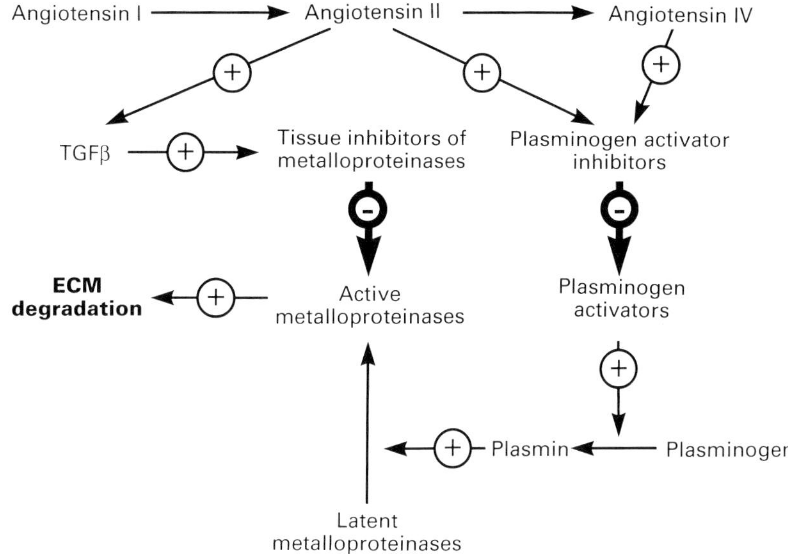

Fig. 6.14 The role of the renin–angiotensin system in the regulation of extracellular matrix degradation. See text for details.

metalloproteinases thereby promoting matrix degradation. Thus, the net effect of angiotensins are to reduce plasmin and metalloproteinase activity and this is prevented by ACE inhibition. Also important in the regulation of matrix degradation are the family of TIMPs. Evidence suggests that angiotensin II increases TIMP levels via a TGF-β-dependent process and this contributes to angiotensin II-associated inhibition of ECM degradation [97].

Angiotensin as a modulator of apoptosis

As function declines in chronic renal disease, kidneys shrink and become fibrotic. Recent data [104] suggest that the apparent increase in scar tissue in end-stage kidneys from animals with interstitial nephritis largely results from dropout of normal cells and collapse and consolidation of existing matrix rather than from the accumulation of excess matrix. Although the process responsible for dropout of normal kidney cells in chronic renal disease is still uncertain, morphologic evidence of cell necrosis is rare. On the other hand, increased apoptotic cell death is observed in both glomerular [105] and interstitial [106] disease and it is likely that many renal cells die by this process.

Apoptosis is an active, highly orchestrated event and the renin–angiotensin system may participate in its regulation. The relationship between angiotensin II and apoptosis has been examined in kidneys subjected to unilateral ureteral obstruction [107]. This maneuver induces apoptosis in renal epithelial cells as well as increased expression of the anti-apoptotic protein, clusterin. Evidence suggests that activation of the renin–angiotensin system suppresses clusterin expression thereby favoring apoptotic cell death. Angiotensin II may also have direct effects on apoptosis that depend on the type of angiotensin II receptor that is expressed. Yamada and coworkers [108] reported that binding of angiotensin II to the AT2 receptor stimulated apoptotic cell death in a rat pheochromocytoma and a mouse fibroblast cell line by a mechanism that involved mitogen-activated protein kinase. On the other hand, in a model of cyclosporin induced interstitial injury, apoptosis was antagonized by blockade of angiotensin II type 1 receptors [109]. These data suggest that angiotensin II can promote apoptosis by binding to AT2 or AT1 receptors in different cell types. As yet, the relevance of these observations to the beneficial effects of renin–angiotensin blocking drugs in chronic renal disease remains to be determined.

Endothelins as mediators of progression of chronic renal disease

Recently reviewed [110], endothelins are a family of predominantly vasoconstrictor peptides that are released by multiple cell types, are independently regulated, and act in an autocrine and paracrine manner to alter kidney function. The renal vasculature is exquisitely sensitive to ET-1 [111], which is released abluminally by endothelial cells to interact with receptors on vascular smooth muscle (VSM) and endothelial cells. There are multiple endothelin receptors; most is known about the endothelin A (ETA) and endothelin B (ETB) receptors which have been cloned and characterized [112,113]. According to the traditional view, ETA receptors, abundant on VSM, have a high affinity for ET-1 and play a prominent part in the pressor response to ET [114]. ETB receptors are present on endothelial cells where they may mediate nitric oxide release and endothelial-dependent relaxation [115]. However, the distribution and function of ETA and ETB receptors varies greatly among species and, in the rat, even according to strain [116]. In the normal rat, endogenous endothelin may actually tonically dilate the afferent arteriole and lower the ultrafiltration coefficient, K_f, via ETB receptors [117]. However, ETB receptors on VSM also mediate vasoconstriction in the rat and this is potentiated in hypertensive animals [116].

Endothelin production is increased in the remnant kidney [118] and blockade of ETA receptors reduces systemic blood pressure as well as glomerular and tubular injury in this setting [119]. Of note, however, ETB receptor gene expression is also enhanced and administration of the mixed ETA and ETB receptor antagonist, bosentan, may be more effective in reducing renal injury than ETA blockade alone [120]. Bosentan also reduced renal injury in an immune model of renal disease [121]. Of note, ET may have multiple non-hemodynamic effects that promote progressive kidney damage. Endothelin is mitogenic for kidney cells [122–124] and its production is increased in human and experimental glomerulonephritis [125–128]. Blockade of endothelin receptors inhibits mesangial cell proliferation [129] and reduces injury in a murine model of lupus nephritis [130]. Endothelins also have direct effects on matrix production and degradation that may promote renal scarring [3]. Endothelins increase matrix production directly [131] and stimulate the release of other cytokines that also promote matrix accumulation. Endothelin also increases levels of tissue inhibitor of metalloproteinases. As discussed above, these substances inhibit the activity of the metalloproteinases that play an important part in ECM degradation. At present, the importance of these various actions of the vascular endothelin system in renal disease progression in humans is still unclear.

Impact of antihypertensive therapy on progression of non-diabetic forms of chronic renal disease: analysis of clinical studies

Essential hypertension

As discussed above, although the vast majority of patients with essential hypertension do not develop clinically important chronic renal disease, epidemiological data suggest that uncontrolled systemic hypertension is a common cause of end-stage renal failure. Although not the primary end-point in most studies, clinical trial data also suggest that antihypertensive therapy can preserve kidney function in this population. For example, in 5000 hypertensives enrolled in the MRFIT study, individuals with a diastolic blood pressure in excess of 95 mmHg experienced a more rapid decline in the reciprocal of serum creatinine (a measure of GFR) than patients with diastolic blood pressure below 95 [132]. In the Hypertension Detection and Follow-up Program trial, subjects randomized to the stepped-care group that had a mean blood pressure of 129/86 had more stable renal function than the referred-care group at a mean pressure of 139/90 [133]. In 12 000 hypertensive men, reducing systolic blood pressure by more than 20 mmHg lessened the likelihood of developing ESRD by almost two-thirds [134]. Smaller decrements in blood pressure were also beneficial. In several smaller studies [135–137], deterioration in renal function was observed despite antihypertensive therapy in patients with diastolic blood pressures in excess of 90 mmHg or MAPs greater than 107 mmHg. Taken together, these data suggest that reducing systolic blood pressure to less than 140 mmHg or MAP to less than 100 mmHg may renal protective in patients with hypertension.

Non-diabetic chronic renal disease

Most patients with chronic kidney disease are hypertensive [1] and numerous studies suggest that reducing blood pressure can slow the rate of decline in renal function. The MDRD study compared the effects of achieving a low versus a more usual blood pressure target on the rate of decline in GFR in 840 patients with an initial GFR between 13 and 55 ml/min [10]. In patients less than 60 years of age, the low and high blood pressure targets were MAPs of 92 and 98 mmHg, respectively, whereas in older patients, MAPs of 107 and 113 mmHg were compared. Patients were treated with a variety of antihypertensive medications with most patients receiving ACE inhibitors or calcium channel blockers alone or in combination with a diuretic. Additional therapies included dietary salt restriction as well as dietary protein restriction in half of the patients. For the group as a whole, no difference in the rate of decline in GFR was observed between patients in the high and low blood pressure groups;

however, only a 4.7 mmHg difference in MAP was achieved between the high and low blood pressure groups and even the usual pressure group had excellent blood pressure control (MAP 97 mmHg). Of note, little disease progression was observed in either the group and this may have resulted from the significant reduction in blood pressure that was achieved in many hypertensive patients. In addition, a relatively high percentage of patients with adult polycystic kidney disease participated in the study and these patients may experience less benefit from aggressive blood pressure lowering than those with other types of renal disease [10].

In fact, secondary analysis suggested that some patients may have benefited from the lower target. For example, there was a trend toward a slower rate of decline in GFR in black patients with renal disease that were randomized to the lower blood pressure target. Unfortunately, only 52 black patients were randomized in this study and that was too few to provide sufficient power to answer this question. On the other hand, more aggressive antihypertensive therapy was associated with a significant reduction in the rate of loss in renal function in proteinuric patients (see Fig. 6.15). This was particularly true for the 55 patients that excreted more than 3 g of protein per day and also observed in those with protein excretion rates between 1 and 3 g/day. A similar conclusion was recently reached by the Northern Italian Cooperative Study Group, who found that reducing MAP to less than 107 mmHg was associated with improved renal survival in proteinuric patients with non-diabetic chronic renal disease [136]. In many chronic renal diseases, heavy proteinuria is associated with a worse prognosis and an increased risk of developing ESRD [138–142]. As discussed above, increased macromolecule filtration may be not only a marker for, but also a cause of glomerular and tubulo-interstitial injury. The data sighted above suggest that aggressive antihypertensive therapy is particularly important for preserving kidney function in this subset of patients.

Of note, rapid normalization of systemic blood pressure may be associated with an initial decline in GFR in patients with hypertension and chronic renal disease. In fact, a sudden, modest initial decline in GFR was observed in the MDRD study in patients randomized to both the usual and low blood pressure groups (see Fig. 6.15). Subsequently, however, the rate of decline in GFR stabilized and no long-term adverse effects of the low blood pressure target were observed. This suggests that low blood pressure targets are safe for the majority of patients with chronic renal disease. In addition, it should be noted that the initial decline in GFR that follows aggressive blood pressure reduction probably results, at least in part, from a decline in glomerular capillary pressure. If so, then a modest initial but non-progressive decline in GFR might actually serve as a marker indicating that one had achieved the desired effect of reducing P_{GC}.

Renal protection: Are all antihypertensive agents created equal?

It has been suggested that drugs that block the renin–angiotensin system may be more effective than other agents in slowing progression of chronic renal disease. A number of clinical trials have examined this question in patients with diabetic and non-diabetic forms of renal disease. For a discussion of the studies involving

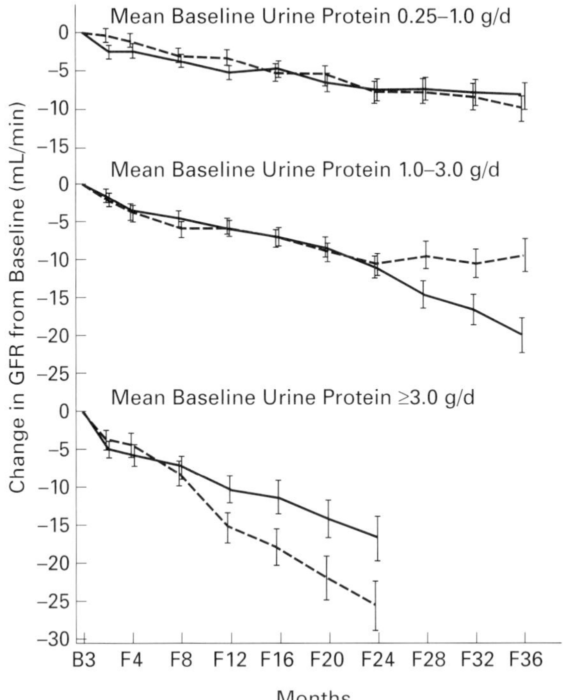

Fig. 6.15 Mean decline in GFR over 24–36 months stratified according to baseline urinary protein excretion rate in patients treated to a traditional (solid line) or low (dashed line) blood pressure target. B3, Third month visit prior to randomization to blood pressure group; F, follow-up visit labeled in terms of the number of months after randomization. GFR at entry was 25–55 ml/min per 1.73 m^2. The number of patients at each level of protein excretion were: 305 patients with 0–250 mg/day; 105 patients with 250 mg–1 g/day; 55 patients with more than 3 g/day. Reproduced from reference 142 with permission.

diabetic patients, the reader is referred to Chapter 7. Discussed above, The REIN trial [32] examined the effects of the ACE inhibitor ramipril on the rate of decline in GFR in 352 patients with chronic nephropathy and persistent proteinuria of at least 1 g/24 h. Patients were stratified according to their baseline protein excretion rate and then randomly assigned to receive ramipril or placebo. Hypertension was present in approximately 75–80% of the patients in both groups and patients were initially treated with increasing doses of study drug to achieve a diastolic blood pressure less than 90 mmHg. If necessary, other blood pressure medications were adjusted, up or down to reach this target. The results of this study are summarized in Fig. 6.16. Higher initial protein excretion rates were associated with a more rapid rate of decline in GFR and this was prevented by administration of ramipril, which also significantly reduced the risk of developing end-stage kidney failure. Of note, follow-up blood pressures were similar in the two groups, averaging 144/88 mmHg

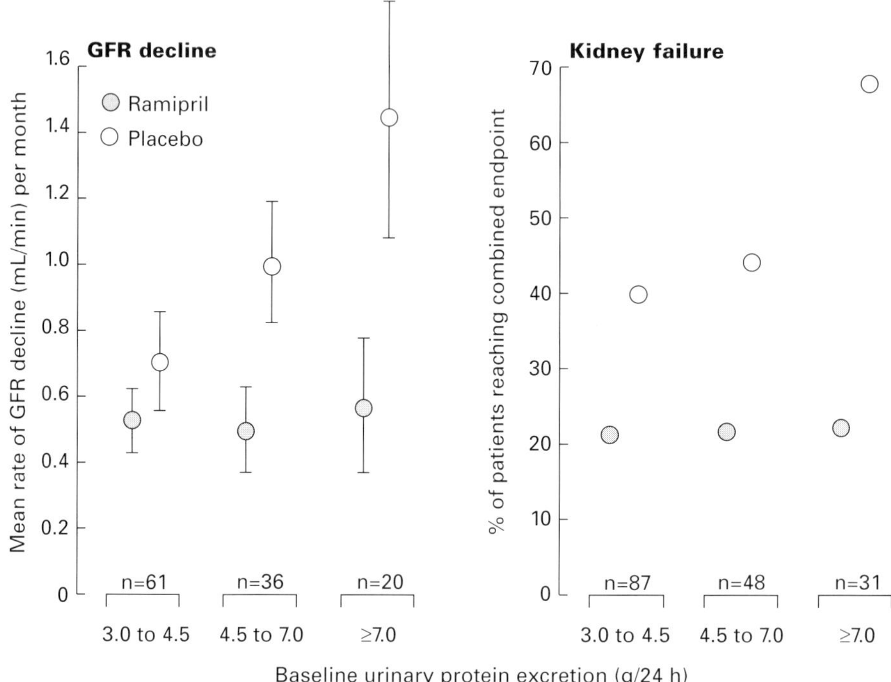

Fig. 6.16 Rate of decline in GFR (top) and the percentage risk of doubling of baseline creatinine or developing end-stage renal disease (bottom) in patients given ramipril or placebo according to baseline protein excretion rate. Patients with greater initial urinary protein excretion rates displayed a more rapid rate of decline in GFR and this was prevented by ramipril. Reproduced from reference 32 with permission.

in the ramipril and 145/89 mmHg in the placebo-treated groups. These data suggest that ACE inhibitors may have blood pressure independent, renal protective effects particularly in patients with heavy proteinuria. However, the average MAP achieved in this study was only 106 mmHg, indicating that, despite treatment, significant hypertension was present in both groups. Whether a particular benefit of ACE inhibitor therapy would still have been observed if MAP had been reduced to <120/80 mmHg (the value associated with optimal preservation of kidney function in proteinuric patients in the MDRD study) is uncertain.

The Angiotensin Converting Enzyme Inhibition in Progressive Renal Insufficiency (AIPRI) study examined 583 patients with chronic renal disease and a GFR between 30 and 60 ml/min as determined by creatinine clearance [11]. Only 21 of the patients had diabetic renal disease. Patients were randomly assigned to receive a fixed dose of the ACE inhibitor benazepril (10 mg/day) or placebo. The end point of the study was either a doubling of serum creatinine or the need for dialysis. Over 80% of the patients were hypertensive, and elevated blood pressure was treated by administration of one of a variety of agents in addition to benazepril or placebo, most often calcium antagonists and/or beta-blockers. In fact, the average patient received two blood pressure medications in addition to the study drug. After 3 years, renal survival was significantly better in patients receiving benazepril as compared with placebo, with the greatest benefit in those patients with substantial proteinuria. However, blood pressure was also significantly lower in the benazepril group and, therefore, the study did not conclusively demonstrate a superiority of ACE inhibition that was independent of blood pressure control. A similar conclusion was recently reached by Giatras *et al.* [143], who performed a meta-analysis of 10 clinical trials that examined the effects of ACE inhibitors on the rate of progression of non-diabetic chronic renal disease. As shown in Fig. 6.17, the authors found that the pooled relative risk of progression was 0.7 in those given ACE inhibitors, consistent with the hypothesis that ACEI lessen injury in patients with hypertension and chronic renal disease. However, as was the case for many of the individual studies,

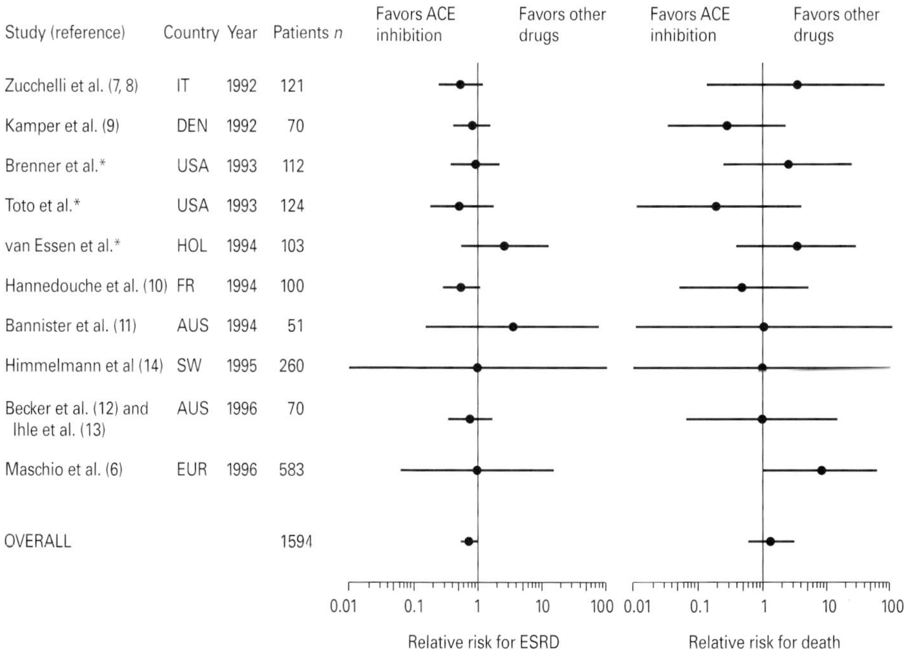

Fig. 6.17 The effect of ACE inhibitor therapy on the risk of ESRD and death in patients with non-diabetic renal disease. The pooled relative risk for the 10 studies that were included in the analysis was 0.70 (95% confidence interval 0.51–0.97), indicating a statistically significant benefit of ACE inhibitor therapy that was also associated with a lower average blood pressure (data not shown). Reproduced from reference 143 with permission. Studies cited refer to reference 143.

in the pooled analysis, weighted mean systolic blood pressure was approximately 5 mmHg less in the ACE inhibitor group, and this may have contributed to the better outcome. In summary, the clinical trials completed to date demonstrate that ACE inhibitors are effective antihypertensive agents in patients with chronic renal disease. In proteinuric patients treated to a target blood pressure of approximately 140/80 mmHg, a two- to three-drug regimen that includes an ACE inhibitor, usually in combination with a diuretic and/or a calcium channel blocker, may be more effective than non-ACE containing regimens is slowing renal disease progression.

As yet, relatively few clinical studies have been conducted to determine whether other classes of antihypertensive agents also have biologically important, blood pressure independent, renal protective effects. As discussed above, experimental evidence suggests that calcium antagonists may slow progression of renal disease in some settings. Consistent with this view, no difference in the rate of decline in GFR was observed in one study in which an ACE inhibitor and a dihydropyridine calcium antagonist were compared [144]. Several large clinical trials are also underway examining the effects of various angiotensin II receptor antagonists on renal injury in patients with type II diabetes. However, as yet, the relative utility of these agents in renal protection has not been adequately examined.

Rational antihypertensive therapy in patients with chronic renal disease

Because all drugs tend to reduce P_{GC} when blood pressure is markedly lowered, it follows that all drugs should be beneficial in preserving kidney function if optimal control of systemic blood pressure is achieved. We have proposed that [145] the apparent superiority of ACE inhibitors in preventing progressive kidney failure may be less evident when patients are treated to a relatively low blood pressure target of <120/80 mmHg. This hypothesis is consistent with available data but has yet to be specifically examined in clinical trials. In fact, the entire debate over which single agent is most effective in slowing progression of chronic renal disease may be somewhat misleading. As discussed above, in virtually every clinical trial that has been performed in patients with hypertension, diabetes, and/or chronic renal disease, blood pressure was rarely adequately controlled by administration of a single agent. For example, in the MDRD study, the average patient in the low blood pressure group received two antihypertensive medications [146]. Similarly, in the AIPRI trial, on average, 1.7 antihypertensive drugs were given in addition to benazepril in order to control blood pressure adequately, indicating that most patients were on triple drug therapy. In the REIN trial [32], 75% of the patients given ramipril were also treated with at least one other antihypertensive medication in order to achieve a diastolic pressure of about 90 mmHg. These data indicate that, when treating patients with hypertension and chronic renal disease, one should expect to prescribe at least two and often three or more antihypertensive medications. In patients with a significant glomerular component to their disease, defined as the excretion of greater than 1 g of protein in 24 h, it makes sense to begin with an ACE inhibitor. Logical drugs to combine with ACE inhibitors in order to achieve a goal blood pressure of <120/80 mmHg in this group include diuretics and/or calcium antagonists. Other agents including beta- and alpha-blockers may also be useful and necessary additions to reduce blood pressure to optimum values. In patients without proteinuria, there is less evidence that specific agents or tight blood pressure control convey additional benefits in terms of preserving kidney function. In this group the major purpose of antihypertensive therapy is to decrease the risk of adverse cardiovascular events. In this setting, blood pressure should be reduced to the more traditional target of <140/90 mmHg. ACE inhibitors may also be useful in these patients because of the potential contribution of inappropriate activation of the renin–angiotensin system to the genesis of hypertension in chronic renal disease. In addition, a recent study in diabetic patients demonstrated that an ACE inhibitor was superior to calcium channel blocker in preventing adverse cardiovascular events [147], and this may also be relevant in patients with non-diabetic forms of renal disease.

Summary

Our understanding of the mechanisms by which the kidney is damaged in patients with systemic hypertension has greatly expanded in the last several years. We now recognize that elevation in systemic blood pressure is a marker for a syndrome which is characterized not only by abnormal hemodynamics, but also by alterations in vascular and renal cellular functions. Nevertheless, elevation is systemic blood pressure is the most easily identified clinical event contributing to progression of chronic renal disease and it should be treated aggressively in all patients. Available clinical trial data suggest that reducing blood pressure treating to the relatively low target of 120/80 mmHg is indicated in proteinuric patients. Most patients with hypertension and chronic renal disease will require combination drug therapy to achieve this goal. In patients that excrete more than 1 g of protein per day, evidence suggests that the prescribed combination of drugs include an ACE inhibitor. Ongoing research in these areas will likely yield novel therapies to preserve kidney function in patients with chronic renal disease even in the absence of systemic hypertension.

Key references

Buckalew VM, Berg RL, Wang S-R *et al.* Prevalence of hypertension in 1795 subjects with chronic renal disease. The Modification of Diet in Renal Disease Study Baseline Cohort. *Am J Kidney Dis* 1996; **28**: 811–821.

Dworkin LD, Brenner BM. The renal circulations. In *The Kidney* (ed Brenner BM and Rector F), pp. 247–285. W.B. Saunders, Philadelphia, 1996.

Preston RA, Singer I, Epstein M. Renal parenchymal hypertension: Current concepts of pathogenesis and management. A summary of the factors that account for the development of hypertension in individuals with chronic renal disease. *Arch Intern Med* 1996; **156**: 602–611.

Walker WG, Neaton JD, Cutler JA, Neuwirth R, Cohen JD. for the MRFIT Research Group. Renal function change in hypertensive members of the multiple risk factor intervention trial. *JAMA* 1992; **268**: 3085–3091.

Weir MR, Dworkin LD. Antihypertensive drugs, dietary salt, and renal protection: How low should you go and with which therapy? *Am J Kidney Dis* 1998; **32**: 1–22.

References

1. Buckalew VM, Berg RL, Wang S-R *et al.* Prevalence of hypertension in 1795 subjects with chronic renal disease. The Modification of Diet in Renal Disease Study Baseline Cohort. *Am J Kidney Dis* 1996; **28**: 811–821.
2. Preston RA, Singer I, Epstein M. Renal parenchymal hypertension: Current concepts of pathogenesis and management. A summary of the factors that account for the development of hypertension in individuals with chronic renal disease. *Arch Intern Med* 1996; **156**: 602–611.
3. Sinclair AM, Isles CG, Brown I, Cameron H, Murray BD, Robertson JWK. Secondary hypertension in a blood pressure clinic. *Arch Intern Med* 1987; **147**: 1289–1293.
4. Joint National Committee. *The Sixth Report of the Joint National Committee on Prevention, Detection Evaluation and Treatment of High Blood Pressure*. NIH Publication no. 98–4080, 1997.
5. Renal Data System. USRDS 1997 Annual Report. Bethesda MDUS. Department of Health and Human Services, National Institute of Diabetes and Digestive and Kidney Disease 1997.
6. Walker WG, Neaton JD, Cutler JA, Neuwirth R, Cohen JD. for the MRFIT Research Group. Renal function change in hypertensive members of the multiple risk factor intervention trial. *JAMA* 1992; **268**: 3085–3091.
7. Klag MJ, Whelton PK, Randall BL, Neaton JD, Braucati FL, Ford CE, Shulman NB, Stamler J. Blood pressure and end-stage renal disease in men. A landmark study that examines the association between elevations in systemic blood pressure and the risk of developing end stage renal disease in man. *N Engl J Med* 1996; **334**: 13–18.
8. Epstein M. Aging and the kidney. *J Am Soc Nephrol* 1996; **7**: 1106–1122.
9. Brazy PC, Stead WW, Fitzwilliam JF. Progression of renal insufficiency: role of blood pressure. *Kidney Int* 1989; **35**: 670–674.
10. Klahr S, Levey AS, Beck GJ, Caggiula AW, Hunsicker L, Kusek JW, Striker G. The effects of dietary protein restriction and blood-pressure control on the progression of chronic renal disease. Modification of Diet in Renal Disease Study Group. *N Engl J Med* 1994; **330**: 877–884.
11. Maschio G, Alberti D, Janin G, Locatelli F, Mann JFE, Motolese M, Ponticelli C, Ritz E, Zucchelli P and the Angiotensin-Converting-Enzyme Inhibition in Progressive Renal Insufficiency Group: Effect of the angiotensin-converting-enzyme inhibitor benazepril on the progression of renal insufficiency. *N Engl J Med* 1996; **334**: 939–945.
12. Hostetter TH, Olson JL, Rennke HG, Venkatachalam MA, Brenner BM. Hyperfiltration in remnant nephrons: a potentially adverse response to renal ablation. *Am J Physiol* 1981; **241**: F85–F93.
13. Dworkin LD, Hostetter TH, Rennke HG, Brenner BM. Hemodynamic basis for glomerular injury in rats with desoxycorticosterone-salt hypertension. *J Clin Invest* 1984; **73**: 1448–1461.
14. Nath KA, Kren SM, Hostetter TH. Dietary protein restriction in established renal injury in the rat: selective role of glomerular capillary pressure in progressive glomerular dysfunction. *J Clin Invest* 1986; **78**: 1199–1205.
15. Dworkin LD, Feiner HD. Glomerular injury in uninephrectomized spontaneously

hypertensive rats: a consequence of glomerular capillary hypertension. *J Clin Invest* 1986; **77**: 797.

16. Anderson S, Meyer T, Rennke HG, Brenner BM. Control of glomerular hypertension limits glomerular injury in rats with reduced renal mass. *J Clin Invest* 1985; **76**: 612–619.
17. Kakinuma Y, Kawamura T, Bills T, Yoshioka T, Ichikawa I, Fogo A. Blood pressure independent effect of angiotensin inhibition on the glomerular and non-glomerular vascular lesions of chronic renal failure. *Kidney Int* 1996; **42**: 46–55.
18. Dworkin LD, Grosser M, Feiner HD, Ullian M, Parker M. Renal vascular effects of antihypertensive therapy in uninephrectomized spontaneously hypertensive rats. *Kidney Int* 1989; **35**: 790–798.
19. Neugarten J, Kaminetsky B, Feiner H, Schacht RG, Liu DT, Baldwin DS. Nephrotoxic serum nephritis with hypertension: amelioration by antihypertensive therapy. *Kidney Int* 1985; **28**: 135–139.
20. Dworkin LD, Feiner HD, Randazzo J. Glomerular hypertension and injury in desoxycorticosterone-salt rats on antihypertensive therapy. *Kidney Int* 1987; **31**: 718–724.
21. Anderson S, Rennke HG, Brenner BM. Therapeutic advantage of converting enzyme inhibitors in arresting progressive renal disease associated with systemic hypertension. *J Clin Invest* 1986; **77**: 1993–2000.
22. Yoshida Y, Kawamura T, Ikoma M, Fogo A, Ichikawa I. Effects of antihypertensive drugs on glomerular morphology. *Kidney Int* 1989; **36**: 626–635.
23. Meyer TW, Anderson S, Rennke HG, Brenner BM. Reversing glomerular hypertension stabilizes established glomerular injury. *Kidney Int* 1987; **31**: 751–759.
24. Dworkin LD, Brenner BM. The renal circulations. In *The Kidney* (ed Brenner BM and Rector F), pp. 247–285. W.B. Saunders, Philadelphia, 1996.
25. Parati G, Omboni S, DiRienzo M, Frattola A, Albini F, Mancia G. Twenty-four hour blood pressure variability: Clinical implications. *Kidney Int* 1992; **41** (Suppl. 37): S24–S28.
26. Griffen KA, Picken M, Bidani AK. Radiotelemetric BP monitoring, antihypertensives and glomeruloprotection in remnant kidney model. *Kidney Int* 1994; **46**: 1010–1018.
27. Dworkin LD, Feiner HD, Parker M, Tolbert E. Effects of nifedipine and enalapril on glomerular structure and function in uninephrectomized spontaneously hypertensive rats. *Kidney Int* 1991; **39**: 1112–1117.
28. Dworkin LD, Tolbert E, Recht PA, Hersch JC, Feiner H, Levin RI. Effects of amlodipine on glomerular filtration, growth, and injury in experimental hypertension. *Hypertension* 1996; **27**: 245–250.
29. Reams GP, Villarreal D, Wu Z, Wang X, Luger AM, Bauer JH. An evaluation of the renal protective effect of manidipine in the uninephrectomized spontaneously hypertensive rat. *Am Heart J* 1993; **125**: 620–625.
30. Griffen KA, Picken MM, Bidani AK. Deleterious effects of calcium channel blockade on pressure transmission and glomerular injury in rat remnant kidneys. *J Clin Invest* 1995; **96**: 793–800.
31. Bidani AK, Schwartz MM, Lewis EJ. Renal autoregulation and vulnerability to hypertensive injury in remnant kidney. *Am J Physiol* 1987; **252**: F1003–F1010.
32. GISEN Group. Randomized placebo-controlled trial of effect of ramipril on decline in glomerular filtration rate and risk of terminal renal failure in proteinuric, non-diabetic nephropathy. *Lancet* 1998; **349**: 1857–1863.
33. Maack T, Park CH, Camargo MJF. Renal filtration, transport, and metabolism of

proteins. In *The Kidney: Physiology and Pathophysiology* (ed. Seldin DW, Giebisch G) pp. 3005–3038. Raven Press, New York, 1992.

34. Wang Y, Chen J, Chen L, Tay YC, Rangan GK, Harris DC. Induction of monocyte chemoattractant protein-1 in proximal tubule cells by urinary protein. *J Am Soc Nephrol* 1997; **10**: 1537–1545.
35. Eddy AA, Giachelli CM, Lombardi D, Pippin J, Gordon K, Alpers CE, Schwartz SM, Johnson RJ. Renal expression of genes that promote interstitial inflammation and fibrosis in rats with protein-overload proteinuria. *Kidney Int* 1995; **47**: 1546–1557.
36. Zoja C, Morigi M, Figliuzzi M, Bruzzi I, Oldroyd S, Benigni A, Rnoco PM, Remuzzi G. Proximal tubule cell synthesis and secretion of endothelin-1 on challenge with albumin and other proteins. *Am J Kidney Dis* 1995; **26**: 934–941.
37. Orisio S, Benigni A, Bruzzi I, Corna D, Perico N, Zoja C, Benatti L, Remuzzi G. Renal endothelin gene expression is increased in remnant kidney and correlates with disease progression. *Kidney Int* 1993; **43**: 354–358.
38. Dulcenombre GG, Largo R, Liu X, Gutierrez S, Lopez-Armada M, Palacios I, Egido J. An orally active Et_A/ET_B receptor antagonist ameliorates proteinuria and glomerular lesions in rats with proliferative nephritis. *Kidney Int* 1996; **50**: 962–972.
39. Benigni A, Zola C, Corna D, Orision S, Facchinetti D, Benati L, Remuzzi G. Blocking both type A and B endothelin receptors in the kidney attenuates renal injury and prolongs survival in rats with remnant kidneys. *Am J Kidney Dis* 1996; **27**: 416–423.
40. Schreiner GF. Renal toxicity of albumin and other lipoproteins. The effects of increased filtration of macromolecules on glomerular cells are reviewed. *Curr Opin Nephrol Hypertension* 1995; **4**: 369–373.
41. Klahr S, Schreiner G, Ichikawa I. The progression of renal disease. A discussion of many of the factors that have been associated with progression of renal disease. *N Engl J Med* 1988; **318**: 1657–1666.
42. Lee H, Lee J, Koh H, Ko KW. Intraglomerular lipid deposition in routine biopsies. *Clin Nephrol* 1991; **36**: 67–75.
43. Grone E, Abboud HE, Hone M, Walli AK, Grone HJ, Stuker D, Robenek H, Wieland E, Seidel D. Actions of lipoproteins in cultured human mesangial cells: modulation by mitogenic vasoconstrictors. *Am J Physiol* 1992; **263**: F686–F696.
44. Wheeler DC, Persaud JW, Fernando R, Sweny P, Varghese Z, Moorhead JF. Effects of low-density lipoproteins in mesangial cell growth and viability in vitro. *Nephrol Dial Transplant* 1990; **5**: 185–191.
45. Sukhatme V. Early transcriptional events in cell growth: the Egr family. *J Am Soc Nephrol* 1990; **1**: 859–866.
46. Rovin BH, Tan LC. LDL stimulates mesangial fibronectin production and chemoattractant expression. *Kidney Int* 1993; **43**: 218–225.
47. Steinberg D, Pathasarathy S, Carew TE, Khoo JC, Witztum JL. Beyond cholesterol. Modifications of low-density lipoprotein that increase its atherogenicity. *N Engl J Med* 1989; **320**: 915–924.
48. Wheeler DC, Chana RS, Topley N, Petersen MM, Davies M, Williams JD. Oxidation of low density lipoprotein by mesangial cells may promote glomerular injury. *Kidney Int* 1994; **45**: 1628–1636.
49. Hostetter TH. Progression of renal disease and renal hypertrophy. The hypertrophic response to renal mass reduction and its role in progression of renal disease are reviewed. *Ann Rev Physiol* 1995; **57**: 263–278.
50. Lax DS, Benstein JA, Tolbert E, Dworkin LD. Effects of salt restriction on renal growth and glomerular injury in rats with remnant kidneys. *Kidney Int* 1992; **41**: 1527–1534.

51. Dworkin LD, Benstein JA, Tolbert E, Feiner HD. Salt restriction inhibits renal growth and stabilizes injury in rats with established renal disease. *J Am Soc Nephrol* 1996; **7**: 437–442.
52. Daniels BS, Hostetter TH. Adverse effects of growth in the glomerular microcirculation. *Am J Physiol* 1990; **258**: F1409–F1416.
53. Dworkin LD, Benstein JA, Parker M, Tolbert E, Feiner HD. Calcium antagonists and converting enzyme inhibitors reduce renal injury in rats with remnant kidneys by different mechanisms. *Kidney Int* 1993; **43**: 808–814.
54. Yoshida Y, Kawamura T, Ikoma M, Fogo A, Ichikawa I. Effects of antihypertensive drugs on glomerular morphology. *Kidney Int* 1989; **36**: 626–635.
55. Yoshida Y, Fogo A, Ichikawa I. Glomerular hemodynamic changes vs. hypertrophy in experimental glomerular sclerosis. *Kidney Int* 1989; **35**: 654–660.
56. Miller PL, Rennke HG, Meyer TW. Glomerular hypertrophy accelerates hypertensive glomerular injury in rats. *Am J Physiol* 1991; **261**: F459–F465.
57. Nagata M, Scharer K, Kriz W. Glomerular damage after uninephrectomy in young rats. I. Hypertrophy and distortion of capillary architecture. *Kidney Int* 1992; **42**: 136–147.
58. Kriz W, Hosser H, Hahnel B, Simons JL, Provoost AP. Development of vascular pole-associated glomerulosclerosis in the Fawn-hooded rat. *J Am Soc Nephrol* 1998; **3**: 381–396.
59. Fine LG, Hammerman MR, Abboud HE. Evolving role of growth factors in the renal response to acute and chronic disease. *J Am Soc Nephrol* 1992; **2**: 1163–1170.
60. Harris RL, Akai Y, Yasuda T, Homma T. The role of physical forces in alterations of mesangial cell function. A summary of a number of studies examining the effects of cyclic stretch on mesangial cell function. *Kidney Int* 1994; **45** (Suppl.): S17–S21.
61. Fries JWU, Sandstrom DJ, Meyer TW, Rennke HG. Glomerular hypertrophy and epithelial cell injury modulate progressive glomerular sclerosis in the rat. *Lab Invest* 1989; **60**: 205–217.
62. Miller PL, Scholey JW, Rennke HG, Meyer TW. Glomerular hypertrophy aggravates epithelial injury in nephrotic rats. *J Clin Invest* 1990; **85**: 1119–1126.
63. Du W, Mills I, Sumpio BE. Cyclic strain causes heterogeneous induction of transcription factors, AP-1, CRE binding protein and NF-κB, in endothelial cells: species and vascular bed diversity. *J Biomechan* 1995; **28**: 1485–1491.
64. Malek AM, Gibbons GH, Dzau VJ, Izumo S. Fluid shear stress differentially modulates expression of genes encoding basic fibroblast growth factor and platelet-derived growth factor B chain in vascular endothelium. *J Clin Invest* 1993; **92**: 2013–2921.
65. Macarthur H, Warner TD, Wood EG, Corder R, Vane JR. Endothelin-1 release from endothelial cells in culture is elevated both acutely and chronically by short periods of mechanical stretch. *Biochem Biophys Res Commun* 1994; **200**: 395–400.
66. Wung BS, Cheng JJ, Chao YJ, Lin J, Shyy YJ, Wang DL. Cyclical strain increases monocyte chemotactic protein-1 secretion in human endothelial cells. *Am J Physiol* 1996; **270**: H1462–H1468.
67. Chien S, Li S, Shyy JYJ. Effects of mechanical forces on signal transduction and gene expression in endothelial cells. A brief review of the effects of mechanical forces on endothelial cell function. *Hypertension* 1998; **31** (2): 162–169.
68. Yasuda T, Kondo S, Homma T, Harris RC. Regulation of extracellular matrix by mechanical stress in rat glomerular mesangial cells. *J Clin Invest* 1996; **98**: 1991–2000.
69. Akai Y, Homma T, Burns KD, Yasuda T, Badr KF, Harris RC. Mechanical

stretch/relaxation of cultured rat mesangial cells induces protooncogenes and cyclo-oxygenase. *Am J Physiol* 1994; **267**: C482–C490.

70. Mattana J, Singhal PC. Applied pressure modulates mesangial cell proliferation and matrix synthesis. *Am J Hypertension* 1995; **8**: 1112–1120.
71. Singhal PC, Sagar S, Garg P. Simulated glomerular pressure modulates mesangial cell 72 kDa metalloproteinase activity. *Connect Tissue Res* 1996; **33**: 257–263.
72. Griffin KA, Picken M, Bidani AK. Method of renal mass reduction is a critical modulator of subsequent hypertension and glomerular injury. *J Am Soc Nephrol* 1994; **4**: 2023–2031.
73. Rosenberg ME, Smith LJ, Correa-Rotter R, Hostetter TH. The paradox of the renin-angiotensin system in chronic renal disease. A discussion of the evidence for and against involvement of the renin-angiotensin system in progression of chronic renal disease. *Kidney Int* 1994; **45**: 403–410.
74. Chanutin A, Ferris EB. Experimental renal insufficiency produced by partial nephrectomy. I. Control diet. *Arch Intern Med* 1932; **49**: 767–787.
75. Bidani AK, Mitchell KD, Schwartz MM, Navar LG, Lewis EJ. Absence of glomerular injury or nephron loss in a normotensive rat remnant kidney model. *Kidney Int* 1990; **38**: 28–38.
76. Edwards RM. Segmental effects of norepinephrine and angiotensin II on isolated renal microvessels. *Am J Physiol* 1983; **244**: F526–F534.
77. MacKenzie HS, Ots M, Farzad Z, Kang-Wook L, Kato S, Brenner BM. Angiotensin receptor antagonists in experimental models of chronic renal failure. *Kidney Int* 1997; **52** (Suppl. 63): S140–S143.
78. Wolf G, Neilson EG. Angiotensin II as a renal growth factor. A review of the effects of angiotensin II on proliferation and hypertrophy of glomerular mesangial and renal tubular cells. *J Am Soc Nephrol* 1993; **3**: 1531–1540.
79. Wolf G, Haberstroh U, Neilson EG. Angiotensin II stimulates the proliferation and biosynthesis of type I collagen in cultured murine mesangial cells. *Am J Pathol* 1992; **140**: 95–107.
80. Anderson PW, Do YS, Hsueh WA. Angiotensin II causes mesangial cell hypertrophy. *Hypertension* 1993; **21**: 29–35.
81. Harris RC, Akai Y, Yasuda T, Homma T. Role of physical factors in the regulation of mesangial cell growth and the interaction with vasoactive agents. *Exp Nephrol* 1994; **2**: 104.
82. Kagami S, Border WA, Miller DE, Noble NA. Angiotensin II stimulates extracellular matrix protein synthesis through induction of transforming growth factor-beta expression in rat glomerular mesangial cells. *J Clin Invest* 1994; **93**: 2431–2437.
83. Schulze-Lohoff E, Kohler M, Fees H, Reindl N, Sterzel RB. Divergent effects of arginine vasopressin and angiotensin II on proliferation and expression of the immediate early genes c-fos, c-jun and Egr-1 in cultured rat glomerular mesangial cells. *J Hypertens* 1993; **11**: 127–134.
84. Yangawa N, Capparell AW, Jo OD, Frieday A, Barrett JD, Eggena P. Production of angiotensinogen and renin-like activity by rabbit proximal tubular cells in culture. *Kidney Int* 1991; **39**: 938–941.
85. Marchetti J, Roseau S, Alhenc-Gelas R. Angiotensin I converting enzyme and kini-hydrolyzing enzyme along the rabbit nephron. *Kidney Int* 1987; **31**: 744–751.
86. Burns KD, Inagami T, Harris RC. Cloning of a rabbit kidney cortex AT1 angiotensin II receptor that is present in proximal tubule epithelium. *Am J Physiol* 1993; **264**: F645–F654.

87. Dulin NO, Ernsberger P, Suciu DJ, Douglas JG. Rabbit renal epithelial angiotensin II receptors. *Am J Physiol* 1994; **267**: F776–F782.
88. Wolf G, Neilson EG. Angiotensin II induces cellular hypertrophy in cultured murine proximal tubular cells. *Am J Physiol* 1990; **259**: F768–F777.
89. Norman J, Badie-Dezfooly B, Nord EP, Kurtz I, Schlosser J, Chaudhari A, Fine LG. EGF-induced mitogenesis in proximal tubular cells: potentiation by angiotensin II. *Am J Physiol* 1987; **253**: F299–F309.
90. Johnson RJ, Alpers CE, Yoshimura A, Lombardi D, Pritzl P, Floege J, Schwartz SM. Renal injury from angiotensin II-mediated hypertension. *Hypertension* 1992; **19**: 464–474.
91. Lafayette RA, Mayer G, Park SK, Meyer TW. Angiotensin II receptor blockade limits glomerular injury in rats with reduced renal mass. *J Clin Invest* 1992; **90**: 766–771.
92. Wolthius A, Boes A, Rodemann HP, Grond J. Vasoactive agents affect growth and protein synthesis of cultured rat mesangial cells. *Kidney Int* 1992; **41**: 124–131.
93. Arai M, Wada A, Isaka Y, Agaki Y, Sugiwa T, Miyazaki M, Moriyana T, Kaneda Y, Naruse K, Naruse M, Orita Y, Ando A, Kanada T, Ueda N, Imai E. In vivo transfection of genes for renin and angiotensinogen into the glomerular cells induced phenotypic change of the mesangial cells and glomerular sclerosis. *Biochem Biophys Res Commun* 1995; **206**: 525–532.
94. Border WA, Ruoslahti E. Transforming growth factor-β in disease: the dark side of tissue repair. *J Clin Invest* 1992; **90**: 1–7.
95. Sharma K, Ziyadeh FN. The emerging role of transforming growth factor-beta and extracellular matrix in kidney diseases. *Am J Physiol* 1994; **266**: F829–F842.
96. Lee LK, Meyer TW, Pollock AS, Lovett DH. Endothelial cell injury initiates glomerular sclerosis in the rat remnant kidney. *J Clin Invest* 1995; **96**: 953–964.
97. Ishidoya S, Morrissey J, McCracken R, Klahr S. Delayed treatment with enalapril halts tubulointerstitial fibrosis in rats with obstructive nephropathy. *Kidney Int* 1996; **49**: 1110–1119.
98. Eddy AA. Molecular insights into renal interstitial fibrosis. In depth review of the pathogenesis of interstitial fibrosis. *J Am Soc Nephrol* 1996; **7**: 2495–2508.
99. Ruiz-Ortega M, Egido J. Angiotensin II modulates cell growth-related events and synthesis of matrix proteins in renal interstitial fibroblasts. *Kidney Int* 1997, **52**. 1497–1510.
100. Ikoma M, Kawamura T, Fogo A, Ichikawa I. Cause of variable therapeutic efficiency of angiotensin converting enzyme inhibitor on glomerular lesions. *Kidney Int* 1991; **40**: 195–202.
101. Ichikawa I. Will angiotensin II receptor antagonists be renoprotective in humans? Review of the effects of AII receptor antagonists on progression of experimental renal disease with a particular emphasis on pathways of matrix production and degradation. *Kidney Int* 1996; **50**: 684–692.
102. Feener EP, Northrup JM, Aiello LP, King GL. Angiotensin II induces plasminogen activator inhibitor-1 and -2 expression in vascular endothelial and smooth muscle cells. *J Clin Invest* 1995; **95**: 1353–1362.
103. Vaughan DE, Lazos SA, Tong K. Angiotensin II regulates the expression of plasminogen activator inhibitor-1 in cultured endothelial cells. A potent link between the renin-angiotensin system and thrombosis. *J Clin Invest* 1995; **95**: 995–1001.
104. Hewitson TD, Darby IA, Jones CL, Becker GJ. Evolution of tubulointerstitial fibrosis in experimental renal infection and scarring. *J Am Soc Nephrol* 1998; **9**: 632–642.

105. Sugiyama H, Kashihara N, Makino H, Yamasaki Y, Ota A. Apoptosis in glomerular sclerosis. *Kidney Int* 1996; **49**: 103–111.
106. Lieberthal W, Levine JS. Mechanisms of apoptosis and its potential role in renal tubular epithelial cell injury. *Am J Physiol* 1996; **271**: F477–F488.
107. Chevalier RL. Growth factors and apoptosis in neonatal ureteral obstruction. *J Am Soc Nephrol* 1996; **7**: 1098–1105.
108. Yamada T, Horiuchi M, Dzau VJ. Angiotensin II type 2 receptor mediates programmed cell death. *Proc Natl Acad Sci USA* 1996; **93**: 156–160.
109. Thomas SE, Andoh TF, Pichler RH, Shankland SJ, Couser WG, Bennett WM, Johnson RJ. Accelerated apoptosis characterizes cyclosporin-associated interstitial fibrosis. *Kidney Int* 1998; **53**: 897–908.
110. Kohan DE. Endothelins in the normal and diseased kidney. *Am J Kidney Dis* 1997; **29**: 2–26.
111. Madeddu P, Troffa C, Glorioso N, Pazzola A, Soro A, Nanunta P, Tonolo G, Demontis MP, Varoni MV, Anania V. Effect of Endothelin on regional hemodynamics and renal function in awake normotensive rats. *J Cardiovasc Pharmacol* 1989; **14**: 818–825.
112. Arai H, Hori S, Aramori I, Ohkubo H, Nakanishi S. Cloning expresssion if a cDNA encoding an endothelin receptor. *Nature London* 1990; **348**: 730–732.
113. Sakurai T, Yanagisawa Y, Takuwa H, Miyazaki S, Kimura S, Goto K, Masaki T. Cloning of a cDNA encoding a non-isopeptide selective subtype of the endothelin receptor. *Nature London* 1990; **348**: 732–735.
114. Ihara M, Noguchi K, Saeki T, Fukuroda T, Tsuchida S, Kimura S, Fukami T, Ishikawa K, Nishikibe M, Yano M. Biological profiles of highly potent novel endothelin antagonists selective for the ET_A receptor. *Life Sci* 1992; **50**: 247–255.
115. Fujitani Y, Unda H, Okada T, Urade Y, Karaki H. A selective agonist of endothelin type B receptor, IRL 1620, stimulates of cyclic GMP increase via nitric oxide formation. *J Pharmacol Exp Ther* 1993; **267**: 683–689.
116. Gellai M, DeWolf R, Pullen M, Nambi P. Distribution and functional role of renal ET receptor subtypes in normotensive and hypertensive rats. *Kidney Int* 1994; **46**: 1287–1294.
117. Qui C, Samsell L, Baylis C. Actions of endogenous endothelin on glomerular hemodynamics in the rat. *Am J Physiol* 1995; **269**: R469–R473.
118. Orisio S, Benigni A, Bruzzi I, Corna D, Perico N, Zoja C, Benatti L, Remuzzi G. Renal endothelin gene expression is increased in remnant kidney and correlates with disease progression. *Kidney Int* 1993; **43**: 354–358.
119. Benigni A, Zoja C, Corna D, Orisio S, Longaretti L, Bertani T, Remuzzi G. A specific endothelin subtype A receptor antagonist protects against injury in renal disease progression. *Kidney Int* 1993; **44**: 440–444.
120. Benigni A, Zoja C, Corna D, Orisio S, Facchinetti D, Benatti L, Remuzzi G. Blocking both type A and B endothelin receptors in the kidney attenuates renal injury and prolongs survival in rats with remnant kidneys. *Am J Kidney Dis* 1996; **27**: 416–423.
121. Dulcenombre GG, Largo R, Liu X, Gutierrez S, Lopez-Armada M, Palacios I, Egidio J. An orally active Et_A/ET_B receptor antagonist ameliorates proteinuria and glomerular lesions in rats with proliferative nephritis. *Kidney Int* 1996; **50**: 962–972.
122. Bakris GL, Re RN. Endothelin modulates angiotensin II-induced mitogenesis of human mesangial cells. *Am J Physiol* 1993; **264**: F937–F942.
123. Kohno M, Horio T, Yokokawa K, Yasunari K, Kurihara N, Takeda T. Endothelin

modulates the mitogenic effect of PDGF on glomerular mesangial cells. *Am J Physiol* 1994; **266**: F894–F900.

124. Nitta K, Uchida K, Kimata N, Kawashima A. Endothelin-1 mediates erythropoietin stimulated glomerular endothelial cell-dependent proliferation of mesangial cells. *Eur J Pharmacol* 1995; **293**: 491–494.
125. Yoshimura A, Iwasaki S, Inui K, Ideura S, Koshikawa S, Yanagisawa M, Masaki T. Endothelin-1 and endothelin B type receptor are induced in mesangial proliferative nephritis in the rat. *Kidney Int* 1995; **48**: 1290–1297.
126. Murer L, Zacchello G, Basso G, Scarpa A, Montini G, Chiozza ML, Zacchello F. Immunohistochemical distribution of endothelin in biopsies of pediatric nephrotic syndrome. *Am J Nephrol* 1994; **14**: 157–161.
127. Nakamura T, Ebihara I, Fukai M, Osada S, Tomino Y, Masaki T, Goto K, Furuichi Y, Koide H. Modulation of glomerular endothelin and endothelin receptor gene expression in aminonucleoside-induced nephrosis. *J Am Soc Nephrol* 1995; **5**: 1585–1590.
128. Roccatello D, Mosso R, Ferro M, Polloni R, DeFilippi PG, Quattrocchio G, Bancale E, Cesano G, Sena LM, Piccoli G. Urinary endothelin in glomerulonephritis patients with normal renal function. *Clin Nephrol* 1994; **41**: 323–330.
129. Fukuda K, Okuda S, Tamaki K, Yanagida T, Ando T, Fujishima M. The role of endothelin-1 as a mitogen on experimental glomerulonephritis in rats. *J Am Soc Nephrol* 1995; **6**: 865, (Abstr.).
130. Nakamura T, Ebihara I, Tomino Y, Koide H. Effect of a specific endothelin A receptor antagonist on murine lupus nephritis. *Kidney Int* 1995; **47**: 481–489.
131. Ruiz-Ortega M, Gomez-Garre D, Alcazar R, Palacios I, Bustos C, Gonzalez S, Plaza JJ, Gonzalez E, Egidio J. Involvement of angiotensin II and endothelin in matrix protein production and renal sclerosis. *J Hypertens* 1994; **12**: 551–558.
132. Walker GW, Neaton JD, Cutler JA, Neuwirth R, Cohen JD. for the MRFIT Research Group: Renal function change in hypertensive members of the Multiple Risk Factor Intervention Trial: Racial and treatment effects. *JAMA* 1992; **268**: 3085–3091.
133. Shulman NB, Ford CE, Hall WD, Blaufox MD, Simon D, Langford HG, Schneider KA. Prognostic value of serum creatinine and effect of treatment of hypertension on renal function. Results from the hypertension detection and follow-up program. The Hypertension Detection and Follow-Up Program Cooperative Group. *Hypertension* 1989; **13** (Suppl. 1): 80–93.
134. Perry HM Jr, Miller JP, Fornoff JR, Baty JD, Sambhi MP, Rutan G, Moskowitz DW, Carmody SE. Early predictors of 15-year end-stage renal disease in hypertensive patients. *Hypertension* 1995; **25**: 587–594.
135. Brazy PC, Fitzwilliam JF. Progressive renal disease: Role of race and antihypertensive medications. *Kidney Int* 1990; **37**: 1113–1119.
136. Locatelli F, Marcelli D, Comelli M, Alberti D, Graziani G, Buccianti G, Redaelli B, Giangrande A. Proteinuria and blood pressure as causal components of progression to end-stage renal failure. *Nephrol Dial Transplant* 1996; **11**: 461–467.
137. Rostand SG, Brown G, Kirk KA, Rutsky EA, Dustan HP. Renal insufficiency in treated essential hypertension. *N Engl J Med* 1989; **320**: 684–688.
138. Rydel JJ, Korbet SM, Borok RZ, Schwartz MM. Focal segmental glomerular sclerosis in adults: Presentation, course, and response to treatment. *Am J Kidney Dis* 1995; **25**: 534–542.
139. Pei Y, Cattran D, Greenwood C. Predicting chronic renal insufficiency in idiopathic membranous glomerulonephritis. *Kidney Int* 1992; **42**: 960–966.

140. Neelakantappa K, Gallo G, Baldwin DS. Proteinuria in IgA nephropathy. *Kidney Int* 1988; **33**: 716–721.
141. Narvate J, Prive M, Saba SR, Ramirez G. Proteinuria in hypertension. *Am J Kidney Dis* 1987; **10**: 408–416.
142. Peterson JC, Adler S, Burkart JM, Greene T, Hebert LA, Hunsicker LG, King AJ, Klahr S, Massry SG, Seifter JL. Blood pressure, proteinuria, and the progression of renal disease. The Modification in Diet Renal Disease Study. *Ann Intern Med* 1995; **123**: 754–762.
143. Giatras I, Lau J, Levey AS. For the Angiotensin-Converting-Enzyme Inhibition in Progressive Renal Disease Study Group: Effect of angiotensin-converting-enzyme inhibitors on the progression of nondiabetic renal disease: a meta-analysis of randomized trials. *Ann Intern Med* 1997; **127**: 337–345.
144. Zucchelli P, Zuccala A, Borghi M, Fusaroli M, Sasdelli M, Stallone C, Sanna G, Gaggi R. Long-term comparison between captopril and nifedipine in the progression of renal insufficiency. *Kidney Int* 1992; **42**: 452–458.
145. Weir MR, Dworkin LD. Antihypertensive drugs, dietary salt, and renal protection: How low should you go and with which therapy? *Am J Kidney Dis* 1998; **32**: 1–22.
146. Lazarus JM, Bourgoignie J, Buckalew V, Greene T, Levey A, Milas NC, Paranandi L, Peterson J, Porush J, Rauch S, Soucie JM, Stollar C for the Modification of Diet in Renal Disease Study Group. Achievement and safety of a low blood pressure goal in chronic renal disease. *Hypertension* 1997; **29**: 641–650.
147. Estacio RO, Jeffers BW, Hiatt WR, Biggerstaff SL, Gifford N, Schrier RW. The effect of nisoldipine as compared with enalapril on cardiovascular outcomes in patients with non-insulin-dependent diabetes and hypertension. *N Engl J Med* 1998; **338**: 645–654.

7

Diabetic nephropathy: natural history and management

Carl Erik Mogensen

Persistently good metabolic control is of major importance for the prevention and postponement of renal disease [1,2], as well as other microvascular complications in patients with type 1 [3] as well as type 2 diabetes mellitus (DM) [4]. Later, several factors appear to affect progression of renal disease of which hypertension seems the most important [5,6]. Similarly, in type 2 DM, hypertension, along with dyslipidemia and hyperglycemia appear to be risk factors for the development of macrovascular complications [7]. Incipient renal disease in diabetes, as judged by the occurrence of microalbuminuria, is frequently characterized by elevation or at least progressively increasing blood pressure. The increase, however, is often subtle and may only be detectable by careful monitoring, e.g. 24 h ambulatory recordings [8–11]. Elevation of blood pressure is found in both types of diabetes, but there appear to be several distinctions between type 1 and type 2 diabetes; some of these are clearly explained by the different aetiology and nature of the diabetic state. In type 2 diabetic patients, higher age, increased body weight, as well as insulin resistance and hyperinsulinemia related to syndrome X [12,13] are important factors. Although hypertension secondary to renal impairment is also frequently seen in type 2 diabetic patients, the renal genesis of hypertension is much more common in the relatively younger type 1 diabetic patients [14], where parental predisposition to hypertension seems to play some part [15,16]. However, differences between type 1 and type 2 regarding the nephropathy are less pronounced than originally thought [17]. Dietary protein intake may also be a modulating factor [18,19], but further studies on intervention are needed [20,21]. Thus, metabolic control, blood pressure elevation and to some extent dietary proteins, and the possibility of modification by treatment [22,23], will be the main issues addressed in this chapter.

Blood pressure, glomerular pressure and genetic factors

In the past decades, there has been a growing interest in the nature of diabetic renal disease, mainly focusing on blood pressure, glomerular capillary pressure, and protein leakage in diabetes [24–27]. The reason is clear: in general two or more risk factors must coincide to provoke serious organ damage. In terms of diabetic nephropathy this means that some degree of poor glycaemic control may not always be noxious *per se*, unless some other risk factor, such as genetic elements and/or elevated blood pressure coexists [28]. However, increased glomerular capillary pressure seems to be a decisive factor, regardless of whether caused by hyperglycemia, systemic hypertension or dietary proteins. In particular, the loss of glomerular autoregulation, induced by hyperglycemia and/or a high protein intake, allows the unopposed transmission of systemic hypertension to the glomerular capillaries [29, 30]. Other risk factors may contribute to renal and especially vascular damage in diabetes, e.g. smoking, lipid abnormalities, or obesity, again highlighting the importance of the metabolic syndrome, or syndrome X [12,7]. It is not difficult to see how these various hemodynamic and metabolic risk factors would interact to make the glomerular capillary injury more progressive.

Diabetic renal disease tends to cluster in families, possibly partly reflecting poor metabolic control, which also predominates in certain families [31,32]. This could be related to angiotensin-converting enzyme (ACE) gene polymorphism, but any association to diabetic renal disease and its progression has recently been challenged. From a clinical viewpoint, ACE genotyping is usually not relevant [28,33,34,35]. Tarnow *et al.* [36] concluded based on a meta-analysis, that the ACE/ID polymorphism contributes to the genetic susceptibility to diabetic nephropathy in Japanese type 2 diabetic patients, but does not play a major part in the initiation of diabetic nephropathy in Caucasians with type 2 diabetes. In Caucasians with type 1 DM, comparison of data is complicated by differences between study populations, but a trend towards a protective effect of the II genotype on the development of microalbuminuria was observed.

Comparing the different risk factors—apart from poor metabolic control—blood pressure elevation, seems to be not only the most important index of organ damage, but also the most readily measurable as well as modifiable risk factor. Virtually all studies agree that standard medical antihypertensive treatment is able to reduce blood pressure in diabetes [24,26] and many studies [2,24,37] have confirmed the original observations of a beneficial impact of antihypertensive treatment on the course of renal disease, both in incipient and overt type 1 diabetic patients [38,39]. Interestingly, ACE inhibitors may be particularly beneficial [26,37,40], although this has been questioned by some [24,41]. Certainly, the side-effect profiles, favour the use of these agents often combined with diuretics especially in incipient nephropathy [24,5,6]. These considerations also apply to cardiovascular events in hypertensive type 2 diabetic patients [42]. Where combination therapy often has to be used to control hypertension [43].

Cumulative incidence of diabetic nephropathy

The cumulative incidence of diabetic nephropathy used to be high (≈35%) but seems to decline over the years, especially in a study from Sweden where only very few patients in a given recent cohort developed nephropathy [44]. However, this observation could not be confirmed by the group at the Steno Hospital in Copenhagen [45]. The explanation is not clear, but certainly the so-called natural history may be considerably modified by more intensive interventions throughout the course of diabetes. This relates to a large extent to metabolic control and blood pressure elevation as major factors, but also other issues are of importance, e.g. smoking. Also race is of importance. Diabetic nephropathy is more commonly seen in African-Americans, and indeed new studies among the Pima Indians (unpublished observation) suggest that with long follow-up periods practically all patients will develop renal disease. This information is important because it has been suggested that there may be important susceptibility factors that could relate to genetics. Comparison has been made with diabetic retinopathy where practically all patients sooner or later develop lesions. However, there are important modifications as usually renal disease is judged by proteinuria and not by biopsies and, in fact the cumulative incidence of diabetic retinopathy and nephropathy may be very similar, if histological or ophthalmologic examinations are used. It has also been discussed why some diabetics seem immune to nephropathy even if they had poor glycaemic control. A likely explanation is that two factors must coexist; namely systemic hypertension as well as hyperglycemia to produce important clinical disease. If the combination of high blood pressure and high blood glucose is present the clinical experience is that practically all patients will develop clinically relevant nephropathy and retinopathy.

New studies emphasize the role of good metabolic control in advanced nephropathy. This has been documented in a study by Breyer and co-workers [46], and recently by Mulec *et al.* [47]. These results are in agreement with information from the Steno Diabetes Centre, London and also from Gothenburg [2,48,34]. Clearly with advanced nephropathy, elevated blood pressure is of importance, and combining the two risk factors in overt nephropathy may have a major impact on progression. With poor control of glycemia and poor blood pressure control the fall rate in glomerular filtration rate (GFR) is high (≈8 ml/min per year). Conversely, with efficient control of blood glucose and blood pressure, the decline in GFR may be close to 1–2 ml/min per year (personal communication, H. H. Parving). Obviously, it is not possible to obtain perfect metabolic control in all patients, especially in those at risk or with nephropathy because the very background for developing complications is the poor control which may not be easy to modify even after the development of complications. This is exemplified in a study from the UK, The Microalbuminuria Collaborative Study, where systemic hypertension, rather than the control of glycemia, seemed to be the predominant factor in the progression of diabetic nephropathy [49].

In summary, one could argue that the concept of natural history of diabetic nephropathy may only be observed in patients with poor metabolic control. However, if risk factors such as hyperglycemia and blood pressure elevation can be controlled, very few patients may actually develop proteinuria and eventually end-stage renal disease both in type 1 and type 2 diabetes. Also with advanced nephropathy glycaemic control seems very important [50]. This was further highlighted by the recent United Kingdom Prospective Diabetes Study (UKPDS) data suggesting an important contribution of good metabolic and blood pressure controls to the reduction of microvascular complications, including microalbuminuria, in type 2 diabetics [171–173].

However, such a strategy of metabolic and hemodynamic controls requires considerable resources not only from the health-care providers but also from patients. In this respect, it is of interest to know that a low socio-economic class is an important risk factor for the development of diabetic complications (Ingrid Mülhaüser, personal communication). This may partly explain difficulties in obtaining sufficiently good metabolic control. It may be easier to implement treatment with ACE inhibitors, even in normoalbuminuric patients, as recently proposed by Ravid and co-workers [51], thus controlling one of the two major cofactors implicated in the development of diabetic nephropathy. However, both strategies should be exercised in the clinical setting as discussed below.

The major risk factors

Hyperglycemia

Perfect metabolic control, that is blood glucose as well as concentrations of other metabolites and hormones within normal range, is presently almost impossible to obtain in diabetic patients. Even in the Diabetes Control and Complications Trial (DCCT) [52] optimized management in type 1 diabetic patients did only rarely result in perfect glycaemic control. Under standard care conditions, HbA_{1C} values may be 50% or most often even higher than normal reference values in most patients. However, good metabolic control remains a key factor in preventing nephropathy [52,53] and its progression [2,34]. Further long-term studies are needed in type 2 diabetic patients but the same relation seems to exist here, especially early in the course of the renal disease [4,54]. The recently published UKPDS suggests that glycemia and blood pressure controls are the cornerstone of the management of type 2 diabetic patients with microvascular complications such as nephropathy and retinopathy [171–173]. In this study, tight glycaemic control reduced the progression of microalbuminuria, although the effect of declining renal function was less obvious [171].

Hypertension

Nowadays very high blood pressure levels are rarely observed in well-managed diabetic patients in organized clinics. Such high pressures are most often encountered in populations without any structured care for complications including hypertension. With appropriate antihypertensive management programmes the degree of elevation of blood pressure is usually not very pronounced as compared with the past [5,55,56]. This is for instance corroborated by new studies where 24-h blood pressure recordings in diabetics are carefully compared with non-diabetics [8]. When diabetics without antihypertensive treatment are selected, it is obvious that blood pressure elevation is not pronounced, about 5 mmHg on average in microalbuminuric patients [8]. Clearly such data may be biased, because patients already in treatment are excluded. On the other hand, even minor blood pressure elevation may lead to vascular and glomerular damage, especially when accompanied by other risk factors, e.g. hyperglycemia. A correlation exists between albuminuria and blood pressure and the association is highlighted when 24 ambulatory blood pressure values are used rather than conventional blood pressure measurements [8]. Diabetic patients may be exquisitely susceptible to systemic blood pressure elevation because the normal protection exerted by the afferent renal arteriolar vasculature is likely to be compromised in diabetic patients with consequent loss of glomerular autoregulation [29,30,57,58].

In the past, blood pressure elevation was usually much higher [5,55,56]. Thus a very pronounced fall in recorded blood pressure has been observed in the diabetes clinics during the last decades, as evidenced by a study from the Steno Diabetes Center, where blood pressure levels in cohorts of patients in the sixties were compared with patients in the eighties [55].

Important differences exist between the two types of diabetes. In type 1 diabetes, the prevalence of hypertension is clearly associated with the degree of albuminuria [59]. With normal albumin excretion rate, blood pressure is close to normal [8]. This has been confirmed in recent studies using 24-h blood pressure recordings [8]. With the occurrence of microalbuminuria there is a considerable increase in the prevalence of elevated blood pressure, and even more marked changes are seen in patients with overt diabetic nephropathy. Thus, a clear relationship between blood pressure and renal damage exists in type 1 diabetes.

In type 2 diabetes, the picture is less clear, although there is usually some association between the degree of albuminuria and blood pressure [60–62]. However, the correlation is weaker, and it is also important to recognize that the prevalence of blood pressure elevation is much higher in the elderly type 2 diabetic patients; at the time of clinical diagnosis about 30–40% of patients have elevated blood pressure or receive antihypertensive treatment [61,62]. In a control population without diabetes this figure may be 20% [60]. Interestingly, the blood pressure elevation in type 2 diabetic patients is usually of a systolic nature [63,64], meaning that effective treatment may be difficult with high initial values and therapeutic goals should be modified [22,23], with a stepwise reduction in blood pressure.

Without treatment the rate of increase in blood pressure with time is high in type 1 diabetic patients with microalbuminuria or overt proteinuria [65–67], supporting the idea that a self-perpetuating process exists. This increase is most pronounced in type 1 diabetic patients. Clear data are more difficult to obtain in type 2 diabetes, because so many patients are treated with antihypertensive drugs and the discontinuation of treatment is not justifiable. Still, an increase in blood pressure levels is often observed in these patients, especially with 24 h blood pressure monitoring [68–71]. In type 1 diabetes, blood pressure may increase by 3–4 mmHg/year with microalbuminuria [72], and about 6 mmHg/year with overt renal disease [66]. Such data may be difficult to reproduce today, simply because so many patients are treated early and effectively.

Twenty-four-hour ambulatory blood pressure recordings

Recent studies suggest that the transition from normoalbuminuria to microalbuminuria is associated in most cases with an increase in blood pressure [9]. However, this small increase in blood pressure is not easily detectable and may be missed if clinic, rather than ambulatory, recordings are used [8]. The clear association between the rise in albuminuria, from normoalbuminuria to microalbuminuria, and the rise in blood pressure can only be documented by the simultaneous measurement of UAE in several samples and 24 h ambulatory blood pressure recordings. However, in general practice it is not feasible to monitor 24 h blood pressure in clinic settings, and therefore, on the basis of these new results, close monitoring of microalbuminuria may be sufficient. This will disclose the development of kidney damage. Importantly, all evidence suggests that the reduction of blood pressure, for example, with ACE inhibitors, will also reduce microalbuminuria and if early treatment is implemented a reduction to normoalbuminuria may even be possible [125]. Such treatment could even be initiated in seemingly normotensive microalbuminuric patients.

Dietary protein

With some variation from country to country, traditional diabetic dietary management often results in a high protein intake [19] (sometimes 50% higher than the average background population). This may not be an appropriate strategy because such a dietary pattern may aggravate the course of renal disease [20,73,74]. Indeed indirect evidence link the level of protein intake in diabetic patients with the development of microalbuminuria. Indeed, the EURODIAB study of complications in type I diabetic patients showed that those whose protein consumption exceeds 20% of their total energy intake had microalbuminuria while those consuming less protein had an AER <20 μg/min [174]. Of interest, the trend to increased albuminuria with increased protein intake was more marked in diabetic patients with hypertension and/or elevated HbA1c levels. This supports the hypothesis of synergism between dietary protein, hyperglycemia and systemic hypertension. With that in mind, the Diabetes and Nutrition Study Group of the European Association for the Study of Diabetes and the American Diabetes Association recommend a protein intake between 10 and 20% of the patient's total energy consumption [175]. They consequently advise diabetic patients to reduce their protein intake to 0.7–0.9 g/kg per day as they felt that was no conclusive evidence to recommend a lower protein intake.

Progression markers and end-points

Microalbuminuria

A key question in clinical management, is to define and elaborate on parameters that can be considered important markers, in terms of disease activity and prognosis (see Table 7.1). This is of special importance in intervention trials, but also in the everyday treatment of patients, where results from clinical trials are rapidly reflected in practical management [6]. An outline of the natural history of renal disease in type 1 diabetic patients is given in Table 7.2.

Table 7.1 The end-point: glomerular filtration rate (GFR) fall rate related to intermediary end-points in diabetic patients

Intermediary end-points	GFR fall (young type 1 diabetic patients)	GFR fall (middle-aged type 2 diabetic patients)
Microalbuminuria* (20–200 µg/min)	Fall in GFR* only seen with progression to proteinuria	Fall rate of GFR* usually not significantly different from normoalbuminuria
Proteinuria** (macroalbuminuria, >200 µg/min)	Clear fall in GFR** (reduced by antihypertensive treatment)	Clear fall in GFR***. High mortality
Elevated blood pressure or hypertension**	Controversy exist, but a clear risk factor with coexisting abnormal albuminuria	Controversy exist, but a clear risk factor with coexisting abnormal albuminuria

Related to future mortality and ESRD with increasing power (*)(**)(***).

It has been known for many years that hypertensive proteinuric diabetic patients carry a poor prognosis [31]. It has also become clear that microalbuminuria [(20–200 µg/min) is an important long-term predictor for poor outcome [75–79]. A decisive parameter is the rate of fall of GFR as measured by exact and reproducible techniques [37,80]. Doubling of serum creatinine has also been used [40]. Obviously, an even more solid end-point is end-stage renal failure (ESRF) and/or death [40,55], but in patients with early clinical proteinuria or microalbuminuria, this is (fortunately) a distant end-point as the development of ESRF may last at least one or two decades, especially after it has been shown that antihypertensive treatment postpones end-stage renal disease [55].

Strong evidence suggests that abnormal albuminuria (even slight elevation) [76,79] is a key parameter and an important intermediary end-point in the monitoring of all diabetic patients; not only because it relates so closely to the more advanced end-points, but also because this parameter can be used both in treatment strategies in controlled clinical trials, and in the day-to-day management of patients [14,27,81,82]. Importantly, glomerular structural damages can be arrested by antihypertensive treatment (β-blockers or ACE inhibitors) in microalbuminuric patients [83].

Albuminuria/hypertension and decline in glomerular filtration rate

It is evident from many studies that patients with normal albumin excretion rate preserve normal renal function in the long term [75], although follow-up has been limited (≈20 years); there may, however, be a small, probably age-related, reduction in GFR [14,76]. Also patients with persistent microalbuminuria usually maintain intact renal function, although a subsequent fall in GFR can be predicted, with progression to macroalbuminuria, possibly partly as a consequence of initial

Table 7.2 Stages in the development of renal changes and lesions in diabetes mellitus (type 1)

Stage		Chronology	Main structural changes or lesions	Glomerular filtration rate	Albumin excretion* (e.g. overnight UAE)	Blood pressure	Reversible by strict insulin treatment	Arrestable or reversible by antihypertensive treatment**
1	Acute renal hypertrophy-hyperfunction	Present at diagnosis of diabetes (reversible with good control)	Increased kidney size. Increased glomerular size	Increased by 20–50%	May be increased, but reversible	Normal	Yes	No hypertension present. Microcirculatory changes modifiable?
2	Normoalbuminuria (<20 μg/min)	Almost all patients normoalbuminuric in first 5 years	On renal biopsy, increased BM thickness after 2 years	Increased by 20–50%, related to HbA_{1C}	Normal by definition (15–20 μg/min may be abnormal)	Normal (BP as in background population) Increase by 1 mmHg/year	Hyperfiltration reduced	Filtration fraction and UAE may be reduced
3	Incipient diabetic nephropathy	After 6–15 years (in ≈35% of patients)	Further BM thickness, mesangial expansion, especially of matrix	Still supra-normal values, predicted to decline with development of proteinuria	20–200 μg/min (increase: ≈20%/year), of glomerular origin	Incipient increase, ≈3 mmHg/year (if untreated)	Microalbuminuria stabilized, GFR also stable, if HbA_{1C} is reduced.	Microalbuminuria reduced. Prevention of fall in GFR likely
4	Proteinuria, clinical overt diabetic nephropathy	After 15–25 years (in ≈35% of patients)	Clear and pronounced abnormalities	Decline ≈10 ml/min/year with clear proteinuria***	Progressive clinical proteinuria*** of glomerular origin	High BP, increase by ≈5 mmHg/year (if untreated)	Higher fall in GFR with poor control	Progression reduced (aiming at 135/85 mmHg)
5	End-stage renal failure	Final outcome, after 25–30 years or more	Glomerular closure	<10 ml/min	Often some decline due to nephron closure	High (if untreated)	No	No

BM, Basement membrane; UAE, Urinary albumin excretion rate.
* The best marker of early renal involvement; ** mostly ACE inhibition + diuretics; *** without antihypertensive treatment.

hyperfiltration [14,67]. In most patients, a decline in GFR is only noted when proteinuria (macroalbuminuria) takes place [14,84–87,103]. It should be noted that antihypertensive treatment may reduce or even normalize albumin excretion (and lead to misclassification), with albuminuria rising again when the antihypertensive treatment is stopped [88]. Feldt-Rasmussen *et al.* [84] observed a significant drop in GFR with the development of clinical nephropathy (UAE >300 mg/24 h) but most of their patients received antihypertensive treatment which modifies the level of UAE and is thus a confounding factor. In patients with more advanced renal disease it was documented long ago that the rate of fall of GFR is at an average of 10 ml/min per year; however, most of these patients had a poorly controlled hypertension [85]. This study also suggested that glomerular hyperfiltration was still present in microalbuminuric type 1 patients, without any time-dependent decline in GFR [85].

In type 1 diabetic patients with elevated blood pressure, but normal albumin excretion rate, Nørgaard *et al.* [89] documented well-preserved renal function. It is postulated that these patients may have essential hypertension along with DM. This suggests that the degree of elevation of blood pressure per se (≈150/95 mmHg) is not an early independent risk factor for the decline in GFR in patients without microalbuminuria or overt diabetic nephropathy. It should be noted that most hypertensive patients were under treatment which was discontinued 4 weeks before investigation [89], another confounding factor.

In conclusion, it is likely that abnormal albuminuria is the main predictor—or perhaps even a determinant—of future decline in renal function [57]. The precise mechanisms of diabetic albuminuria remain to be defined although changes in the glomerular permeability to proteins is likely to play an important part. The mechanism underlying microalbuminuria-induced renal damage may either be an increased transglomerular traffic of proteins leading to further glomerular damage or an increased tubular reabsorption of albumin. The latter may cause interstitial damage, which in turn, may lead to secondary structural damage to the glomeruli. Further, a good correlation has been shown in diabetic patients between the severity of tubulo-interstitial changes and GFR. Another hypothesis for this self-perpetuating process involves glomerular hyperfiltration. Patients with a decline in GFR due to nephron closure are likely to show single nephron hyperfiltration in the remaining glomeruli (the mechanism of hyperfiltration-induced glomerulosclerosis is discussed in Chapter 3). Abnormal albuminuria is clearly associated with vascular damage in other organs [90–101] and is associated with a higher cardiovascular morbidity and mortality.

Pathogenesis of hypertension in diabetes mellitus

Renal dysfunction

There is compelling evidence that elevated blood pressure in type 1 diabetes is related to impaired renal function. Blood pressure rises at the microalbuminuria stage [8]. There is some controversy regarding the transition from normoalbuminuria to microalbuminuria. Some groups suggested that elevated blood pressure is important in this transition process [25], while new studies using 24 h ambulatory recordings suggest that blood pressure increases only after or along with the occurrence of microalbuminuria [8,9]. However, it is clear that blood pressure elevation tends to be aggravated with progressive microalbuminuria. With overt proteinuria clear-cut hypertension is generally present [24,66].

The exact mechanism behind the increase in blood pressure and renal impairment is not clear. It is well established that blood pressure increases with reduction of GFR in most glomerular diseases, but in diabetic patients elevated blood pressure is detected prior to the reduction of renal function [2,75]. It is possible that the mesangial expansion observed in diabetic nephropathy, already at the microalbuminuria stage, is of importance, but this remains to be confirmed [102]. The blood pressure elevation may also relate to the sodium retention associated with renal disease [84,103]. In type 2 diabetics, the relationship between elevated blood pressure and impaired renal function is also present, but less conspicuous due to many confounding factors. Usually there is a correlation between the mainly systolic blood pressure elevation and the degree of albuminuria but the correlation is not always very strong [63].

Sodium retention

There is an association between exchangeable sodium and elevated blood pressure in microalbuminuric patients suggesting that sodium excess may be of importance [84,103]. The sodium excess may be explained by increased tubular reabsorption of sodium, possibly stimulated by exogenous or endogenous hyperinsulinemia [104,105]. However, the association is mainly empirical and there may be common underlying mechanisms that explain both sodium retention and elevated blood pressure.

General systemic hyperperfusion

There is some evidence of increased cardiac contractility in diabetes, which may produce increased output and thus contribute to hyperperfusion in diabetes [106]. Interestingly, in type 1 diabetes there is a correlation between cardiac contractility and the degree of microalbuminuria. However, with the transition to overt proteinuria a decrease in contractility is observed [106]. Besides generalized hyperperfusion, there may be evidence of increased localized pressure not only in the kidney, but also in the peripheral circulation as recently demonstrated by Sandeman *et al.* [107]. This abnormality may possibly parallel the increase in glomerular pressure, but it is not observed in type 2 diabetes [108], where some degree of hyperfiltration exists.

Large vessel disease

In type 2 diabetes, there is evidence of increased arterial stiffness [63]. This phenomenon may explain why the blood pressure elevation, in these patients, is predominantly systolic in nature [63]. Diastolic pressure is usually also elevated, but often to a lesser extent unless overt renal damage is present. The hypothesis that large vessel disease generates systolic hypertension, which in turn increases albuminuria, and provokes renal damage is intriguing. Blood pressure reduction may reduce albuminuria but may also provoke ischemia in other organs, e.g. the brain or the heart. Treatment, therefore, is often difficult and a stepwise reduction in blood pressure is recommended [22,23]. These limitations clearly support the concept of early antihypertensive treatment in these individuals, e.g. in patients with microalbuminuria with marginal blood pressure elevation. This was supported by the blood pressure study of the UKPDS which showed marked reduction in microvascular complications with tight blood pressure control (144/82 mmHg) compared with less tight control (154/87 mmHg). A new concept in the treatment of diabetes may involve starting antihypertensive treatment in all microalbuminuric patients even those with who are normotensive [172].

Hyperinsulinemia

Of note, patients with essential hypertension do show insulin resistance and/or hyperinsulinemia [12]. As insulin resistance is a mechanism involved in the pathogenesis of type 2 diabetes, insulin resistance may also contribute to blood pressure elevation in diabetes. Indeed, elevated blood pressure is found early in the course of type 2 diabetes right from the time of diagnosis [61,62], when insulin resistance is probably an important phenomenon [12]. However, there are some controversy regarding this concept, because insulin itself may not necessarily induce hypertension [109]. Also the correlation between insulin resistance and elevated blood pressure is relatively weak, as numerous factors are likely to be involved in the control of blood pressure [12,29,110]. There are other abnormalities that may be involved in the genesis of hypertension in diabetes, such as increased sympathetic nervous activity producing increased vascular reactivity [111]. This may also be related to obesity. However, as these phenomena may not point clearly to specific modalities of treatment, they will not be discussed further [112].

Mechanisms of hypertension and choice of therapy

Based upon the known mechanisms operating in the genesis of hypertension some interesting concepts regarding selection of antihypertensive treatment are evolving in diabetes. The abnormalities in renal function where hyperperfusion, hyperfiltration, and increased glomerular capillary pressure (hypertension) may be important mediators, favour the use of ACE inhibitors, as these agents tend to reduce efferent glomerular resistance [113]. This effect, operating by reducing glomerular hypertension, may be protective to some extent independently of changes in systemic hypertension [75,113–115]. The sodium retention evident in both type 1 and 2 diabetes, supports the use of diuretics or sodium restriction in antihypertensive programmes in diabetes [84,103–105]. The early cardiac hyperfunction in microalbuminuric patients may suggest the use of cardioselective β-blockers [106]. Obviously, the generalized blood pressure reduction seen with all these agents may be of prime importance, but additional considerations highlighted above may favour the use of combination therapy including ACE inhibitors, diuretics, and possibly β1-blockers (or other agents) [116] (Table 7.3). Calcium-channel blockers reduce blood

Table 7.3 How antihypertensive agents may be combined in diabetes

β-blockers	Yes (diuretics often required)			
ACE inhibition	Yes (diuretics often required)	Yes	Yes (theoretically interesting combination, results promising)	
Ca-blockers*	Yes (diuretics often required)	Yes (rarely used)	Yes (rarely used)	Yes (often used, also with diuretics)
	Diuretics	β-blockers	β-blockers + diuretics	ACE inhibition

Careful clinical metabolic and blood pressure monitoring always required, including control of serum-electrolytes and serum-creatinine or GFR index (combination therapy used in more than 50% of patients).
* New results suggest that cardiovascular long-term effects are less favourable than with ACE inhibition in type 2 diabetes [42].

pressure, but there is mounting evidence of unfavourable effects on the cardiovascular system of hypertensive type 2 diabetes [42,117]. This was recently shown in the Appropriate Blood Pressure Control in Diabetes (ABCD) trial where nisoldipine, a short acting calcium-channel blocker, led to increased fatal and non-fatal myocardial infarction compared with the ACE inhibitor enalapril [42].

Obviously, from a theoretical point of view, potential additional beneficial effect should be considered (see Table 7.4). For instance, ACE inhibitors may specifically reduce the increased capillary pressures seen in these patients, as suggested in animal studies [113]. This is usually associated with an antiproteinuric effect also due to ACE inhibitor-induced changes in glomerular size permselectivity. The presence of edema would favour the use of diuretics. It is suggested that arrythmias may play a part in early diabetic mortality, especially in type 2 diabetic patients. The observation that in post myocardial infarction trials, β-blockers are especially effective in diabetic patients [118,119], points to additional beneficial effects of β-blockers in the management of hypertension in diabetics where silent myocardial infarctions are not uncommon.

Clearly, side effects are important and these are usually dose-related. For instance, the well-known diabetogenic effect of diuretics may be dose-dependent with sufficient blood pressure reduction achievable with low doses [120] which are not diabetogenic. Potassium loss is important but can readily be restored by potassium supplementation or by the use of ACE inhibition. Also low-dose diuretic therapy may not impair lipid metabolism [120]. A side-effect that has caused some concern is hypoglycemic unawareness. This was previously reported with unselective β-

Table 7.4 Diabetes-related side-effects and favourable effects related to antihypertensive treatment in diabetics (mainly type 1 diabetes)

	Diuretics (Thiazide or loop)	Non-cardioselective β-blockers	Cardioselective β-blockers	ACE inhibitors diuretic	Triple treatment: diuretic β1-blockers/ ACE inhibitors	Calcium blockers	β-blocker
Glucose intolerance	Yes, type 2, but related strongly to hypokalemia)	No problem	No problem	No side-effects Insulin sensitivity not changed clinically	Limited or no change (with moderate dosages)	No	No
Hypoglycaemic masking	No	Yes, mainly in type 1 diabetes	A problem, but limited, seen in few patients	Not seen	Limited or no change (with small dosages)	No	No
Unfavourable lipid profits	Yes, but not with small doses	Likely	Limited	No side-effects	?	No	No
Other unfavourable effects	May cause sodium depletion	Less physical exercise capacity	Less physical exercise capacity	Cough and drug-related side-effects	Limited (with moderate dosages)	Foot edema seen in few patients.	No
Favourable effects (apart from blood pressure reduction)	Elimination of edema	Reduction of cardiovascular morbidity/ mortality? Normalization of cardiac arrhythmias?	Reduction of cardiovascular morbidity/ mortality? Normalization of cardiac arrhythmias?	Elimination sodium excess and possibly restoration of glomerular pressure gradients	Probably also combination of favourable effects (stable GFR?)	No potentiation of peripheral ischemia?	?
Reduction of albuminuria	Not well documented	Not well documented	Yes, but relatively few studies exist	Very consistent finding	Addition of ACE inhibition reduces abnormal albuminuria	Not a consistent finding	?
Reducing fall rate of GFR	Not documented	Not documented	Yes	Yes	GFR stable on this programme	Not documented	?

blockers but is only of minor importance with cardioselective β-blockers. Furthermore, this phenomenon is of less relevance in type 2 diabetics who may specifically benefit from cardioprotection. Most ACE inhibitors do not have diabetogenic effects [121]. Thus they do not have a detrimental effect on glucose metabolism or lipid homeostasis; whereas a positive effect has in fact been observed in some studies [122]. This positive or neutral metabolic profile may therefore favour the use of ACE inhibitors in diabetic patients. Cough as a side-effect is surprisingly rare in diabetic patients, possibly due to diabetic neuropathic changes. The new angiotensin II receptor (AT_1R) antagonists could be considered as an alternative to ACE inhibitors when side-effects preclude their use [123,124].

Evaluation of antihypertensive treatment

Evaluation of treatment effect has to be differentiated depending on the degree of albuminuria. Type 1 diabetic patients with normoalbuminuria rarely need antihypertensive treatment. In patients with persistent microalbuminuria (incipient nephropathy) there is well preserved renal function and thus the effect-parameter is the reduction of albuminuria, but during long-term follow-up the effect-parameter is the prevention of a fall in GFR. In patients with overt nephropathy the main effect-parameter is the fall rate of GFR [37] (or clear change in serum creatinine) [40], with reduction in albuminuria [127] as a secondary but more easily measurable and modifiable parameter.

Intervention trials in normoalbuminuria

Even in type 1 diabetic patients with normal blood pressure and normal albumin excretion, renal hemodynamics may be beneficially influenced by ACE inhibition [73]. This study was of an experimental nature and treatment of such individuals cannot be recommended, although a trial should be conducted in high-risk normoalbuminuric patient [high normal UAE (>12 μg/min), high HbA_{1C} (>9–10%)]. However, the EUCLID study did not document a clear effect in a 2-year trial [128], but longer intervention is likely to be needed.

Intervention trials in microalbuminuria

Several intervention studies have been published, some with self-controlled or cross-over design, some double-blinded without being long-term and some long-term and randomized without being blinded [14,24,39,86,129–137]. All these trials showed a reduction or stabilization in microalbuminuria. In a recent randomized double-blind large-scale placebo-controlled study [135,138], the effect of an ACE inhibitor (Captopril) was investigated with respect to progression to clinical nephropathy in normotensive type 1 diabetic patients with microalbuminuria. The major end-point was the progression to persistent proteinuria (UAE >200 μg/min). In this large study, treatment delayed the progression to overt renal disease in normotensive, type 1 diabetic patients with microalbuminuria.

Interestingly, in all these studies from 1985 to 1998, patients were included purely on the basis of microalbuminuria and with the exclusion of hypertensive patients.

Therefore, in most studies blood pressure was close to normal, and in some of the patients the blood pressure was in the middle of the range seen in healthy young individuals with (mean arterial pressure of ≈90 mmHg) [139]. However, there seems to be a tendency towards a correlation between the reduction in blood pressure and decreased albuminuria. A recent analysis concluded that about 50% of the anti-albuminuric effect in one long-term study [86] could be secondary a reduction in blood pressure [75].

The clinical consequence is that the indication for antihypertensive treatment should be microalbuminuria (as in these clinical trials) rather than some elevation of blood pressure (Table 7.5). Obviously, any elevation of blood pressure or any increasing blood pressure would further strengthen the indication, because there is a correlation between rate of progression of microalbuminuria and blood pressure [139]. The conclusion from these studies suggests that antihypertensive treatment should be initiated whenever microalbuminuria is consistently found regardless of blood pressure levels (Fig 7.1). A more cautious view would be to start antihypertensive treatment if microalbuminuria is clearly increasing (5–10% per year), but the variability in UAE makes this approach somewhat difficult in the everyday clinical setting. All studies document a reduction or stabilization of microalbuminuria, irrespective of the treatment used; however, most studies were conducted with ACE inhibitors as the principal agent with few or no side-effects. Diuretics were systematically added in one important study [86]. Thus the scenario for the use of antihypertensive treatment, in particular ACE inhibitors, is moving away from the indication of elevated blood pressure to the indication of increased/increasing UAE as proposed in recently published guidelines [140]. Combination therapy is also very useful in such patients as discussed above [114].

In type 2 diabetic patients, microalbuminuria can be reduced by ACE inhibition [133,134,142–144] and two long-term studies suggest a beneficial effect on GFR [143,144]. The rate of fall of GFR correlates with blood pressure levels [70]. This important topic has recently been reviewed by Cooper and McNally [88]. However, in these patients who often suffer from diffuse atherosclerosis a cautious use of ACE inhibitors is advised as these drugs could precipitate renal insufficiency in susceptible individuals, in particular those with renovascular disease.

Table 7.5 Observed effects of ACE inhibitors in type 1 diabetic patients

1	No trials in newly diagnosed patients
2	Normoalbuminuria reduced; BP not significantly changed; Filtration fraction reduced
3	Microalbuminuria reduced; BP reduced (diastolic and systolic); Fall in GFR prevented (7–8-year follow-up)
4	Proteinuria reduced; BP reduced (diastolic and systolic); Fall rate of GFR reduced
5	End-stage renal disease and mortality postponed

Stages as described in Table 7.2.

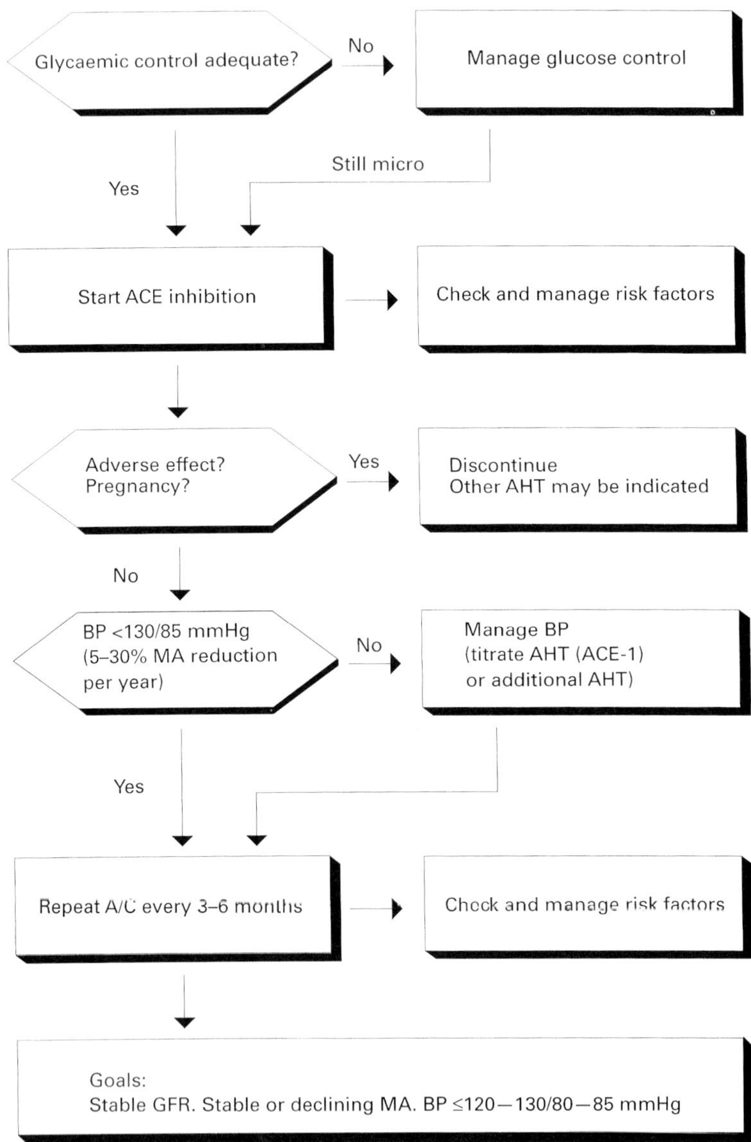

Fig. 7.1 Microalbuminuria in diabetes. Microalbuminuria type 1 patients below 60 years of age. New studies suggest similar effects in the relatively young and lean type 2 diabetic patients. MA, microalbuminuria; A/C, albumin/creatinine ratio; AHT, antihypertensive treatment. Modified from Mogensen *et al.* 1995 [140].

Intervention trials in patients with proteinuria/overt diabetic nephropathy

In untreated patients, there is a correlation between the rate of fall of GFR and blood pressure [85], but interestingly the correlation between GFR and albuminuria is equally strong [85]. It has been suggested that a pronounced fall in proteinuria after the start of antihypertensive treatment predicts a more benign course of renal disease in type 1 diabetic patients [127], compatible with an important role for albuminuria in the progression of diabetic renal disease [75]. Several studies have documented that antihypertensive treatment unequivocally reduces the fall of GFR. This is invariably accompanied by a reduction of albuminuria [37,38,40,145,146]. Therefore antihypertensive treatment is the major therapeutic option for these patients. The use of ACE inhibitors (with diuretics) is popular, although antihypertensive programmes, e.g. with β_1-blocker have been reported to be equally effective [24,41], but possibly with more side-effects [24]. The recent important study by Lewis *et al.* [40] showed that the number of patients with doubling of serum creatinine could be reduced by ACE inhibition [40] confirming earlier studies. Pregnant diabetic patients require special attention [147,148] and ACE inhibitors are strictly contraindicated here.

In proteinuric type 2 diabetic patients, it has also been shown that during antihypertensive treatment there is a correlation between blood pressure elevation and the rate of decline in GFR [126,149,150], suggesting that elevated blood pressure in type 2 diabetic patients is also important for the rate of progression of renal disease. When these patients exhibit overt proteinuria, they generally have a poor prognosis [126]. A long-term intervention trial over several years with the fall of GFR as the end-point have been conducted recently in type 2 diabetes [24]. The rate of fall of GFR is general high, in some patient dramatic, and ACE inhibition and β-blockers seem to have a similar effect on outcome [151]. This was also the conclusion of the blood pressure arm of the UKPDS study who showed an advantage for tight blood pressure control but no difference in the protective effect of ACE inhibition and β-blockade [172]. Important large-scale studies are now ongoing using angiotensin II receptor antagonist and results are keenly available in this high risk population. Finally, one long-term study compared an ACE inhibitor (lisinopril), a long-acting non-dihydropyridine calcium antagonist (Diltiazem) and a β-blocker (atenolol) inpatients with type 2 diabetes and progressive nephropathy [176]. It showed equal protection for lisinopril and diltiazem along with a significant reduction in proteinuria. The effect of atenolol on blood pressure, proteinuria and the progression of renal insufficiency was weaker.

Effect of antihypertensive treatment on renal death

The recent study by Lewis *et al.* documented a beneficial effect of ACE inhibition in this respect as combined ESRF and death were postponed [40]. Thus, ACE inhibitors are effective at all stages of diabetic renal disease (Table 7.5).

Optimized glycaemic control

In the last few years, it has become increasing clear that good glycaemic control is of utmost importance in the prevention and postponement of diabetic renal disease. As documented in the DCCT, good glycaemic control is able to reduce the number of patients who develop microalbuminuria and overt renal disease. Improved metabolic control seems also to protect against the deterioration in renal function in patients with microalbuminuria [84,103]. However, it is important to stress that it is quite often difficult to obtain good metabolic control, especially in patients with incipient or overt renal disease. There is no formalized long-term trial with a sufficient number of patients on the effect on optimized diabetes care in patients with overt renal disease. However, new studies strongly suggest a correlation between the progression of renal disease, as measured by the rate of fall of GFR and the level of HbA_{1C}. If HbA_{1C} is satisfactory, with values of about 8% (reference value 5.5%) progression is slow [2]. This observation was recently confirmed by Björck *et al.* [34] and Alaveras *et al.* [48]. In patients with type 2 diabetes, progression can be reduced by early intervention [4]. With overt nephropathy there is no correlation between progression and HbA_{1C} [126]. The value of good glycaemic control has also been highlighted in the UKPDS study where glycemia control with either insulin or sulphonylureas led to improved outcome with a reduction in microvascular complications [171].

Protein-reduced diet

In normoalbuminuric type 1 diabetic patients, renal hyperfiltration can be reduced by normalizing dietary protein intake, a potential beneficial effect [18].

Studies suggests that microalbuminuria can be reduced on a 2-year intervention basis by a low protein diet [74,152], but so far, no long-term results are available, and compliance may pose a problem.

In diabetic nephropathy, new data have recently been published indicating that the rate of decline of GFR can be reduced by a low protein diet [74]. Patients were monitored on their usual dietary intake of proteins and thereafter patients were put on a low-protein diet. A remarkable reduction in the rate of fall of GFR was observed, although the response varied considerably. Patients served as their own controls without a parallel non-treated group and it cannot be excluded that late or long-term action of antihypertensive treatment may explain at least part of the observed beneficial effect. Zeller *et al.* [153] in a randomized parallel study also documented beneficial effect on the fall rate of GFR in these patients. However, in this study patients on the control diet had higher albuminuria rate at the onset possibly biasing the results. The MDRD study was not convincingly positive but this trial only included few diabetics [154]. Nyberg *et al.* [155,156] did not find correlation between dietary protein intake and status of renal disease in type 1 diabetic patients. A meta-analysis of low protein diet studies in diabetic nephropathy, suggested some benefit [20]. This was also implied by a second meta-analysis of similar trials where diabetic patients may have benefited more from dietary protein restriction when compared with non-diabetic patients with progressive renal insufficiency [177].

At this point in time [22,23], the general consensus may be to prescribe a protein intake of approximately the adult recommended dietary allowance of 0.8 g/kg per day (~10% of daily calories) in the patient with overt nephropathy. However, it has been suggested that once the GFR begins to fall, further restriction to 0.6 g/kg per day may prove useful in slowing the decline of GFR in selected patients. On the other hand, nutrition deficiency may occur in some individuals and may be associated with muscle weakness. Protein-restricted meal plans should be designed by a registered dietician familiar with all components of the dietary management of diabetes.

Summary

This chapter clearly documents that excess albuminuria, often accompanied by increased blood pressure, is associated with factual or subsequent organ damage, not only in the kidney but also in other organs, especially the eyes and the heart. In the kidney, abnormal albuminuria, starting in the microalbuminuric range, reflects more advanced glomerular structural lesions, although the exact location of the permeability defect has not been defined at an ultrastructural level. Blood pressure elevation may not initiate the glomerular permeability defect but high systemic blood pressure aggravates the course of established lesions and clinical disease. Transition from microalbuminuria to macroalbuminuria is associated with a reduction in GFR, the key parameter in evaluation of renal function.

Biochemical and hemodynamic hypotheses have been put forward supported by animal models, but these notions are difficult to substantiate in humans, where isolated phenomena cannot be studied, and direct measurement of parameters such as glomerular wall charge and intraglomerular pressure is not possible. A unifying concept would be attractive, comprising biochemical aberrations, such as charge defects [157–160], changes in enzymatic activities [161,162], and glycation phenomena [163] as well as hemodynamic changes such as hyperfiltration with elevated glomerular capillary pressure [164], aggravated by early systemic hypertension [2,55]. This may be seen along with vascular and endothelial changes [165], reflected by increases in von Willebrand factor [166,167], circulating prorenin [168] as well as increased transcapillary escape rate of albumin [72] and dyslipidemia [169]. Antioxidant status may also play a part [170]. A common pathway explaining all or most of these abnormalities should be pursued, with the basis in prolonged hyperglycemia [52] and related biochemical changes, characteristic for the diabetic state.

However, when diabetic complications are evolving increasing blood pressure remains a decisive factor in promoting organ damage in the kidney, and antihypertensive treatment seems to be the therapeutic cornerstone of ameliorating the deterioration in organ function. A low protein diet may also reduce albuminuria and the fall in GFR. However, strict antihypertensive therapy may limit the need for any dramatic reduction of the protein content of the diet and along with tight glycemia control may achieve the desired goal of preventing or retarding diabetic microvascular complications including nephropathy.

Key references

Chaturvedi N and the EUCLID Study Group. ACE inhibitors for protection against microvascular complications in patients with type 1 diabetes. *Nephrol Dialysis Transplant* 1998; 13: 1064.

The Diabetes Control and Complications Trial Research Group. The effect of intensive treatment of diabetes on the development and progression of long-term complications in insulin-dependent diabetes mellitus. *N Engl J Med* 1993; **329**: 977–986.

Mogensen CE. Combined high blood pressure and glucose in type 2 diabetes: double jeopardy. *Br Med J* 1998; **317**: 693–694.

Mogensen CE. Microalbuminuria, blood pressure and diabetic renal disease: origin and development of ideas. *Diabetologia* 1999; **42**: 263–285.

Lewis EJ, Hunsicker LG, Bain RP, Rhode RD. The effect of angiotensin-converting-enzyme inhibition on nephropathy. *N Engl J Med* 1993; **329**: 1456–1462.

Stephenson JM, Fuller JH, Viberti GC, Sjolie AK, Navalesi R, EURODIAB IDDM Complications Study Group. Blood pressure, retinopathy and urinary albumin excretion in IDDM. the EURODIAB IDDM Complications Study. *Diabetologia* 1995; **38**: 599–603.

UK Prospective Diabetes Study (UKPDS) Group. Intensive blood-glucose with sulphonylureas or insulin compared with conventional treatment and risk of complications in patients with type 2 diabetes (UKPDS33). *Lancet* 1998; **352**: 837–853.

References

1. Mogensen CE. Microalbuminuria, blood pressure and diabetic renal disease: origin and development of ideas. *Diabetologia* 1999; **42**: 263–285.
2. Parving H-H, Rossing P, Hommel E, Smidt UM. Angiotensin converting enzyme inhibition in diabetic nephropathy: ten years experience. *Am J Kidney Dis* 1995; **26**: 99–107.
3. Tattersall RB. The quest for normoglycemia: a historical perspective. *Diabetic Med* 1994; **11**: 618–635.
4. Gaster B, Hirsch IB. The effects of improved glycemic control on complications in type 2 diabetes. *Arch Intern Med* 1998; **158**: 134–140.
5. Mogensen CE. Diabetic renal disease: The quest for normotension—and beyond. *Diabetic Med* 1995; **12**: 756–769.
6. Mogensen CE. Management of early nephropathy in diabetic patients. With emphasis on microalbuminuria. *Annu Rev Med* 1995; **46**: 79–94.
7. Turner RC, Millns H, Neil HAW, Stratton IM, Manley SE, Matthews DR, Holman RR for the United Kingdom Prospective Diabetes Study Group. Risk factors for coronary artery disease in non-insulin dependent diabetes mellitus: United Kingdom Prospective Diabetes Study (UKPDS. 23). *Br Med J* 1998; **316**: 823–828.
8. Hansen KW, Poulsen PL, Mogensen CE. Ambulatory blood pressure and abnormal albuminuria in type 1 diabetic patients. *Kidney Int*, 1994; **45** (Suppl. 45): S134–S140.
9. Poulsen PL, Hansen KW, Mogensen CE. Ambulatory blood pressure in the transition from normo- to microalbuminuria. A longitudinal study in IDDM patients. *Diabetes* 1994; **43**: 1248–1253.
10. Poulsen PL, Ebbehøj E, Hansen KW, Mogensen CE. High normo- or low microalbuminuria. Basis for intervention in insulin-dependent diabetes mellitus. *Kidney Int* 1997; **52** (Suppl. 63): S15–S18.
11. Poulsen PL, Bek T, Ebbehøj E, Hansen KW, Mogensen CE. 24-h ambulatory blood pressure and retinopathy in normoalbuminuric IDDM patients. *Diabetologia* 1998; **41**: 105–110.

12. Ferrannini E. The metabolic syndrome. In *Target Organ Damage in the Mature Hypertensive* (ed. CE Mogensen), pp. 2.31–2.49. Science Press, London, 1993.
13. Reaven GM, Lithell H, Landsberg L. Hypertension and associated metabolic abnormalities—the role of insulin resistance and the sympathoadrenal system. *N Engl J Med* 1996; **334**: 374–381.
14. Mogensen CE, Damsgaard EM, Frøland A, Hansen KW, Nielsen S, Mau Pedersen M, Schmitz A, Thuesen L, Østerby R. Reduced glomerular filtration rate and cardiovascular damage in diabetes: a key role for abnormal albuminuria. *Acta Diabetologica* 1992; **29**: 201–213.
15. Fagerudd JA, Tarnow L, Jacobsen P, Stenman S, Nielsen FS, Pettersson-Fernholm KJ, Grönhagen-Riska C, Parving H-H, Groop P-H. Predisposition to essential hypertension and development of diabetic nephropathy in IDDM patients. *Diabetes* 1998; **47**: 439–444.
16. Roglic G, Colhoun HM, Stevens LK, Lemkes HH, Manes C, Fuller JH, the EURODIAB IDDM, Complications Study Group. Parental history of hypertension and microvascular complications in insulin-dependent diabetes mellitus: the EUORDIAB IDDM complications study. *Diabetic Med* 1998; **15**: 418–426.
17. Ritz E. Nephropathy in type 2 diabetes. *J Int Med* 1999; **245**: 111–126.
18. Mau Pedersen M, Mogensen CE, Schønau Jørgensen F, Møller B, Lykke G, Pedersen O. Renal effects of from limitation of high dietary protein in normoalbuminuric insulin-dependent diabetic patients. *Kidney Int* 1989; **36** (Suppl. 27): S115–S121.
19. Toeller M, Klischan A, Heitkamp G, Schumacher W, Milne R, Buyken A, Karamanos B, Gries FA, the EURODIABIDDM, Complications Study Group. Nutritional intake of 2968 IDDM patients from 30 centres in Europe. *Diabetologia* 1996; **39**: 929–939.
20. Pendrini MT, Levey AS, Lau J, Chalmers TC, Wang PH. The effect of dietary protein restriction on the progression of diabetic and non-diabetic renal disease: a meta-analysis. *Ann Intern Med* 1996; **124**: 627–632.
21. Parving H-H. Effects of dietary protein in renal disease (letter). *Ann Intern Med* 1997; **126**: 330–331.
22. American Diabetes Association. Standards of medical care for patients with diabetes mellitus. *Diabetes Care* 1999; **22** (Suppl. 1): S32–S41.
23. American Diabetes Association. Diabetic nephropathy. *Diabetes Care* 1999; **22** (Suppl. 1): S66–S69.
24. Parving H-H, Rossing P. The use of antihypertensive agents in prevention and treatment of diabetic nephropathy. *Current Opinion Nephrol Hypertension* 1994; **3**: 292–300.
25. Viberti GC, Messent J. Introduction: Hypertension and diabetes. Critical combination for micro- and macrovascular disease. *Diabetes Care* 1991; **14** (Suppl. 4): 4–7.
26. Bennett PH, Haffner S, Kasiske BL, Keane WF, Mogensen CE, Parving H-H, Steffes MW, Striker GE. Screening and management of microalbuminuria in patients with diabetes mellitus—recommendations to the scientific advisory board of the national kidney foundation from an Ad Hoc Committee of the Council on Diabetes Mellitus of the National Kidney Foundation. *Am J Kidney* 1995; **25**: 107–112.
27. Mogensen CE. Definition of diabetic renal disease in insulin-dependent diabetes mellitus based on renal function tests. In *The Kidney and Hypertension in Diabetes Mellitus* (ed. CE Mogensen), pp. 17–30. Kluwer, Boston, 1998.
28. Jacobsen P, Rossing K, Rossing P, Tartow L, Mallet C, Poirier O, Cambien F, Parving H-H. Angiotensin converting enzyme gene polymorphism and ACE inhibition in diabetic nephropathy. *Kidney Int* 1998; **53**: 1002–1006.

29. Parving H-H, Kastrup J, Smidt UM, Andersen AR, Feldt-Rasmussen B, Christiansen JS. Impaired autoregulation of glomerular filtration rate in type 1 (insulin-dependent) diabetics with diabetic nephropathy. *Diabetologia* 1984; **27**: 547–552.
30. Christensen PK, Hansen HP, Parving H-H. Impaired autoregulation of GFR in hypertensive non-insulin dependent diabetic patients. *Kidney Int* 1997; **52**: 1369–1374.
31. Borch-Johnsen K. Incidence of nephropathy in insulin-dependent diabetes mellitus as related to mortality. Cost and benefits of early intervention. In *The Kidney and Hypertension in Diabetes Mellitus* (ed. CE Mogensen), pp. 163–170. Kluwer, Boston, 1998.
32. Pettitt DJ, Knowler WC, Nelson RG. Familial factors in diabetic nephropathy. In *The Kidney and Hypertension in Diabetes Mellitus* (ed. CE Mogensen), pp. 103–111. Kluwer, Boston, 1998.
33. Marre M, Bouhanick B. Genetics and diabetic nephropathy. In *The Kidney and Hypertension in Diabetes Mellitus* (ed. CE Mogensen), pp. 113–122. Kluwer, Boston, 1998.
34. Björck S, Blohmé G, Sylvén C, Mulec H. Deletion insertion polymorphism of the angiotensin converting enzyme gene and progression of diabetic nephropathy. *Nephrol Dialysis Transplant* 1997; **12** (Suppl. 2): 67–70.
35. Schmidt S, Ritz E. Angiotensin I converting enzyme gene polymorphism and diabetic nephropathy in type II diabetes. *Nephrol Dialysis Transplant* 1997; **12** (Suppl. 2): 37–41.
36. Tarnow L, Gluud C, Parving H-H. Diabetic nephropathy and the insertion/deletion polymorphism of the angiotensin-converting enzyme gene. *Nephrology Dialysis Transplant* 1998; **13** (5): 1125–1130.
37. Mogensen CE. Angiotensin converting enzyme inhibitors and diabetic nephropathy (editorial). *Br Med J* 1992; **304**: 227–228.
38. Mogensen CE. Long-term antihypertensive treatment inhibiting progression of diabetic nephropathy. *Br Med J* 1982; **285**: 685–688.
39. Christensen CK, Mogensen CE. Effect of antihypertensive treatment on progression of incipient diabetic nephropathy. *Hypertension* 1985; **7** (Suppl. II): II-109–13.
40. Lewis EJ, Hunsicker LG, Bain RP, Rhode RD. The effect of angiotensin-converting-enzyme inhibition on nephropathy. *N Engl J Med* 1993; **329**: 1456–1462.
41. Sawicki PT. Do ACE inhibitors offer specific benefits in the antihypertensive treatment of diabetic patients? 17 years of unfulfilled promises. *Diabetologia* 1998; **41**: 598–602.
42. Estacio RO, Jeffers BW, Hiatt WR, Biggerstaff SL, Gifford N, Schrier RW. The effect of nisoldipine as compared with enalapril on cardiovascular outcomes in patients with non-insulin-dependent diabetes and hypertension. *N Engl J Med* 1998; **338**: 645–652.
43. Hansen L, Zanchetti A, Carruthers SG, Dahlöf B, Elmfeldt D, Julius S, Ménard J, Rahn KH, Wedel H, Westerling S for the HOT Study Group. Effects of intensive blood-pressure lowering and low-dose aspirin in patients with hypertension: principal results of the Hypertension Optimal Treatment (HOT) randomised trial. *Lancet* 1998; **351**: 1755–62.
44. Bojestig M, Arnquist HJ, Hermansson G, Karlberg B, Ludvigsson J. Declining incidence of nephropathy in insulin-dependent diabetes mellitus. *N Engl J Med* 1994; **330**: 15–18.
45. Rossing P, Rossing K, Jacobsen P, Parving H-H. Unchanged incidence of diabetic nephropathy in IDDM patients. *Diabetes* 1995; **4**: 739–743.
46. Breyer JA, Raymond PB, Evans JK, Nahman NS, Lewis EJ, Cooper M, McGill J, Berl T and the Collaborative Study Group. Predictors of the progression of renal insufficiency in patients with insulin-dependent diabetes and overt diabetic nephropathy. *Kidney Int* 1996; **50**: 1651–1658.
47. Mulec H, Blohmé G, Grände B, Björck S. The effect of metabolic control on rate of

decline in renal function in insulin-dependent diabetes mellitus with overt diabetic nephropathy. *Nephrology Dialysis Transplant* 1998; **13**: 651–655.

48. Alaveras EAG, Thomas SM, Sagriotis A, Viberti GC. Promotors of progression of diabetic nephropathy: the relative roles of blood glucose and blood pressure control. *Nephrol Dialysis Transplant* 1997; **12** (Suppl. 2): 71–74.
49. Microalbuminuria Collaborative Study Group UK. Intensive therapy and progression to clinical albuminuria in patients with insulin dependent diabetes mellitus and microalbuminuria. *Br Med J* 1995; **311**: 973–977.
50. Wu M-S, Yu C-C, Yang C-W, Wu C-H, Haung J-Y, Hong J-J, Chiang FC-Y, Huang C-C, Leu M-L. Poor pre-dialysis glycaemic control is a predictor of mortality in type II diabetic patients on maintenance hemodialysis. *Nephrol Dialysis Transplant* 1997; **12**: 2105–2110.
51. Ravid M, Brosh D, Levi Z, Bar-Dayan Y, Ravid D, Rachmani R. Use of enalapril to attenuate decline in renal function in normotensive patients with type 2 diabetes mellitus. A randomized controlled trial. *Ann Intern Med* 1998; **128**: 982–988.
52. The Diabetes Control and Complications Trial Research Group. The effect of intensive treatment of diabetes on the development and progression of long-term complications in insulin-dependent diabetes mellitus. *N Engl J Med* 1993; **329**: 977–986.
53. Krolewski AS, Laffel LMB, Krolewski M, Quinn M, Warram JH. Glycosylated hemoglobin and the risk of microalbuminuria in patients with insulin-dependent diabetes mellitus. *N Engl J Med* 1995; **332**: 1251–1255.
54. Ohkubo Y, Kishikawa H, Araki E, Miyata T, Isami S, Motoyoshi S, Kojima Y, Furuyoshi N, Shichiri M. Intensive insulin therapy prevents the progression of diabetic microvascular complications in Japanese patients with non-insulin-dependent diabetes mellitus: a randomized prospective 6-year study. *Diabetes Res Clin Prac* 1995; **28**: 103–117.
55. Mathiesen ER, Borch-Johnsen K, Jensen DV, Deckert T. Improved survival in patients with diabetic nephropathy. *Diabetologia* 1989; **32**: 884–886.
56. Viberti GC, Keen H, Wiseman MJ. Raised arterial pressure in parents of proteinuric insulin-dependent diabetics. *Br Med J* 1987; **295**: 515–517.
57. Østerby R. Lessons from kidney biopsies. *Diabetes/Metabolism Rev* 1996; **12**: 151–174.
58. Østerby R, Schmitz A, Nyberg G, Asplund J. Renal structural changes in insulin-dependent diabetic patients with albuminuria. Comparison of cases with onset of albuminuria after short or long duration. *APMIS* 1998; **106**: 361–370.
59. Nørgaard K, Feldt-Rasmussen B, Borch-Johnsen K, Sælan H, Deckert T. Prevalence of hypertension in Type 1 (insulin-dependent) diabetes mellitus. *Diabetologia* 1990; **33**: 407–410.
60. Damsgaard EM, Mogensen CE. Microalbuminuria in elderly hyperglycaemic patients and controls. *Diabetic Med*, 1986; **3**: 430–435.
61. United Kingdom Prospective Diabetes Study. A Multicenter Study. III. Prevalence of hypertension and hypotensive therapy in patients with newly diagnosed diabetes. *Hypertension* 1985; **7** (Suppl. II): II-8–13.
62. Olivarius NF, Andreasen AH, Keiding N, Mogensen CE. Epidemiology of renal involvement in newly-diagnosed middle-aged and elderly diabetic patients. Cross-sectional data from the population-based study ‘Diabetes Care in General Practice’, Denmark. *Diabetologia* 1993; **36**: 1007–1016.
63. Schmitz A. The kidney in non-insulin-dependent diabetes. Studies on glomerular structure and function and the relationship between microalbuminuria and mortality. *Acta Diabetologica* 1992; **29**: 47–69.
64. Schmitz A. Microalbuminuria, blood pressure, metabolic control, and renal involve-

ment. Longitudinal studies in white non-insulin-dependent diabetic patients. *Am J Hypertension* 1997; **10**: 189–197.

65. Feldt-Rasmussen B, Mathiesen ER, Deckert T. Effect of two years of strict metabolic control on the progression of incipient nephropathy in insulin-dependent diabetes. *Lancet* 1986; **ii**: 1300–1304.
66. Parving H-H, Smidt UM, Andersen AR, Svendsen P, Aa. Early aggressive antihypertensive treatment reduces rate of decline in kidney function in diabetic nephropathy. *Lancet* 1983; **i**: 1175–1179.
67. Mogensen CE. Hyperfiltration, hypertension, and diabetic nephropathy in IDDM patients. *Diabetes Nutr Metab* 1989; **2**: 227–244.
68. Nielsen S, Schmitz A, Poulsen PL, Hansen KW, Mogensen CE. Changes in 24 hour ambulatory blood pressure related to albuminuria in NIDDM patients without proteinuria. *Diabetes Care* 1995; **18**: 1434–1441.
69. Schmitz A, Væth M, Mogensen CE. Systolic blood pressure relates to the rate of progression of albuminuria in NIDDM. *Diabetologia* 1994; **37**: 1251–1258.
70. Nielsen S, Schmitz A, Rehling M, Mogensen CE. Systolic blood pressure relates to the rate of decline of glomerular filtration rate in Type 2 diabetes. *Diabetes Care* 1993; **16**: 1427–1432.
71. Nielsen S, Schmitz A, Rehling M, Mogensen CE. The clinical course of renal function in NIDDM patients with normo- and microalbuminuria. *J Intern Med* 1997; **241**: 133–141.
72. Feldt-Rasmussen B. Increased transcapillary escape rate of albumin in type 1 (insulin-dependent) diabetic patients with microalbuminuria. *Diabetologia* 1986; **29**: 282–286.
73. Mau Pedersen M, Schmitz A, Pedersen EB, Danielsen H, Christiansen JS. Acute and long-term renal effects of angiotensin converting enzyme inhibition in normotensive, normoalbuminuric insulin-dependent diabetics. *Diabetic Med* 1988; **5**: 562–569.
74. Walker JD. Non-glycaemic intervention in diabetic nephropathy: the role of dietary protein intake. In *The Kidney and Hypertension in Diabetes Mellitus* (ed. CE Mogensen), pp. 443–453. Kluwer, Boston, 1998.
75. Mogensen CE, Østerby R, Hansen KW, Damsgaard EM. Blood pressure elevation versus abnormal albuminuria in the genesis and prediction of renal disease in diabetes. *Diabetes Care* 1992; **15**: 1192–1204.
76. Mau Pedersen M, Christensen CK, Mogensen CE. Long-term (18 year) prognosis. for normo- and microalbuminuric type 1 (insulin-dependent) diabetic patients (Abstract). *Diabetologia* 1992; **35**: A60.
77. Messent JWC, Elliott TG, Hill RD, Jarrett RJ, Keen H, Viberti GC. Prognostic significance of microalbuminuria in insulin-dependent diabetes mellitus: a twenty-three year follow-up study. *Kidney Int* 1992; **41**: 836–839.
78. Rossing P, Hougaard P, Borch-Johnsen K, Parving H-H. Risk factors for mortality in IDDM patients, a 10 years observational follow up study. *Br Med J* 1996; **313**: 779–784.
79. Dinneen SF, Gerstein HC. The association of microalbuminuria and mortality in non-insulin-dependent diabetes mellitus. A systematic overview of the literature. *Arch Intern Med* 1997; **157**: 1413–1418.
80. Mogensen CE, Hansen KW, Nielsen S, Mau Pedersen M, Rehling M, Schmitz A. Monitoring diabetic nephropathy: Glomerular filtration rate and abnormal albuminuria in diabetic renal disease—reproducibility, progression, and efficacy of antihypertensive intervention. *Am J Kidney Dis* 1993; **22**: 174–187.
81. Mogensen CE, Mau Pedersen M, Hansen KW, Christensen CK. Micro-albuminuria

and the organ-damage concept in antihypertensive therapy for patients with insulin-dependent diabetes mellitus. *J Hypertension* 1992; **10** (Suppl. 1): S43–S51.

82. Mogensen CE, Vestbo E, Poulsen PL, Christiansen C, Damsgaard E, Eiskjær H, Frøland A, Hansen KW, Nielsen S, Mau Pedersen M. Microalbuminuria and potential confounders. A review and some observations on variability of urinary albumin excretion. *Diabetes Care* 1995; **18**: 572–581.
83. Rudberg S, Østerby R, Bangsted H-J, Dahlquist G, Persson B. Effect of angiotensin converting enzyme inhibitor or betablocker on glomerulopathy in young microalbuminuric IDDM patients. *Diabetelogia* 1998; in press.
84. Feldt-Rasmussen B, Mathiesen ER, Jensen T, Lauritzen T, Deckert T. Effect of improved metabolic control loss of kidney function in type 1 (insulin-dependent) diabetic patients: an update of the Steno studies. *Diabetologia* 1991; **34**: 164–170.
85. Mogensen CE. Progression of nephropathy in long-term diabetics with proteinuria and effect of initial anti-hypertensive treatment. *Scand J Clin Lab Invest* 1976; **36**: 383–388.
86. Mathiesen ER, Hommel E, Giese J, Parving H-H. Efficacy of captopril in postponing nephropathy in normotensive insulin-dependent diabetic patients with microalbuminuria. *Br Med J* 1991; **303**: 81–87.
87. Mathiesen ER, Hommel E, Hansen HP, Smidt UM, Parving H-H. Randomised controlled trial of long term efficacy of captopril on preservation of kidney function in normontensive patients with insulin dependant diabets and microalbuminuria. *Br Med J* 1999; **319**: 24–25.
88. Cooper ME, McNally PG. Antihypertensive treatment in NIDDM, with special reference to abnormal albuminuria. In *The Kidney and Hypertension in Diabetes Mellitus* (ed. CE Mogensen), pp. 419–434. Kluwer, Boston, 1998.
89. Nørgaard K, Rasmussen E, Jensen T, Giese J, Feldt-Rasmussen B. Essential hypertension and type 1 diabetes. *Am J Hypertension* 1993; **6**: 830–836.
90. Mogensen CE, Vigstrup J, Ehlers N. Microalbuminuria predicts proliferative diabetic retinopathy. *Lancet* 1985; **ii**: 1512–1513.
91. Klein R, Moss SE, Klein BEK. Gross proteinuria predicts the incidence of proliferative diabetic retinopathy. *Diabetes* 1992; **41** (Suppl. 1): Abstract 129.
92. Nørgaard K, Feldt-Rasmussen B, Deckert T. Is hypertension a major independent risk factor for retinopathy in Type 1 diabetes? *Diabetic Med* 1991; **8**: 334–337.
93. Stephenson JM, Fuller JH, Viberti GC, Sjolie AK, Navalesi R, EURODIAB IDDM Complications Study Group. Blood pressure, retinopathy and urinary albumin excretion in IDDM. the EURODIAB IDDM Complications Study. *Diabetologia* 1995; **38**: 599–603.
94. Knowler WC, Bennett PH, Ballintine EJ. Increased incidence of retinopathy in diabetics with elevated blood pressure. A six-year follow-up study in Pima Indians. *N Engl J Med* 1980; **302**: 645–650.
95. Casale PN, Devereux RB, Milner M. Value of echocardiographic measurement of left ventricular mass in predicting cardiovascular morbid events in hypertensive men. *Ann Intern Med* 1986; **105**: 173–178.
96. Thuesen L, Christiansen JS, Mogensen CE, Henningsen P. Echocardiographic-determined left ventricular wall characteristics in insulin dependent diabetic patients. *Acta Med Scand* 1988; **224**: 343–348.
97. Gilbert RE, Tsalamandris C, Allen TJ, Colville D, Jerums G. Early nephropathy predicts vision-threatening retinal disease in patients with type 1 diabetes mellitus. *J Am Soc Nephrol* 1998; **9**: 85–89.
98. Chaturvedi N, Sjolie A-K, Stephenson JM, Abrahamian H, Keipes M, Castellarin A,

Rogulja-Pepeonik Z, Fuller JH, the EUCLID, Study Group. Effect of lisinopril on progression of retinopathy in normotensive people with type 1 diabetes. *Lancet* 1998; **351**: 28–31.

99. Chaturvedi N and the EUCLID Study Group. ACE inhibitors for protection against microvascular complications in patients with type 1 diabetes. *Nephrol Dialysis Transplant* 1998; **13**: 1064.
100. Nielsen FS, Alo S, Rossing P, Bang LE, Svendsen TL, Gall M-A, Smidt UM, Kastrup J, Parving H-H. Left ventricular hypertrophy in non-insulin-dependent diabetic patients with and without diabetic nephropathy. *Diabetic Med* 1997; **14**: 538–546.
101. Brocco E, Fioretto P, Mauer M, Saller A, Carraro A, Frigato F, Chiesura- Corona M, Bianchi L, Baggio B, Maioli M, Abaterusso C, Velussi M, Sambataro M, Virgili F, Ossi E, Nosadini R. Renal structure and function in non-insulin dependent diabetic patients with microalbuminuria. *Kidney Int* 1997; **52** (Suppl. 63): S40–S44.
102. Bangstad H-J. Østerby R. Dahl-Jørgensen K. Berg KJ. Hartmann A, Hanssen KF. Improvement of blood glucose control in iddm patients retards the progression of morphological changes in early diabetic nephropathy. *Diabetologia* 1994; **37**: 483–490.
103. Feldt-Rasmussen B, Nørgaard K, Jensen T, Deckert T. Microalbuminuria, clinical nephropathy and hypertension in diabetes. *J Hum Hypertension* 1991; **5**: 255–263.
104. Weidmann P, Ferrari P. Central role of sodium in hypertension in diabetic subjects. *Diabetes Care* 1991; **14**: 220–232.
105. Weidmann P, Boehlen LM, de Courten M. Effects of different antihypertensive drugs on human diabetic proteinuria. *Nephrol Dialysis Transplantation* 1993; **8**: 582–584.
106. Thuesen L, Christiansen JS, Mogensen CE, Henningsen P. Cardiac hyperfunction in insulin-dependent diabetic patients developing microvascular complications. *Diabetes* 1988; **37**: 851–856.
107. Sandeman DD, Shore AC, Tooke JE. Relation of skin capillary pressure in patients with insulin-dependent diabetes mellitus to complications and metabolic control. *N Engl J Med* 1992; **327**: 760–764.
108. Shore AC, Jaap AJ, Tooke JE. Capillary pressure in non-insulin-dependent diabetes mellitus. *Diabetes* 1994; **43**: 1198–1202.
109. Gans ROB, Bilo HJG, Nauta JJP, Heine RJ, Donker AJM. Acute hyperinsulinemia induces sodium retention and a blood pressure decline in diabetes mellitus. *Hypertension* 1992; **20**: 199–209.
110. Ferrannini E. Effect of insulin on the kidney and the cardiovascular system. In *The Kidney and Hypertension in Diabetes Mellitus* (ed. CE Mogensen), pp. 131–140. Kluwer, Boston, 1998.
111. Daly PA, Landsberg L. Hypertension in obesity and NIDDM. Role of insulin and sympathetic nervous system. *Diabetes Care* 1991; **14**: 240–248.
112. Yki-Järvinen H, Utriainen T. Insulin-induced vasodilatation: physiology or pharmacology. *Diabetologia* 1998; **41**: 369–379.
113. Anderson S. Pathogenesis of diabetic glomerulopathy: The role of glomerular hemodynamic factors. In *The Kidney and Hypertension in Diabetes Mellitus* (ed. CE Mogensen), pp. 297–306. Kluwer, Boston, 1998.
114. Mogensen CE. Renoprotective role of ACE inhibitors in diabetic nephropathy. *Br Heart J* 1994; **72** (Suppl. 38): 45.
115. Mogensen CE. Introduction. *Nephrol Dialysis Transplant* 1998; **13**: 1056–1079.

116. Mogensen CE, Mau Pedersen M, Ebbehøj E, Poulsen PL, Schmitz A. Combination therapy in hypertension-associated diabetic renal disease. *Int J Clin Prac Suppl* 1997; **90**: 52–58.
117. Pahor M, Psaty BM, Furberg C. Treatment of hypertension patients with diabetes. *Lancet* 1998; **351**: 689–690.
118. Malmberg K, Herlitz J, Hjalmarson Å, Rydén L. Effects of metoprolol on mortality and late infarction in diabetics with suspected acute myocardial infarction: retrospective data from two large studies. *Eur Heart J* 1989; **10**: 423–428.
119. Kjekshus J, Gilpin E, Cali G, Blackey AR, Henning H, Ross JJr. Diabetic patients and β-blockers after acute myocardial infarction. *Eur Heart J* 1990; **11**: 43–50.
120. Carlsen J, Køber C, Torp-Pedersen C, Johansen P. Relation between dose of bendrofuazide antihypertensive effect and adverse biochemical effect. *Br Med J*, 1990; **300**: 975–978.
121. Thürig CH, Böhlen L, Schneider M, de Courten M, Shaw SG, Riesen W, Weidmann P. Lisinopril is neutral to insulin sensitivity and serum lipoproteins in essential hypertensive patients. *Eur J Clin Pharmacol* 1995; **49**: 21–26.
122. Torlone E, Britta M, Rambotti AM, Perriello G, Santeusanio F, Brunetti P, Bolli GB. Improved insulin action and glycemic control after long-term angiotensin-converting enzyme inhibition in subjects with arterial hypertension and type II diabetes. *Diabetes Care* 1993; **16**: 1347–1355.
123. Forsblom C, Trenkwalder P, Dahl K, Mulder H on behalf of the Multicenter Study Group. Angiotensin II receptor blockers in type 2 diabetic patients with microalbuminu ria. *Nephrol Dialysis Transplant* 1998; **13**: 1069.
124. Chan JCN, Critchley JAJH, Cockram CS. Antihypertensive treatment in microalbuminuric type 2 diabetic patients. *Nephrol Dialysis Transplant* 1998; **13**: 1059.
125. Hansen KW, Poulsen PL, Ebbehøj E. Blood pressure elevation in diabetes: the results from 24-h ambulatory blood pressure recordings. In *The Kidney and Hypertension in Diabetes Mellitus* (ed. CE Mogensen), pp. 335–356. Kluwer, Boston, 1998.
126. Gall M-A, Nielsen FS, Smidt UM, Parving H-H. The course of kidney function in Type 2 (non-insulin-dependent) diabetic patients with diabetic nephropathy. *Diabetologia* 1993; **36**: 1071–1078.
127. Rossing P, Hommel E, Smidt UM, Parving H-H. Reduction in albuminuria predicts a beneficial effect on diminishing the progression of human diabetic nephropathy during antihypertensive treatment. *Diabetologia* 1994; **37**: 511–516.
128. The EUCLID, Study Group. Randomised placebo-controlled trial of lisinopril in normotensive patients with insulin-dependent diabetes and normoalbuminuria or microalbuminuria. *Lancet* 1997; **349**: 1789–1792.
129. Marre M, Chatellier G, Leblanc H, Guyenne T-T, Ménard J, Passa PH. Prevention of diabetic nephropathy with Enalapril in normotensive diabetics with microalbuminuria. *Br Med J* 1988; **297**: 1092–1095.
130. Marre M, Hallab M, Billiard A, Le Jeune JJ, Bled F, Girault A, Fressinaud Ph. Small doses of ramipril to reduce microalbuminuria in diabetic patients with incipient nephropathy independently of blood pressure changes. *J Cardiovascular Pharmacol* 1991; **18** (Suppl. 2): S165–S168.
131. Rudberg S, Aperia A, Freyschuss U, Persson B. Enalapril reduces microalbuminuria in young normotensive type 1 (insulin-dependent) diabetic patients irrespective of its hypotensive effect. *Diabetologia* 1990; **33**: 470–476.
132. Cook JJ, Daneman D, Spino M, Sochett E, Perlman K, Balfe JW. Angiotensin convert-

ing enzyme inhibitor therapy to decrease microalbuminuria in normotensive children with insulin-dependent diabetes mellitus. *J Pediatr* 1990; **117**: 39–45.

133. Melbourne Diabetic Nephropathy Study Group. Comparison between perindopril and nifedipine in hypertensive and normotensive diabetic patients with microalbuminuria. *Br Med J* 1991; **302**: 210–216.
134. Hallab M, Gallois Y, Chatellier G, Rohmer V, Fressinaud P, Marre M. Comparison of reduction in microalbuminuria by enalapril and hydrochlorothiazide in normotensive patients with insulin dependent diabetes. *Br Med J* 1993; **306**: 175–182.
135. Viberti GC, Mogensen CE, Groop LC, Pauls JF for the European Microalbuminuria Captopril Study Group. Effect of captopril on progression to clinical proteinuria in patients with insulin-dependent diabetes mellitus and microalbuminuria. *J Am Med Assoc* 1994; **271**: 275–279.
136. Crepaldi G, Carta Q, Deferrari G, Mangili R, Navalesi R, Santeusanio F, Spalluto A, Vanasia A, Nosadini R and The Italian Microalbuminuria Study Group in IDDM. Effects of Lisinopril and nifedipine on the progression to overt albuminuria in IDDM patients with incipient nephropathy and normal blood pressure. *Diabetes Care* 1998; **21**: 104–110.
137. Ravid M, Lang R, Rachmani R, Lishner M. Long-term renoprotective effect of angiotensin-converting enzyme inhibition in non-insulin-dependent diabetes mellitus. A 7-year follow-up study. *Arch Intern Med* 1996; **156**: 286–289.
138. The Microalbuminuria Captopril Study Group. Captopril reduces the risk of nephropathy in IDDM patients with microalbuminuria. *Diabetologia* 1996; **39**: 587–593.
139. Mogensen CE, Hansen KW, Mau Pedersen M, Christensen CK. Renal factors influencing blood pressure threshold and choice of treatment for hypertension in IDDM. *Diabetes Care* 1991; **14** (Suppl. 4): 13–26.
140. Mogensen CE, Keane WF, Bennett PH, Jerums G, Parving H-H, Passa P, Steffes MW, Striker GE, Viberti GC. Prevention of diabetic renal disease with special reference to microalbuminuria. *Lancet* 1995; **346**: 1080–1084.
141. Chan JCN, Cockram CS, Nicholls MG, Cheung CK, Swaminathan R. Comparison of enalapril and nifedipine in treating non-insulin dependent diabetes associated with hypertension: one year analysis. *Br Med J* 1992; **305**: 981–985.
142. Lacourcière Y, Nadeau A, Poirier L, Tancrède G. Captopril or conventional therapy in hypertensive type II diabetics. Three-year analysis. *Hypertension* 1993; **21**: 786–794.
143. Ravid M, Savin H, Jutrin I, Bental T, Katz B, Lishner M. Long-term stabilizing effect of angiotensin-converting enzyme inhibition on plasma creatinine and on proteinuria in normotensive type II diabetic patients. *Ann Intern Med* 1993; **118**: 577–581.
144. Lebovitz HE, Wiegmann TB, Cnaan A, Shahinfar S, Sica DA, Broadstone V, Schwartz SL, Mengel MC, Segal R, Versaggi JA, Bolton WK. Renal protective effects of enalapril in hypertensive NIDDM. Role of baseline albuminuria. *Kidney Int* 1994; **45** (Suppl. 45): S150–S155.
145. Parving H-H, Andersen AR, Schmidt UM, Hommel E, Mathiesen ER, Svendsen P. Aa. Effect of antihypertensive treatment on kidney function in diabetic nephropathy. *Br Med J* 1987; **294**: 1443–1447.
146. Björck S, Mulec H, Johnsen SA, Nordén G, Aurell M. Renal protective effect of enalapril in diabetic nephropathy. *Br Med J* 1992; **304**: 339–343.
147. Mogensen CE, Klebe JG. Microalbuminuria and diabetic pregnancy. In *The Kidney and Hypertension in Diabetes Mellitus* (ed. CE Mogensen), pp. 455–462. Kluwer, Boston, 1998.
148. Kitzmiller JL, Combs CA. Diabetic nephropathy and pregnancy. In *The Kidney and*

Hypertension in Diabetes Mellitus (ed. CE Mogensen), pp. 463–474. Kluwer, Boston, 1998.

149. Baba T, Murabayashi S, Tomiyama T, Takebe K. Uncontrolled hypertension is associated with rapid progression of nephropathy in type 2 diabetic patients with proteinuria and preserved renal function. *Tohoku J Exp Med* 1990; **161**: 741–748.
150. Biesenbach G, Janko O, Zazgornik J. Similar rate of progression in the predialysis phase in type I and type II diabetes mellitus. *Nephrol Dialysis Transplant* 1994; **9**: 1097–1102.
151. Nielsen FS, Rossing P, Gall M-A, Skott P, Smidt UM, Parving H-H. Long-term effect of lisinopril and atenolol on kidney function in hypertensive NIDDM subjects. With diabetic nephropathy. *Diabetes* 1997; **46**: 1182–1188.
152. Dullaart RPF, Beusekamp BJ, van Meijer S, Doormaal JJ, Sluiter WJ. Long-term effects of protein-restricted diet on albuminuria and renal function in IDDM patients without clinical nephropathy and hypertension. *Diabetes Care* 1993; **16**: 483–492.
153. Zeller K, Whittakerm E, Sullivan L, Raskin P, Jacobson HR. Effect of restricting dietary protein on the progression of renal failure in patients with insulin-dependent diabetes mellitus. *N Engl J Med* 1991; **324**: 78–84.
154. Klahr S, Levey AS, Beck GJ, Caggiula AW, Hunsicker L, Kusek JW, Striker G for the Modification of Diet in Renal Disease Study Group. The effects of dietary protein restriction and blood-pressure control on the progression of chronic renal disease. *N Engl J Med* 1994; **330**: 877–884.
155. Nyberg G, Nordén G, Attman P-O, Aurell M, Uddebom G, Lenner RA, Isaksson B. Diabetic nephropathy: Is dietary protein harmful? *J Diabetic Complications* 1987; **1**: 37–40.
156. Nyberg G, Blohmé G, Nordén G. Impact of metabolic control in progression of clinical diabetic nephropathy. *Diabetologia* 1987; **30**: 82–86.
157. Kofoed-Enevoldsen A. The Steno hypothesis and glomerular basement membrane biochemistry in diabetic nephropathy. In *The Kidney and Hypertension in Diabetes Mellitus* (ed. CE Mogensen), pp. 281–288. Kluwer, Boston, 1998.
158. Raats CJI, Van Den Borden J, Berden J. Significance of heparan sulfate altertions for the development of proteinuria. *Nephrol Dialysis Transplant* 1998; **13**: 1057.
159. van der Pijl JW, van der Woude FJ, Geelhoed-Duijvestijn PHLM, Frölich M, van der Meer FJM, van Lemkes HHPJ, Es LA. Danaparoid sodium lowers proteinuria in diabetic nephropathy. *J Am Soc Nephrol* 1997; **8**: 456–462.
160. van der Woude FJ, Det NF. Heparan sulphate proteoglycans and diabetic nephropathy. *Exp Nephrol* 1997; **5**: 180–188.
161. Shah VO, Dorin RI, Sun Y, Braun M, Zager PG. Aldose reductase gene expression is increased in diabetic nephropathy. *J Clin Endocrinol Metab* 1997; **82**: 2294–2298.
162. Cohen MP. General aspects of aldose reductase inhibition. In *Pharmacology of Diabetes Present Practice and Future Perspectives* (eds CE Mogensen, E Standl), pp. 181–91. Walter de Gruyter, Berlin, 1991.
163. Cooper M, Jerums G. Advanced glycation end-products, diabetic renal disease. In *The Kidney and Hypertension in Diabetes Mellitus* (ed. CE Mogensen), pp. 257–262. Kluwer, Boston, 1998.
164. Cortes P, Riser BL. The nature of the diabetic glomerulus: pressure-induced and metabolic aberrations. In *The Kidney and Hypertension in Diabetes Mellitus* (ed. CE Mogensen), pp. 7–16. Kluwer, Boston, 1998.
165. Gazis A, Page SR, Cockcroft JR. ACE inhibitors, diabetes and cardiovascular disease. *Diabetologia* 1998; **41**: 595–597.

166. Stehouwer CDA, Stroes ESG, Hackeng WHL, Mulder PGH, den Ottolander GJH. Von Willebrand factor and development of diabetic nephropathy in IDDM. *Diabetes* 1991; **40**: 971–976.
167. Stehouwer CDA, Nauta JJP, Zeldenrust GC, Hackeng WHL, Donker AJM, den Ottolander GJH. Urinary albumin excretion, cardiovascular disease, and endothelial dysfunction in non-insulin-dependent diabetes mellitus. *Lancet* 1992; **340**: 319–323.
168. Franken AAM, Derkx FHM, Man in't Veld AJ, Hop WCJ, van Rens GH, Peperkamp E, de Jongm PTVM, Schalekamp MADH. High plasma prorenin in diabetes mellitus and its correlation with some complications. *J Clin Endocrinol Metab* 1990; **71**: 1008–1015.
169. Alberti KGMM. Lipids and diabetes: a fatal combination? *Diabetic Med*, 1998; **15**: 359.
170. Maxwell SRJ, Thomason H, Sandler D, Leguen C, Baxter MA, Thorpe GHG, Jones AF, Barnett AH. Antioxidant status in patients with uncomplicated insulin-dependent and non-insulin-dependent diabetes mellitus. *Eur J Clin Invest* 1997; **27**: 484–490.
171. UK Prospective Diabetes Study (UKPDS) Group. Intensive blood-glucose with sulphonylureas or insulin compared with conventional treatment and risk of complications in patients with type 2 diabetes (UKPDS33). *Lancet* 1998; **352**: 837–853.
172. UK Prospective Diabetes Study Group. Tight blood pressure control and risk of macrovascular and microvascular complications in type 2 diabetes: UKPDS38. *Br Med J* 1998; **317**: 703–712.
173. Mogensen CE. Combined high blood pressure and glucose in type 2 diabetes: double jeopardy. *Br Med J* 1998; **317**: 693–694.
174. Toeller M, Buyken A, Heitkamp G *et al.* Protein intake and urinary albumin excretion rates in the EURODIAB IDDM Complications Study. *Diabetologia* 1997; **40**: 1219–1226.
175. Diabetes Nutrition Group of the European Association for the Study of Diabetes. Recommendations for the nutritional management of patients with diabetes mellitus. *Diabetes Nutr Metab* 1995; **8**: 186–189.
176. Bakris GL, Copley JB, Vicknair N, Sadler R, Leurgans S. Calcium channel blockers versus other antihypertensive therapies on progression of NIDDM associated nephropathy. *Kidney Int* 1996; **50**: 1641–1650.
177. Kasiske BL, Lakatua JDA, Ma JZ, Louis TA. A meta-analysis of the effects of dietary protein restriction on the rate of decline in renal function. *Am J Kidney Dis* 1998; **31**: 954–961.

8

Natural history and prognosis of chronic primary glomerulonephritis

Giuseppe D'Amico

Among the various idiopathic glomerulonephritides with a chronic course and a potential progression toward renal failure, four major types, on which we will focus our attention in this chapter, have been identified because of their distinctive morphological and clinical features:

1. Mesangioproliferative glomerulonephritis (GN) with immunoglobulin A (IgA) deposits [(IgA nephropathy (IgAN)].
2. Membranous nephropathy (MN).
3. Membranoproliferative (or mesangiocapillary) GN (MPGN).
4. Focal segmental glomerulosclerosis (FSGS).

Factors affecting the natural course of chronic glomerular diseases and its study

Numerous studies have been performed in these last 30 years in different geographical areas, to try to define the natural history and prognosis of these diseases, but the results have been conflicting, because many factors, that we will briefly analyze, may influence the clinical course and be responsible for completely different outcomes in different patients with the same clinicomorphological type of GN.

Pathogenetic factors

We do not yet know what the initial pathogenetic event which induces the glomerular injury and damage in the four types of chronic GN is. We cannot even exclude, at this point of our knowledge, that each of them is in fact a syndrome, with possibly variable pathogenetic mechanisms. Moreover, even if we postulate a common pathogenetic mechanism in a group of patients with comparable histologic features, we must take into account that in the single patients severity and duration of the injuring insult may vary markedly.

In chronic diseases, in which we believe that the injury persists through time, the damage induced may differ greatly according to its discontinuous or continuous nature: in the former case, the clinical course of the disease will be characterized by episodes of recurrence, with stages of relapse, while in the latter case a more or less rapid but relentless course, with progressive damage, can be hypothesized.

Another variable, which can explain different severity of the damage and trend to progression in different patients, even when the injuring mechanism is similar, is a different genetic background: it is now universally accepted that the molecular mechanisms responsible for the progression of an immunologically and non-immunologically mediated damage are more intensely activated when deleterious environmental factors interact with a 'susceptible' genetic set-up, especially in polygenic disorders such as the glomerular diseases we are considering.

Effect of therapeutic interventions

Owing to our persisting ignorance on the relevant pathogenetic mechanisms responsible for each of the four types of chronic GN, the therapeutic approach has been hitherto extremely variable, aspecific anti-inflammatory and/or immunodepressive drugs (steroids and/or cytotoxic agents) being the most frequently used remedy with markedly variable schedules. Moreover, while some nephrologists have chosen an aggressive approach, in administering high doses of these drugs to the totality of their patients, others have privileged a more conservative attitude, reserving treatment to those with a more severe clinical picture (nephrotic or nephritic syndrome, rapidly developing renal insufficiency). Whatever the choice has been, in the majority of cases the therapeutic protocol has not been a controlled one, and it is still difficult to say if, and to what extent, therapy has favorably influenced the natural history of the disease. As a consequence, we suspect that the many surveys reporting on the natural history of the four chronic glomerular diseases have been more or less biased by the effect of treatment in a variable percentage of the patients studied, but we are not in a position to assess the degree in which the above confounding factor interfered with the 'natural' history of the disease. Undoubtedly, the overall prognosis of all the four types of idiopathic GN has improved over the last 20 years, since steroids and cytotoxic drugs have been more frequently and aggressively used by the clinical nephrologist, but other therapeutic measures permitting a better control of clinical complications such as arterial hypertension and edema meantime became concomitantly available, and it is therefore difficult to evaluate the specific role of immunosupressive therapy on the improved prognosis.

Difficulties in performing correct retrospective studies on the clinical course of chronic glomerular diseases.

The factors analyzed in the previous paragraphs tremendously influence the results of all studies performed, especially over the last 10–15 years, on sufficiently large cohorts of patients. Many of these studies: (a) have analyzed selected populations (this bias is particularly evident for diseases whose histological diagnosis depends on the different local policy as to the indications of biopsy, the less severe patients being biopsied in some places, but not in others; (b) have used more or less restrictive criteria in enrolling the patients to be studied, both in terms of histological and immunohistological parameters and of clinical features; (c) have restricted the study to too limited a period of time; (d) have combined treated and untreated patients in the studied population; (e) have singled out different morphological and/or clinical parameters for the statistical study of the influence of histological and clinical factors on renal survival (prognostic indicators), using different semiquantitative histological grading of lesions.

In the next pages we will review and comment on the results of a retrospective analysis of the most recent literature dealing with the clinical course and prognosis of the four glomerular diseases indicated above, and the predictive value of some clinical and histological features present at onset or at the time of biopsy on said prognosis.

We will hold good our previous 1992 survey [1], in which we selected, among the hundreds of published retrospective studies, only those that fit the following qualifying requirements: (a) large cohorts of patients as non-selected as possible, including those observed in an early stage of disease; (b) definite histological and clinical criteria for the diagnosis and the outcome of the idiopathic type of the four diseases; and (c) reasonably complete (small percentages of patients lost to observation) and prolonged (at least 5 years on average) follow-ups.

Natural history and prognosis of IgA nephropathy

The disease occurs at all ages, but most commonly in young adults and children. Males predominate over females in the reports from all parts of the world, except Japan, with ratios between 2:1 and 4:1. It is more frequently found in white people and Asians, and less commonly in black people.

In almost 50% of patients, the clinical presentation is an episodic, macroscopic hematuria, often coincident with an upper respiratory tract infection (or, less commonly, gastroenteritis), which is frequently recurrent. The presenting clinical sign in the remaining patients is the finding of urinary abnormalities, characterized by persistent microscopic hematuria, associated with a proteinuria which is usually mild (or even absent, in more than 10% of our patients) and is frequently discovered by a chance urinalysis. Obviously, the asymptomatic urinary abnormalities of this large subgroup are frequently overlooked in geographical areas or institutions with restrictive biopsy policies, with consequent 'selection' of the population whose clinical course is monitored. This phenomenon of selection may probably explain why in some surveys severe proteinuria with nephrotic syndrome is reported in a consistent percentage of cases, while in less selected populations it is of rare occurrence: nephrotic syndrome was present at onset in only 3.3 of the 487 IgA patients studied by the Research Group on Progressive Renal Disease in Japan [2], and proteinuria >3.0 g/24 h was detected in only 6.9% of the 374 patients studied in Milan [3].

The most common clinical course is an indolent one, a slow progression to renal insufficiency manifesting in some, but not all, patients. However, in a small percentage of cases (about 4%), rather prolonged remission of all clinical signs has been reported, even without any treatment, although concomitant disappearance of IgA deposits has been an exceptional phenomenon. A clinical course characterized by more rapid progression is also reported in a few cases, usually associated with the presence of marked extracapillary proliferation and/or segmental necrotizing lesions of the capillary loops.

Overall renal survival

As listed in Table 8.1, actuarial renal survival analyses on sufficiently large populations have been reported in the literature since 1984, from different countries. As shown in the table, some of the survival curves have been calculated from the time of first diagnosis or onset of urinary abnormalities, while the time of biopsy represented the starting point for some other surveys. With the exception of the data reported by Alamartine *et al.* [10] in Europe and Ibels and Györy [13] in Australia, indicating a particularly good prognosis (respectively, 94% and 93% at 10 years from the first clinical manifestation), other studies from all over the world, except the USA, agree in estimating an actuarial renal survival at 10 years ranging between 80% and 87% from apparent onset. A definitely poorer renal survival was reported in all three studies from the USA (in two of them, calculated from the time of biopsy), and probably refer to cohorts of more severely ill symptomatic patients, due to the restrictive policy of biopsy.

How much the calculated survival has been influenced by the treatment is difficult to establish, because the efficacy of steroids and immunosuppressive drugs in IgA nephropathy has been disputed until very recently (reviewed in [21]) and many nephrologists did not treat at all the large majority of their patients, the only exception being the generalized use of angiotensin-converting enzyme (ACE) inhibitors in these last years. However, the results of the very recent Italian multicenter controlled trial, carried out on a relatively small population of patients with proteinuria >1 g/24 h, suggest that a 6-month course of steroid treatment can protect against deterioration in renal function [22].

The possible influence of treatment on survival was not analyzed in any of the 18 studies listed in Table 8.1.

Prognostic indices

Among the very numerous studies on the clinical and histological predictors of an unfavorable outcome, we selected, according to the criteria previously mentioned, the studies already listed in Table 8.1 (except those of Velo *et al.* and Rekola *et al.*) plus those of Chida *et al.* [23], Frimat *et al.* [24], and Kobayashi *et al.* [25].

In all 19 studies, an univariate analysis of several clinical and histological parameters, each independently considered, has been performed. In only 13 of them [2,4,5,8,10,11,13,16,17,19,20,24,25] a multivariate survivorship analysis of the most significant independent risk factors was also associated. While the different studies were comparable for the selection of the clinical parameters analyzed in the statistical analyses, the histological parameters selected by the different investigators varied widely (semiquantitative grading of individual features or cumulative grading of

Table 8.1 Actuarial renal survival in idiopathic IgA nephropathy

Authors	No. of patients	Mean age at onset (years)	Mean follow-up (months)	Actuarial renal survival at 10 years
Europe				
D'Amico *et al.* (1986) Italy [4]	365	29	79	85%*
Beukhof *et al.* (1986) The Netherlands [5]	75	24	92	84%*
Noel *et al.* (1987) France [6]	280	—	>60	85%*
Velo *et al.* (1987) Spain [7]	153	22	>60	81%*
Bogenschutz *et al.* (1990) Germany [8]	239	—	59	81%‡
Rekola *et al.* (1990) Finland [9]	209	25	76	83%†
Alamartine *et al.* (1991) France [10]	282	28	96	94%*
Johnston *et al.* (1992) UK [11]	220	30	65	83%†
Australia				
Nicholls *et al.* (1984) [12]	244	32	60	87%†
Ibels *et al.* (1994) [13]	121	39	107	93%*
Asia				
Woo *et al.* (1987) Singapore [14]	151	27	65	82%*
Kusumoto *et al.* (1987) Japan [15]	86	27	114	80%*
Katafuchi *et al.* (1994) Japan [16]	225	32	48	74%†
Yagame *et al.* (1996) Japan [17]	206	30	110	87%†
Koyama *et al.* (1997) Japan [2]	448	>10 years in 95%	142	85%*
USA				
Wyatt *et al.* (1984) [18]	58	27	>60	78%*
Radford *et al.* (1997) [19]	148	39	45	67%†
Haas *et al.* (1997) [20]	109	~40	>18	57%†

* After the first manifestations; † After the biopsy; ‡ Not specified.

several histological features to give multiple scores of severity), making a reliable comparison more difficult.

In the last few years, four studies on long-term prognosis of sufficiently large populations of pediatric patients have been published from the USA [26,27], Europe [28], and Japan [29]. They indicate that renal survival and risk factors are no different from those of adult patients.

The results of these statistical analyses of retrospective data are summarized in Table 8.2. We have separated the risk factors for which there was substantial agreement among the various investigators, from those with a weaker or less concordant statistical significance. For the histological parameters, we selected those which, when separately evaluated, where significantly associated with a worse prognosis. As we said, some investigators [8,16,17,19,20,23–25] used, especially for the multivariate survivorship analysis, stages of morphological classifications, or global scores inclusive of all histological features, or separate scores for the glomerular, tubulo-interstitial, and vascular features evaluated semiquantitatively. These features were differently associated and graded in the various studies, a different role being attributed to the proliferative component as a marker of more severe and progressive disease (see Kurt Lee's editorial, [30]).

Glomerular sclerosis (both global and segmental), as well as interstitial damage (both leukocyte infiltration and fibrosis), are universally accepted as the most powerful risk factors, while three more (extension of IgA deposits into the walls of peripheral capillary loops and/or segmental thickening of glomerular basement membrane, marked extracapillary proliferation, and marked arterial hyalinosis) have also emerged as significant risk factors in some of the statistical multivariate analyses.

The fact that interstitial damage, including leukocyte infiltration, is a powerful independent prognostic factor in this disease, as well as in the other types of chronic

Table 8.2 Clinical and histological risk factors in IgAN, according to the most accurate studies of the literature (see text)

Significant by multivariate analysis in almost all studies
- Elevated serum creatinine at presentation
- Severe proteinuria at presentation and/or during the follow-up
- Arterial hypertension at presentation
- Global sclerosis of many glomeruli and/or widespread segmental glomerulosclerosis
- Marked tubulo-interstitial lesions (mainly interstitial infiltration and/or fibrosis)

Significant by multivariate or univariate analysis in some studies
- Older age at presentation
- Absence of any history of recurrent macroscopic hematuria
- Extension of IgA deposits into the walls of peripheral capillary loops and/or segmental thickening of GBM
- Marked arteriolar hyalinosis
- Diffuse mesangial hypercellularity and/or expansion
- Marked extracapillary proliferation and/or segmental necrosis of the capillary wall

GN that we will take into consideration (see below), emphasizes the role of the tubulo-interstitial lesions in the progression of all glomerular diseases. The emerging correlation between such lesions and the extent of the urinary protein loss (another powerful prognostic indicator, as shown in Table 8.2), suggest that the injuring effect of proteinuria on the reabsorbing tubular cells might be the mediator between glomerular and tubulo-interstitial damage [31]. As shown in Table 8.2, among the morphological features of glomerular damage, extracapillary proliferation is a significant prognostic indicator. We have recently stressed the fact that, at least in some patients with IgAN, such proliferation might be the marker of a vasculitic damage, although it is infrequent to find in the biopsy specimen the segmental lesion which is the hallmark of the capillaritis so frequently found in Henoch–Schönlein syndrome.

The only immunohistological parameter of unfavorable prognosis is the presence of immune deposits outside the mesangial area into the walls of the peripheral capillary loops. This finding, together with the finding that glomerular basement membrane lesions seen by light microscopy are also a risk factor, indicates that the disease is more severe and more likely to progress when the deposits and the damage they induce are less restricted to the mesangial area. The cause of this involvement of the peripheral capillary loops is still unknown. It could be due either to a more sustained and prolonged overload of immune reactants in the mesangium, with its consequent engulfment and the overflow of complexes to the peripheral capillary walls, or to the arrival at the glomerular level of immune complexes of different physicochemical characteristics which favor entrapment on the subendothelial side of the capillary walls.

As for the clinical prognostic factors, the existence of a functional impairment at presentation, a long-lasting severe proteinuria, and an arterial hypertension at presentation have been indicated by multivariate analysis in all the studies as the most significant (Table 8.2). All of them appear to be rather non-specific, and we will see them to be risk factors also in the other types of chronic GN (see below).

Large consensus, although not unanimous, exists on the assumption that progression is less frequent and rapid in patients with recurrent episodes of macroscopic hematuria than in those with less evident acute clinical signs (persistent microscopic hematuria with proteinuria). We already emphasized [32] that there are two possible explanations for this: (a) IgAN with and without recurrent macroscopic hematuria are two different diseases, with a different severity [this possibility was brought up by Beukhof *et al.* back in 1986 [5]], and (b) in the two subgroups, the damaging mechanism is the same, but in patients with recurrent macroscopic hematuria it acts discontinuously (perhaps triggered by exogenous antigens coming intermittently from the mucosal surfaces?), while in patients without recurrent macroscopic hematuria some less evident but continuously acting immunological mechanism, perhaps endogenous antigens (dietary antigens, autoantigens), induces more severe and progressive damage with time.

We have stressed in the past [32], in agreement with other investigators, that unfortunately even those prognostic indicators that appear to be significant in the retrospective statistical analysis of a large population of patients are not always reliable for predicting the outcome for a single patient. In other words, some patients with rather marked proteinuria and/or severe histological lesions at the time of biopsy can have quite favorable courses, and some patients with moderate proteinuria and/or mild histological lesions may have rapidly progressive courses in the following years. Even when some impairment of renal function has already developed, and glomerular sclerosis is severe, the speed of progression to end-stage renal failure (ESRF) is quite variable.

We think that this wide variability in the clinical course of IgAN, probably more unpredictable than that of many other immune-mediated primary chronic glomerulonephritides, is due to the heterogeneity of this disease, the fact that what we call IgAN is a range of diseases having a common pathogenetic marker, the mesangial deposition of IgA immune complexes, but probably different, still unknown mechanisms of immunological and non-immunological damage. We suspect that the possible sudden changes in the natural history of what we call idiopathic IgAN is due to the fact that all these still obscure immunological events (IgA mediated and non-IgA dependent) may act discontinuously, at least in a subgroup of patients.

Natural history and prognosis of idiopathic membranous nephropathy

It is quite probable that treatment with steroids, especially when they are associated with immunosuppressive drugs (chlorambucil, cyclophosphamide, cyclosporine), has changed the clinical course of the disease and has improved the prognosis of idiopathic MN. Therefore, only the few retrospective or prospective studies describing the clinical course of sufficiently large cohorts of untreated patients allow evaluation of the 'natural' history of this disease [33–38].

Membranous nephropathy occurs at all ages, but especially in adults and the elderly, where it represents the most common cause of nephrotic syndrome. Male gender is prevalent, with a ratio of approximately 2 : 1 [39]. Nephrotic syndrome is found at presentation in about 80% of patients, although lower percentages (as low as 63%) have been reported. A marked non-selective proteinuria in non-nephrotic range is present in the remaining patients. Microscopic hematuria is associated to proteinuria in more than 50% of cases. Arterial hypertension and/or impairment of renal function are present already at presentation in variable percentages of patients.

The clinical course and outcome are rather variable. As indicated in Table 8.3, almost complete disappearance of proteinuria within 4–5 years occurs in between 20% and 25% of untreated patients with nephrotic syndrome at presentation. Although relapse has been reported, these patients usually do not progress to renal insufficiency. Deterioration of renal function occurs, usually during the first 5 years of follow-up, in some of the patients in whom the nephrotic syndrome persists, or, less frequently, in those in whom a partial remission, with proteinuria <2 g/day, has developed. However, some other patients with persisting nephrotic syndrome do not develop renal insufficiency for very long periods of time. Obviously, complications due to the persistent massive loss of proteins, with consequent dyslipidemia, may occur in these patients. Patients with MN and persistent nephrotic syndrome are

Table 8.3 Actuarial renal survival in non-treated idiopathic membranous nephropathy

Authors	No. of patients	Mean age at presentation (years)	% of patients with nephrotic syndrome at presentation	Mean duration of follow up (months)	% of patients with complete clinical remission during follow-up	Actuarial renal survival	
						At 5 years	At 10 years
Noel *et al.* 1979 [33]	116	38	76%	54	23%	87%	76%
Radaelli *et al.* 1988 [36]	85	51	74%	58	20%	81%	66%
Schieppati *et al.* 1993 [38]	100	51	63%	52	24%	88%	74%*

* Survival at 8 years.

particularly exposed to the risk of thomboembolic events, especially renal vein thrombosis [an incidence up to 29%, according to Bellomo and Atkins [40]].

Overall renal survival

The data on actuarial renal survival at 5 and 10 years reported in the literature are listed in Table 8.3 for the three European studies on populations of untreated patients and in Table 8.4 for the studies performed on mixed populations of treated and untreated patients in different geographical areas.

It is evident that the calculated renal survival has been rather variable, even in the studies referring to units in which it is an established policy not to treat patients with MN. Renal survival at 10 years in the three European studies on untreated patients varied between 66% and 76% (Table 8.3), and was somewhat worse than in the three European studies on mixed populations of treated and untreated patients (Table 8.4). Table 8.4 shows also that renal survival was particularly favorable, higher than 90% at 10 years, in both studies performed in Japan. Even on the basis of the recent pooled analysis of all the studies [39] the majority of which are not listed in Table 8.4 because they are not sufficiently accurate or complete, it is now accepted that prognosis of idiopathic MN is better in this Asian country, as well as in Australia. This pooled analysis of all data of the literature up to 1993, for a total of 1189 patients [39], indicated a renal survival outcome of 86% at 5 years, and 65% at 10 years, definitely lower than that of the few selected studies listed in our Table 8.4. The results listed in Table 8.4, as well as the conclusion of the pooled analysis of all the randomized trials performed by Hogan *et al.* [39], do not support any significant improvement of renal survival with glucocorticoids or alkylating agents, the two categories of drugs which were more widely tested. However, performing a more focused meta-analysis on the results of the best controlled trials, these investigators,

Table 8.4 Actuarial renal survival in cohorts including treated and untreated patients with membranous nephropathy

Authors	No. of patients	Mean age (years)	% with nephrotic syndrome at presentation and with clinical remission (%)	Mean duration of follow up (months)	Actuarial renal survival at 10 years	Better renal survival in treated patients[‡] (from comparison of survival curves)
Europe						
Honkanen *et al.* 1986 (Finland) [41]	67	39	75% (25%)	80	83% (*)	No
Zucchelli *et al.* 1987 (Italy) [42]	82	47	100% (24%)	127	82%	Yes
Wehrmann *et al.* 1989 (Germany) [43]	334	36	73% (—)	62	77%	No
USA						
Donadio *et al.* 1988 [35]	140	50	83% (41%)	74	58%	No
Australia						
Murphy *et al.* 1988 [44]	139	36	54% (33%)	52	81%	No
Japan						
Kida *et al.* 1986 [45]	104	40	60% (40%)	138	90%	No
Abe *et al.* 1986 [46]	89	39	75% (37%)	72	96%	No[†]

* Overall survival (including non-renal deaths).
† Calculated as % of clinical remission at long-term follow-up.
‡ Retrospective analysis of non-randomized subgroups of patients (except for the study of Zucchelli *et al.*).

as well as Couchoud *et al.* [47], Imperiale *et al.* [48], and Cattran [49], concluded that alkylating agents, given alone or in association with steroids, as well as cyclosporine in selected patients, seem to reduce the risk of renal function deterioration and to increase the occurrence of complete and partial remission. All these reviews of pooled data stress the fact that the evaluation of any tested treatment is difficult, as the clinical course of patients with idiopathic MN is quite variable, the chance of spontaneous remission rather high, and the possibility of spontaneous relapses of the nephrotic syndrome after remission not negligible. A very recent methodologic meta-analysis [50], after an accurate selection of the 26 best reports of the literature on the natural history of MN and the effect of the various therapeutic regimens, emphasizes that some important basic methodological principles, which are accurately commented, have been partially disregarded even in these selected published studies.

Prognostic indices

In the majority of the published studies the same methodologic biases apply to the evaluation of the clinical and histological factors which may influence the outcome of the disease. They explain why, even when selecting, as we did, the 28 most accurate retrospective or prospective studies, there is no agreement on the statistical significance of the single factors, considered in the univariate analysis [33–38,41,43–46,51–67], and even more so in the multivariate analysis (13 studies).

In Table 8.5, we summarize the results of these selected studies, distinguishing once again between those prognostic indicators accepted by the majority of investigators and those as to which there is less concordance. However, at variance with the studies on risk factors in IgAN reported in Table 8.2, none of the clinical or histologic factors included in the multivariate statistical analysis appeared to be a significant prognostic index in the great majority of these studies. Sufficient agreement, with many exceptions, is had among the different investigators for the

Table 8.5 Clinical and histological risk factors in idiopathic membranous nephropathy, according to the most accurate studies of the literature (see text)

Significant by multivariate analysis in many studies
Elevated serum creatinine at presentation
Proteinuria in the nephrotic range at presentation
Marked tubulo-interstitial lesions
Significant by multivariate or univariate analysis in some studies
Male sex
Older age at presentation
Stage of the glomerular lesions

elevated serum creatinine and the massive proteinuria at presentation as clinical risk factors, while the prognostic value of interstitial damage was confirmed in all the four studies in which this parameter was analyzed [36,42,66,67]. The value of male gender, older age, and stage of the glomerular lesions is more controversial.

Very recently, in Canada, Cattran and his associates [68] focused their attention on the prognostic value of severe proteinuria, and tested a predictive model based on the calculated 'highest sustained six-month period of proteinuria'. This parameter appeared to be a better prognostic index than the degree of proteinuria checked at presentation. Introducing this factor in the multiple logistic modelling for 184 Canadian patients, the only additional prognostic variables of importance were the initial creatinine clearance and the rate of change in function over the same 6-month interval with the most sustained average level of proteinuria. The same predictive model was tested also in 101 Italian patients and 78 Finnish patients. In all the three countries accuracy of prediction was ≥85%.

Natural history and prognosis of idiopathic type I membranoproliferative glomerulonephritis

Although this glomerular disease is becoming very rare in the developed countries [69,70], it is still rather frequent in the less-developed countries of Africa, Asia, and Latin-America, and it has therefore been included in our review.

It affects children and adolescents more frequently than adults: it rarely occurs before the age of 5 and after the sixth decade. There is no gender predominance. In type I, characterized by the presence of electron-dense subendothelial deposits, the clinical presentation is a nephrotic syndrome in about 60% of cases, usually accompanied by microscopic hematuria. Acute nephritic syndrome may be the presenting feature in 15–20% of cases; recurrent macroscopic hematuria is occasionally seen. The remaining patients present with less evident, usually asymptomatic proteinuria and microscopic hematuria. Reduced serum levels of the early components of the classic pathway of complement activation are frequently present in type I MPGN.

The clinical course of untreated patients is characterized by spontaneous variations in severity of proteinuria and variable rate of deterioration of renal function, with periods of prolonged remission in many patients (total remission being reported in 7–10% of patients), or episodes of acute deterioration of renal function and/or rapid variation of the severity of proteinuria, which can occur without any obvious triggering events.

Overall renal survival

The outcome of type I MPGN, documented in a number of small cohorts during the 1970s, was reviewed by Cameron in 1979 [71]. Ten-year actuarial survival of renal function varied from 40% to 70%. More recently, four studies of long-term treatment of small populations of patients were reviewed in 1989 by Donadio and Offord [72], who calculated 10-year renal survivals ranging from 60% to 85%. However, these studies did not fit our requirements.

Table 8.6 summarizes data from two studies in the UK [73] and Spain [74] of relatively small populations of patients with type I MPGN, and of two more recent multicenter studies from Germany [75] and Italy [76] which both refer to large mixed cohorts of treated and untreated patients, comparable for the total number of patients, their mean age, percentage with nephrotic syndrome at presentation, and duration of follow-up. The reported renal survivals 10 years after onset were 64% and 60% in the two large populations [75,76], 62% in the patients from London [73], and 54% in those from Barcelona [74]. In three of the four studies, survival curves of treated and untreated patients did not show better survival in treated patients [74–76], the treatment consisting of steroids, eventually associated with cytotoxic agents (cyclophosphamide), or antiplatelet agents.

Prognostic indices

Only the four rather recent studies listed in Table 8.6, fitting our criteria, give some indications as to the clinical and histological prognostic indicators, and in only two of them, the multicenter studies from Germany [75] and Italy [76], a multivariate survivorship analysis was carried out. Both of these two large studies showed that impairment of renal function and arterial hypertension at presentation negatively influenced renal survival.

The Italian study, although not the German one, confirmed the adverse prognostic significance of the nephrotic syndrome, already stressed by other investigators, including Cameron's group [73] and the group from Barcelona [74], listed in Table 8.6. The English study also confirmed the importance of renal hypertension, but not of impaired renal function at presentation. Only in the Italian study [76] was multivariate analysis performed, and it showed that reduced glomerular filtration rate, severe proteinuria, and arterial hypertension at presentation were significant independent risk factors. As for the histological prognostic indices, in both the large

Table 8.6 Actuarial renal survival in idiopathic type I membrano-proliferative GN

Authors	No. of patients	Mean age at presentation (years)	% of patients with nephrotic syndrome	Renal survival at 10 years	Better survival in treated patients* (from comparison of survival curves)
Cameron *et al.* 1983 (UK) [73]	69	26	48%	62%	—
Valles Prats *et al.* 1985 (Spain) [74]	72	25	84%	54%	No
Schmitt *et al.* 1990 (Germany) [75]	220	36	75%	64%	No
Italian Study Group 1990 [76]	259	34	70%	60%	No

* Retrospective analysis of non-randomized subgroups of patients.

multicenter studies tubulo-interstitial damage appeared to be the most powerful risk factor. The classification of the glomerular damage was different in the two studies: In the German one [75], the total damage was graded from I (segmental form) to IV (lobular) and V (crescents), while in the Italian study [76], a separate classification was used for the subgroup with nodular lesions (thought to be a microaneurismic type of lesion similar to that of diabetic glomerulosclerosis). In both studies, the presence of crescents and, in the Italian one, the presence of nodular segmental lesions, were indicators of poor prognosis, while the severity of the mesangial proliferation and peripheral interposition did not influence renal survival. Survivorship analysis was also used in the study of Cameron *et al.* [73] to evaluate the prognostic role of the presence of crescents, and the results were in accordance with the previous two studies. In the Italian study, the prognostic role of arteriolar damage was also evaluated, and it appeared to be a significant risk factor even by multivariate analysis, as was interstitial damage. These data are summarized in Table 8.7.

Natural history and prognosis of idiopathic focal segmental glomerulosclerosis

It is widely known in large renal units that the incidence of primary FSGS in adult patients is progressively increasing, this disease now being in many institutions the most frequent diagnosis following native kidney biopsies of patients with idiopathic nephrotic syndrome, especially black people. At Columbia-Presbyterian Medical Center in New York, an approximately sevenfold increase from 1974 to 1993 has been reported [77]. Similarly, at the University of Chicago a retrospective analysis of all adult renal biopsies for the same range of years revealed that the yearly incidence of FSGS increased from 4.0% during the period between 1974 and 1979 to 12.2% during the period from 1987 to 1993, while the odds of a diagnosis of MN (mean yearly incidence, 9.5%) did not vary significantly over the study period [78].

The disease affects children and adults of both sexes, and is particularly frequent in black adults. Presentation and clinical course can be different in children and adults: children appear to present more frequently with the nephrotic syndrome [79], are more likely to respond to therapy and progress to renal insufficiency less rapidly than adults. Even in adult patients, proteinuria in the nephrotic range represents the

Table 8.7 Clinical and histological risk factors in patients with idiopathic type I membranoproliferative GN, according to the four most accurate studies of the literature (see text)

Significant by multivariate analysis in almost all studies
Elevated serum creatinine at presentation
Severe proteinuria at presentation
Arterial hypertension at presentation
Marked tubulo-interstitial lesions

must frequent characterizing clinical feature already at presentation, occurring in 65–75% of patients (68% of 492 patients, according to the review of Korbet *et al.* [79]), and becomes even more frequent during the subsequent course, occurring in some of the patients presenting at onset with a non-nephrotic proteinuria. Microscopic hematuria is almost constantly present at onset, representing a useful sign to differentiate FSGS from minimal change nephropathy, a disease to which it is frequently related. Hypertension is found rather frequently at presentation (usually in more than half of the patients), and some impairment in renal function can be found in a less consistent percentage of cases.

A progressive clinical course, with frequent occurrence of renal failure, is characteristic of patients showing a nephrotic syndrome at presentation or developing it subsequently. Although in a single patient proteinuria may have large fluctuations, spontaneous remission of nephrotic syndrome is a very rare phenomenon (between 1.5 and 3.0%). As we will see, the clinical course is definitely more favorable in untreated patients who not develop nephrotic syndrome.

Overall renal survival

While old reports suggested that treatment with steroids, and/or cytotoxic drugs induced little benefit in terms of induced remission and outcome, and documented higher than 50% progression to ESRF at 10 years in patients with nephrotic syndrome [80], it is now evident than more vigorous and protracted therapy with these drugs (up to 4–6 months) or with cyclosporine may induce complete or partial remission in a good percentage of cases (ranging from 30% to 50% in the different reports of the most recent literature, and, even more interestingly, may completely change prognosis in responders to treatment [79,81–94]. Responders only exceptionally progress to chronic renal failure, while many among non-responders develop ESRF, usually within the first 5 years from onset. After prolonged treatment, a remission probably related to its effect can even manifest many months after withdrawal of the therapy: consequently, prolonged treatment is appropriate even when it does not seem to promptly influence the severity of proteinuria. Although relapses may occur in patients who have remission of the nephrotic syndrome after treatment (such relapses are less frequent when cytotoxic drugs are associated with steroids), sustained complete remission is rather frequent in the long run, even in patients having had one or more relapses.

Only five recent studies, listed in Table 8.8, have reported curves of actuarial renal survival in adult patients. Renal survival at 10 years was between 56 and 58% in patients with nephrotic syndrome, while it was higher than 90% in those who did not develop this syndrome; it was also very good (>95%) in patients with nephrotic syndrome who responded to treatment, while it was poor (<40%) in patients with nephrotic syndrome and no response to treatment; it was also very poor (28%) in patients with the histological variant of the disease called 'collapsing FSGS' in the only study in which survival curves were separately obtained for this variant [87]. As the table indicates, complete treatment-induced clinical remission ranged between 33% and 52%, but was definitely lower in patients with the

Table 8.8 Actuarial renal survival in idiopathic focal segmental glomerulosclerosis

Authors	No. of patients	Mean age at presentation (years)	Mean duration of follow-up (months)	% of patients with nephrotic syndrome at onset or during follow-up	% of nephrotic treated patients achieving complete clinical remission	Actuarial renal survival at 10 years (%)			
						Patients with nephrotic syndrome	Patients without nephrotic syndrome	Patients responders to treatment	Patients non-responders to treatment
Wehrmann *et al.* 1990 [85]	250	32	55	66%		56%	94%	—	—
Pei *et al.* 1987 [81]	93	35	61	78% in adults 95% in children	39% in adults 44% in children	79	(96%)	96%	30%
Banfi *et al.* 1991 [82]	59	35	75	100%‡	52%	58%	—	98%	28%
Rydel *et al.* 1995 [86]	81	40	>12 in 80%	74%	33%	57%	92%	100%	38%
Valeri *et al.* 1996 [87]	50 43*	33 32	61 32	60% 91%	33% 10%	66%† 28%†			

* Patients with the collapsing variant; † Renal survival at 3 years; ‡ Only patients with nephrotic syndrome have been included in the study.

collapsing variant of the disease. It is worth emphasizing that all studies showed that even partial clinical remission (proteinuria <2 g/day) induced by treatment improves the prognosis in comparison with non-response: Korbet *et al.* [79], summarizing data of the literature on the outcome of 233 adult patients with FSGS, reported that ESRF occurred, after an average follow-up of 5.5 years, in 3% of the 78 patients with complete clinical remission, in 25% of the 32 patients with partial remission, and in 60% of the 123 patients who did not respond to treatment. According to the same review, outcome was somewhat more favorable in the 243 children included, as only 37% of the 161 patients with no response to treatment developed ESRF after a mean follow-up of 6.1 years. Unfortunately, there are no recent studies on the natural history of pediatric cohorts reporting detailed life table analysis of actuarial renal survival.

Prognostic indices

In these last 10 years, a sufficiently accurate statistical evaluation (which also includes a multivariate analysis of all the potential risk factors) of the role of clinical and histological factors on the prognosis, has only been carried out by a limited number of investigators [81,82,84–88]. Many other previous studies [89–99] had considered only single risk factors, using different statistical methodologies. The results of these studies are summarized in Table 8.9. They confirm that development of nephrotic syndrome at some time during the clinical course, as well as lack of response to treatment, represent, together with the existence of a deterioration of renal function at presentation, the most powerful clinical predictors of unfavorable prognosis. Some, but not all, studies showed the prognostic value of three more clinical variables: age, sex, and blood pressure.

As for histological factors, once again the severity of the tubulo-interstitial involvement appeared to be the most powerful risk factor.

Still more controversial was the role as prognostic indicators of the morphological variants of FSGS (prevalence of glomerular sclerosis at the tubular pole or 'tip lesions'; presence of 'diffuse mesangial cellularity'; presence of endocapillary and extracapillary hypercellularity with focal segmental distribution, or 'cellular variant'; glomerulomegaly; collapse of the glomerular capillaries, or 'collapsing variant'). There is almost universal agreement that the collapsing variant, frequent in black patients, and usually associated with severe tubulo-interstitial damage, has a worse prognosis in comparison with all other morphological types [87,100,101], while the initial statement that the 'tip variant' has a particularly favorable prognosis [102] has not been subsequently confirmed [77,98,103].

Special attention has been given over the last few years to the role of increased diameter of glomeruli (glomerular hypertrophy, glomerulomegaly), after the study of Fogo *et al.* [104], showing that glomerular hypertrophy in pediatric patients with apparent minimal change nephropathy could predict subsequent development of FSGS. Some investigators [84,105,106] have reported that an increased mean diameter of glomeruli in patients with FSGS is a significant risk factor, even at the multivariate analysis [84].

Table 8.9 Clinical and histological risk factors in patients with idiopathic focal segmental glomerulosclerosis, according to the most recent studies, including five reports with multivariate survivorship analysis (see text)

Significant for the majority of investigators
Elevated serum creatinine at presentation
Nephrotic syndrome at presentation or during the follow-up
No response to prolonged treatment with steroids and cytotoxic drugs
Marked tubulo-interstitial lesions
Collapsing variant
Significant only in some studies
Older age at presentation
Male sex
Arterial hypertension at presentation
Increased mean glomerular diameter at biopsy
More advanced glomerular lesions

Conclusions

Our survey of the major studies on the natural history and prognosis of four types of chronic progressive idiopathic primary GN (IgAN, MN, MPGN, and FSGS) enables us to draw the following conclusions:

1. The average trend of developing ESRF is different for each of the four diseases, actuarial renal survival at 10 years from apparent onset ranging from 85–90% in patients with IgAN, to 65–75% in patients with MN, to 60–65% in patients with MPGN, to 55–60% in patients with FSGS and nephrotic syndrome.
2. For each of the four types of idiopathic GN there is an extreme variability of the rate of progression, deterioration of renal function, even after long periods of observation, occurring only in a subset of patients; it is therefore of paramount importance to define, with a correct methodology and on sufficiently large cohorts of patients, the clinical and histological features which are associated with a less favorable outcome, the so-called 'risk-factors'.
3. Clinical and histological factors which appear at the actuarial survival analysis, either univariate or multivariate, the most powerful indicators of unfavorable outcome, are basically the same for all the four types of GN: severity of proteinuria (especially if it is evaluated not only at presentation, but at the subsequent follow-up as well), and existence of a deterioration of renal function at the time of presentation are the most powerful clinical risk-factors, while the extent of tubulo-interstitial involvement (mainly interstitial leukocyte infiltration and/or fibrosis) is the common histological hallmark of more probable and more rapid progression. Even though more severe interstitial lesions are often associated with more severe glomerular involvement (especially in IgAN), this is not always the case (especially in MN and FSGS), explaining why, in a multivariate analysis of

large populations of patients, extent of glomerular damage is not a significant prognostic indicator.

4. There is now sufficient evidence that in two of the four diseases, MN and FSGS, when nephrotic syndrome is present, treatment with steroids associated with cytotoxic drugs, especially if protracted, may favorably influence the prognosis, even in patients in whom no improvement of urinary protein loss and/or renal function occurs during its administration: therefore, up to 6 months of protracted therapy is justified in these patients, regardless of apparent lack of response. More controversial is the effectiveness of any immunosuppressive therapy in IgAN and MPGN. Obviously, there is the rationale for giving ACE inhibitors to all proteinuric patients when arterial hypertension is present, but also (at reduced doses) even in the absence of blood pressure elevation.
5. None of the many studies on the prognosis of the four glomerular diseases that we have reviewed, including the most recent ones, fulfills the criteria of excellence and the data summarized in our Tables 8.2, 8.5, 8.7, and 8.9 are not definitive. Consequently, none of the many controlled trials on the effect of therapy carried out, even in the last decade, can be considered sufficiently accurate, in view of the inaccuracy of the criteria of selection of the enrolled patients: the patients enrolled in the 'treatment' group or in the 'control' group should have had a comparable probability to progress toward renal insufficiency, if none of them had been treated, and we still are not in a position to predict progression in the single patient. In our opinion, the methodological advice of Marx and Marx [50] may help to better define prognosis in future studies, and therefore to design more accurate protocols for controlled therapeutic trials.

Key references

Cattran DC. Cytotoxic, cyclosporine and membranous nephropathy. *Curr Op Nephrol Hypert* 1996; **5**: 427–436.

D'Amico G. Epidemiological, clinical and prognostic indices in IgA nephropathy. *Nephrology* 1997; **3**: 13–17.

Donadio JV Jr, Offord KP. Reassessment of treatment results in membranoproliferative glomerulonephritis, with emphasis on life-table analysis. *Am J Kidney Dis* 1989; **14**: 445–451.

Koyama A, Igarashi M, Kobayashi M, *et al.* Natural history and risk factors for immunoglobulin A nephropathy in Japan. *Am J Kidney Dis* 1997; **29**: 526–532.

Pei Y, Cattran D, Delmore T, *et al.* Evidence suggesting under-treatment in adults with idiopathic focal segmental glomerulosclerosis. *Am J Med* 1987; **82**: 938–944.

Ponticelli C, Zucchelli P, Passerini P, *et al.* A randomized trial of methylprednisolone and chlorambucil in idiopathic membranous nephropathy. *N Engl J Med* 1989; **320**: 8–13.

Schieppati A, Mosconi L, Perna A, *et al.* Prognosis of untreated patients with idiopathic membranous nephropathy. *N Engl J Med* 1993: **329**: 85–89.

References

1. D'Amico G. Influence of clinical and histological features on actuarial renal survival in adult patients with idiopathic IgA nephropathy, membranous nephropathy, and

membranoproliferative glomerulonephritis: survey of the recent literature. *Am J Kidney Dis* 1992; **4**: 315–323.

2. Koyama A, Igarashi M, Kobayashi M, *et al.* Natural history and risk factors for immunoglobulin A nephropathy in Japan. *Am J Kidney Dis* 1997; **29**: 526–532.
3. D'Amico G, Imbasciati E, Barbiano di Belgioioso G, *et al.* Idiopathic IgA mesangial nephropathy. Clinical and histological study of 374 patients. *Medicine* 1985; **64**: 49–60.
4. D'Amico G, Minetti L, Ponticelli C, *et al.* Prognostic indicators in idiopathic IgA mesangial nephropathy. *Q J Med* 1986; **59**: 363–378.
5. Beukhof JR, Kardaun O, Schaafsma W, *et al.* Toward individual prognosis of IgA nephropathy. *Kidney Int* 1986; **29**: 549–556.
6. Noel LH, Droz D, Gascon M, *et al.* Primary IgA nephropathy: from the first described cases to the present. *Semin Nephrol* 1987; **7**: 351–354.
7. Velo M, Lozano L, Egido J, *et al.* Natural history of IgA nephropathy in patients followed up for more than ten years in Spain. *Semin Nephrol* 1987; **7**: 346–350.
8. Bogenschütz O, Bohle A, Batz C, *et al.* IgA nephritis: on the importance of morphological and clinical parameters in the long-term prognosis of 239 patients. *Am J Nephrol* 1990; **10**: 137–147.
9. Rekola S, Bergstrand A, Bucht H. Development of hypertension in IgA nephropathy as a marker of a poor prognosis. *Am J Nephrol* 1990; **10**: 290–295.
10. Alamartine E, Sabatier JC, Guerin C, *et al.* Prognostic factors in mesangial IgA glomerulonephritis: an extensive study with univariate and multivariate analysis. *Am J Kidney Dis* 1991; **18**: 12–19.
11. Johnston PA, Brown JS, Braumholtz DA, *et al.* Clinico-pathological correlations and long-term follow-up of 253 United Kingdom patients with IgA nephropathy. A report from the MRC glomerulonephritis Registry. *Q J Med* 1992; **84**: 619–627.
12. Nicholls KM, Fairley KF, Downling JP, *et al.* The clinical course of mesangial IgA associated nephropathy in adults. *Q J Med* 1984; **53**: 227–250.
13. Ibels LS, Györy AZ. IgA nephropathy: analysis of the natural history, important factors in the progression of renal disease, and a review of the literature. *Medicine* 1994; 73: 79–102.
14. Woo KT, Edmondson RPS, Wu AYT, *et al.* The natural history of IgA nephritis in Singapore. *Clin Nephrol* 1986; **25**: 15–21.
15. Kusumoto Y, Takebayashi S, Taguchi T, *et al.* Long-term prognosis and prognostic indices of IgA nephropathy in juvenile and adult Japanese. *Clin Nephrol* 1987; **28**: 118–124.
16. Katafuchi R, Oh Y, Hori K, *et al.* An important role of glomerular segmental lesions on progression of IgA nephropathy: a multivariate analysis. *Clin Nephrol* 1994; **41**: 191–198.
17. Yagame M, Suzuki D, Jinde K, *et al.* Value of pathological grading in prediction of renal survival in IgA nephropathy. *Nephrology* 1996; **2**: 107–117.
18. Wyatt RJ, Julian BA, Bhathena DB, *et al.* IgA nephropathy: presentation, clinical course, and prognosis in children and adults. *Am J Kidney Dis* 1984; **4**: 192–200.
19. Radford MG, Donadio JV, Bergstralh EJ, *et al.* Predicting renal outcome in IgA nephropathy. *J Am Soc Nephrol* 1997; **8**: 199–207.
20. Haas M. Histologic subclassification of IgA nephropathy: a clinicopathologic study of 244 cases. *Am J Kidney Dis* 1997; 29: 829–842.
21. D'Amico G. Treatment of IgA nephropathy: an overview. *Nephrology* 1997; **3S2**: S725–S30.
22. Pozzi C, Bolasco PG, Fogazzi GB, *et al.* Corticosteroids in IgA nephropathy: a randomised controlled trial. *Lancet* 1999; **353**: 883–837.

23. Chida Y, Tomura S, Takeuchi J, *et al.* Renal survival rate of IgA nephropathy. *Nephron* 1985; **40**: 189–194.
24. Frimat L, Briançon S, Hestin D, *et al.* IgA nephropathy: prognostic classification of end-stage renal failure. *Nephrol Dial Transplant* 1997; **12**: 2569–2575.
25. Kobayashi Y, Kokubo T, Horii A, *et al.* Prognostic prediction of long-term clinical courses in individual IgA nephropathy patients. *Nephrology* 1997; **3**: 35–40.
26. Hogg RJ, Silva FG, Wyatt RJ, *et al.* Prognostic indicators in children with IgA nephropathy. Report of the Southwest Pediatric Nephrology Study Group. *Pediatr Nephrol* 1994; **8**: 15–20.
27. Wyatt RJ, Kritchevsky SB, Woodford SY, *et al.* IgA nephropathy: Long-term prognosis for pediatric patients. *J Pediatr* 1995; **127**: 913–919.
28. Berg UB. Long term follow up of renal function in IgA nephropathy. *Arch Dis Childhood* 1991; **66**: 588–592.
29. Yoshikawa N, Ito H, Nakamura H. Prognostic indicators in childhood IgA nephropathy. *Nephron* 1992; **60**: 60–67.
30. Kurt Lee SM. Prognostic indicators of progressive renal disease in IgA nephroparthy: emergence of a new histologic grading system. *Am J Kidney Dis* 1997; **29**: 953–958.
31. D'Amico G. Tubulo-interstitial damage in glomerular diseases: its role in the progression of the renal damage. 1998; **13 S1**: S80–S5.
32. D'Amico G. Epidemiological, clinical and prognostic indices in IgA nephropathy. *Nephrology* 1997; **3**: 13–17.
33. Noel LH, Zanetti M, Droz D, *et al.* Long-term prognosis of idiopathic membranous glomerulonephritis. *Am J Med* 1979; **66**: 82–90.
34. Davison AM, Cameron JS, Kerr DNS, *et al.* The natural history of renal function in untreated idiopathic membranous glomerulonephritis in adults. *Clin Nephrol* 1984; **22**: 61–67.
35. Donadio JV Jr, Torres VE, Velosa JA, *et al.* Idiopathic membranous nephropathy: the natural history of untreated patients. *Kidney Int* 1988; **33**: 708–715.
36. Radaelli L, Confalonieri R, Macaluso M, *et al.* La glomerulonefrite membranosa: evoluzione e prognosi di 85 pazienti non trattati. *G It Nefrol* 1988; **5**: 17–22.
37. Durin S, Barbanel C, Landais P, *et al.* Evolution à long terme des glomérulonéphrites extra-membraneuses idiopathiques: etude des facteurs prédictifs de l'insuffisance rénale terminale chez 82 malades non traités. *Néphrologie* 1990; **11**: 67–71.
38. Schieppati A, Mosconi L, Perna A, *et al.* Prognosis of untreated patients with idiopathic membranous nephropathy. *N Engl J Med* 1993: **329**: 85–89.
39. Hogan SL, Muller KE, Jennette JC, *et al.* A review of therapeutic studies of idiopathic membranous glomerulopathy. *Am J Kidney Dis* 1995; **25**: 862–875.
40. Bellomo R, Atkins RC. Membranous nephropathy and thromboembolism: is prophylactic anticoagulation warranted? *Nephron* 1993; **63**: 249–253.
41. Honkanen E. Survival in idiopathic membranous glomerulonephritis. *Clin Nephrol* 1986; **25**: 22-28.
42. Zucchelli P, Ponticelli C, Cagnoli L, *et al.* Long-term outcome of idiopathic membranous nephropathy with nephrotic syndrome. *Nephrol Dial Transplant* 1987; **2**: 73–78.
43. Wehrmann M, Bohle A, Bogenschütz O, *et al.* Long-term prognosis of chronic idiopathic membranous glomerulonephritis. An analysis of 334 cases with particular regard to tubulo-interstitial changes. *Clin Nephrol* 1989; **31**: 67–76.
44. Murphy BF, Fairley KF, Kincaid-Smith PS, *et al.* Idiopathic membranous glomerulonephritis: long-term follow-up in 139 cases. *Clin Nephrol* 1988; **30**: 175–181.

45. Kida H, Asamoto T, Yokoyama H, *et al.* Long-term prognosis of membranous nephropathy. *Clin Nephrol* 1986; **25**: 64–69.
46. Abe S, Amagasaki Y, Konishi K, *et al.* Idiopathic membranous glomerulonephritis: aspects of geographical differences. *J Clin Pathol* 1986; **39**: 1193–1198.
47. Couchoud C, Laville M, Boissel JP, *et al.* Treatment of membranous nephropathy: a meta-analysis. *Nephrol Dial Transplant* 1994; **9**: 469–470.
48. Imperiale TF, Goldfarb S, Berns JS. Are cytotoxic agents beneficial in idiopathic membranous nephropathy? A meta-analysis of the controlled trials. *J Am Soc Nephrol* 1995; **5**: 1553–1558.
49. Cattran DC. Cytotoxic, cyclosporine and membranous nephropathy. *Curr Op Nephrol Hypert* 1996; **5**: 427–436.
50. Marx BE, Marx M. Prognosis of idiopathic membranous nephropathy: a methodologic meta-analysis. *Kidney Int* 1997; **51**: 873–879.
51. Ehrenreich T, Porush JG, Churg J, *et al.* Treatment of idiopathic membranous nephropathy. *N Engl J Med* 1976; **295**: 741–746.
52. Collaborative Study of the Adult Idiopathic Nephrotic Syndrome. A controlled study of short-term prednisone treatment in adults with membranous nephropathy. *N Engl J Med* 1979; **301**: 1301–1306.
53. Hopper J Jr, Trew PA, Biava CG. Membranous nephropathy: its relative benignity in women. *Nephron* 1981; **29**: 18–24.
54. Ponticelli C, Zucchelli P, Imbasciati E, *et al.* Controlled trial of methylprednisolone and chlorambucil in idiopathic membranous nephropathy. *N Engl J Med* 1984; **310**: 946–950.
55. Tu WH, Petitti DB, Biava CG. Membranous nephropathy: predictors of terminal renal failure. *Nephron* 1984; **36**: 118–124.
56. Shearman JD, Geng Yin Z, Aarons I, *et al.* The effect of treatment with prednisolone or cyclophosphamide-warfarin-dipyridamole combination on the outcome of patients with membranous nephropathy. *Clin Nephrol* 1988; **30**: 320–329.
57. Abe S, Amagasaki Y, Iyori S, *et al.* Significance of tubulointerstitial lesions in biopsy specimens of glomerulonephritic patients. *Am J Nephrol* 1989; **9**: 30–37.
58. Cattran DC, Delmore T, Roscoe J, *et al.* A randomized controlled trial of prednisone in patients with idiopathic membranous nephropathy. *N Engl J Med* 1989; **320**: 210–215.
59. Ponticelli C, Zucchelli P, Passerini P, *et al.* A randomized trial of methylprednisolone and chlorambucil in idiopathic membranous nephropathy. *N Engl J Med* 1989; **320**: 8–13.
60. Cameron JS, Hearly MJR, Adu D, *et al.* The Medical Research Council Trial of short-term high-dose alternate day prednisolone in idiopathic membranous nephropathy with nephrotic syndrome in adults. *Q J Med* 1990; **74**: 133–156.
61. Hay NM, Bailey RR, Lynn KL, *et al.* Membranous nephropathy: a 19 years prospective study in 51 patients. *N Z Med J* 1992; **105**: 489–491.
62. Pei Y, Cattran D, Greenwood C. Predicting chronic renal insufficiency in idiopathic membranous glomerulonephritis. *Kidney Int* 1992; **42**: 960–966.
63. Ponticelli C, Zucchelli P, Passerini P, *et al.* Methylprednisolone plus chlorambucil as compared with methylprednisolone alone for the treatment of idiopathic membranous nephropathy. *N Engl J Med* 1992; **327**: 599–603.
64. Lee HS, Koh HI. Nature of progressive glomerulosclerosis in human membranous nephropathy. *Clin Nephrol* 1993; **39**: 7–16.
65. Honkanen E, Törnoroth T, Grönhagen-Riska C, *et al.* Long-term survival in idiopathic membranous glomerulonephritis: can the course be clinically predicted? *Clin Nephrol* 1994; **41**: 127–134.

66. Toth T, Takebayashi S. Factors contributing to the outcome in 100 adult patients with idiopathic membranous glomerulonephritis. *Int Urol Nephrol* 1994; **26**: 93–106.
67. Ponticelli C. Prognosis and treatment of membranous nephropathy. *Kidney Int* 1986; **29**: 927–940.
68. Cattran DC, Pei Y, Greenwood CMT, *et al.* Validation of a predictive model of idiopathic membranous nephropathy: its clinical and research implications. *Kidney Int* 1997; **51**: 901–907.
69. Barbiano di Belgioioso G, Baroni M, Pagliari B, *et al.* Is membranoproliferative glomerulonephritis really decreasing? A multicenter study of 1548 cases of primary glomerulonephritis. *Nephron* 1985; **40**: 380–381.
70. Jungers P, Forget D, Droz D, *et al.* Reduction in the incidence of membranoproliferative glomerulonephritis in France. *Proc Eur Dial Transplant Assoc* 1985; **22**: 730–735.
71. Cameron JS. The natural history of glomerulonephritis. In *Progress in glomerulonephritis* (ed. Kincaid-Smith P, D'Apice ASF, Atkins RC) Wiley, New York, 1979; 1.
72. Donadio JV Jr, Offord KP. Reassessment of treatment results in membranoproliferative glomerulonephritis, with emphasis on life-table analysis. *Am J Kidney Dis* 1989; **14**: 445–451.
73. Cameron JS, Turner DR, Heaton J, *et al.* Idiopathic mesangiocaphillary glomerulonephritis. Comparison of types I and II in children and adults and long-term prognosis. *Am J Med* 1983; **74**: 175–192.
74. Valles Prats M, Espinel Garuz E, Alloza JL, *et al.* Glomerulonefritis mesangiocapilar idiopatica. Estudio de 72 casos. *Nefrologia* 1985; **5**: 17–23.
75. Schmitt H, Bohle A, Reineke T, *et al.* Long-term prognosis of membranoproliferative glomerulonephritis type I. Significance of clinical and morphological parameters: an investigation of 220 cases. *Nephron* 1990; **55**: 242–250.
76. D'Agati V. The many masks of focal segmental glomerulosclerosis. *Kidney Int* 1994; **46**: 1223–1241.
77. Gruppo Italiano di Immunopatologia Renale. Le glomerulonefriti membranoproliferative. *G It Nefrol* 1990; **7**: 67–102.
78. Haas M, Spargo BH, Coventry S. Increasing incidence of focal-segmental glomerulosclerosis among adult nephropaties: a 20-year renal biopsy study. *Am J Kidney Dis* 1995; **26**: 740–750.
79. Korbet SM, Schwartz MM, Lewis EJ. Primary focal segmental glomerulosclerosis: clinical course and response to therapy. *Am J Kidney Dis* 1994; **23**: 773–783.
80. Schena FP, Cameron JS. Treatment of proteinuric idiopathic glomerulonephritides in adults: a retrospective survey. *Am J Med* 1988; **85**: 315–326.
81. Pei Y, Cattran D, Delmore T, *et al.* Evidence suggesting under-treatment in adults with idiopathic focal segmental glomerulosclerosis. *Am J Med* 1987; **82**: 938–944.
82. Banfi G, Moriggi M, Sabadini E, *et al.* The impact of prolonged immunosuppression on the outcome of idiopathic focal segmental glomerulosclerosis with nephrotic syndrome in adults. *Clin Nephrol* 1991; **36**: 53–59.
83. Agarwal SK, Dash S, Tiwari S, *et al.* Idiopathic adult focal segmental glomerulosclerosis: a clinicopathological study and response to steroid. *Nephron* 1993; **63**: 168–171.
84. Shiiki H, Nishino T, Uyama H, *et al.* Clinical and morphological predictors of renal outcome in adult patients with focal and segmental glomerulosclerosis (FSGS). *Clin Nephrol* 1996; **46**: 362–368.
85. Wehrmann M, Bohle A, Held H, *et al.* Long-term prognosis of focal sclerosing glomerulonephritis. An analysis of 250 cases with particular regard to tubulointerstitial changes. *Clin Nephrol* 1990; **33**: 115–122.
86. Rydel JJ, Korbet SM, Borok RZ, *et al.* Focal segmental glomerular sclerosis in

adults: presentation, course, and response to treatment. *Am J Kidney Dis* 1995; **25**: 534–542.

87. Valeri A, Barisoni L, Appel GB, *et al.* Idiopathic collapsing focal segmental glomerulosclerosis: a clinicopathologic study. *Kidney Int* 1996; **50**: 1734–1746.
88. Mongeau JG, Robitaille PO, Clermont MJ, *et al.* Focal segmental glomerulosclerosis (FSG) 20 years later. From toddler to grown up. *Clin Nephrol* 1993; **40**: 1–6.
89. Newman WJ, Tisher CC, McCoy RC, *et al.* Focal glomerulosclerosis contrasting clinical patterns in children and adults. *Medicine* 1976; **55**: 67–87.
90. Cameron JS, Turner DR, Ogg CS, *et al.* The long-term prognosis of patients with focal and segmental glomerulosclerosis. *Clin Nephrol* 1978; **10**: 213–218.
91. Arbus GS, Powell S, Bacheyie GS, *et al.* Focal segmental glomerulosclerosis with idiopathic nephrotic syndrome: Three types of clinical response. *J Pediatr* 1982; **101**: 40–45.
92. Kleinknecht C, Gubler MC. Nephrose. *Nephrologie pediatrique*, 3rd edn. (ed. Royer P, Mathieu H, Habib R, Broyer M) Flammarion Médicine Science, Paris, 1983; 274.
93. Velosa JA, Holley KE, Torres VE, *et al.* Significance of proteinuria on the outcome of renal function in patients with focal segmental glomerulosclerosis. *Mayo Clin Proc* 1983; **58**: 568–577.
94. Tejani A, Nicastri A, Sen D, *et al.* Long-term evaluation of children with nephrotic syndrome and focal segmental glomerular sclerosis. *Nephron* 1983; **35**: 225–231.
95. Southwest Pediatric Nephrology Study Group. Focal segmental glomerulosclerosis in children with idiopathic nephrotic syndrome. A report of the Southwest Pediatric Nephrology Group. *Kidney Int* 1985; **27**: 442–449.
96. Lee HS, Spargo BH. Significance of renal hyaline arteriosclerosis in focal segmental glomerulosclerosis. *Nephron* 1986; **41**: 86–93.
97. Habib R. Immunopathological findings in idiopathic nephrosis: clinical significance of glomerular 'immune deposits'. *Pediatr Nephrol* 1988; **2**: 402–408.
98. Morita M, White RHR, Coad NAG, *et al.* The clinical significance of the glomerular location of segmental lesions in focal segmental glomerulosclerosis. *Clin Nephrol* 1990; **33**: 211–219.
99. Nagai R, Cattran DC, Pei Y. Steroid therapy and prognosis of focal segmental glomerulosclerosis in the elderly. *Clin Nephrol* 1994; **42**: 18–21.
100. Weiss MA, Daquioag E, Margolin EG, *et al.* Nephrotic syndrome progressive renal failure, and glomerular 'collapse': a new clinicopathologic entity? *Am J Kidney Dis* 1986; **7**: 20–28.
101. Detwiler RK, Falk RJ, Hogan SL, *et al.* Collapsing glomerulopathy: a clinically and pathologically distinct variant of focal segmental glomerulosclerosis. *Kidney Int* 1994; **45**: 1416–1424.
102. Howie AJ, Brenner DB. The glomerular tip lesions: a previously undescribed type of segmental glomerular abnormality. *J Pathol* 1984; **142**: 205–220.
103. Schwartz MM, Korbet SM, Rydell J, *et al.* Primary focal segmental glomerular sclerosis in adults: prognostic value of histologic variants. *Am J Kidney Dis* 1995; **25**: 845–852.
104. Fogo A, Hawkins EP, Berry PL, *et al.* Glomerular hypertrophy in minimal change disease predicts subsequent progression to focal glomerular sclerosis. *Kidney Int* 1990; **38**: 115–123.
105. Onetti Muda A, Feriozzi S, Cinotti GA, *et al.* Glomerular hypertrophy and chronic renal failure in focal segmental glomerulosclerosis. *Am J Kidney Dis* 1994; **23**: 237–241.
106. Lee S, Lim SD. The significance of glomerular hypertrophy in focal segmental glomerulosclerosis. *Clin Nephrol* 1995; **44**: 349–355.

9

The natural history and management of renovascular disease

John E. Scoble

Introduction

In the recent past the natural history of major renal diseases would not have included a chapter on renovascular disease. The presentations of renovascular disease are diverse and complex (Table 9.1), and this chapter represents a recognition of renovascular disease as a major cause of acute [1] and chronic renal failure [2]. Renovascular disease is important in the pediatric population as a cause of hypertension [3] but the importance of the atherosclerotic renal artery stenosis (ARAS) as a cause of end-stage renal failure in the older population becomes clearer with each year [4–6]. It possibly now represents the single most common cause of end-stage renal failure in patients over the age of 60 years [5,6]. The pathophysiology has previously been dominated by research from animal models where the alteration in renal blood flow was the single and potentially reversible element. This was enshrined in the definition of Jacobson in 1988 when he described 'a clinically significant reduction in glomerular filtration rate in patients with hemodynamically significant obstruction to renal blood flow in the renal artery of solitary kidney or in both renal arteries if two kidneys are present' [7]. However, since then other authors including Jacobson have removed the requirement for the lesion to be hemodynamically significant [8,9]. The processes involved in the pathophysiology of renovascular disease we now realize are shared with other renal diseases and not just a simple response to a diminution of renal blood flow. However, lesions such as atheroembolic disease, for which ARAS is a marker [10], are unique to ARAS [11]. The other feature which is potentially different from other forms of renal disease is that it is theoretically possible to reverse the insult to the ischaemic kidney by the restoration of a normal renal blood flow [12].

Although all forms of renovascular disease will be discussed in this chapter the major discussion will be of ARAS as this is now recognized as a vital clinical problem. ARAS can present in many ways ranging from an incidental finding at angiography with no symptoms to bilateral total occlusion and renal failure. There is controversy over whether treatment is worthwhile in ARAS, what the goals of treatment should be, and whether the diagnosis is worth making at all [13]. ARAS can be an important diagnosis to make as intervention in selected patients has been shown to improve

Table 9.1 Renovascular disease

Presentation of renovascular disease
Hypertension
Flash pulmonary edema
Progressive renal impairment
Acute renal impairment ± ACEI
As part of widespread vascular disease
Incidental finding at angiography for other diseases
Significance of renovascular disease
Treatable cause of hypertension
Treatable cause of end-stage renal failure
Marker for atheroembolic disease in ARAS
Marker for increased mortality in ARAS

renal function [14]. However, without an understanding of the natural history of ARAS it is difficult to draw firm conclusions on these issues. In other forms of renovascular disease the indications for intervention are clearer as discussed below. This chapter attempts to describe the natural history of renovascular disease and suggest areas where intervention may be profitable in the future.

Incidence

The incidence of renovascular disease is very dependent on the clinical setting, although the most common cause of renovascular disease is atherosclerosis. Since the work of Goldblatt renal artery stenosis has been associated with hypertension [15]. The presentation of fibromuscular dysplasia causing renal artery stenosis is invariably associated with hypertension [16]. In our experience this is, however, a rare condition when compared with ARAS. It is difficult to determine the incidence of ARAS in patients with hypertension as no large study with angiography of all patients has been completed (Table 9.2). The Co-operative Study on Renovascular Hypertension which reported in 1972 [17] attempted to answer this question. However, their conclusion of a rate of 36% for renovascular disease as a cause of hypertension was an estimate without angiography in all patients and the patients studied were those who had been referred to the specialist hypertension clinics taking part in the study. The patients in the series from Ying *et al.* [12] and Carmichael *et al.* [18] all had angiograms because there was significant clinical suspicion of renal artery stenosis necessitating referral to those units (Table 9.2). In patients with hypertension and renal impairment reported by Ying *et al.* [12] the incidence was higher than in hypertension alone. It is interesting to note that in the published data on patients referred to these two specialist hypertension clinics an incidence of 35% for renal artery stenosis was consistent. Swartbol [19] has shown that in patients found at angiography for peripheral vascular disease to have ARAS 20% were not hypertensive. Thus the incidence of ARAS in the hypertensive community is unclear

Table 9.2 Incidence of artherosclerotic renal artery stenosis (ARAS)

Author	Association	% (total number)
Schwartz *et al.* 1964 [22]	Post mortem	24 (154)
Sawicki *et al.* 1991 [23]	Post mortem	
	all	4.3 (5194)
	diabetes	8.3
Maxwell *et al.* 1972 [17]	Hypertension	36 (2442)*
Ying *et al.* 1984 [12]	Hypertension	37 (106)
	Hypertension + renal impairment	48 (21)
Carmichael *et al.* 1986 [18]	Hypertension	36 (235)
Ramirez *et al.* 1987 [150]	Coronary angiography	14 (102)
Harding *et al.* 1992 [21]	Coronary angiography	30 (1235)
Rackson *et al.* 1990 [26]	Aortic dissection	16 (63)†
Olin *et al.* 1990 [24]	Abdominal aortic aneurysm	38 (109)‡
Olin *et al.* 1990 [24]	Aorto-occlusive disease	33 (21)‡
Valentine *et al.* 1993 [25]	Aneurysmal or occlusive vascular disease	28 (346)‡
Dustan *et al.* 1964 [27]	Peripheral vascular disease	37 (149)‡
Olin *et al.* 1990 [24]	Peripheral occlusive vascular disease	39 (189)‡
Wilms *et al.* 1990 [29]	Peripheral vascular disease	22 (100)‡
Choudhri *et al.* 1990 [28]	Peripheral vascular disease	59 (100)
Swartbol *et al.* 1992 [19]	Peripheral vascular disease	49 (450)
Missouris *et al.* 1994 [30]	Peripheral vascular disease	45 (127)
Wachtell *et al.* 1996 [151]	Peripheral vascular disease	31 (100)
		14 (100)‡
Meyrier *et al.* 1988 [4]	Renal failure	
	Retrospective	0.3 (5891)
	Prospective	1.4 (1087)
Scoble *et al.* 1989 [5]	Renal failure (over 50 years of age)	14 (71)
Kalra *et al.* 1990 [1]	Acute renal failure	16 (600)
Mailloux *et al.* [152]	Chronic renal failure	
	Age 15–40	1 (175)
	Age 41–61	5 (237)
	Age 61+	25 (271)§
O'Neil *et al.* 1992 [114]	Chronic renal failure, non-dialysis dependent.	14 (21)¶
Vidt *et al.* 1988 [10]	Renal cholesterol emboli	79 (24)

* An estimate with incomplete angiographic data.
† Stenosis diagnosed if above 70% of diameter.
‡ Stenosis diagnosed only if above 50%.
§ Diagnosed on clinical suspicion without angiographic corroboration.
¶ Stenosis diagnosed by renal duplex sonography.

and ARAS may occur in the absence of hypertension. The data from angiographic studies discussed later suggest that hypertension alone is not a good discriminant factor for ARAS. However, in younger adult patients with hypertension fibromuscular disease is an important consideration in the United Kingdom [3] but in Japan the most important diagnosis to be entertained would be Takayasu's syndrome [20]. This is also true in the pediatric population where conditions such as the middle aortic syndrome are important [3].

Atherosclerosis is a widespread vasculopathy unlike fibromuscular dysplasia. Because angiography is used in the diagnosis of vascular lesions in other vascular beds it is possible to get a more precise estimate of the incidence of ARAS in patients with atherosclerosis. The best study for the incidence of ARAS in patients undergoing coronary angiography was that of Harding *et al.* [21] This was a very large prospective study and gave an overall incidence of 30% for any form of ARAS with 15% of patients having greater than 50% luminal stenosis and 15% less than 50% stenosis. Other studies have excluded ARAS with a stenosis of less than 50% diameter as being insignificant as shown in Table 9.2. Because of the risk of progression and the association with atheroembolic disease we believe that any lesion should be considered potentially 'significant'. This will be discussed in detail in the section on progression. The predictive factors for the presence of ARAS which Harding *et al.* [21] found were age, severity of coronary artery disease, congestive heart failure, female gender, and peripheral vascular disease. Hypertension was not an associated variable in keeping with the post-mortem studies [22,23]. The incidence of ARAS in abdominal aneurysmal [24,25], aortic occlusive disease [24,25], and aortic dissection [26] is considerable, although once more some lesions have been excluded because they were less than 50% of the luminal diameter (Table 9.2). In overall terms a third of patients with any of these conditions could be expected to have ARAS in keeping with the proportion for patients undergoing coronary angiography. The proportion of patients with ARAS though is highest in patients undergoing angiography for peripheral vascular disease [19,24,27–30]. As can be seen from Table 9.2 the proportion from both retrospective and prospective studies was that 50% of these patients had ARAS which in most cases was unsuspected. Missouris *et al.* [30] also demonstrated two other features. The first was that the presence of ARAS correlated with the severity of the peripheral vascular disease. The second was that patients with ARAS had a increased mortality from operative intervention for peripheral vascular disease compared with patients without renal artery involvement. Thus the highest proportion of patients with ARAS occurs in the patients with peripheral vascular disease and in patients undergoing coronary angiography peripheral vascular disease is a powerful predictor of the presence of ARAS.

Is the natural history of ARAS changing or is it becoming increasingly recognized (Table 9.2)? It is probable that with an increasingly aged population the diagnosis will become more common. the use of angiotensin-converting enzyme inhibitors (ACEI) may have brought to medical attention patients whom would not otherwise have been diagnosed [31] and may accelerate the rate of decline of function in the affected kidney [1,5].

At the present time angiography, as discussed below, represents the best and most widely agreed method for definitively diagnosing ARAS as discussed below. This is an invasive procedure and no 'normal' population has been, or probably will be screened, with this investigation. The most obvious method for diagnosis of ARAS is at post mortem. The disadvantage of this method of assessment is that post mortems are carried out in only a small proportion of patients and these patients are not representative of the population as a whole. Both studies which have looked at this in detail have been on patients who have died in hospital and this represents a small proportion of deaths. The first data by Schwartz and White [22] as shown in Table 9.3, gave an overall incidence of 24% in the 154 post mortems studied. This was a prospective study and in this study 87% of post mortems on patients over the age of 75 years revealed ARAS. They, however, found no consistent relationship between the presence and severity of the renal artery stenosis at post mortem and the diastolic blood pressure recorded premortem. The study of Sawicki *et al.* [23] was a retrospective study and found a lower overall incidence than Schwartz and White [22]. Both Sawicki *et al.* and Schwartz and White found that in the majority of patients the renal artery stenosis was undiagnosed premortem [22,23]. Both of these studies illustrate the underdiagnosis of ARAS by clinicians and that hypertension alone is not a good predictive feature of its presence. Schwartz and White also illustrated that ARAS is a disease whose incidence markedly increases with age [22]. In the future non-invasive tests may become available which could be used to screen an asymptomatic population safely [32,33], but until that is achieved no precise incidence can be determined. However, that does not mean that an attempt cannot be made to estimate the incidence of ARAS in the general population and more precisely in clinical subgroups. ARAS does not occur in the absence of atherosclerotic disease elsewhere and estimations based on the incidence in patients with other atherosclerotic involvement may be very close to the real incidence. Table 9.2 shows the available data on the incidence of ARAS in various clinical settings.

Atheroembolic renal disease is a common accompaniment of ARAS [10], although rarely diagnosed. Many case reports illustrate its occurrence as reviewed by Lye *et al.* [34] Vidt *et al.* [10] have reported that in patients with renal cholesterol emboli

Table 9.3 Incidence of ARAS in a post mortem study

Age	<55% total ($n = 26$)	55–64% total ($n = 29$)	65–74% total ($n = 48$)	75+% total ($n = 45$)
No stenosis	69	31	27	13
Moderate stenosis, unilateral or bilateral	19	38	46	44
Severe unilateral stenosis	12	31	6	22
Severe bilateral stenosis	0	0	21	20

The data of Schwartz and White [22].

at the Cleveland Clinic 79% had ARAS, although the overall numbers were small. Meyrier *et al.* [4] reported cholesterol embolization in eight patients with ARAS and two with aortic disease not affecting the renal artery. These two studies demonstrate that in the majority of cases of patients with proven renal cholesterol embolization ARAS will be the cause. The incidence of atheroembolic disease which so often coexists with ARAS is difficult to estimate but any estimate is likely not to reflect the true nature of the problem. The findings from post mortems of patients with abdominal aortic disease suggest a very high incidence whether or not the patient undergoes surgery [35]. The interesting work in renal biopsies in patients over the age of 65 years suggests that atheroembolic disease is common but usually presents as an insidiously progressive decline in renal function [36]. The common conception of atheroembolic disease is of a rapid decline in renal function after intra-arterial instrumentation, thrombolysis, or anticoagulation [37]. If, however, a cholesterol cleft is found on renal biopsy then there is an 85% chance of that kidney being supplied by stenosed renal artery [10]. Figure 9.1 is a histological slide of the aorta of a patient with ARAS and illustrates the cholesterol-rich lining which can detach and shower lower vessels.

Thus ARAS may present in many different ways. Is it possible to estimate its incidence in the general population? The strongest associations are with angiography for peripheral vascular and coronary artery disease (Table 9.2). The proportion of these patients with ARAS in these groups was approximately 50% for peripheral vascular disease and 30% for coronary artery disease (Table 9.2). In the United Kingdom General Practitioners are responsible for the health care of specific groups of patients and are a reliable source of information on medical events occurring within this group. We collaborated with one rural practice with a stable patient population of 14 300 [2]. No patients were known within the practice to suffer from ARAS but we

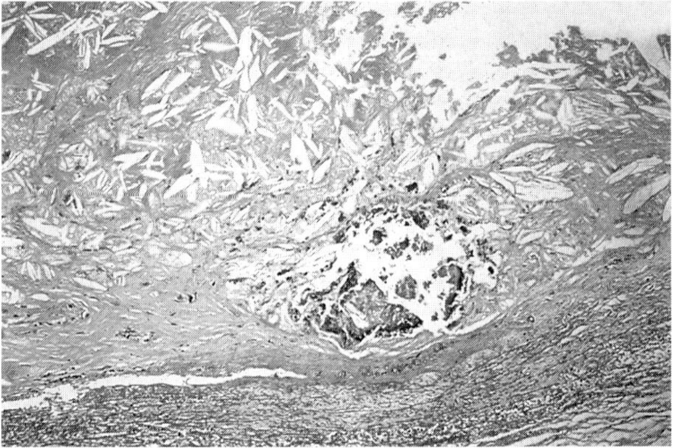

Fig. 9.1 This shows the extent of the cholesterol deposition in the aorta of a patient with renal artery stenosis [Hartely, in press]. Reproduced by courtesy of the *British Journal of Renal Medicine*.

posed the question of how many patients had angiography for either coronary artery or peripheral vascular disease in a 12-month period? In this practice three patients had angiography for peripheral vascular disease and none for coronary artery disease. Using the incidence data available this would suggest at least 1.5 new patients with ARAS in this practice per year. If factored up this would represent a minimum of 105 new patients with ARAS per million population per year. These calculations are somewhat speculative but are almost certainly an underestimate of the condition within the community.

The renal damage in a kidney with ARAS may be multifactorial leading to interstitial damage which may be independent of the degree of stenosis.

The pathobiology of renovascular disease

Renal blood supply

An understanding of the renal blood supply is paramount in the understanding of renovascular disease. This is especially important as renal artery stenosis and occlusion may be asymptomatic until late in the process or not at all. In atherosclerotic disease it has been shown that renal artery occlusion is not associated with any symptoms [38]. In other vascular territories such as the heart occlusion is associated with abrupt and often fatal results [39]. In humans, however, there are extensive collateral blood vessels to the kidneys [40]. In addition there may be multiple renal arteries to either side and the position of the renal ostia may be different in conditions such as horseshoe kidney. In general the renal artery origin is on the posterior aspect of the aorta and an anterior–posterior radiological study may not demonstrate the origin of the artery. The collateral vessels can occur from the adrenal, lumbar, gonadal and ureteric arteries [41]. These may not be important when the renal arteries are patent but in the presence of complete occlusion they can support renal function. In the examination of single kidney glomerular filtration rates (SKGFR) it has been found that a kidney with total renal artery occlusion was able to filter at a rate of 12 ml/min [42]. In the dog it can be demonstrated that the collateral supply is sufficient to maintain viability beyond 3 h of complete arterial occlusion, although progressive loss of renal function may occur after this [40]. Yune and Klatte reviewed 301 aortograms to examine the renal blood supply [41] to kidneys with renal artery stenosis. The most common collateral supply in kidneys with renal artery stenosis was the adrenal and lumbar arteries rather than the peri-ureteric vessels [41]. They also observed intrarenal collateral vessels. These findings have led to the observation that renal revascularization may be significantly delayed if progressive renal artery narrowing has occurred prior to occlusion [43]. As discussed later prolonged renal artery occlusion and anuria have been followed by successful revascularization and recovery of function. In fact a case has been made that urgent revascularization is not required in renal artery occlusion [43]. In many respects the process of renal artery occlusion might be thought of as paralleling coronary artery occlusion. However, they are very different in that acute occlusion in the coronary is usually associated with degrees of occlusion of less than 50% of the cross-sectional area of the coronary artery [39] whereas the evidence in all forms of renovascular disease is that the lesion is progressive with no sudden occlusion [44]. In the myocardium no delay in revascularization can be allowed after occlusion as shown by the efficacy of early thrombolysis. In the renal artery spontaneously revascularization may occur and an important role for thrombolysis alone is uncertain except after angioplasty to the renal artery [45].

Acute renal artery occlusion

This chapter reviews in depth the causes of chronic progressive renal artery narrowing which constitutes the vast majority of renovascular disease leading to progressive renal insufficiency. Occlusion of a stenosed renal artery is a final event of progressive renal narrowing. However, acute blockage of a normal renal artery is rare [46] and unlike the coronary circulation renal artery occlusion is usually on the background of high renal artery stenosis [38,44,47]. Acute occlusion may be associated with embolization from a central source [48,49], trauma [50,51], or clotting abnormalities [52–55]. Recent descriptions have suggested that spontaneous renal artery thrombosis can occur frequently in the primary antiphospholipid syndrome [52–55]. This is probably the single most common cause of spontaneous thrombosis of a normal renal artery and may result in renal infarction [54]. It is fascinating to examine the literature on spontaneous renal artery occlusion and observe that there is no record of the antiphospholipid syndrome in early reports and yet it is a common description in later reports. Renal artery thrombosis has been described in the presence of ACEI [56,57] and with membranous glomerulonephritis and the nephrotic syndrome [58]. Retrograde occlusions of the renal arteries after aortic thrombosis has been described [59] but there is considerable discussion as to whether this will only occur if there is renal artery stenosis already present [60]. However, cases of spontaneous renal artery thrombosis in the absence of a specific cause have also been described [61,62].

In acute renal artery thrombosis there have been several reports of good long-term function following complete or partial renal artery occlusion treated with surgery, anticoagulation or angioplasty [48,51,63–78], The longest reported delay for revascularization was of 42 days in an anuric patient with renal artery occlusion who had been on an ACEI. Surgery produced complete resolution of renal function [57]. In one case renal function was documented to have been preserved for at least 9 years after surgery for occlusion of a single anuric kidney [66]. These cases, however, must be distinguished from progressive renal artery occlusion, which is painless [38] and results in loss of function in that kidney.

Acute infarction

This process is common in any organ which has been deprived of its blood flow. As discussed above due to the collateral blood flow renal function may remain viable for considerable periods in the presence of renal artery occlusion. The process of infarction will result in the loss of cellular integrity and cannot be reversed once initiated.

Unlike coronary disease infarction is a relatively uncommon event in the kidney where the report of acute loin pain and haematuria are rare [38] and associated with occlusion of a normal renal artery. Weibull *et al.* have shown that occlusion of a stenosed renal artery is asymptomatic [38]. With progressive renal narrowing collateral blood supply often will have time to develop considerably and prevent acute infarction when the renal artery eventually occludes.

Ischemia and fibrosis

The nature of the underlying process has been discussed in Chapter 6. It is, however, interesting to find that the original Goldblatt canine experiments contained a description of the histology in the kidneys with renal artery stenosis imposed [15]. They described '*diffuse parenchymatous degeneration, most severe in the proximal tubules*' and '*diffuse increase in connective tissue*'. These are the changes which we now recognize in renal ischemia in general and have been described by subsequent authors [79,80]. However, the issue in the kidney is at what stage these changes become irreversible? There is an implicit presumption among many clinicians that the kidney with renal artery stenosis is viable and only needs the removal of the stenosis to perform normally again. Jacobson [7] has defined ischaemic nephropathy as discussed previously with the implication that reversal of the impediment to renal artery flow may improve the renal function. Recent evidence suggests that the processes within the kidney with renal artery stenosis are complex [81]. Truong *et al.* [82] have shown that in an experimental model of renal artery stenosis the stenosed kidney exhibited marked interstitial damage and many other features consistent with acute cellular allograft rejection! There was a chronic interstitial nephritis with marked tubulitis but the glomeruli were well preserved. It is well known that such interstitial damage correlates better with long-term function than glomerular damage in a wide variety of conditions [83–85]. Grone *et al.* [86] have shown in a single clip model treated with Enalapril that there was a loss of kidney length. The renal blood flow decreased to 39% of normal and the glomerular filtration to 3% of normal. This was associated with a reduction in activity of cathepsin B and L and the Na-K-ATPase. The tubular cells were atrophic but not necrotic. All these changes were reversible after removal of the clip. The authors postulated a process suggested in cardiac disease of hibernation [86]. They did not, however, establish a process for deciding between reversible and irreversible changes secondary to ischemia. It is fascinating that removal of the normal kidney induces resolution of atrophy in the stenosed kidney. In fact it has been shown that contralateral nephrectomy at the time of clipping of a kidney will abrogate the atrophy in that kidney [87]. Marcussen [80] has shown that this experimental work is mirrored in human kidneys where there was severe atrophy of the tubular compartment but only shrinkage of glomeruli in kidneys with renal artery stenosis. The volume fraction of the proximal and distal tubules was severely contracted with only a small change in the glomerular volume fraction. Jackson *et al.* [88] in an animal model of experimental renal artery stenosis have shown that changes in the stenotic kidney are severely magnified by the use of an ACEI. In their single clip hypertension model blood pressure control was the achieved with and without an ACEI. The animals receiving an ACEI had such severe atrophy in the stenotic kidney that the authors described the changes as pharmacological nephrectomy! ACEI have also been reported as being associated with acute renal artery thrombosis in stenotic arteries [56,57]. The cellular mechanisms which produce the ischaemic renal damage are the subject of considerable research but are outside the remit of this review. The hemodynamic changes as a consequence of renal artery stenosis may lead to severe irreversible structural changes and this may be exacerbated by the use of ACEI. The exact point at which irreversible fibrosis is initiated is unclear. The experiments of Gobe *et al.* [87] used a single clip model but instead of reversing the process by removal of the clip they removed the normal unclipped kidney! They examined the clipped kidneys and found atrophy. The removal of the contralateral kidney stimulated renal hyperplasia and increased clusterin expression. There was also an increase in apoptotic cell death in the stenosed kidney which seems destined to progress to fibrosis. In this model there was de-differentiation of tubular cells but no fibrosis in the stenosed kidney prior to removal of the contralateral kidney but there was no fibrosis. In clinical practice the presence of interstitial fibrosis is taken by many investigators to indicate irreversible renal damage which will not be reversed by revascularization. The difficulty in determining at what point irreversible renal damage has occurred is illustrated in Fig. 9.2. In this patient with a cadaveric renal transplant and a plasma creatinine of 300 μmol/l renal artery stenosis was thought to have been excluded and a renal biopsy was performed. The changes were non-specific and chronic graft damage was suspected. However, following a further decline in renal function to the point where the patient was dialysis dependent a renal angiogram was performed which showed renal artery stenosis. Angioplasty was performed and a dramatic improvement in renal function was observed to a point where the plasma

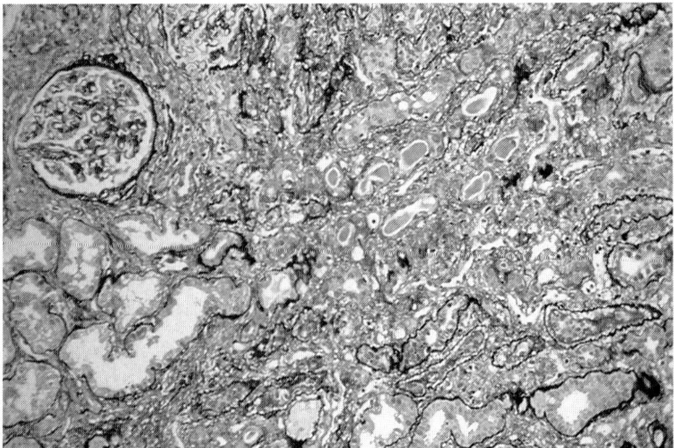

Fig. 9.2 This shows the renal histology of a renal transplant with a plasma creatinine of 300 μmol/l. After further deterioration in renal function to dialysis dependence renal artery stenosis was diagnosed and the plasma creatinine after angioplasty was 150 μmol/l. The histology is reproduced by courtesy of Dr B. Hartley, Guy's Hospital, London.

creatinine was 150 μmol/l. The features of ischaemic nephropathy were non-specific in the renal biopsy and did not predict the potential renal function after angioplasty. The changes of renal ischemia are non-specific with no glomerular changes or antibody deposition demonstrable on immunofluorescence. This illustrates the lack of specific histological features of reversible renal ischemia. The features of irreversible renal ischemia are probably those of interstitial fibrosis described by Risdon *et al.* in [83] in all forms of renal disease. It is now accepted that analysis of the tubulo-interstitial compartment is the only dependable indicator of renal function [83–85].

This process of renal fibrosis would be expected to lead to loss of renal volume. This has been related to the degree of renal artery stenosis in two studies from the Seattle group [89,90]. They have shown that the progressive loss of renal length is related to the degree of initial renal artery narrowing. However, they also noted that the rate of loss of renal length both in the kidneys with renal artery stenosis and those without was related to the systolic blood pressure. These studies were not functional but they did note that there was a correlation in the rate of atrophy and a rise in plasma creatinine. As will be discussed later there is evidence that the changes in atherosclerotic disease are not precisely related to a diminution of renal size as in other glomerular diseases [42].

Hypertensive nephrosclerosis

This has been discussed in detail in Chapter 6. The importance of renovascular disease as a cause of hypertension was recognized after the work of Goldblatt *et al.* [15] This has been demonstrated to be clinically important in fibromuscular dysplasia as discussed later. It is interesting to see that in atherosclerotic disease the close linkage has not been established. In a study of patient with proven ARAS demonstrated on angiography for peripheral vascular disease 25% of patients with this were not hypertensive [19]. In the large study of patients undergoing angiography for coronary artery disease it was found that hypertension was not a predictive factor for the presence of ARAS which occurred in 30% of these patients [21]. This has been reinforced by the data which has accumulated in older patients showing a lack of efficacy of revascularization in the cure of hypertension. This is in marked contrast to the excellent results obtained in the fibromuscular patients [91]. In the older patients hypertensive nephrosclerosis may play a part in the pathological process but the hypertension may be primary rather than secondary to the renal artery stenosis. This is supported by the observation of Swartbol *et al.* who found that 25% of cases of renal artery stenosis were normotensive [92] and the analysis of Harding *et al.* who found that hypertension was not a predictive factor in patients with coronary artery disease who were found to have renal artery stenosis [21].

Atheroembolic disease

This process is achieving greater importance in the understanding of the processes of renal disease associated with atherosclerosis [11,93]. The original work of Flory

[94] showed that in experimental animals infusion of atherosclerotic material and more specifically the cholesterol crystals can induce severe organ damage. The case reports since that time have been frequent but the varied clinical presentations have suggested that this condition can be considered as the 'Cinderella of renal pathology' [95]. This is because in many cases the specific diagnosis and the variable clinical findings find difficulty in being brought together as with the slipper in Cinderella! This is because the specific lesion is the cholesterol cleft. The cholesterol crystal causes occlusion of the small artery. However, if the cholesterol crystal is not seen then the changes in the surrounding tissue are those of interstitial fibrosis (Fig. 9.3). The cholesterol cleft is easily seen but if the microscopy field did not include this the surrounding areas are not specific for any process causing renal fibrosis. The best data on the incidence of atheroembolic disease comes from post-mortem specimens where the histologist has the ability to search for the lesion. In the routine renal biopsy specimen sampling error can easily cause the diagnosis not to be made.

The clinical manifestation of atheroembolic disease are very similar to those of a systemic vasculitis. This may explain the distant effects of atheroembolic disease. The patients have eosinophilia and eosinophiluria and the plasma complement levels may fall [96]. The result is an insidious decline in renal function with a very poor overall prognosis [34]. The finding of renal fibrosis in kidneys with renal artery stenosis may be as much from atheroembolic disease as from ischemia produced by a reduction in renal blood flow. This process results in severe interstitial as well as arterial fibrosis. Lye *et al.* [34] have reviewed the published series of renal cholesterol embolic disease. In 40% of cases the presentation was with acute renal failure and the overall mortality of all cases was 64%. This probably overemphasizes acute embolic rather than the chronic disease. We have seen cholesterol clefts in renal

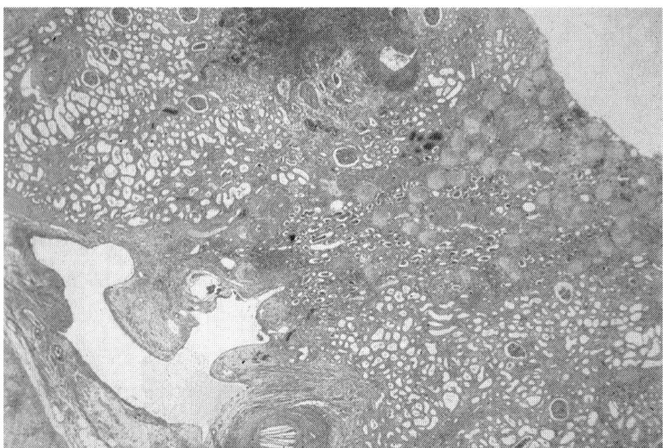

Fig. 9.3 Cholesterol embolus and fibrosis. This shows the extent of the fibrosis associated with the cholesterol embolus seen as a cleft in the renal arteriole. Reproduced by courtesy Dr O'Donnell, Guy's Hospital London.

biopsies of patients with chronic renal impairment where no previous instrumentation had occurred nor was there an acute illness. In ARAS the atheroma is often not related to the renal artery *per se* but renal involvement occurs as a result of spill-over of atheromatous disease from the aorta into the renal ostium. In many respects ARAS could be thought of as a marker of aortic disease. Certainly, with an atherosclerotic lesion at the ostium it would be surprising if embolization did not occur. Although much is made of the 50% reduction in diameter as being 'significant renal artery stenosis' the ostial changes may lead to cholesterol embolization at any degree of stenosis. This is illustrated by the cholesterol crystals in the aortic wall next to a stenosed renal artery (Fig. 9.1). Vidt *et al.* [10] have shown that in documented cases of renal cholesterol embolization all had aortic atheroma and 79% had ARAS as discussed earlier. Thus renal cholesterol embolization may be an underestimated cause of damage in kidneys with ARAS and the damage may not correlate with the degree of anatomical occlusion [42].

Focal segmental glomerulosclerosis

Although this is a distinct histological entity the clinical characteristics can be very variable [97]. In some cases it is as a response to obesity whereas in others a circulating factor has been implicated [97]. Thadhani *et al.* [98] have presented data to suggest that in patients over the age of 65 years 30% of patients with focal segmental glomerulosclerosis have renal artery stenosis which is atherosclerotic in aetiology. It has been long recognized that renal artery stenosis can be associated with proteinuria and there have been cases of nephrotic range proteinuria which have been cured by renal revascularization (Table 9.4). Unfortunately, proteinuria has been described with atheroembolic disease which is also a correlate of ARAS.

Proteinuria in atherosclerotic nephropathy

Many of the processes of progressive renal dysfunction in this book are associated with proteinuria. In the past this has been thought of as indicating specific glomerular diseases. The differential diagnosis of the nephrotic syndrome is wide but does not often include renovascular disease. Proteinuria has been recognized as an important predictor of renal dysfunction in the best studied progressive renal disease, namely diabetic nephropathy [99]. Less obvious from the data has been that the presence of proteinuria has been a poor prognostic feature in patients without diabetes. In fact in some studies the magnification of risk by proteinuria is as great in the non-diabetic group, as in those with diabetes, although in the latter group the initial risks is greater [100]. Proteinuria is common in many forms of atherosclerotic nephropathy (Table 9.4). The importance of proteinuria as a marker of diabetic nephropathy rather than atherosclerotic nephropathy in older patients is open to question at the present time. It is possible that in many cases it is a marker of atherosclerotic rather than diabetic renal disease because there are no data on screening of these patients for the renovascular disease which they obviously have.

In fact proteinuria in atherosclerotic renal disease is often described on an

Table 9.4 Proteinuria and atherosclerotic nephropathy

Author	No. of patients	Comments	Nephrotic range (>3 g/24 h)	Mean proteinuria (g/24 h)
Renal artery stenosis				
Montoliu *et al.* [153]	1	Normal renal biopsy in unaffected kidney, cured by nephrectomy	1	13–31
Takeda *et al.* [154]	1	Improved with Captopril	1	
Eiser *et al.* [155]	1	Nephrectomy cured hypertension and proteinuria	1	3.4–3.6
Adams *et al.* [156]	83	'Abnormal urinalysis' in 36% with worse response to intervention		
Martinez Vea *et al.* [79]	1	Cured by nephrectomy, reduced by Captopril	1	16.2
Sato *et al.* [157]	1	Normal biopsy in unaffected kidney, cured by vein bypass to one kidney	1	4–7
Chen *et al.* [101]	1	Proteinuria cured by nephrectomy	1	11.6
Thadhani *et al.* [98]	8	Associated with FSGS, 24-h protein in only 7/8 patients	4.4	
Mikhail *et al.* [102]	3	Patients with progressive dysfunction after angioplasty	0	0.7
Atheroembolic disease				
Greendyke and Akamatsu [158]	3	1–3+protein in the patients		
Snyder and Shapiro [159]	1	2–3+protein on Dipstix testing		
Moldveen-Geronimus and Marriam [160]	2	1–3+protein		
Harrington *et al.* [161]	2	1–3+protein		
Dalakos *et al.* [162]	1	0.9 g/l, no total given		
Regester [163]	1			1.8
Varanasi *et al.* [164]	1			0.3
Smith *et al.* [165]	4	1+protein in 2/4		
Cosio *et al.* [96]	7	1–2+protein in 4/7		

Table 9.4 *(Cont.)*

Author	No. of patients	Comments	Nephrotic range (>3 g/24 h)	Mean proteinuria (g/24 h)
Hannedouche *et al.* [166]	1	Necrotizing glomerulonephritis		2
Schwartz and McDonald [167]	2	2+protein in 1/2		
Hyman *et al.* [168]	1	2+protein		
Fine *et al.* [169]	63	54% (34) had >1+ proteinuria (Review)	3	
Aujla *et al.* [170]	1	Renal transplant proteinuria	2	
Mannesse *et al.* [171]	4		2	3.95
Case record *New England Journal of Medicine* [172]	1		1	3.5
Wilson *et al.* [173]	9	1–3+in 7/9		
Bendixen *et al.* [174]	1	2+protein		
Sheehan *et al.* [175]	1	2+protein		
Blakely *et al.* [176]	1	Nephritic urinary sediment		1.1
Thadhani *et al.*[177]	52	63% had >1+urine protein	2	
Haqqie *et al.*[178]	4		4	8.3
Case record *New England Journal of Medicine*[179]	1		1	3.1
Greenberg *et al.*[180]	24	FSGS in 15 patients	9	

anecdotal basis (Table 9.4). Nephrotic range proteinuria has been cured by nephrectomy of a kidney with a renal artery occlusion [101]. However, the precise importance of renin-mediated proteinuria vs. the association with atheroembolic disease in unclear (Table 9.4). It may be that the processes are similar or common. It is interesting to surmise that in fact proteinuria in patients with ARAS may be the rule rather than the exception. It may also indicate processes which will not be reversed by restoration of renal blood flow as shown in the progressive renal dysfunction seen after renal angioplasty [102].

Angiotensin-converting enzyme inhibitor-induced renal dysfunction

This is an area which has only been recognized since the vitally important observation of Hricik *et al.* in 1983 [31]. These authors reported the deleterious effect of ACEI of renal function in patients with renal artery stenosis. Early work has shown that blood flow in an artery is maintained until the luminal diameter is reduced by 70% of its original size [103]. In the kidney below this homeostatic mechanisms involving Angiotensin II and the constriction of the efferent arteriole maintain the glomerular filtration even below this level. This has been used in the Captopril DTPA scan which uses the differences in renal scan before and after administration of Captopril [104]. The importance of the stenosis is illustrated by the fact that after successful angioplasty the DTPA scan is relatively unchanged after Captopril administration [46,104]. The work on the long-term effects of ACEI on renal function are controversial. An initial paper suggested that long-term ACEI in the presence of renal artery stenosis led to a 'pharmacological nephrectomy' [88]. In this paper using a single clip rat model for hypertension blood pressure was controlled with either Minoxidil or an ACEI. In the Minoxidil-treated animals there was preservation of the parenchyma of the kidney with the clip whereas in the animals on an ACEI there was a dramatic loss of renal volume. Others have not confirmed these experiments and suggested that the only feature controlling the loss of renal parenchyma is the degree of renal perfusion distal to the clip [105] It is unclear what the effect of dramatically decreased filtration is on a kidney independent of any effect of decreased tubular perfusion pressure. In the only other clinical scenario which has absent filtration, urinary obstruction, the effects of no filtration are profound.

Recent evidence for the recognition of the entity of 'atherosclerotic nephropathy'

It can be seen from the descriptions above that patients with ARAS may have a number of processes in progress at any one time. The focus previously has been on the importance of the narrowing of the renal artery. The paper by Jacobson in 1988 [7] was a seminal one and defined reversible renal dysfunction due to renal artery narrowing as '*Ischaemic Nephropathy*'. It is now recognized that there are many components to '*Atherosclerotic Nephropathy*' as discussed above. The lesions secondary to atherosclerotic aortic disease can be diverse and multiple. The analogy has been drawn with lupus nephritis [42] where the actual histological features can be of any sort but all are compatible with the single diagnosis of systemic lupus erythematosus. The importance of a specific manifestation of atherosclerotic nephropathy will determine the treatment. If the major cause of a decline in renal function in a kidney is atheroembolic disease then any change in the renal artery diameter may not produce an improvement in renal function.

We have combined two universally used tests by the technique of single kidney glomerular filtration to estimate the individual kidney function in patients with atherosclerotic disease. A ^{99m}Technetium dimercaptosuccinic acid (DMSA) scintigraphy scan [106] to determine relative renal function and ^{51}Chromium ethylenediamine tetra-acetic acid (EDTA) glomerular filtration rate [107] to determine overall renal function (Figs 9.4–9.8). Both of these tests have been widely validated in renal disease and their use has significant implications for the understanding of renovascular disease [42]. In these cases the renal length by ultrasound has been compared with the renal function in that kidney. The renal arteries were defined as the following. *Normal*, these were kidneys where either: (a) there was no stenosis on

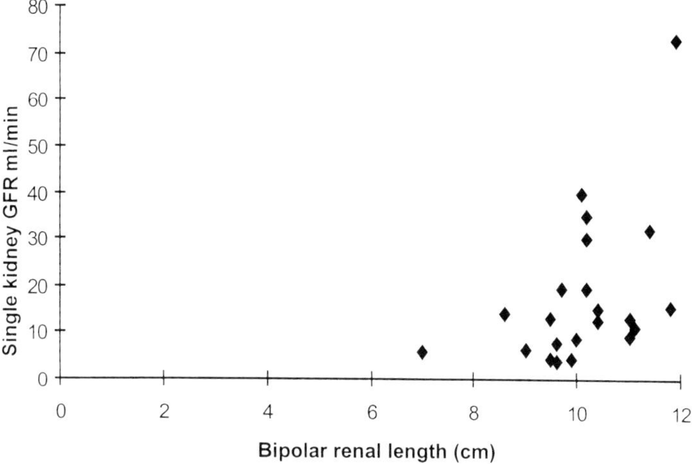

Fig. 9.4 Renal function and length in 'normal kidneys'. Correlation coefficient $r = 0.457$; $p < 0.05$, $n = 22$ [44].

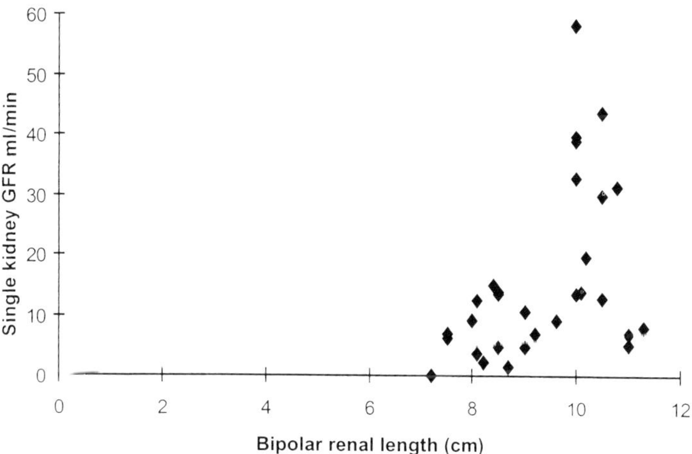

Fig. 9.5 Renal function and length in kidneys with renal artery stenosis. Correlation coefficient $r = 0.477$; $p < 0.05$, $n = 26$ [44].

angiography but the contralateral kidney was either occluded or had renal artery stenosis, or (b) no renal artery stenosis was demonstrated but aortography revealed widespread atheromatous disease (Fig. 9.4). *Stenosis*, these were kidneys where there was a stenosis of 50% or greater of the luminal diameter. These kidneys had not undergone angioplasty (Fig. 9.5). *Occluded*, these were kidneys where angiography failed to show a patent renal artery (Fig. 9.6). *Angioplasty*, these were kidneys where previously a renal angioplasty had been performed for renal artery stenosis (Fig. 9.7).

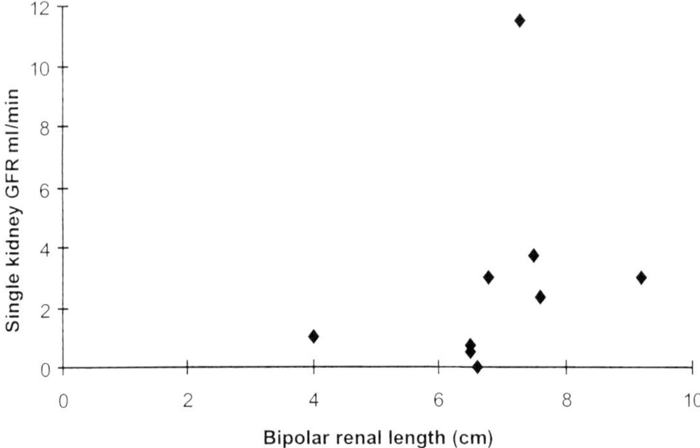

Fig. 9.6 Renal function and length in kidneys with renal artery occlusion. Correlation coefficient $r = 0.595$; $p > 0.05$, $n = 8$ [42].

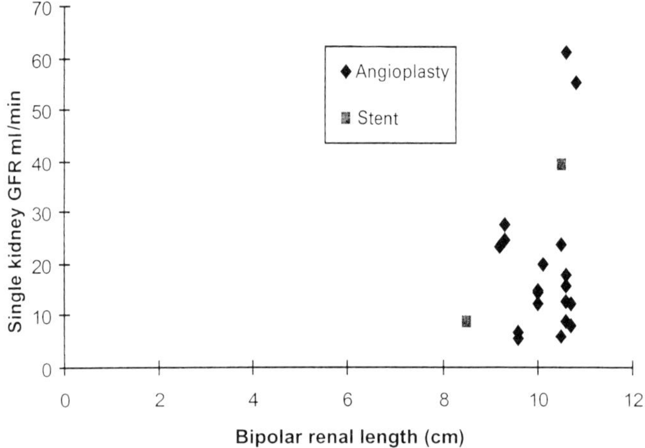

Fig. 9.7 Renal function and length in kidneys following angioplasty or endovascular stenting. Correlation coefficient $r = 0.123$; $p > 0.05$, $n = 15$ [44].

Stent, these were kidneys where an endovascular stent had been inserted at angioplasty (Fig. 9.7).

The most interesting feature is that the 'normal' kidneys show the same splay of function in relationship to length. Figure 9.8 demonstrates that in patients with unilateral renal artery stenosis the renal function may be better in the kidney with renal artery stenosis rather than the contralateral kidney with the 'normal' renal artery. However, both lie downstream from an atheromatous aorta which can lead to atheroembolic disease (Fig. 9.1).

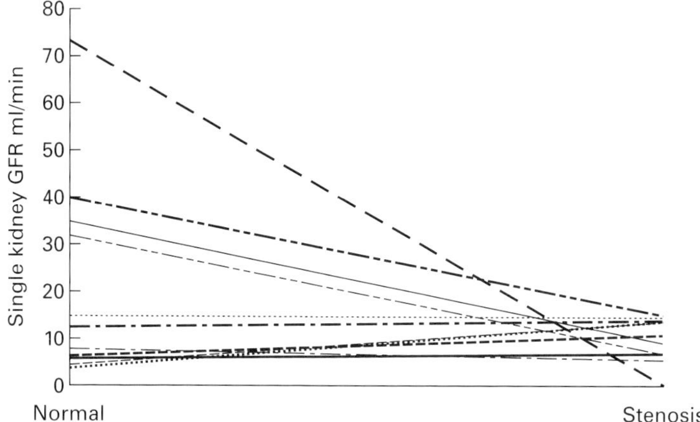

Fig. 9.8 Comparison of SKGFR in paired kidneys with normal and stenosed renal arteries [44].

These data support the view that the presence of ARAS is a marker of renal disease in both kidneys. This suggests that both kidneys are undergoing a process which is causing a decline in renal function which may not be reversed by the relief of the renal artery stenosis [102]. We would term this process *'atherosclerotic nephropathy'*.

Investigations in renovascular disease

The investigations in renovascular disease must try and establish both the anatomical and the physiological lesion. Table 9.5 gives the advantages and disadvantages of the various techniques. The important issue is that each give different information which is often complementary rather than exclusive. Previous techniques such as the observation of a delayed dense nephrogram using an intravenous urogram are now of purely historical interest. The gold standard investigation at the time of writing is the intra-arterial digital subtraction angiogram [108]. As with all gold standards its absolute nature is illusory. This methodology only gives a two-dimensional assessment of the renal artery narrowing. Some centres have tried to reduce the risk of contrast nephrotoxicity by the introduction of carbon dioxide angiography and this has proven useful. Unfortunately, the equipment to effectively use carbon dioxide is expensive to obtain the optimum images [109]. Spiral computed tomography (CT) scanning may provide an important step forward in the assessment of renal artery narrowing and some authors believe that it is the optimum method [110]. The advantage is that there is no aortic instrumentation and thus risk of atheroembolic disease. The disadvantage of spiral CT scanning is the large contrast load and the postacquisition interpretation of the images. Magnetic resonance imaging may give the best possible compromise for imaging of the renal arteries and replace angiography in the near future [32]. As can be seen in Fig. 9.9 the images may be

Table 9.5 Investigation of renovascular disease

Method	Advantages	Disadvantages
Post mortem	Absolute test with direct measurement of stenosis Possible	Not applicable *in vivo*
IVP	None	Not used
Intra-arterial angiography	The gold standard for diagnosis	Contrast load, risk of atheroembolism, only gives two-dimensional assessment of renal artery narrowing
Captopril DTPA scan	Non-invasive	Not useful in renal impairment or bilateral diseases
Spiral CT scanning	Non-invasive	Contrast load, post acquisition interpretation
MRI scanning	Non-invasive	Long acquisition time but may replace diagnostic angiography in immediate future
Doppler ultrasound	Non-invasive, excellent for renal transplants	Difficult to routinely use for native kidneys. May improve with new contrast agents
Intra-arterial Doppler ultrasound	Invasive and requires catheter to pass stenosis	Gives absolute assessment of stenosis

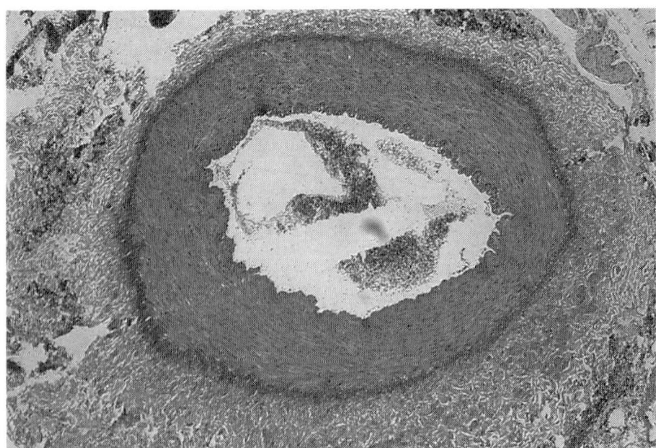

Fig. 9.9 This shows the medial hyperplasia of a renal artery removed from a patient with fibromuscular dysplasia. The specimen was taken after the affected kidney was removed and the patient cured of her hypertension. Reproduced by courtesy of Dr R. Hartely, Guy's Hospital London.

recognizable to the clinician as providing similar information as an intra-arterial digital subtraction angiogram. Doppler ultrasound has provided an important research method of investigation of renal artery stenosis [33]. In clinical practice the renal transplant artery is relatively superficial and without bowel gas interposed. Excellent reproducible results can be obtained in this situation by this excellent non-invasive test. However, in the native kidneys it has proven possible only for the premier units such as those of Strandness in Seattle to provide reproducible results [33] due to the difficulty of direct imaging of the renal arteries. Indirect measures using the renal arterial waveform have been proposed by various authors but are not widely accepted [33]. It is possible that in the future that contrast agents may improve the resolution of these techniques. Captopril DTPA scanning has achieved an important status in the functional diagnosis of renal artery disease [104]. The important issue to understand is that this test determines hemodynamically significant narrowing. In this situation it is important in determining whether renal artery dilatation or surgery will cure hypertension. As has been observed by Ramsay and Waller [91] this question is much more important in hypertension in younger patients. In the diagnosis of fibromuscular dysplasia this is important but the use of the test in ARAS is less clear. In these patients as discussed elsewhere the renal artery narrowing is a marker of disease rather the absolute cause of renal dysfunction. The findings in patients with atherosclerotic disease and renal impairment has been disappointing [111].

The view of the author is that for the anatomical definition of renal artery stenosis intra-arterial digital subtraction angiography in experienced hands provides an accurate, quick, and low morbidity outpatient investigation.

Clinical features of renal artery stenosis

Fibromuscular dysplasia

This condition represents the purest form of renal artery stenosis [16]. The early series from the Mayo Clinic is an excellent indication of the nature of the disease. The male to female ratio was 7 : 1 with the patients being significantly younger than the patients with ARAS [112]. This patient presented with hypertension and successful angioplasty cured the hypertension. Disease other than in the renal artery is described but rare especially when compared with the pan-vasculopathy in atherosclerotic disease [16]. Figure 9.9 illustrates the renal artery changes in a middle-aged woman with troublesome hypertension and a small right kidney. After nephrectomy the hypertension was cured needing no further drug treatment. Follow-up studies using SKGFR at Guy's Hospital have shown stable renal function in both the kidney which has undergone angioplasty and the contralateral kidney in a very different pattern to that seen in ARAS. Renal dysfunction will occur if there is untreated bilateral disease or there is untreated hypertension. However, even the early Mayo Clinic series suggested an excellent outcome for these patients [112]. In the era of successful interventional radiology it should prove possible to improve the renal artery anatomy and improve if not cure the hypertension [91].

Takayasu's syndrome

This disease is common in Asia but relatively rare in Europe. Intriguingly, the disease is also rare in individuals of Asian descent living in South Africa! This would suggest some environmental factor in the pathobiology of this disease. Although known as Takayasu's syndrome, Takayasu only described some ocular manifestations which in retrospect were realized to be part of a systemic illness [20]. The disease is one of a progressive larger vessel vasculitis and it has been termed the 'pulseless disease'. Many arteries are involved and the renal problems may be only part of a much larger problem. From the renal perspective it produces progressive renal artery ostial stenosis with hypertension and declining renal function. Therapy is targeted at dampening down the underlying vasculitis and then attempting angioplasty. It is unwarranted to intervene until the erythrocyte sedimentation rate has been normalized [20], although this has been characterized as a large vessel vasculitis there is no suggestion of any intrinsic renal vasculitis such as in polyarteritis nodosa.

Middle aortic syndrome

This is a rare disease predominantly affecting a pediatric population. It involves narrowing of the abdominal aorta and stenosis of the arteries arising from this area. Unlike fibromuscular dysplasia there is aortic involvement but unlike Takayasu's syndrome this is smooth and does not appear to be inflammatory. Its presentation is usually with hypertension but it may lead to renal failure if intervention is unsuccessful [3,113]. Once more there is no suggestion of any intrinsic renal dysfunction and the pathological process is that of ischaemic nephropathy. There does not appear to be an inflammatory component to this condition but the aortic fibrosis is progressive and interventions may not be as successful as in fibromuscular dysplasia [3,113].

Atherosclerotic renal artery stenosis (ARAS)

As discussed above the clinical features of ARAS are related to the other clinical manifestations of the a atherosclerotic disease. Renal failure has been recognized as a consequence of ARAS and Table 9.2 show the data for the incidence of ARAS in acute and chronic renal failure. The studies by Meyrier *et al.* [4] and Scoble *et al.* [5] studies had widely different rates of ARAS in chronic renal failure. Both studies had similar indications for angiography and ARAS was found in a similar proportion of patients angiogrammed (15 of 31 Meyrier *et al.* [4], 10 of 24 Scoble *et al.* [5]) but the two major differences were in the number of angiograms performed compared with the patient pools and in the duration of study (31 of 1087 over 52 months [4], 24 of 71 over 18months [5]). The difference in incidence between the two studies may represent a different population composition but also may reflect a higher index of suspicion in the latter study where the diagnosis of ARAS was actively being sought. O'Neil *et al.* [114] randomly selected patients from a nephrology clinic with impaired renal function, but not dialysis dependent, and found ARAS in three of the 21 patients screened by renal duplex sonography. of the three patients identified all had been assigned diagnoses other than ischaemic nephropathy prior to renal duplex sonography. The study by Kalra *et al.* [1] study showed a similar incidence of ARAS as the cause of acute renal failure to the study by Scoble *et al.* [5] for chronic renal failure. Kalra *et al.* [1] paper suggested that in a third of patients with ARAS causing acute renal failure ACEI treatment contributed to the decline in renal function. In other studies we have reported that 38–50% of all patients diagnosed as having ARAS were on ACEI at the time of diagnosis with the diagnosis being unsuspected [5,115,116]. These data illustrate that ARAS is an increasingly recognized and common cause of both acute and chronic renal failure. Evidence suggests that end-stage ARAS is a potentially reversible cause of renal failure and so it is a diagnosis that ought to be sought [117,118]. At the present moment there are no randomized trials with drug therapy that demonstrate a change in the rate of progression of renal impairment or of the lesion itself, although they do exist for atheromatous lesions in other vascular territories [119]. The challenge for the future is to identify patients with asymptomatic disease and to halt the progression of the atheromatous lesions rather than intervene with end-stage atherosclerotic renal disease when some devastating complication such as renal failure has occurred.

Although we can demonstrate a renal artery narrowing at investigation it is important to consider in ARAS that both the lesion and the accompanying atherosclerotic problems are progressive. There are two forms of progression to be considered. The first is progression of the degree of anatomical stenosis leading to ischemia as discussed above. The second is the progression of renal impairment in the stenosed kidney. Both of these play an important part in the final outcome for a patient with ARAS.

Anatomical progression of the lesion in ARAS has been established since the early studies including that of Hunt and String [112]. The absence of a prospective study of the renal artery anatomy has meant that it is difficult to be precise on the rate of progression. Lack of clinical signs may not preclude progression as an important feature of ARAS as in most instances progression is painless and without symptoms. Weibull *et al.* [38] have shown that in angiographically documented ARAS progression to occlusion was only associated with a slight change in plasma creatinine without any symptoms or signs. Postma *et al.* [120] in a small retrospective study have shown that occlusion is more likely to occur in patients treated with an ACEI and diuretic. Although progression to bilateral occlusion may be associated with severe impairment in renal function the only conclusive way of diagnosing progression is repeat angiography. There has been no prospective study published of repeat angiography in all patients previously diagnosed as having ARAS. Schreiber *et al.* [121] have shown that in a retrospective analysis the ARAS progressed in 44% of patients at re-angiography which included progression to occlusion in 16% with a mean follow-up of 52 months. These authors also showed that the higher the degree of initial stenosis the higher the probability of progression to occlusion.

Progression in terms of worsening function in the individual kidney has less clinical data except in the experimental models discussed in the section on mechanisms of renal damage. Dean *et al.* [122] showed that in 46% of patients the serum creatinine increased by over 25% and the glomerular filtration rate fell by more than 25% in 29% of patients in a follow-up period ranging from 6 to 78 months. Dean *et al.* later demonstrated that the rate of decline of overall renal function was more rapid in patients with bilateral vs. patients with unilateral disease. In terms of overall renal function we have also shown that the functional outcome is dependent on the initial angiographic findings [116]. Survival of renal function sufficient to remain off dialysis was 97% for patients with unilateral stenosis, 82% for patients with bilateral stenosis and 45% for those with unilateral occlusion and occlusion or stenosis on the contralateral side at 2 years. Thus not surprisingly progression in terms of renal function is related to the initial degree of stenosis.

As shown in Table 9.1 progression of the renal artery narrowing may lead to other clinical features of which the most important is 'flash pulmonary edema'. Pickering *et al.* [123] were the first to describe as acute unprovoked pulmonary edema as a presentation of ARAS. Messina *et al.* [124] have suggested that the 'flash pulmonary edema' is a marker of bilateral renal artery stenosis but we have found that in our series it has been associated with renal artery occlusion [116]. Missouris *et al.* [30] have suggested that ARAS must be considered in patients with chronic congestive heart failure as excellent therapeutic results occurred in two patients with revascularization. There are no data on the incidence of ARAS in patients presenting in acute or chronic left ventricular failure. However, preliminary results suggest that this is very common, and up to 30% of patients referred to a general medical clinic with this problem with a plasma creatinine of less than 300 μmol/l were found to have ARAS [125]. The clinical syndrome of 'flash pulmonary edema' does, however, appear to be a clear manifestation of ARAS and this diagnosis must be considered in these cases as the results from revascularization have been excellent [123].

What is the clinical outcome for patients with ARAS? The most important consideration is the morbidity and mortality of the individual patient with ARAS. Patient survival has been shown to be diminished in patients with ARAS [115,116,126,127]. The original data from Hunt and String [112] showed that a third of patients would be dead at 5 years. We have compared the survival of patients at the Royal Free Hospital [115] with those published for peripheral vascular disease from San Diego [128]. The initial mortality is much higher in patients presenting with renal impairment but the survival is very similar to that for severe peripheral vascular disease at 5 years. We have shown that patient survival correlated with the initial angiographic finding [116]. It is probable that the different angiographic findings at presentation in our study relate to different stages in the progression of ARAS. Mailloux *et al.* [127] have shown that patient survival once on dialysis is worse than any other cause of chronic renal failure with a 5-year survival on dialysis of only 12%. The presence of ARAS confers on to patients a worse prognosis when compared with patients with peripheral vascular disease or with other dialysis patients.

Treatment of renal artery stenosis

Potential therapeutic measures

The potential interventions depend on the processes present in the kidney supplied by a stenosed renal artery. In the case of experimentally induced renal artery stenosis the removal of the clip may improve the renal function. This is probably the case with fibromuscular dysplasia of the renal artery [91]. However, as discussed above, the processes in atherosclerotic disease may be more complex. The methods for revascularization of the kidney are divided into surgical and interventional radiology. Surgical intervention will be discussed first as historically it was the first used, although at present interventional radiology is the initial modality preferred by centres interested in the disease in the first instance.

Surgery for renovascular disease

There are a large number of extensive surgical series encompassing one case where a 100% improvement in renal function was demonstrated in anuric renal failure after successful surgery [63–65,129]. However, the situation was altered by the paper of Bengtsson *et al.* [130] in 1974 where they demonstrated impressive results in half their patients but also a 50% mortality. Novick at the Cleveland Clinic has been in the forefront of surgery for renal revascularization [131]. The techniques have evolved to use visceral arteries instead of major aortic surgery in these patients. On the right the gastroduodenal artery can be used and on the left the splenic artery can be used. The result of these procedures for patients with end-stage renal failure are impressive in experienced hands [14,122,131–135]. In selected cases surgical intervention can produce dramatic results in dialysis-dependent renal atherosclerotic disease. Weibull *et al.* [136] have tried to compare the efficacy of angioplasty and surgery in patients who were suitable for both procedures. They concluded that, although the primary patency rate was lower in the angioplasty group, the overall outcome in both groups after secondary intervention was the same. In most situations renal angioplasty was the modality preferred in the first instance. It is important to state that this study did not include any renal artery stents as it was undertaken before widespread use of this procedure.

Renal angioplasty

Renal angioplasty is now in widespread use for renal artery stenosis [137]. There have been many studies following the clinical course of patients who have undergone renal angioplasty but there have been no randomized trials to compare intervention with a placebo group. The technical success of the procedures is high in experienced centres. The Glasgow group have presented compelling retrospective data to suggest that progressive renal dysfunction can be prevented by renal artery stenting [138]. However, it is unclear what the long-term outcome of intervention is and we have demonstrated that there can be progressive renal dysfunction in spite of a patent renal artery after angioplasty [102]. In fact Strandness and his collaborators in Seattle have shown that the rate of progression of renal artery stenosis after angioplasty is the same as preangioplasty [47]. This would suggest that angioplasty without stenting reverses the renal artery narrowing but in itself does not alter the underlying progressive decline in luminal surface area. A reasonable synthesis of the presently available data is that renal angioplasty is effective treatment in resetting the renal artery diameter but is less good at altering the process of renal artery narrowing. As the degree of stenosis predicts the likelihood of renal artery occlusion angioplasty represents a method of making renal artery occlusion less likely. It is important to observe that in a group with a horrendous 2-year mortality this form of treatment may be sufficient for the lifespan of most patients with ARAS [116]. The relief of obstruction in ARAS has had a disappointing effect on hypertension which represent a poor indication for intervention in this disease [91].

Although the progressive nature of ARAS is recognized the evidence for improvement in outcome with revascularization is limited as recently reviewed by Textor [139]. There have been no studies to examine medical management which could decrease the rate of occlusion of renal arteries with atheroma as there have been with peripheral and coronary vascular disease [119]. Interventions with revascularization by angioplasty and surgery have shown disappointing results when hypertension is considered [140,141]. Two recent randomized trials have not shown a dramatic benefit of hypertension over conventional medical therapy [142,143]. Treatment of renal artery stenosis to improve renal function is controversial [144]. Dialysis-dependent patients who become independent of dialysis represent a small but important group [131] where intervention is of undoubted value. Novick *et al.* suggested that there was a better prognosis for patients who became dialysis independent when compared with patients with ARAS who remained on dialysis [131]. The clearest indication for intervention is 'flash pulmonary edema' where revascularization can abolish the problem [123]. At the present time there are specific indications for revascularization in end-stage ARAS but no evidence that we can otherwise alter its natural history.

Future strategies

These are without any basis in published data, although some have speculated as to the possibilities [145]. It must be presumed that the very high mortality of patients with ARAS must indicate a potential use of 3-hydroxy-3-methylglutaryl coenzyme A enzyme inhibitors, the statins. Compared with published data in patients with coronary artery disease where an impressive reduction in mortality has been observed [146,147] patients with atherosclerotic renovascular disease must offer an excellent opportunity for lipid lowering therapy [116,127]. No randomized trial has been undertaken but in the United Kingdom the recent advice from the Chief Medical Officer that patients with a total plasma cholesterol of greater than 5.5 mmol/l and peripheral vascular disease should receive lipid lowering therapy encompasses most patients with ARAS. More intriguingly there are anecdotal reports in which lipid lowering has altered the course of atheroembolic disease [148]. If this is the case it may be possible to alter the progress of atherosclerotic nephropathy. Whether aggressive ACEI use or AII blocking will alter the process leading to proteinuria in atherosclerotic nephropathy remains unclear but a tantalizing possibility.

Progress in interventional radiology will enable the renal blood flow to be improved in most cases. As discussed above this may in itself not prevent progressive renal dysfunction in these patients. However, in fibromuscular hyperplasia it is unlikely in the future that anything other than interventional radiology will be needed except in the most complex cases. The difficulty in dealing with ARAS is that those most at risk of end-stage renal failure are also those with the highest mortality [116,127,149]. If two studies are combined this illustrates the case. Connolly *et al.* [116] have shown that the 2-year mortality with unilateral occlusion and occlusion or stenosis is approximately 50%. One could use these data to suggest the same mortality would apply to patients with unilateral stenosis and contralateral occlusion where the majority of the function came from the kidney with the stenosis. If one also presumes that occlusion would lead to loss of function then this can be compared with the data from the Seattle group who suggest 2-year occlusion rate of 10% in severely stenotic lesions [44]. That is of an original 100 patients with severe renovascular disease after 2 years 50 would have died. However, because the overall rate of occlusion was 10% and half the patients had died in fact only five patients would progress to renal failure. It is interesting to speculate that an improvement in mortality in these high-risk patients by aggressive lipid lowering therapy may in fact increase the rate of end-stage renal failure due to renovascular disease if the lipid lowering does not halt the progression of the renal artery lesions. As discussed below the effect of lipid lowering therapies on coronary artery narrowing has been much less clear than its effect on overall mortality.

It is interesting to compare the possibilities of procedures and treatments applied to the coronary and renal arteries. Although similar in occurring often in the same patient the processes have a number of differences. As shown in larger studies the disease in the kidney is related to the first centimetre of renal artery [21]. Diffuse disease can occur but is rarer and more commonly seen after intervention. This is obviously different to the heart where multiple lesions not related to the ostia of the coronary arteries are seen. Although regression trials have been performed in the coronary circulation [119] it has only been the recent mortality studies that have clarified the role of lipid lowering therapy [146,147]. This is in keeping with the observations discussed earlier that coronary artery occlusion usually occurs in arteries with less than 50% reduction in surface area. This has been interpreted as suggesting that plaque stabilization is more important than actual regression of the stenotic lesion in preventing occlusion [39]. It is going to be a significant challenge to renal physicians to decide which measures useful in other vascular territories will be efficacious in the renal artery.

Conclusions

The natural history of renovascular disease depends very much on the cause of the renal artery narrowing. In cases of pure renal artery disease such as fibromuscular dysplasia the clinical course will mirror the renal disease. For more complex disease such as atherosclerosis the clinical course may be determined by arterial involvement in other organs. The renal changes in renovascular disease may be purely related to ischemia or may involve other processes such as atheroembolic disease. Much remains to be understood in renovascular disease and the concept of treatment being related purely to improvement in renal blood flow is one which cannot be held at this time.

Key references

Flory CM. Arterial occlusions produced by emboli from eroded aortic atheromatous plaques. *American Journal of Pathology* 1945; **21**: 549–565.

Harden PN, MacLeod MJ, Rodger RSC, *et al.* Effect of renal-artery stenting on progression of renovascular renal failure. *Lancet* 1997; **349**: 1133–1136.

Hricik DE, Browning PJ, Kopelman R, Goorno WE, Madias NE, Dzau VJ. Captopril-induced functional renal insufficiency in patients with bilateral renal-artery stenoses or renal-artery stenosis in a solitary kidney. *New England Journal of Medicine* 1983; **308**: 373–376.

Novick A, Scoble J, Hamilton G, eds. *Renal Vascular Disease*. London: W.B. Saunders.

Scoble JE, Maher ER, Hamilton G, Dick R, Sweny P, Moorhead JF. Atherosclerotic renovascular disease causing renal impairment—a case for treatment. *Clinical Nephrology* 1989; **31**: 119–122.

Wollenweber J, Sheps SG, Davis GD. Clinical course of atherosclerotic renovascular disease. *American Journal of Medicine* 1968; **21**: 60–70.

Ying CY, Tifft CP, Garvas H, Chobanian AV. Renal revascularisation in the azotemic hypertensive patient resistant to therapy. *New England Journal of Medicine* 1984; **311**: 1070–1075.

References

1. Kalra PS, Mamtora H, Holmes AM, Waldek S. Renovascular disease and renal complications of angiotensin-converting enzyme inhibitor therapy. *Quarterly Journal of Medicine* 1990; **282**: 1013.
2. Scoble JE. The epidemiology and clinical manifestations of atherosclerotic renal disease. In: Novick A, Scoble J, Hamilton G, eds. *Renal Vascular Disease*. London: W.B. Saunders, 1995: 303–314.
3. Dillon MJ, Deal JE. Renovascular hypertension in children. In: Novick A, Scoble J, Hamilton G, eds. *Renal Vascular Disease*. London: W.B. Saunders, 1995: 235–244.
4. Meyrier A, Buchet P, Simon P, Fernet M, Rainfray M, Callard P. Atheromatous renal disease. *American Journal of Medicine* 1988; **85**: 139–146.
5. Scoble JE, Maher ER, Hamilton G, Dick R, Sweny P, Moorhead JF. Atherosclerotic renovascular disease causing renal impairment—a case for treatment. *Clinical Nephrology* 1989; **31**: 119–122.
6. Mailloux LU, Napolitano B, Belluci AG, Vernace M, Wilkes BM, Mossey RT. Renal vascular disease causing end-stage renal disease, incidence, clinical correlates and outcomes: a 20-year clinical experience. *American Journal of Kidney Disease* 1994; **24**: 622–629.
7. Jacobson HR. Ischemic renal disease: an overlooked clinical entity? *Kidney International* 1988; **34**: 729–743.

8. Breyer J, Jacobson H. Ischemic nephropathy. *Current Opinions in Nephrological Hypertension* 1993; **2**: 216–224.
9. Greco BA, Breyer JA. Atherosclerotic ischaemic renal disease. *American Journal of Kidney Disease* 1997; **29**: 167–187.
10. Vidt DG, Eisele G, Gephardt GN, Tubbs R, Novick AC. Atheroembolic renal disease: association with renal artery stenosis. *Cleveland Clinic Journal of Medicine* 1989; **56**: 407–413.
11. Phinney MS, Smith MC. Atheroembolic renal disease. In: Novick A, Scoble J, Hamilton G, eds. *Renal Vascular Disease*. London: W.B. Saunders, 1995: 63–74.
12. Ying CY, Tifft CP, Garvas H, Chobanian AV. Renal revascularisation in the azotemic hypertensive patient resistant to therapy. *New England Journal of Medicine* 1984; **311**: 1070–1075.
13. Scoble JE. Is the 'wait and see' approach justified in atherosclerotic renal artery stenosis? *Nephrology Dialysis Transplantation* 1995; **10**: 588–589.
14. Novick AC, Pohl MA, Schreiber M, Gifford RY, Vidt DG. Revascularization for preservation of renal function in patients with atherosclerotic renovascular disease. *Journal of Urology* 1983; **129**: 907–911.
15. Goldblatt H, Lynch J, Hanzal RF, Summerville WW. The production of persistent elevation of systolic blood pressure by means of renal ischemia. *Journal of Experimental Medicine* 1934; **59**: 347–378.
16. Stanley JC. Renal artery fibrodysplasia. In: Novick A, Scoble J, Hamilton G, eds. *Renal Vascular Disease*. London: W.B. Saunders, 1995: 21–33.
17. Maxwell MH, Bleifer KH, Franklin SS, Varady PD. Co-operative study of renovascular hypertension: demographic analysis of study. *Journal of the American Medicine Association* 1972; **220**: 1195–1204.
18. Carmichael DJS, Mathias CJ, Snell ME, Peart S. Detection and investigation of renal artery stenosis. *Lancet* 1986; **i**: 667–670.
19. Swartbol P. Renal artery stenosis in patients with peripheral vascular disease and its correlation to hypertension. A retrospective study. *International Angiology* 1992; **11**: 195–199.
20. Toma H. Takayasu's arteritis. In: Novick A, Scoble J, Hamilton G, eds. *Renal Vascular Disease*. London: W.B. Saunders, 1995: 47–62.
21. Harding MB, Smith LR, Himmelstein SI, *et al.* Renal artery stenosis: prevalence and associated risks factors in patients undergoing routine cardiac catheterization. *Journal of the American Society of Nephrology* 1992; **2**: 1608–1616.
22. Schwartz CJ, White TA. Stenosis of renal artery: an unselected necropsy study. *British Medicine Journal* 1964; **2**: 1415–1421.
23. Sawicki PT, Kaiser S, Heinemann L, Frenzel H, Berger M. Prevalence of renal artery stenosis in diabetes mellitus—an autopsy study. *Journal of Internal Medicine* 1991; **229**: 489–492.
24. Olin JW, Melia M, Young JR, Graor RA, Risius B. Prevalence of atherosclerotic renal artery stenosis in patients with atherosclerosis elsewhere. *American Journal of Medicine* 1990; **88**: 1-46N–1-51N.
25. Valentine RJ, Clagett GP, Miller GL, Myers SI, Martin JD, Chervu A. The coronary risk of unsuspected renal artery stenosis. *Journal of Vascular Surgery* 1993; **18**: 433–439.
26. Rackson ME, Lossef SV, Sos TA. Renal artery stenosis in patients with aortic dissection: increased prevalence. *Radiology* 1990; **177**: 555–558.
27. Dustan HP, Humphries AW, De Wolf VG, Page IH. Normal arterial pressure in patients

with renal arterial stenosis. *Journal of the American Medicine Association* 1964; **187**: 1028–1029.

28. Choudhri AH, Cleland JGF, Rowlands PC, Tran TL, McCarthy M, Al-Kutoubi MA. Unsuspected renal artery stenosis in peripheral vascular disease. *British Medicine Journal* 1990; **301**: 1197–1198.
29. Wilms G, Marchal G. The angiographic incidence of renal artery stenosis in the arteriosclerotic population. *European Journal of Radiology* 1990; **10**: 195–197.
30. Missouris CG, Buckenham T, Cappucio FP, MacGregor GA. Renal artery stenosis: a common and important problem in patients with peripheral vascular disease. *American Journal of Medicine* 1994; **96**: 10–14.
31. Hricik DE, Browning PJ, Kopelman R, Goorno WE, Madias NE, Dzau VJ. Captopril-induced functional renal insufficiency in patients with bilateral renal-artery stenoses or renal-artery stenosis in a solitary kidney. *New England Journal of Medicine* 1983; **308**: 373–376.
32. Gedroyc W. Magnetic resonance angiography of the renal arteries. In: Novick A, Scoble J, Hamilton G, eds. *Renal Vascular Disease*. London: W.B. Saunders, 1995: 91–106.
33. Strandness DE. Duplex ultrasound scanning. In: Novick A, Scoble J, Hamilton G, eds. *Renal Vascular Disease*. London: W.B. Saunders, 1995: 119–133.
34. Lye WC, Cheah JS, Sinniah R. Renal cholesterol embolic disease. *American Journal of Nephrology* 1993; **13**: 489–493.
35. Thurlbeck WM, Castleman B. Atheromatous emboli to the kidneys after aortic surgery. *New England Journal of Medicine* 1957; **257**: 442–447.
36. Preston RA, Stemmer CL, Materson BJ, Perez-Stable E, Pardo V. Renal biopsy in patients 65 years of age or older. *Journal of the American Geriatrics Society* 1990; **38**: 669–674.
37. Gaines PA, Cumberland DC, Kennedy A, Welsh CL, Moorhead P, Rutley MS. Cholesterol embolisation: a lethal complication of vascular catheterisation. *Lancet* 1988; **i**: 168.
38. Weibull H, Bergqvist D, Andersson I, Choi DL, Jonsson K, Bergentz SE. Symptoms and signs of thrombotic occlusion of atherosclerotic renal artery stenosis. *European Journal of Vascular Surgery* 1990; **15**: 161–165.
39. Ross R. The pathogenesis of atherosclerosis: a perspective for the 1990s. *Nature* 1993; **362**: 801–809.
40. Lohse JR, Shore RM, Belzer FO. Acute renal artery occlusion. *Archives of Surgery* 1982; **117**: 801–804.
41. Yune HY, Klatte EC. Collateral circulation to an ischemic kidney. *Radiology* 1976; **119**: 539–546.
42. Scoble JE, Mikhail A, Reidy J, Cook GJR. Individual kidney function in atherosclerotic renal-artery disease. *Nephrology Dialysis Transplantation* 1998; **13**: 1048–1049.
43. Higgins RM, Goldsmith DJA, Ashleigh R, Venning MC, Ackrill P. Elective rather than emergency intervention for acute renal artery occlusion with anuria. *Nephron* 1994; **68**: 265–267.
44. Zierler RE, Bergelin RO, Isaacson JA, Strandness DE. Natural history of atherosclerotic renal artery stenosis: a prospective study with duplex ultrasonography. *Journal of Vascular Surgery* 1994; **19**: 250–258.
45. Hamilton G. Fibrinolytic therapy in renovascular disease. In: Novick A, Scoble J, Hamilton G, eds. *Renal Vascular Disease*. London: W.B. Saunders, 1995: 417–430.
46. Scoble JE. Ischaemic renal disease. In: Davison, Cameron, Grunfeld, Kerr, Ritz,

Winearls, eds. *Oxford Textbook of Clinical Nephrology*. Oxford: Oxford University Press, 1998: 1679–1687.

47. Tullis MJ, Zierler RE, Glickerman DJ, Bergelin RO, Cantwell-Gab K, Strandness DE. Results of percutaneous transluminal angioplasty for atherosclerotic renal artery stenosis: a follow-up study with duplex ultrasonography. *Journal of Vascular Surgery* 1997; **25**: 46–54.
48. Pilmore HL, Walker RJ, Solomon C, Packer S, Wood D. Acute bilateral renal artery occlusion: successful revascularization with streptokinase. *American Journal of Nephrology* 1995; **15**: 90–91.
49. Perkins RP, Jacobsen DS, Feder FP, Lipchik EO, Fine PH. Return of renal function after late embolectomy. *New England Journal of Medicine* 1967; **276**: 1194–1195.
50. Brunetti DR, Harviel JD, Sasaki TM, *et al.* Successful renal autotransplantation in patient with bilateral renal artery thrombosis. *Urology* 1993; **43**: 235–237.
51. Klink BK, Sutherin S, Heyse P, McCarthy MC. Traumatic bilateral renal artery thrombosis diagnosed by computed tomography with successful revascularization. *Journal of Trauma* 1992; **32**: 259–262.
52. Balligand JL, Lefebvre C, Zenagui D, Coche E. Cerebral and renal arterial thromboses in systemic lupus erythematosus with antiphospholipid antibodies: a report of two cases. *Acta Clinica Belgica* 1990; **45**: 372–378.
53. Ames PRJ, Cianciaruso B, Bellizzi V, *et al.* Bilateral renal artery occlusion in a patient with primary antiphospholipid antibody syndrome: thrombosis, vasculitis or both? *Journal of Rheumatology* 1992; **19**: 1802–1806.
54. Poux JM, Boudet R, Lacroix P, *et al.* Renal infarction and thrombosis of the infrarenal aorta in a 35-year-old man with primary antiphospholipid syndrome. *American Journal of Kidney Disease* 1996; **27**: 721–725.
55. Ostuni PA, Lazzarin P, Pengo V, Ruffatti A, Schiavon F, Gambari P. Renal artery thrombosis and hypertension in a 13 year old girl with antiphospholipid syndrome. *Annals of Rheumatic Disease* 1990; **49**: 184–187.
56. Hannedouche T, Godin M, Fries D, Fillastre JP. Acute renal thrombosis induced by angiotensin-converting enzyme inhibitors in patients with renovascular hypertension. *Nephron* 1991; **57**: 230–231.
57. Pontremoli R, Rampoldi V, Morbidelli A, Fiorini F, Ranise A, Garibotto G. Acute renal failure due to acute bilateral renal artery thrombosis: successful surgical revascularization after prolonged anuria. *Nephron* 1990; **56**: 322–324.
58. Shibasaki T, Ishimoto F, Kodama K, Ohno I, Sakai O. Renal artery thrombosis in a patient with membranous glomerulonephritis. *Internal Medicine* 1992; **31**: 294–297.
59. Streather C, Wlodarczyk ZC, Sneddon F, *et al.* Progression of occlusive renal vascular disease and axillo-femoral bypass grafts. *Nephrology Dialysis Transplantation* 1993; **8**: 1186–1187.
60. Ligush J, Criado E, Burnham SJ, Johnson G, Keagy BA. Management and outcome of chronic atherosclerotic infrarenal aortic occlusion. *Journal of Vascular Surgery* 1996; **24**: 394–405.
61. Theiss M, Wirth MP, Dolken W, Frohmuller HG. Spontaneous thrombosis of the renal vessels. Rare entities to be considered in differential diagnosis of patients presenting with lumbar flank pain and haematuria. *Urological International* 1992; **48**: 441–445.
62. Campbell JP, Lane PW. Spontaneous renal artery thrombosis associated with altered mental status. *Annals of Emergency Medicine* 1992; **21**: 1505–1507.
63. Castillo PA, Barrera F. Human hypertension due to thrombotic occlusion of both renal arteries. *American Heart Journal* 1958; **56**: 769–775.

64. Moyer JD, Rao CN, Widrich WC, Olsson CA. Conservative management of renal artery embolus. *Journal of Urology* 1973; **109**: 138–143.
65. Smith SP, Hamburger RJ, Donohue JP, Grim CE. Occlusion of the artery to a solitary kidney. *Journal of the American Medicine Association* 1974; **230**: 1306–1307.
66. Schonwald HN, Campbell EW, Galleher EP. Anuria secondary to renal artery obstruction in a solitary kidney: 9 year follow-up. *Journal of Urology* 1978; **120**: 618–619.
67. Wasser WG, Krakoff LR, Haimov M, Glabman S, Mitty HA. Restoration of renal function after bilateral renal artery occlusion. *Archives of Internal Medicine* 1981; **141**: 1647–1651.
68. Flye MW, Anderson RW, Fish JC, Silver D. Successful surgical treatment of anuria caused by renal artery occlusion. *Annals of Surgery* 1982; **195**: 346–353.
69. Williams B, Feehally J, Attard AR, Bell PRF. Recovery of renal function after delayed revascularisation of acute occlusion of the renal artery. *British Medicine Journal* 1988; **296**: 1591–1592.
70. Mugge A, Gilba DC, Frei U, *et al.* Renal artery embolism: thrombolysis with recombinant tissue-plasminogen activator. *Journal of Internal Medicine* 1990; **228**: 279–286.
71. Letsou GV, Gusberg R. Isolated bilateral renal artery thrombosis: an unusual consequence of blunt abdominal trauma. *Journal of Trauma* 1990; **30**: 509–511.
72. Kennedy JS, Gerety BM, Silverman R, Pattison ME, Siskind MS, Popnd GD. Simultaneous renal arterial and venous thrombosis associated with idiopathic nephrotic syndrome: treatment with intra-arterial urokinase. *American Journal of Medicine* 1991; **90**: 124–127.
73. Takeda M, Katayama Y, Saito K, Tsutsui T, Komeyama T. Successful fibrinolytic therapy using tissue plasminogen activator in acute renal failure due to acute thrombosis of bilateral renal arteries. *Urological International* 1993; **51**: 177–180.
74. Salam TA, Lumsden AB, Martin LG. Local infusion of fibrinolytic agents for acute renal artery thromboembolism: report of ten cases. *Annals of Vascular Surgery* 1993; **7**: 21–26.
75. Boyer L, Ravel A, Boissier A, *et al.* Percutaneous recanalization of recent renal artery occlusions: report of 10 cases. *Cardiovascular Interventional Radiology* 1994; **17**: 258–263.
76. Braun DR, Sawczuk IS, Axelrod SA. Idiopathic renal infarction. *Urology* 1995; **45**: 142–145.
77. Le Goff C, Ryckelynck Levaltier B, Henri P, Lobbedez T, de Hurault Ligny B. Reversible acute renal failure following aortic thrombosis inducing bilateral renal-artery occlusive disease. *Nephrology Dialysis Transplantation* 1995; **10**: 879–881.
78. Mikhail A, Reidy J, Taylor PR, Scoble JE. Renal artery embolisation after back massage in a patient with aortic occlusion. *Nephrology Dialysis Transplantation* 1997; **12**: 797–798.
79. Martinez Vea A, Garcia Ruiz C, Carrera M, Oliver JA, Ricjart C. Effect of Captopril in nephrotic-range proteinuria due to renovascular hypertension. *Nephron* 1987; **45**: 162–163.
80. Marcussen N. Atubular glomeruli in renal artery stenosis. *Laboratory Investigations* 1991; **65**: 558–565.
81. Shanley PF. The pathology of chronic renal ischemia. *Seminars in Nephrology* 1996; **16**: 21–32.
82. Truong LD, Farhood A, Tasby J, Gillum D. Experimental chronic renal ischemia: morphologic and immunologic studies. *Kidney International* 1992; **41**: 1676–1689.
83. Risdon RA, Sloper JC, de Wardener HE. Relationship between renal function and

histological changes found in renal biopsy specimens from patients with persistent glomerular nephritis. *Lancet* 1968; **ii**: 363–366.

84. Bohle A, Mackensen-Haen S, Gise HV. Significance of tubulointerstitial changes in the renal cortex for the excretory function and concentration ability of the kidney: a morphometric contribution. *American Journal of Nephrology* 1987; **7**: 421–433.
85. Bohle A, Wehrmann M, Bogenschutz O, Batz C, Muller CA, Muller GA. The pathogenesis of chronic renal failure in diabetic nephropathy. *Pathological Research Practice* 1991; **187**: 251–259.
86. Grone HJ, Warnecke E, Olbricht CJ. Characteristics of renal tubular atrophy in experimental renovascular hypertension: a model of kidney hibernation. *Nephron* 1996; **72**: 243–252.
87. Gobe GC, Buttyan KRL, Ethridge MR, Smith PJ. Clusterin expression and apoptosis in tissue remodelling associated with renal regeneration. *Kidney International* 1995; **47**: 411–420.
88. Jackson B, Franze L, Sumithran E, Johnston CI. Pharmacological nephrectomy with chronic angiotensin converting enzyme inhibitor treatment in renovascular hypertension in the rat. *Journal of Laboratory Clinical Medicine* 1990; **115**: 21–27.
89. Guzman RP, Zierler RE, Isaacson JA, Bergelin RO, Strandness DE. Renal atrophy and arterial stenosis: a prospective study with duplex ultrasound. *Hypertension* 1994; **23**: 346–350.
90. Caps MT, Zierler RE, Polisssar NL, *et al.* Risk of atrophy in kidneys with atherosclerotic renal artery stenosis, *Kidney International* 1998; **53**: 735–742.
91. Ramsay LE, Waller PC. *Blood Pressure Response to Percutaneous Transluminal Angioplasty for Renovascular Hypertension:* an overview of published series, *British Medical Journal* 1990; **300**: 569–572.
92. Swartbol P, Parsson H, Thorvinger B, Norgren L. To what extent does peripheral vascular disease and hypertension predict renal artery stenosis. *International Angiology* 1994; **13**: 109–114.
93. Vidt DG. Cholesterol emboli; a common cause of renal failure. *Annual Review of Medicine* 1997; **48**: 375–385.
94. Flory CM. Arterial occlusions produced by emboli from eroded aortic atheromatous plaques. *American Journal of Pathology* 1945; **21**: 549–565.
95. Scoble JE, O'Donnell PJO. Renal atheroembolic disease: the Cinderella of nephrology? *Nephrology Dialysis Transplantation* 1996; **11**: 1516–1517.
96. Cosio FG, Zager RA, Sharma HM. Atheroembolic disease causes hypocomplementemia. *Lancet* 1985; **ii**: 118–121.
97. Cameron JS. The enigma of focal segmental glomerulosclerosis. *Kidney International* 1996; **50**: S119–S131.
98. Thadhani R, Pascual M, Nickeleit V, Tolkoff-Rubin N, Colvin R. Preliminary description of focal segmental glomerulosclerosis in patients with renovascular disease. *Lancet* 1996; **347**: 231–233.
99. Alzaid AA. Microalbuminuria in patients with NIDDM. an overview. *Diabetes Care* 1996; **19**: 79–89.
100. Damsgaard EM, Froland A, Jorgensen OD, Mogensen CA. Eight to nine year mortality in known non-insulin dependent diabetics. *Kidney International* 1992; **41**: 731–735.
101. Chen R, Novick AC, Pohl M. Reversible renin mediated massive proteinuria successfully treated by nephrectomy. *Journal of Urology* 1995; **153**: 133–134.
102. Mikhail A, Cook GJR, Reidy J, Scoble JE. Progressive renal dysfunction despite successful renal artery angioplasty in a single kidney. *Lancet* 1997; **349**: 926.

103. May AG, De Weese JA, Rob CG. Hemodynamic effects of arterial stenosis. *Surgery* 1963; **53**: 513–524.
104. Nally JV. Captopril renography. In: Novick A, Scoble J, Hamilton G, eds. *Renal Vascular Disease*. London W.B. Saunders, 1995: 195–203.
105. Veniant M, Heudes D, Clozel JP, Bruneval P, Menard J. Calcium blockade versus ACE inhibition in clipped and unclipped kidneys of 2K–1C rats. *Kidney International* 1994; **46**: 421–429.
106. Maisey M, Britton KE. Nuclear imaging in nephrology. In: Davison AM, Cameron JS, Grunfeld JP, Kerr DNS, Ritz E, Winerals CG, eds. *Oxford Textbook of Clinical Nephrology*. Oxford: Oxford University Press, 1998: 137–149.
107. Cameron JS, Greger R. Renal function and testing of function. In: Davison AM, Cameron JS, Grunfeld JP, Kerr DNS, Ritz E, Winerals CG, eds. *Oxford Textbook of Clinical Nephrology*. Oxford: Oxford University Press, 1998: 39–69.
108. Reidy J. Contrast arteriography. In: Novick A, Scoble J, Hamilton G, eds. *Renal Vascular Disease*. London: W.B. Saunders, 1995: 77–90.
109. Kerns SR, Hawkins IF. Carbon dioxide angiography. In: Novick A, Scoble J, Hamilton G, eds. *Renal Vascular Disease*. London: W.B. Saunders, 1995: 107–117.
110. Olbricht CJ, Galanski M, Chavan A, Prokop M. Spiral CT angiography—can we forget about arteriography to diagnose renal artery stenosis? *Nephrology Dialysis Transplantation* 1996; **11**: 1227–1231.
111. Scoble J, McLean A, Stansby G, Sweny P, Hilson, A. The use of Captopril-DTPA scanning in the diagnosis of atherosclerotic renal artery stenosis in patients with impaired renal function. *American Journal of Hypertension* 1991; **4**: S721–S723.
112. Hunt JC, String CG. Renovascular hypertension: mechanisms, natural history and treatment. *American Journal of Cardiology* 1973; **32**: 562–574.
113. Panayiotopoulos YP, Tyrell MR, Koffman G, Reidy JF, Haycock GB, Taylor PR. Mid-aortic syndrome presenting in childhood. *British Journal of Surgery* 1996; **83**: 235–240.
114. O'Neil EA, Hansen KJ, Canzanello VJ, Pennell TC, Dean RH. Prevalence of ischemic nephropathy in patients with renal insufficiency. *American Surgeon* 1992; **58**: 485–490.
115. Scoble JE, Sweny P, Stansby G, Hamilton G. Patients with atherosclerotic renovascular disease presenting to a renal unit: an audit of outcome. *Postgraduate Medicine Journal* 1993; **69**: 461–465.
116. Connolly JO, Higgins RM, Walters HL, *et al.* Presentation, clinical features and outcome in different patterns of atherosclerotic renovascular disease. *Quarterly Journal of Medicine* 1994; **87**: 413–421.
117. Kaylor WM, Novick AC, Ziegelbaum M, Vidt DG. Reversal of end stage renal failure with surgical revascularization in patients with atherosclerotic renal artery occlusion. *Journal of Urology* 1989; **141**: 486–488.
118. Pattison JM, Reidy JF, Rafferty MJ, *et al.* Percutaneous transluminal renal angioplasty in patients with renal failure. *Quarterly Journal of Medicine* 1992; **85**: 883–888.
119. Brown G, Albers JJ, Fischer LD, *et al.* Regression of coronary artery disease as a result of intensive lipid-lowering therapy in men with high levels of apolipoprotein B. *New England Journal of Medicine* 1990; **323**: 1289–1298.
120. Postma CT, Hoefnagels WHL, Barentsz JO, de Boo T, Thien T. Occlusion of unilateral stenosed renal arteries—relation to medical treatment. *Journal of Human Hypertension* 1989; **3**: 185–190.
121. Schreiber MJ, Pohl MA, Novick AC. The natural history of atherosclerotic and fibrous renal artery disease. *Urological Clinics North America* 1984; **11**: 383–392.

122. Dean RH, Tribble RW, Hansen KJ, O'Neil E, Craven TE, Redding JF. Evolution of renal insufficiency in ischemic nephropathy. *Annals of Surgery* 1991; **213**: 446–456.
123. Pickering TG, Herman L, Devereux RB, *et al.* Recurrent pulmonary edema in hypertension due to bilateral renal artery stenosis: treatment by angioplasty or surgical intervention. *Lancet* 1988; **2**: 551–552.
124. Messina LM, Zelenock GB, Yao KA, Stanley JC. Renal revascularization for recurrent pulmonary edema in patients with poorly controlled hypertension and renal insufficiency: a distinct subgroup of patients with arteriosclerotic renal artery occlusive disease. *Journal of Vascular Surgery* 1992; **15**: 73–78.
125. MacDowall P, Kalra PA, O'Donoghue DJ, Waldeck S, Mamotora H. A study of the prevalence of occult renovascular disease (RVD) in an elderly population with cardiac failure. *Journal of the American Society of Nephrology* 1996; **7**: 1393.
126. Wollenweber J, Sheps SG, Davis GD. Clinical course of atherosclerotic renovascular disease. *American Journal of Medicine* 1968; **21**: 60–70.
127. Mailloux LU, Bellucci AG, Mossey RT, *et al.* Predictors of survival in patients undergoing dialysis. *American Journal of Medicine* 1988; **84**: 855–862.
128. Criqui MH, Langer RD, Fronek A, *et al.* Mortality over a period of 10 years in patients with peripheral arterial disease. *New England Journal of Medicine* 1992; **326**: 381–386.
129. Sheil AGR, May J, Stokes GS, Johnson JR, Tiller DJ, Stewart JH. Reversal of renal failure by revascularization of kidneys with thrombosed renal arteries. *Lancet* 1973; **ii**: 865–866.
130. Bengtsson U, Bergentz SE, Norback B. Surgical treatment of renal artery stenosis with impending uremia. *Clinical Nephrology* 1974; **2**: 222–229.
131. Novick AC, Textor SC, Bodie B, Khauli RB. Revascularization to preserve renal function in patients with atherosclerotic renovascular disease. *Urological Clinics North America* 1984; **11**: 477–490.
132. Novick AC. Alternative bypass techniques for renal revascularization. In: Novick A, Scoble J, Hamilton G, eds. *Renal Vascular Disease*. London: W.B. Saunders, 1995: 465–480.
133. Novick AC. Extracorporeal microvascular reconstruction and autotransplantation for branch renal artery disease. In: Novick A, Scoble J, Hamilton G, eds. *Renal Vascular Disease*. London: W.B. Saunders, 1995: 497–509
134. Stansby GP, Scoble JE, Hamilton G. Use of hepatic arterial circulation for renal revascularisation. *Annals of Royal College Surgeons England* 1992; **74**: 260–264.
135. Hansen KJ, Thomason RB, Craven TE, *et al.* Surgical management of dialysis-dependent ischemic nephropathy. *Journal of Vascular Surgery* 1995; **21**: 197–211.
136. Weibull H, Bergqvist D, Bergentz SE, Jonsson K, Hulthen L, Manhem P. Percutaneous transluminal renal angioplasty versus surgical reconstruction of atherosclerotic renal artery stenosis: a prospective randomized study. *Journal of Vascular Surgery* 1993; **18**: 841–852.
137. Geyskes GG. Percutaneous transluminal angioplasty in atherosclerosis. In: Novick A, Scoble J, Hamilton G, eds. *Renal Vascular Disease*. London: W.B. Saunders, 1995: 385–401.
138. Harden PN, MacLeod MJ, Rodger RSC, *et al.* Effect of renal-artery stenting on progression of renovascular renal failure. *Lancet* 1997; **349**: 1133–1136.
139. Textor SC. Revascularization in atherosclerotic renal artery disease. *Kidney International* 1998; **53**: 799–811.
140. Marshall FI, Hagen S, Mahaffy RG, *et al.* Percutaneous transluminal angioplasty for

atheromatous renal artery stenosis-blood pressure response and discriminant analysis outcome predictors. *Quarterly Journal of Medicine* 1990; **75**: 483–489.

141. Morin JE, Hutchinson TA, Lisbona R. Long term prognosis of surgical treatment of renovascular hypertension: a fifteen year experience. *Journal of Vascular Surgery.* 1986; **3**: 545–549.
142. Webster J, Marshall F, Abdalla M, *et al.* Randomised comparison of percutaneous angioplasty vs continued medical therapy for hypertensive patients with renal artery stenosis. *Journal of Human Hypertension* 1998; **12**: 329–335.
143. Plouin PF, Chatellier G, Darne B, Raynaud A. Blood pressure outcome of angioplasty in atherosclerotic renal artery stenosis. *Hypertension* 1998; **31**: 823–829.
144. Kremer Hovinga TK, de Jong PE, van der Ham GK, de Zeeuw D. Relief of renal artery stenosis: a tool to improve or preserve renal function in renovascular disease? *Nephrology Dialysis Transplantation* 1990; **5**: 481–488.
145. Zuccala A, Zucchelli P. Atherosclerotic renal artery stenosis—when is intervention by PTA or surgery justified? *Nephrology Dialysis Transplantation* 1995; **10**: 585–587.
146. Shepherd J, Cobbe SM, Ford I, *et al.* Prevention of coronary heart disease with Pravastatin in men with hypercholesterolemia. *New England Journal of Medicine* 1995; **333**: 1301–1307.
147. Scandinavian, Simvastatin Survival Group. Randomised trial of cholesterol lowering in 4444 patients with coronary heart disease: the Scandinavian Simvastatin Survival Study. *Lancet* 1994; **344**: 1383–1389.
148. Cabili S, Hochman I, Goor Y. Reversal of gangrenous lesions in the blue toe syndrome with lovastatin. *Angiology* 1993; **44**: 821–825.
149. Conlon PJ, Athirakul K, Schwab SJ, Crowley J, Stack R, Albers F. Long term follow-up of asymptomatic renal vascular disease. *Journal of the American Society of Nephrology* 1996; **7**: 1384.
150. Ramirez G, Bugni W, Farber SM, Curry AJ. Incidence of renal artery stenosis in a population having cardiac catheterization. *Southern Medicine Journal* 1987; **80**: 734–737.
151. Wachtell K, Ibsen H, Olsen MH, Christoffersen JK, Norgaard H, Mantoni M. Prevalence of renal artery stenosis in patients with peripheral vascular disease and hypertension. *Journal of Human Hypertension* 1996; **10**: 83–85.
152. Mailloux LU, Belluci AG, Napolitano B, Mossey T, Wilkes BM, Bluestone PA. Survival estimates for 683 patients starting dialysis from 1970 through 1989 identification of risk factors for survival. *Clinical Nephrology* 1994; **42**: 127–135.
153. Montoliu J, Botey A, Torras A, Darnell A, Revert L. Renin-induced massive proteinuria in man. *Clinical Nephrology* 1979; **11**: 267–271.
154. Takeda Morimoto S, Uchida K, Kigoshi Sumitani T, Matsubara F. Effects of Captopril on both hypertension and proteinuria. *Archives of Internal Medicine* 1980; **140**: 1531–1533.
155. Eiser AR, Katz SM, Swartz C. Reversible nephrotic range proteinuria with renal artery stenosis: a clinical example of renin-associated proteinuria. *Nephron* 1982; **30**: 374–377.
156. Adams MB, Harris SS, Kauffman HM, Towne JB. Effect of primary renal disease in patients with renovascular insufficiency. *Journal of Vascular Surgery* 1984; **1**: 482–486.
157. Sato H, Saito T, Kasai Y, Abe K, Yoshinaga K. Massive proteinuria due to renal artery stenosis. *Nephron* 1989; **51**: 136–137.
158. Greendyke RM, Akamatsu Y. Atheromatous embolism as a cause of renal failure. *Journal of Urology* 1960; **83**: 231–237.
159. Snyder HE, Shapiro JL. A correlative study of atheromatous embolism in human beings and experimental animals. *Surgery* 1961; **49**: 195–204.

160. Moldveen-Geronimus M, Merriam JC. Cholesterol embolization. *Circulation* 1967; **35**: 946–953.
161. Harrington JT, Sommers SC, Kassirer JP. Atheromatous emboli with progressive renal failure. *Annals of Internal Medicine* 1968; **68**: 152–160.
162. Dalakos TG, Streeten DHP, Jones D, Obeid A. 'Malignant' hypertension resulting from atheromatous embolization predominantly of one kidney. *American Journal of Medicine* 1974; **57**: 135–138.
163. Regester RF. Renal failure secondary to spontaneous atheromatous microembolism. *Journal of the Tennessee Medical Association* 1979; 328–330.
164. Varanasi UR, Moorthy AV, Beirne GJ. Spontaneous atheroembolic disease as a cause of renal failure in the elderly. *Journal of the American Geriatrics Society* 1979; **27**: 407–409.
165. Smith MC, Ghose MK, Henry AR. The clinical spectrum of renal cholesterol embolization. *American Journal of Medicine* 1981; **71**: 174–189.
166. Hannedouche T, Godin M, Courtois H, *et al.* Necrotizing glomerulonephritis and renal cholesterol embolization. *Nephron* 1986; **42**: 271–272.
167. Schwartz MW, McDonald GB. Cholesterol embolization syndrome. *Journal of the American Medicine Association* 1987; **258**: 1934–1935.
168. Hyman BT, Landas SK, Ashman RF, Schelper RL, Robinson RA. Warfarin-related purple toes syndrome and cholesterol microembolization. *American Journal of Medicine* 1987; **82**: 1233–1237.
169. Fine M, Kapoor W, Falanga V. Cholesterol crystal embolization: a review of 221 cases in the English literature. *Angiology* 1987; **38**: 769–784.
170. Aujla ND, Greenberg A, Banner BF, Johnston JR, Tzakis AG. Atheroembolic involvement of renal allografts. *American Journal of Kidney Disease* 1989; **13**: 329–332.
171. Mannesse CK, Blankestijn PJ, Veld AJM, Schalekamp MADH. Renal failure and cholesterol crystal embolization. *Clinical Nephrology* 1991; **36**: 240–245.
172. Case, records of *et al.* Case 2–1991. *New England Journal of Medicine* 1991; **324**: 113–120.
173. Wilson DM, Salazer TL, Farkouh ME. Eosinophiluria in atheroembolic renal disease. *American Journal of Medicine* 1991; **91**: 186–189.
174. Bendixen BH, Younger DS, Hair LS, *et al.* Cholesterol emboli neuropathy. *Neurology* 1992; **42**: 428–430.
175. Sheehan MG, Condemi JJ, Rosenfeld SI. Position dependent livedo reticularis in cholesterol emboli syndrome. *Journal of Rheumatology* 1993; **20**: 1973–1974.
176. Blakely P, Cosby RL, McDonald BR. Nephritic urinary sediment in embolic renal disease. *Clinical Nephrology* 1994; **42**: 401–403.
177. Thadhani RI, Camargo CA, Xavier RJ, Fang LST, Bazari H. Atheroembolic renal failure after invasive procedures. *Medicine* 1995; **74**: 350–358.
178. Haqqie SS, Urizar RE, Singh J. Nephrotic-range proteinuria in renal atheroembolic disease: report of four cases. *American Journal of Kidney Disease* 1996; **4**: 493–501.
179. Case records of New England Journal of Medicine. Case 11–1996. *New England Journal of Medicine* 1996; **334**: 973–979.
180. Greenberg A, Bastacky SI, Iqbal A, Borochovitz D, Johnson JP. Focal segmental glomerulosclerosis associated with nephrotic syn¡drome in cholesterol atheroembolism: clinicopathological correlations. *American Journal of Kidney Disease* 1997; **29**: 334–344.

10

Chronic tubulo-interstitial nephropathy

R. M. Smith and C. R. V. Tomson

Introduction

It has long been known that histological changes in the tubulo-interstitial compartment of the kidney are far more predictive of subsequent changes in renal function than glomerular changes [1–6]. These findings have focused attention on the importance of the interstitial compartment in the progression of glomerular disease. Paradoxically, however, in diseases in which the pathogenesis is largely within the interstitium, glomerular changes and the accompanying proteinuria appear to be more predictive of outcome—for instance, in reflux nephropathy. Tubulo-interstitial diseases also pose challenges for the hyperfiltration theory of progression—why, for instance, is proteinuria so rare in polycystic kidney disease despite progressive loss of functioning nephrons?—and why is progressive renal failure so rare after relief of obstruction, even in patients who are left with severe renal impairment? Perhaps the type of scarring, rather than simply the number of nephrons lost, is a determinant of progression. This disparate group of diseases teach us that there are numerous contributing factors to progressive renal disease, many of which remain ill understood.

Autosomal dominant polycystic kidney disease

Definition

The differential diagnosis of cystic diseases of the kidney has been reviewed recently [7]. The hallmark of autosomal dominant polycystic kidney disease (ADPKD) is the presence of numerous bilateral fluid-filled cysts scattered diffusely throughout renal cortex and medulla. A minimum of three cysts distributed bilaterally in the presence of an autosomal dominant family history has been validated as a diagnostic criterion for patients under 18 years of age [8] and has been adopted in many adult studies [9]. Using this criterion Parfrey *et al.* [10] reported no false positives in 126 patients with a 50% risk of PKD-1 mutations. However, the increased incidence of simple cysts with advancing age makes this criterion less useful in the adult patient. Ravine *et al.* [11] have demonstrated that in kindreds with PKD-1 mutations two cysts are sufficient for a diagnosis of ADPKD in individuals less than 30 years. From 30 to 59 years they suggested at least two cysts in each kidney to be required compared with at least four cysts in each kidney in patients aged 60 years and above. Further studies are needed to validate these criteria for non-PKD-1 linked ADPKD. Renal cysts may be demonstrated by intravenous urography, ultrasound scanning (USS), computed tomography (CT), or magnetic resonance imaging. USS is readily available, safe and is superior to urography/tomography in cyst detection, particularly in early cases [12]. CT is more sensitive for cyst detection than USS [12] and may be of use in equivocal cases.

Pathogenesis

Elucidation of the pathogenetic mechanisms operating in ADPKD is central to development of rational interventions to prevent onset and progression of renal impairment. The pathogenesis of ADPKD may be considered under three headings: genetics and biochemistry, cell biology of cyst formation, and pathogenesis of renal impairment.

Genetics and biochemistry

ADPKD is the second most common inherited monogenic disorder with a gene frequency of 1:400–1:1000 [13–15]. It is an autosomal dominant trait with almost complete penetrance but variable expressivity [13,14]. The *PKD-1* gene has been localized to chromosome 16p13.3 [16–18] and accounts for approximately 85–90% of ADPKD [19,20]. The *PKD-2* gene, localized to chromosome 4q21 accounts for the majority of the rest of cases [19,21–24]. A number of families with ADPKD not linked to 16p13 or 4q21 have been described [25–27].

The *PKD-1* gene encodes a 4304 amino acid protein (polycystin) within which are a number of recognisable sub-units allowing the properties of the protein to be predicted and discussion of how this genetic defect may give rise to the phenotype of ADPKD [20,28] (discussed below). The *PKD-2* gene encodes an integral membrane protein of 968 amino acids with homology to the $\alpha_{1E\text{-}1}$ subunit of a voltage-activated calcium channel [29].

The autosomal dominant pattern of inheritance of ADPKD predicts that all renal epithelial cells will initially carry one normal and one abnormal allele. Two *general* theories may explain how such a defect gives rise to a pathological phenotype: a dominant negative effect or loss of function effect. The dominant negative mechanism requires the abnormal allele to code for a 'gain of function' which in turn suppresses the activity of the normal allele or other genes. Such a dominant negative effect of the PKD-1/PKD-2 mutations should have equal effect in all tubules and would thus need to interact with additional environmental or genetic factors in order to produce the variable clinical picture seen in ADPKD and to be consistent with the finding that in ADPKD less than 1% of tubules are affected [30]. Conversely, a loss of function mechanism proposes that the mutant allele is non-functional, resulting in a reduced 'dose' of activity encoded at the locus in question. Structural analyses of the PKD-1 and PKD-2 gene products argue against a dominant negative effect of pathogenetic mutations and would be more in favour of a loss of function mechanism [20,28]. The loss of 50% of activity at the PKD-1 or PKD-2 loci due to loss of one allele may itself be pathogenetic. However, if loss of a single allele alone caused ADPKD, as argued above for a dominant negative effect, all tubules would be affected and the variable tubular involvement and variable clinical picture would require interaction with additional environmental or genetic factors. Two observations have suggested that random acquisition of somatic mutations at the PKD-1 or PKD-2 loci may be the additional genetic factor producing sufficient loss of function to produce disease. Cystic epithelia have been demonstrated to show loss of the region of chromosome 16p13 containing the PKD-1 gene [31] and a high degree of clonality within individual cysts supporting derivation of these cysts from a single mutated 'parent' cell [32]. Such a model has been termed the 'two-hit' (one inherited and one acquired) model and is attractive as it incorporates a random component in pathogenesis predicting both variability between individuals and focal 'loss of function' and cyst generation. Thus, the onset of cyst development would be timed by the second somatic mutation in renal epithelial cells and the random nature of this event would account for the Gaussian distribution of difference in age of onset of end-stage renal disease (ESRD) between parent and offspring found by Geberth *et al.* [33]. This model would also accommodate variation in disease expression within families [34] and between twins who share the same inherited mutation [35,36]. Given the high penetrance and large number of cysts seen in ADPKD the two-hit model would require a high mutation rate at the ADPKD loci. The lack of a founder effect, the high percentage of individuals who represent 'new mutations' and the large number of different mutations demonstrated in the PKD-1 gene would support the suggestion that the ADPKD loci are mutational hot spots. Further, supporting the two-hit model of pathogenesis, in contrast to the clonality demonstrated within individual cysts, different mutations have been demonstrated in different cysts of the same individual and cells in a single cyst have been demonstrated to have two different mutations of the two PKD-1 alleles. The unique structure of the PKD-1 gene has been proposed as an explanation for this high mutation rate. In keeping with this Watnick *et al.* [37] found clustering of base pair substitutions in exons 23 and 25 of the PKD-1 gene suggesting unique structural features predisposing to mutations at these sites. Such clustering has, however, not been universally found. The finding that most cyst epithelia retain immunoreactivity for polycystin requires that most cysts carry a mis-sense or non-sense 'second hit' mutation in the 'normal' allele preserving polycystin expression but inhibiting normal function [38,39]. Although this high percentage of mis-sense mutations has been suggested by some workers to be unlikely and accordingly has been used to argue against a 'two-hit' loss of function model, there is a precedent in the mutation of the ATM gene in the pathogenesis of T-cell prolymphocytic leukemia [40]. The technique used to detect mutations may bias against detection of non-terminating lesions and analysis of the Cardiff database demonstrates a large number of mutations in the PKD-1 gene which would be predicted to preserve polycystin expression but inhibit function.

Cell biology of cyst formation

Cysts are homogeneously distributed throughout the cortex and medulla and arise from Bowman's capsule, proximal and distal tubules, and collecting ducts. Abnormal renal tubular epithelial cell growth, abnormalities of the tubular basement membrane, abnormal localization of Na+/K+ ATPase (possibly giving rise to abnormal fluid secretion) and deranged extracellular matrix composition are all implicated in cystogenesis (reviewed in [9]). Cystic epithelia have been demonstrated to secrete fluid by an adenylate cyclase and chloride channel dependent mechanism [41,42]. The predicted structure of the PKD-1 protein includes multiple extracellular domains capable of mediating protein–protein and protein–carbohydrate interactions suggesting that the primary defect in ADPKD is an abnormal interaction of tubular epithelial cells with the extracellular matrix and cell membrane bound ligands leading to an inability to maintain tubular differentiation [20,28]. This undifferentiated state then results in the abnormalities described above and hence the pathological phenotype. Furthermore, the PKD-2 protein has significant homology with voltage-gated ion channels [29] and has been shown to interact with polycystin. The finding that polycystin has significant homology with a sea urchin sperm membrane protein which acts as a receptor for egg jelly triggering the acrosome reaction through regulation of ion channels [38], suggests that PKD-1 and PKD-2 may act in tandem as a cell surface complex [43,44] also regulating ion channel activity and explaining why defects in either gene give rise to a similar clinical phenotype. However, structural analysis of conservation between the Puffer fish and human PKD-2 genes shows the intracytoplasmic C-terminal domain which has been suggested to interact with polycystin-1 to be poorly conserved arguing against this portion of the molecule having a critical function (D. Sandford, personal communication).

Pathogenesis of renal impairment

Loss of function of cystic tubules cannot alone account for renal impairment in ADPKD as less than 1% of tubules become cystic [30]. Cysts above 200 μm do not communicate with tubules and it is therefore suggested that continued fluid production causes cyst expansion leading to compression of surrounding tissue and renal impairment [30,45]. Cyst fluid from patients with ADPKD has been shown to stimulate renal epithelial cell fluid secretion [46] and a low molecular weight lipid molecule responsible for this activity has been isolated [47]. Thus, once established, cyst expansion would be progressive and the potential for encroachment upon adjacent normal tissue great. Alternatively, in common with other forms of chronic tubulo-interstitial nephropathy (TIN), the histopathology of ADPKD is characterized by interstitial fibrosis and the expression of proinflammatory chemokines (e.g. MCP-1 and osteopontin), growth factors, metalloproteinases, and the deposition of types I and IV collagen, laminin, and fibronectin (reviewed in [48]). The relative contribution of these different pathophysiological mechanisms is unclear.

Natural history

ADPKD accounts for 8–9% of patients with ESRD requiring replacement therapy in Europe [49] and has not changed significantly between 1977 and 1992 [50]. The most recent data from the US Renal Data System (USRDS) shows an incidence of

ADPKD of only 2.7% among patients treated for ESRD between 1991 and 1995 [51].

ADPKD is typified by an initial period with well preserved renal function followed by a rapid fall [52–56]. It has been projected that 100% of carriers will show evidence of disease by 80 years [14], but that significantly fewer will progress to ESRF. In a study of individuals with ultrasonographic, clinical, or genetic evidence of disease from 17 families with PKD-1 linked and non-PKD-1 linked disease, the earliest age at onset of ESRD was 30 years and 25% had ESRD by 47 years, 50% by 59 years and 75% by the age of 70 [10]. The mean age at onset of ESRD was 59.3 yrs. These findings agree well with those of Marcelli *et al.* [53], Gabow *et al.* [57], and Churchill *et al.* [54] except that the latter group found significantly fewer patients with ESRD at 73 years (47%). Finally, the demonstration that interfamilial variation in age of onset of ESRD is greater than intrafamilial variation [58] would seem to support the early suggestion that age at ESRD runs true in families [14]. However, it is now clear that individuals carrying the same genetic defect may vary greatly in disease expression (D. Sandford, personal communication; [10,33,34]). Rarely, onset in infancy and *in utero* has been described, although it has been suggested that the pathogenesis in such cases may be more complex with anticipation being seen and an influence of additional non-PKD loci being demonstrated.

Mean rate of progression

Two studies have used isotope glomerular filtration rate (GFR) measurements to determine rates of progression in large groups of ADPKD patients. The MDRD study found GFR to decrease by a mean of 4.3 ml/min per 1.73 m^2 in 59 patients with a GFR at entry of 13–24 ml/min per 1.73 m^2 and by 5.8 ml/min per 1.73 m^2 in 141 patients with a GFR of 25–55 ml/min per 1.73 m^2 at entry [59]. In the 25–55 ml/min per 1.73 m^2 group only, female patients had a significantly slower rate of decline. Choukron *et al.* [55] reported similar rates of decline [5.3 ml/min per 1.73 m^2] in patients with GFR at entry of 50–60 ml/min per 1.73 m^2. For patients with GFR at entry of 30–50 ml/min per 1.73 m^2 male patients again showed a more rapid decline in GFR (6.4 ml/min per 1.73 m^2) than female patients (5.0 ml/min per 1.73 m^2).

A number of trials have presented data on the rate of progression of renal failure in ADPKD and compared the rate of progression in ADPKD with chronic renal failure (CRF) in general. Results are conflicting with both faster [59,60] and slower [55,61,62] progression as compared with CRF in general reported.

Prognostic factors

There may be considerable variation in the manifestation of the same genetic defect within a given family [34] and even between monozygotic twins. Elucidation of the factors responsible both for this variation and for the variation between unrelated individuals may suggest therapeutic strategies for prevention of progression of renal impairment in ADPKD.

Hypertension and left ventricular hypertrophy

Hypertension and left ventricular hypertrophy (LVH) are frequently seen in ADPKD [63–65]. Hypertension often precedes renal failure [66,67] and is the presenting feature in 13–20% of patients [56,68]. Hypertension becomes more common as function deteriorates, 82% of patients with ESRD being hypertensive [53,69].

A number of studies have suggested that hypertension in ADPKD is associated with a more rapid decline in renal function. Gabow *et al.* [57] reported the experience of the University of Colorado in 301 subjects. Hypertensive subjects ($n = 197$) reached a serum creatinine of 130 μmol/l (1.5 mg/dl) at a mean age of 47 years as opposed to 66 years in normotensive subjects. This effect was not attributable to the greater incidence of hypertension in male subjects. Importantly, left ventricular mass showed a similar correlation with a worse renal outcome. The Northern Italian Co-operative Study Group analysed 74 patients with ADPKD [53] finding those patients with a mean resting blood pressure below 107 mmHg (with or without antihypertensive therapy) to have a slower rate of progression than those with a mean blood pressure above this value (relative risk 1.26, 90% confidence interval 0.99–1.61 $p < 0.05$). It has been suggested that a linear regression model is inadequate for analysis of the relationship between blood pressure and progression of renal impairment. In 26 patients Gonzalo *et al.* [70] found no correlation between mean arterial pressure (MAP) and rate of deterioration of renal function. However, using a polynomial regression it was found that a MAP lower than 105 mmHg or higher than 120 mmHg is associated with a more rapid progression of renal impairment. Finally, in a retrospective study of 157 patients (109 reaching ESRD and 48 dialysis independent) Choukron *et al.* [55] found no influence of blood pressure at enrolment on progression rate. It is important here to remember that association does not prove causality, and hypertension and a faster rate of progression may both be markers for more severe disease. Only intervention studies can definitively address this question.

In ADPKD there is evidence for increased activity of the renin–angiotensin system even prior to development of renal impairment (reviewed in [69,71–74]). Renal ischemia secondary to cyst expansion has been suggested to be important in driving this increased renin release [66,75,76]. This increased renin release may be directly responsible for LVH rather than indirectly through generation of systemic hypertension [77].

Angiotensin-converting enzyme and angiotensin II receptor polymorphism

Given the central role of the renin–angiotensin system in glomerular physiology and the evidence for increased activity of the renin–angiotensin system in ADPKD, the description of functionally significant polymorphisms of the angiotensin-converting enzyme (ACE) gene [78], angiotensinogen and AT1 receptor [79] is of great interest when considering prognostic factors in ADPKD (reviewed in [80]). DD homozygotes for the insertion/deletion polymorphism of the ACE gene have higher circulating [81] and tissue [82] levels of ACE. In a wide range of chronic renal diseases the DD genotype has been suggested to correlate with more rapid progression of renal impairment although not all reports have confirmed these findings (reviewed in [80]). In a study of 189 individuals from 46 families, PKD-1 patients with the DD genotype have been shown to have worse renal survival than patients with either the DI or II genotypes [83]. There was no detectable effect of the ATG M235T polymorphism or the AT1 receptor A1166C polymorphism on age of onset of renal disease and, in contrast to studies of myocardial infarction, no synergism of these polymorphisms with the ACE gene polymorphism.

Proteinuria

Heavy proteinuria is sufficiently uncommon in ADPKD that any polycystic patient with heavy proteinuria should be investigated for alternative causes [84]. At the levels most often encountered (300 mg/day or less) authors differ on whether urinary protein excretion is [59] or is not [55] associated with a more rapid rate of progression of renal impairment in ADPKD. This effect if present is relatively small.

Genetic defect

For PKD-1 the mean age of onset of ESRD is 53–59 years and for non-PKD-1 it is 69–73 years in a number of studies where direct comparisons have been made [10,57,85–88]. PKD-2 has a lower prevalence of hypertension at younger ages [87]; however, both PKD-1 and PKD-2 mutations may be associated with severe extrarenal manifestations and disease due to a PKD-2 mutation may be indistinguishable from the typical course for PKD-1 disease [67,89]. The finding that a large deletion of the PKD-1 gene associated with tuberous sclerosis is associated with unusually severe polycystic disease of the kidneys suggested that the nature of the ADPKD gene mutation may determine severity of disease [18]. However, mechanistically this is difficult to envisage and subsequent analyses have demonstrated large deletions associated with mild disease.

Family history

Two aspects of the family history have been suggested to allow prediction of likely course of disease when faced with an individual patient. In contrast to the initial description by Dalgaard [14] it is now recognized that there may be significant intrafamilial variation in disease expression [34,88]. Cairns [90] first suggested that younger generations of families with polycystic kidney disease have earlier onset disease. This was rejected by Dalgaard [14]. This idea of anticipation was revived by Fick *et al.* [91] who found evidence of progressively earlier onset of renal disease in 54% of 94 informative families. Torra *et al.* [58] studied 76 offspring/parent pairs finding 33 having onset of ESRD at least 10 years earlier for offspring than parent, 22 pairs have offspring onset 2–9 years earlier than parent, and 21 offspring with ESRD later than their parent. Prompted by this report Geberth *et al.* [33] carried out a detailed study of their ADPKD population analysing 74 parent–offspring pairs from 148 families. They provide strong evidence against anticipation, the difference in age at ESRD between parent and offspring being normally distributed. This would be in keeping with structural analyses as in conditions where anticipation is seen this may be explained by inherent instability of the gene in question (e.g. myotonic dystrophy or fragile X syndrome [92,93]). No such structural instability is evident in the PKD-1 or PKD-2 genes. The data of Geberth *et al.* argue for a random genetic or environmental event determining the age at renal death as discussed above and makes the family history of little help in predicting the course of disease in an individual patient. Importantly juvenile or neonatal onset ADPKD may differ in this respect forming a subgroup of patients with an additional genetic locus influencing manifestation of disease. In this group of patients anticipation may be seen.

Genetic imprinting

It has been suggested that the gender of the transmitting parent influences the prognosis in ADPKD. Bear *et al.* [88] studied 10 PKD-1 families finding that the mean age of onset of ESRD for patients with maternal inheritance was 50.5 years as opposed to patients with paternal inheritance who had a mean age of onset of 64.8 years ($p = 0.004$). Although an early report from the University of Colorado found no effect of gender of the transmitting parent [57] these workers subsequently noted a predominance of mothers as the transmitting parent when the age of onset for offspring was less than the parent [91]. Choukron *et al.* [55] found no significant effect of sex of carrier on rate of progression even when subdividing male and female patients. However, the onset of ESRD was sooner in male but not female patients when the disease was transmitted by mother as opposed to father (46.3 versus 54.1 years $p < 0.01$).

Race

In non-polycystic disease the MDRD study found a more rapid decline in GFR in African-American patients ($n = 53$, 19 ml/min over 3 years) versus non-African-American patients ($n = 525$, 11 ml/min over 3 years $p = 0.02$) [59]. This finding has been confirmed for ADPKD particularly in the presence of sickle cell disease (mean age of onset of ESRD black versus white patients 43.2 versus 55.4 years) [94].

Gender

Many, but not all [88], studies have demonstrated male gender to be associated with a worse prognosis in ADPKD [14,55,57,95–97]. Early studies did not control for differences in blood pressure raising the possibility that gender was acting as a determinant of blood pressure [96]. However, subsequent studies have excluded this possibility [57]. The data of the Colorado group suggested that the rate of progression of renal impairment once established is equivalent for male and female patients, the worse prognosis in male patients being secondary to earlier-onset disease [57]. The MDRD study confirmed this, demonstrating that females have a slower rate of decline than males in early renal insufficiency but that once GFR fell below 25 ml/min per 1.73 m^2 the rate of decline was equivalent in both sexes [59]. Studies in Han:SPRD-Cy/Cy rats have directly implicated testosterone in this effect [98]. In considering how testosterone may mediate this effect it is of interest that testosterone increases intrarenal mRNA for components of the renin–angiotensin system [99].

Others

Glomerular hyperfiltration is a normal accompaniment of pregnancy. As this may be deleterious to glomerular function the effect of parity on progression of renal disease in ADPKD is of interest. In 580 subjects from 194 families Gabow *et al.* [57] found that women having three or more pregnancies reached a serum creatinine of 130 μmol/l by a mean age of 51 years whereas those with fewer pregnancies reached this level by a mean age of 59. Bear *et al.* [88] could find no effect of parity on disease progression in 17 families studied. In addition to prognostic factors already discussed Gabow *et al.* [57] reported worse renal function at a given age with hepatic cysts in women, urinary tract infections in men, and one or more episodes of gross haematuria in either sex.

Effect of intervention

Consideration of pathogenetic mechanisms and factors associated with a poor prognosis suggests strategies for intervention in the development of ESRD in ADPKD. Theoretically, it may be possible to intervene at each stage of the pathogenetic process outlined above. At present our understanding of the pathogenesis of ADPKD is incomplete and interventions in the development of cysts are restricted to the laboratory. These will be reviewed briefly. However, following development of renal impairment it is important to ask whether control of exacerbating factors slows the rate of deterioration in renal function as in other forms of chronic tubulo-interstitial nephritis.

Cystogenesis

With cloning of the PKD-1 and PKD-2 genes and characterization of the gene products intervention at this basic level may ultimately be possible. However, the mechanism by which the genetic defect generates disease will ultimately determine what therapeutic options are possible. A dominant negative effect would require a gene therapy approach aimed at inactivating the deleterious gene. However, if, as seems probable, a loss of function model explains development of disease then delivery of a normal copy of the defective gene to renal epithelia might effect a cure. Given the small percentage of tubules which need to develop cysts in order to cause disease a normal allele would need to be delivered to a high percentage of epithelial cells in order to be effective. To achieve this in a stable manner with such a large gene is technically impossible at present.

Cyst expansion

Three aspects of cyst expansion may theoretically provide targets for intervention; increased cell proliferation, increased fluid secretion, and extracellular membrane abnormalities [100]. Paclitaxel blocks cell division through inhibition of microtubule polymerization. Woo *et al.* [101] demonstrated that paclitaxel slowed the progression of renal disease in C57BL/6J-*cpk*/*cpk* mice. The Han:SPRD-Cy/Cy rat model is considered a useful model for study of ADPKD [102], although the genetic defect is not in the rat homologue of the PKD-1 gene [103]. Martinez *et al.* [104] confirmed the findings of Woo *et al.* in *cpk* mice but not in Han:SPRD-Cy/Cy rats or DBA/2FG-pcy/pcy mice. They also found significant toxicity associated with paclitaxel administration. Hydroxymethylglutaryl CoA reductase inhibitors have the potential to inhibit fluid secretion and cellular proliferation. In the Han:SPRD-Cy/Cy rat lovastatin reduced the severity of disease in male but not female animals [105]. These findings await clinical evaluation. If cyst expansion is central to development of renal impairment, decompression of cysts may be expected to slow progression. Elzinga *et al.* [106] reported on the effects of cyst decompression in 30 patients. Although pain was relieved progression of disease was unaffected. Of particular interest were 19 patients who underwent unilateral decompression. Split function isotope scans did not show any change in the division of renal function after surgery. The percentage of cysts remaining intact is, however, central to determining whether this study refutes the suggestion that cyst expansion is central to the development of renal impairment. A further study reported laparoscopic marsupialization of cysts to be effective also in relieving pain [107]. This study used CT to assess the percentage of cysts decompressed but reported only small numbers of patients some of whom had simple cysts rather than ADPKD. Importantly, recurrence of cysts was noted.

Exacerbating factors

Hypertension

Of the interventions demonstrated to be effective in preventing progression of chronic renal impairment in general, treatment of hypertension is of particular interest in ADPKD as it has been identified as a prognostic indicator and a high frequency of polycystic patients are hypertensive. Only two prospective randomized controlled trials have reported data on an informative subgroup of patients with ADPKD. They concur, with no benefit on progression of disease [108,109]. However, the commonest cause of death in ADPKD is cardiovascular disease [13,110–112]. Thus the recommendations from the MDRD study are in keeping with this literature as a whole: blood pressure should be lowered to relevant national guideline levels to prevent cardiovascular morbidity and mortality but this or further reduction in blood pressure is not beneficial to the rate of progression of renal impairment [113].

It is of interest to consider why no benefit of treatment of hypertension was seen given the association between more progressive ADPKD and hypertension. When considering the effect of hypertension in the progression of ADPKD it is particularly worth reiterating that association does not prove causality. In an elegant study Geberth *et al.* [114] found that patients with ADPKD with a non-affected parent who had essential hypertension had a worse prognosis than patients with a non-affected parent who was spontaneously normotensive. Thus, an inherited deleterious trait may independently determine progression of renal disease and systemic hypertension.

Two studies have compared ACEI directly with other antihypertensives in non-diabetic CRF of diverse aetiology finding that ACEI had an effect over and above that of other antihypertensives producing a similar level of blood pressure control [115,116]. In a further prospective randomized placebo-controlled trial a benefit of enalapril over and above control of hypertension was suggested [117]. A fourth trial comparing benazepril with placebo found similar results but has been criticized for monitoring renal function by creatinine clearance [109]. In contrast Zucchelli *et al.* [118] found nifedipine and captopril to be equally effective but calcium channel blockers have themselves been suggested to have a renoprotective effect. Importantly, ACEI have been shown to inhibit proteinuria independent of an effect on systemic blood pressure [119]. Thus, data from these trials would be consistent with this slowing of progression being secondary to beneficial effects on glomerular hemodynamics and reduction of proteinuria rather than to the reduction in systemic MAP. As most ADPKD patients do not have significant proteinuria (only one in the >3 g/24 h group reported so far from the Gruppo Italiano di Studi Epidemiologici in Nefrologia (GISEN) study) it is not surprising that no effect of antihypertensive treatment or ACEI has been seen in this disease. The influence on progression of renal disease of genetic polymorphisms affecting components of the renin–angiotensin system is relevant to this discussion. Such effects may be particularly marked in ADPKD where abnormal activation of the renin–angiotensin system appears to be central to the development of hypertension. In keeping with this, inhibition of ACE specifically inhibits progression of renal disease in the Han:SPRD-Cy/Cy rat [120]. However, preliminary data presented by a number of workers at the 1997 American Society of Nephrology was conflicting with regard to ACE genotype as a predictor of progression of renal disease and development of hypertension in ADPKD. Two questions remain. First, it is unclear at what level of proteinuria treatment is indicated. This question will be addressed specifically by the GISEN study which has stratified patients to 1–3 g or >3 g and is ongoing. Second, it is not clear what dose of ACEI may be optimal in slowing progression in chronic renal disease associated with proteinuria. This is of particular relevance to ADPKD where over-activity of the renin–angiotensin system is suggested. Further studies using higher doses of ACEI may thus be of interest. Care should be taken as in any type of chronic renal disease as ADPKD patients showing acute reversible deterioration of renal function following commencement of ACEI have been described.

In their retrospective study of 174 patients with advanced chronic renal impairment Hannedouche *et al.* [61] found patients who were spontaneously normotensive to have a slower rate of progression than patients who achieved the same level of systemic blood pressure on antihypertensive treatment. This group contained 42 patients with ADPKD and the authors state that the results were similar when corrected for type of nephropathy. However, as would be expected, only 7% of the ADPKD group were spontaneously normotensive and it is therefore difficult to believe that this subgroup analysis is truly informative.

Protein intake

In animal models protein restriction slows progression of polycystic kidney disease [98]. Of the five prospective randomized controlled trials which have examined the effect of dietary protein restriction on progression of renal disease, three of these trials cannot be considered informative with respect to ADPKD as one did not report subgroup analyses [121] and in two [122–124] the ADPKD group was small. Locatelli *et al.* [125] and the MDRD study [59] reported 74 and 200 patients with ADPKD respectively. These studies showed no statistically significant effect of restricted protein intake on actuarial renal survival or mean progression rate in ADPKD.

Conclusions

Treatment options to slow the progression of renal impairment are becoming apparent for many patients with CRF. ADPKD has been particularly unrewarding in this respect. Although we can only speculate as to why, it is likely that the genetic defect and resulting pathophysiology/anatomy are so dominant in progression of disease that interventions aimed at limiting a progressive insult to the interstitium are irrelevant in this condition.

Postinfectious renal scarring, reflux nephropathy, chronic pyelonephritis, and non-cystic renal dysplasia

Reflux nephropathy accounts for up to 10% of patients in ESRD registries in Europe [126] and Australasia [127]. However, the most recent analysis of cause of ESRD from the United States, in which much more detail on primary renal disease was collected, indicated reflux nephropathy as the cause of only 0.5% of the total cases of ESRD, with chronic interstitial nephritis accounting for 2% [51]; and a recent report from Sweden showed no new cases of end-stage renal failure (ESRF) from non-obstructive pyelonephritis in children between 1986 and 1994 [128]. Some of these discrepancies may be due to changes in the diagnostic labels attached to patients with renal failure and focal renal scarring; the European data, in particular, lumps together reflux nephropathy, congenital and acquired obstruction, and a number of other categories [126]. The terms 'chronic atrophic pyelonephritis' and ' reflux nephropathy' have become more or less interchangeable in the vocabularies of many nephrologists, but this hides a great deal of diagnostic confusion. Several different diseases, which may well carry different risks of progressive renal failure, have been lumped together in published studies and registry data. These include postinfectious renal scarring caused by primary vesicoureteric reflux (VUR), renal damage associated with secondary VUR, renal damage associated with urinary tract obstruction, and renal dysplasia. Whether the incidence of serious renal damage associated with any of these diseases is indeed decreasing remains extremely uncertain.

Definition and pathogenesis

Reflux nephropathy: postinfectious focal renal scarring

Reflux nephropathy is the term commonly used for the radiological finding of focal renal scarring, usually confined to the upper and lower poles of one or both kidneys, with distortion (clubbing) of underlying calyces. The conventional view is that this scarring is caused by primary VUR in association with urinary infection. (The more cumbersome term 'postinfectious focal renal scarring' [129] may be more accurate, as there is seldom evidence of ongoing inflammation or infection). The focal scarring is most accurately detected by dimercaptosuccinic acid (DMSA) scanning, although this does not allow detection of the underlying calyceal abnormalities, which are best demonstrated by intravenous urography.

Clinical and experimental observations support the view that intrarenal reflux of infected urine occurs in compound papillae [130] and causes scarring within a few days [131–133]. Early antibiotic treatment can prevent scar formation in this situation, at least in animal models [132]; delay in diagnosis in children is significantly associated with the severity of scarring [134]. Compound papillae occur in the upper and lower poles of the human kidney, hence the distribution of scars. Reflux of sterile urine can, over prolonged periods of time, also cause scarring in pig models [135,136] but has not been shown to be important for the pathogenesis of scarring in humans. VUR is seen in 30–50% of children undergoing investigation for urinary tract infection [137] but is very rare in unselected children [138–140]. Scarring is found in up to 5% of children undergoing investigation for urinary tract infection [141], although this percentage depends on the criteria for referral and investigation of children suspected of having urinary tract infection. The likelihood of new scarring falls with age: most scars are formed within the first year of life, and studies using DMSA scanning show that the likelihood of new scarring after the fourth birthday is very low [142]; studies suggesting new scar formation in children over 5 used intravenous urography, which is less sensitive in detection of early scarring [143]. A follow-up study of children with antenatally diagnosed reflux supported the concept that focal scarring is most likely to be the result of urine infection in postnatal life [144]. Primary VUR is an inherited condition [145–149] which usually resolves in childhood: even if it does not, however, there is very little evidence that scarring results from ascending infection after the age of 5. Reflux nephropathy is an important cause of hypertension in childhood [129,133,150,151] and early adult life [152].

The widespread acceptance of this view of the pathogenesis of reflux nephropathy and its importance as a cause of childhood hypertension and childhood and adult renal failure have led to recommendations for the radiological investigation of all children with urinary infection [153] and of the offspring of parents with reflux nephropathy [154]. The assumption behind these recommendations is that early institution of antibiotic treatment or antireflux surgery will reduce the risk of progressive renal damage. However, there is no conclusive evidence that this assumption is correct, for several reasons:

1. Acute urinary infection can cause transient VUR [155].
2. Classical radiological appearances of reflux nephropathy have been described in children without any history of urinary tract infection [127], although it is impossible to be sure that such scarring is truly 'non-infective' unless regular urine cultures have been performed since birth, given the difficulties of diagnosing urine infection in infants.

3. An association between frequent upper urinary tract infection and renal scarring could be because urine infection with VUR causes scarring, or because VUR and scarring, like other anatomical abnormalities, act as risk factors for persistent urine infection.
4. There are no controlled trials of medical or surgical treatment against placebo in infants with VUR, and nor are there likely to be, as they would widely be considered to be unethical.

In addition to these problems, several different disease processes, each with their own aetiology and natural history may be classified as reflux nephropathy, and this has implications for treatment, including the prevention of progression.

Other causes of cortical scarring with calyceal deformity

Secondary vesicoureteric reflux VUR may be primary, or secondary to bladder disease. In primary VUR, the kidney is exposed to high pressure urine during micturition as a result of anatomical failure of the ureterovesical valve, often associated with ectopic, lateral insertion of the ureters into the bladder [156]. This results in intra-renal reflux, confined to compound papillae, explaining the polar distribution of scars in reflux nephropathy. In VUR secondary, for instance, to neurogenic bladder or to bladder outflow obstruction, the ureterovesical junction may be anatomically normal, but becomes incompetent due to high intravesical pressures. In this situation, the kidneys may be exposed to high pressure for prolonged periods (compared with the transient high pressure associated with primary VUR), converting non-refluxing papillae into refluxing papillae, and allowing widespread scarring to take place, possibly even in the absence of infection. Thus, primary and secondary VUR may carry very different risks of renal scarring, with or without coincident urine infection.

Dysplasia Primary VUR may frequently be associated with other congenital abnormalities, including renal dysplasia, which may cause a small scarred kidney with calyceal deformity indistinguishable from classical reflux nephropathy [135,136,157–160]. In this situation, renal scarring may be the result of dysplasia rather than reflux of infected urine—in which case scarring will not be prevented by early treatment and prophylaxis of urinary tract infections. For instance, radiological abnormalities of the kidneys detected *in utero* seem certain to be due to dysplasia or arrested growth rather than reflux of infected urine. Further evidence of the association between dysplasia and VUR comes from a study of the contralateral urinary tract in patients with unilateral renal dysplasia or agenesis, in whom VUR was present in 43% and 30% respectively [161]. VUR may also occasionally be associated with a small, smooth, unscarred kidney, possibly due to intra-uterine renal growth retardation as a consequence of VUR [159].

Papillary necrosis This may occur in infancy as a result of severe hypovolemia, causing identical radiological appearances [162].

Natural history

Because the diagnosis of chronic pyelonephritis requires radiological imaging, and may not otherwise come to medical attention, there are no data from unselected populations with the disease. All of the available information comes from series of patients known to have renal scarring, usually selected via hospital radiology or out-patient departments. Because of the diagnostic problems outlined above, all the studies in humans probably include a mixture of patients with reflux nephropathy, dysplasia, and other causes of scarring.

Rate of progression

Most studies which have included patients with reflux nephropathy have reported a slower rate of decline in renal function compared with other diagnostic groups [61,62,163–166]. These comparisons are likely to be heavily influenced by the criteria by which patients were selected: for instance, the inclusion of large numbers of patients with reflux nephropathy at low risk of progression would result in this conclusion, given that disease progression in many other diseases (e.g. diabetic nephropathy, polycystic disease) is often inexorable. However, the studies from the Necker Hospital [61,164,165] were all retrospective studies of patients who had already reached end-stage; in these studies patients with reflux nephropathy were included within the 'interstitial nephritis' category and not identified separately. Williams *et al.* studied patients with established renal impairment (serum creatinine >200 μmol/l, or >150 μmol/l and deteriorating), and found a lower rate of deterioration in reflux nephropathy (0.8±0.2 l/mmol per year) than in glomerulonephritis (2.3±0.4 l/mmol per year) and diabetic nephropathy (1.4±0.2 l/mmol per year) but higher than the mean rate in adult polycystic disease (0.5±0.05 l/mmol per year) [62].

Prognostic factors

Proteinuria

Increased excretion of tubular proteins has been reported to be a sensitive marker of tubular damage in children with reflux nephropathy. In one series urinary *N*-acetyl-β-D-glucosaminidase (NAG), retinol-binding protein (RBP), and albumin were measured in 40 children with VUR but no scarring, 93 children with VUR and various degrees of scarring, and 10 children with previous urinary tract infection but no VUR [167]. NAG and RBP excretion correlated well with the severity of scarring, RBP being a better discriminant. Another study has suggested that α_1-microglobulin is more predictive of the later development of decreased DMSA uptake and microalbuminuria: no measurements or estimations of GFR were reported [168]. A proportion of patients (42% in one series) [169] develop glomerular proteinuria, which may reach nephrotic proportions [170–174]. This is associated with glomerular abnormalities on renal biopsy [173–178]. Clinically detectable proteinuria is an important risk marker for subsequent progressive renal failure [62,169,175,179]. Williams *et al.* studied 108 patients with established renal impairment, including 13 with reflux nephropathy: even within this small subgroup there was a significant correlation between progression rate and 24 h protein excretion [62].

Hypertension

Because proteinuria and hypertension occur so frequently together, it is not surprising that, in univariate analysis, hypertension is a powerful predictor of progression in reflux nephropathy, as in other diseases [169,179].

Histological abnormalities

As discussed earlier, the development of glomerular proteinuria in patients with reflux nephropathy is associated with a high risk of progressive renal damage and is usually associated with systemic hypertension. Proteinuria may occasionally reach nephrotic proportions. Renal biopsy studies in such patients show a characteristic combination of focal segmental glomerulosclerosis (FSGS) and hyalinosis and periglomerular fibrosis; in the interstitium a chronic inflammatory cell infiltrate, together with patchy fibrosis, tubular atrophy, and vascular thickening is characteristic [170–178]. El-Khatib *et al.* reported inverse correlations between renal size (measured on urography) and both maximum glomerular size and the proportion of sclerosed glomeruli; the closest correlation with the amount of proteinuria was with the proportion of sclerosed glomeruli [175]. These observations are consistent with the hypothesis that loss of renal mass caused by pyelonephritic scarring results in glomerular hypertrophy and subsequently in progressive glomerulosclerosis, as observed in animal models [180–184] and in humans [185,186]. In a study of renal biopsies from 24 children and adolescents, all with relatively well preserved renal function, only four of whom were hypertensive, glomerular size was twice that of patients with minimal change nephrotic syndrome or normal renal biopsies and correlated directly with the amount of proteinuria and the percentage of segmentally sclerosed glomeruli, and inversely with renal size and GFR. Segmental glomerulosclerosis was of hilar origin (consistent with the classification of focal segmental sclerosis proposed by Howie [187]; marked thickening of hilar arteries was noted, with hyaline deposits within the walls of these vessels [177].

In contrast with these findings, a study of 86 nephrectomy specimens from children with reflux nephropathy failed to find any association between FSGS (present in 18 specimens) and age at nephrectomy, or severity of hypoplasia and/or scarring. FSGS was not present in 18 hypoplastic kidneys or 72 kidneys from children without VUR [188]. One explanation for these findings is that the nephrectomy specimens examined in this study were taken before FSGS had had time to develop in response to reduced nephron mass; no data were given on glomerular morphology.

Radiological findings

Although bilateral scarring is a risk factor for progressive renal failure [169,179] it is not a *sine qua non* for progression, implying that radiologically normal kidneys in patients with contralateral scarring are not normal; a suggestion which is supported by the finding of histological changes characteristic of reflux nephropathy in biopsies of kidneys which are radiologically normal [178]. A close correlation between renal excretory function and renal size has been reported in two studies [175,189]. In the first of these renal size was estimated by comparing the renal area on intravenous urography with the area of the first three lumbar vertebrae [175]. In the second, renal volume measured by CT was closely correlated with GFR in 29 patients with classical reflux nephropathy without hypertension or proteinuria [189].

Gender

A number of studies have reported more rapid progression in males than females in various renal diseases [61,164,165]. Of the studies confined to reflux nephropathy, Arze *et al.* did not examine the effect of gender [169]: Jacobson studied only women [190]; and El-Khatib found that male sex was a risk factor for progression on univariate but not multivariate analysis [179].

Recurrent infection?

As reviewed earlier, most evidence suggests that the acquisition of new scars is extremely rare after the age of 4, and certainly after the age of 10, in patients with primary VUR. However, it remains possible that ascending urinary infection might contribute to progressive renal damage, perhaps by inciting an inflammatory response within existing scars. Observational studies have reached divergent conclusions on this question. A long-term follow-up of 130 patients with classical radiological features of chronic pyelonephritis found repeated urinary infection in 83 of 83 of the patients with stable renal function and only eight of 22 of those with rising serum creatinine [169]. In contrast, a 5-year prospective study of 50 women, of whom five developed ESRD showed a higher rate of decline of GFR in patients with hypertension, bilateral scarring, and in those with an episode of symptomatic urinary tract infection during follow-up [190] although it was not clear whether each of these factors was predictive of progression in multivariate analysis. This is in contrast to a retrospective review of 30 patients followed since childhood reported earlier by the same author in which progression was unrelated to the incidence of urinary infections [129]. Recurrent acute pyelonephritis is more common in women with pyelonephritic scarring when compared with women with recurrent urinary tract infections in childhood who do not have scarring, and it is thus perhaps not surprising that severity of renal scarring is correlated with frequency of pyelonephritic episodes [191]. No relationship was found between recurrent urinary infections and progression in a series of 54 patients studied at the Mayo Clinic [174] Each of these studies suffers from the problems of selective referral; the findings are likely to be biased by the proportion of patients whose scarring was initially detected during investigation of recurrent urinary infection, compared with those who were referred with proteinuria or hypertension, for instance. Also, as discussed earlier, upper tract scarring may be the *cause*, rather than the *result*, of recurrent or persistent urinary tract infection. Clearly, patients with reflux nephropathy who present with symptomatic upper or lower urinary tract infection require prompt treatment, if only to relieve symptoms. Convincing proof that regular urine cultures and aggressive treatment of occult urinary tract infection is of benefit to patients with non-obstructive reflux nephropathy would require a randomized controlled trial. The practice of sending a mid-stream urine culture from such patients on an annual visit to the nephrology clinic has no rational basis at all.

In addition to these studies of patients with established renal scarring, there are a number of studies of the effects of covert bacteriuria in schoolgirls [192–194]. The Cardiff–Oxford group randomized 248 girls aged 5–12 with asymptomatic bacteriuria to antibiotic treatment or no treatment: no difference was found in the frequency of symptomatic urinary infections, development of new radiological scarring, kidney growth, or resolution of VUR [192]. The Newcastle study randomized 211 girls without renal scarring to antibiotic treatment or no treatment. At 5 years, no significant difference was found in renal growth [193]. However, a long-term follow-up at the age of 18 and during subsequent pregnancies showed that those children who had not received antibiotic treatment had a significantly smaller increment in GFR and significantly reduced fractional glucose reabsorption during pregnancy, suggesting impairment of renal functional reserve [194].

Angiotensin-converting enzyme genotype

Two studies have been reported in abstract or letter form. In one, 26 children with grade III or IV VUR were studies. Ten children had no scarring on DMSA scanning; the remaining 16 children had scars, including 13 with impaired renal function. The DD genotype was more common in the latter group (68.8% versus 20%, $p < 0.05$) [195]. In the other study, none of 16 children with scarring had the DD genotype, compared with 17% of children with VUR and no scarring and 18% of controls [196].

Effect of interventions

Antibiotic treatment

There have been *no* placebo-controlled trials of the effect of antibiotic treatment on new scarring, hypertension, or renal impairment, and such trials would now be considered unethical in children. In adults, where there is little convincing evidence that recurrent infections contribute to the risk of progressive renal damage, there would be no ethical reason not to perform a study to ask whether treatment of asymptomatic urine infection altered the risk of progression, but such a study would require large numbers of patients and is unlikely ever to be performed. The trials that do exist are trials comparing medical and surgical treatment of children with grade III and IV reflux: these are described in the following section.

Antireflux surgery

Two large-scale trials of the treatment of reflux nephropathy in children have been performed; the International Reflux study in Children and the Birmingham study [197–200]. The International study compared ureteric reimplantation with long-term antibiotic treatment in children with grade III and IV reflux; in the Birmingham study of children with grade III reflux, children in both groups received antibiotic chemoprophylaxis for 2 years, or for 5 years if significant reflux was still present. In both studies the majority of children had significant radiological scarring at entry, the severity of scarring being correlated with the severity of reflux. In both studies surgery was successful in abolishing reflux and in reducing the rate of acute pyelonephritis; despite this, there was no overall difference in the acquisition of new scars in the medically and surgically treated groups.

Antihypertensive treatment

Insufficient numbers of patients with reflux nephropathy have been included in the major randomized trials of antihypertensive treatment in the progression of non-diabetic renal disease to allow sub-group analysis of the effects of antihypertensive treatment in this diagnostic category. In the AIPRI study it was noted that the proportion of patients with interstitial nephritis was low in both treatment and placebo groups [109]. In a patient with proteinuric progressive renal failure and reflux nephropathy it would appear rational to treat hypertension with an ACE inhibitor, but a trial large enough to prove this is unlikely ever to be performed.

Protein restriction

The only randomized study to report separately on TIN showed no difference in cumulative renal survival between the 'controlled' protein group and the low protein group [125]. Other studies implied either a better [201] or worse [124] response to protein restriction in patients with TIN compared with those with glomerular disease.

Obstructive nephropathy

Urinary tract obstruction can occur at any age, but is important particularly as a cause of renal damage *in utero* and in early infancy, and, as a result of bladder outflow obstruction, in older men. Data on the importance of obstructive uropathy as a cause of end-stage renal failure are scarce. The European Registry reports congenital and acquired obstructive uropathy together with various types of pyelonephritis, which overall were responsible for 16.6% of the 22 489 cases reported [126]. In contrast, the USRDS reported that, together with nephrocalcinosis and so-called 'gouty' nephropathy, obstruction accounted for only 1.2% of the 305 876 patients receiving treatment for ESRD in 1991–1995 [51]. However, acquired obstructive uropathy is an important avoidable cause of acute [202] and chronic [203] renal impairment in older men.

Causes

Congenital

Urinary tract abnormalities account for 30–50% of fetal anomalies and are found in up to eight in every 1000 pregnancies, and carry a poor prognosis for survival, due to renal failure, oligohydramnios and pulmonary hypoplasia, and associated abnormalities when they are part of a malformation syndrome [204–208]. In a prospective study of 100 cases of antenatal hydronephrosis in Bristol, the abnormalities resolved soon after birth in 36 infants. In the remaining 64, 12 of 48 undergoing micturating cystography had unilateral or bilateral VUR, three had pelvi-ureteric junction obstruction, three had non-obstructive megaureter, and two had multicystic dysplastic kidneys. No focal scars were seen on DMSA scanning [208].

Causes of congenital obstruction include posterior urethral valves in males [209], neurogenic bladder (most often associated with spina bifida), pelvi-ureteric junction obstruction, and ureterovesical obstruction [210]. These urological abnormalities are often associated with renal dysplasia or hypoplasia, either because congenital obstruction impairs renal development [211] or because both are inherited together.

Bladder outflow obstruction

Patients with lower urinary tract symptoms are not a homogeneous group. Symptoms commonly referred to as 'prostatism' are not always due to prostatic bladder outflow obstruction, but may be due to detrusor instability or to detrusor underactivity, the distinction between these groups requiring urodynamic assessment [212]. The entity which gives rise to obstructive nephropathy is usually termed 'high pressure chronic retention' [213,214]; this usually presents with enuresis, a tense painless palpable bladder, salt and water retention with hypertension [214], and renal impairment with hydronephrosis. Typical 'obstructive ' symptoms of hesitancy, poor stream, and urinary frequency are often absent [213]. A direct correlation between end filling pressure in the bladder and serum creatinine has been reported [213]. One study has suggested that this syndrome is part of a continuum rather than a distinct entity [215]. Relief of obstruction corrects the hypertension [214] and results in improvements in renal function [216]. Renal impairment has been reported in 8% of patients undergoing prostatectomy, although this may be an underestimate, as a serum creatinine of >200 μmol/l was used as to define renal impairment [217].

Retroperitoneal fibrosis

Renal failure due to retroperitoneal fibrosis is rare, and often reversible. Presentation is usually with flank or abdominal pain and hypertension and occurs most commonly in middle-aged men; an acute phase response is common; and the diagnosis is best confirmed with intravenous urography followed by CT scanning [218]. Significant hydronephrosis may be absent [219,220]. The retroperitoneal inflammation is thought to be caused by an autoimmune response to components of atherosclerotic plaque [221,222]. Surgical ureterolysis followed by corticosteroid treatment, adjusted to suppress the acute phase response, is standard: steroid treatment alone is associated with an increased risk of loss of renal function [218], although a case can be made for a trial of steroid treatment with surgery if obstruction persists [223]. Ureteric stenting combined with steroids would appear sensible, if monitored carefully: the difficulty is in knowing when it is safe to remove the stent, as ureteric obstruction may persist after suppression of inflammation.

Diagnosis

Detection of hydronephrosis by ultrasonography has become widely accepted as the first-line investigation of suspected obstructive uropathy, both *in utero*, in children, and in adults [220]. However, obstructive uropathy can be present in the absence of hydronephrosis, most often as a result of fibrosis or encasement of the collecting systems, for instance in patients with malignant disease or retroperitoneal fibrosis [219,224]. Conversely, the presence of hydronephrosis does not necessarily indicate current obstruction, particularly in patients who have had obstruction in the past, who may be left with permanently 'baggy' collecting systems. Diagnosis of obstruction in such patients requires diuresis renography using Frusemide either 20 min after, or 15 min before the injection of the radiopharmaceutical [225]. Diagnostic accuracy is reduced in patients with a single kidney, in whom no comparison can be made between 'suspect' and 'normal' kidneys; and in patients with renal impairment, in whom the injection of Frusemide results in an attenuated diuretic response, even if the dose is increased [225]. Alternatively, a Whitaker test may be performed, involving measurement of the pressure generated within the renal pelvis during antegrade infusion of saline [226]; this has the advantage that the fine needle used for the antegrade perfusion can, if necessary, be changed for a nephrostomy tube, allowing what is probably the definitive test—waiting to see if direct drainage via the nephrostomy tube improves function. Low compliance of the upper tract during a Whitaker test is associated with low renal plasma flow when compared with obstructed kidneys with high compliance [227]. Resistive index is raised in acute obstructive nephropathy, but although relatively sensitive this finding is not specific [228].

Pathophysiology

Acute obstruction leads rapidly to an acute fall in glomerular filtration as a result in increased hydraulic pressure within the tubules, followed initially by afferent arteriolar vasodilatation and then, within 24 h, by afferent arteriolar vasoconstriction, possibly associated with a decrease in glomerular ultrafiltration coefficient. Numerous vasoactive mediators are involved in causing this vasoconstriction; these include angiotensin II, thromboxane A_2, leukotriene B_4, and endothelins. At the same time, vasodilator prostaglandins (e.g. E_2) and nitric oxide are produced, modulating the effects of vasoconstriction on GFR [229]. These changes are followed by macrophage infiltration, which may be responsible for the rapid development of interstitial fibrosis and tubular atrophy in animal models of obstruction [230]. Angiotensin II also induces fibrosis, *via* increased expression of transforming growth factor (TGF)-β and type IV collagen; in animal models, converting enzyme inhibition decreases macrophage infiltration and halts the development of tubulo-interstitial fibrosis after obstruction [231], even if treatment is delayed until after the insult [232]. Similarly, a thromboxane antagonist ameliorated both the functional and histological effects of transient unilateral ureteral obstruction in the rat when given before and after obstruction [233].

The effects of obstruction on renal function are most pronounced after relief of obstruction, and include distal renal tubular acidosis, impaired sodium reabsorption (partly due to increased atrial natriuretic peptide release as a result of volume retention during obstruction), and impaired water reabsorption [229,234–236]. Ongoing tubular injury can be detected by measurement of urinary *N*-acetyl-β-glucosaminidase [237]; a study in children suggested that this might be useful in predicting whether surgical correction of obstruction was likely to result in improvement of renal function [238], but this suggestion has not been tested prospectively. Post-obstructive diuresis and natriuresis often simply reflect mobilization of retained salt and water, but may continue to cause profound hypovolemia and further renal impairment; this is uncommon in practice, although occasional patients may be left with a permanent salt-wasting state requiring long-term sodium supplementation [239]. The degree to which renal excretory function returns after relief of obstruction is not related to the magnitude of the post-obstructive diuresis [239].

Natural history

Congenital obstructive uropathy

Congenital obstruction (for instance, due to urethral valves), as with congenital reflux, may be associated, either causally or because both are genetically determined, with dysplasia or arrested renal growth *in utero* [211,240]. Congenital unilateral renal dysplasia or aplasia is one of the few situations in which the human equivalent of remnant nephropathy has been described [241–243]. This may be because the growing kidney is more susceptible to development of glomerular hypertrophy and subsequent glomerulosclerosis than that of the adult; it may also be because the remaining kidney is also congenitally abnormal, with growth arrest causing oligomeganephronia. Prune belly syndrome, often cited as a cause of obstructive uropathy in children, is frequently associated with renal dysplasia [244]. Multiple urological abnormalities were noted in one series of 54 children who progressed to ESRF; for instance, VUR or obstruction were commonly seen in association with posterior urethral valves. The mean time from first detection of obstructive uropathy to end-stage was 9 years. At nephrectomy, evidence of hypoplasia or dysplasia was noted in 39 of 41 kidneys; these changes were frequently severe and diffuse, with associated tubulo-interstitial fibrosis and atrophy and glomerulosclerosis in viable glomeruli [210].

Long-term follow-up of boys with posterior urethral valves suggests that the presence of a 'pop-off' mechanism, reducing or preventing the transmission of high pressure to one or both kidneys, might be associated with better preservation of renal function. Three anatomical abnormalities were identified which might provide such protection: unilateral reflux into a dysplastic kidney; large congenital bladder diverticulae; and urinary extravasation with or without urinary ascites. At follow-up only one of 20 boys who had one of these three abnormalities had a serum creatinine above 1.0 mg/dl (88.4 mmol/l), compared with 20 of 51 boys without a 'pop-off' mechanism [245].

Acquired obstructive uropathy

Despite the high prevalence of acute renal failure caused by obstruction [202] and the extensive published literature on the pathophysiology of acute obstructive uropathy, there is surprisingly little information on the long-term outcome of severe obstructive nephropathy. It is well recognized that the degree of functional improvement after relief of obstruction depends on how much parenchymal damage has occurred, and that this is largely related to the time for which obstruction has been present; parenchymal thinning and increased cortical echogenicity are indicative of irreversible damage [246]. The patients reported by Sacks *et al.* who presented with severe renal impairment requiring dialysis had mostly had lower urinary tract symptoms for many years, and even in this group only eight of the 17 survivors required long-term dialysis [203]. Despite careful searching, we have been unable to find any systematic studies of the progression of renal failure after relief of obstruction. We suspect that this is because progression is, in fact, very rare in this situation, even if the patient is left with severe renal impairment. What case reports there are attest not so much to progression, as to recovery of renal function after relief of obstruction, sometimes after weeks to months of apparent complete loss of function [247–250].

Animal studies suggest that transient obstruction results in a permanent loss of filtering nephrons, offset by hyperfiltration in the remaining nephrons [251]. According to the hyperfiltration hypothesis, this would be expected to lead to FSGS and eventual progressive renal failure, if the initial insult were severe enough. However, the authors of one report of FSGS in obstructed kidneys were at pains to point out that this was only seen in areas of the kidney which also showed scarring, with intense interstitial and periglomerular inflammation, and only in one of 44 kidneys was FSGS found remote from the area of chronic inflammation [252]. While it might be argued that this failure to find 'remnant-type' FSGS after obstruction was due to the fact that these samples were from children, in whom FSGS might not yet have had time to develop, there are no studies in the literature to support the notion that FSGS or glomerular proteinuria commonly develop after relief of obstruction, even in patients who are left with severe renal impairment. This suggests to us that obstructive damage, even if causes extensive loss of nephrons, does not cause progressive glomerulosclerosis. Although the acute stage of obstructive nephropathy is an inflammatory process, destruction of nephrons only occurs in the acute 'destructive' phase: evidence of ongoing tubular damage is absent in the stable hydronephrotic phase [237]. FSGS following surgical partial nephrectomy is an 'inflammatory disease mediated by cytokines' [253]. Perhaps the lack of ongoing inflammation after relief of obstruction is the reason for the absence of progression.

Renal dysfunction associated with neurogenic bladder

Some patients with spina bifida or spinal cord injury are at risk of progressive renal injury as a result of sustained high pressure reflux, often exacerbated by ascending infection and/or mechanical obstruction by stones [254]. Those at highest risk are the group whose neurological injury causes uncontrolled reflex contraction of the bladder, associated with detrusor sphincter dyssynergia (contraction of the sphincter during bladder contraction): sustained and uncontrolled bladder contraction causes bladder muscle hypertrophy, trabeculation, high pressure reflux and/or vesicoureteric obstruction and diverticulum formation [255,256]. Patients with normal co-ordination of bladder contraction and those with areflexic, acontractile bladders are at lower risk. Similar abnormalities may be seen in occult spinal dysraphism, which is often associated with anorectal abnormalities [257,258]. Radiological evidence of upper urinary tract changes may be present at birth, or may develop in infants with initially normal upper tracts [259]. Renal parenchymal damage is avoidable with modern investigation and management [260]. Avoidance of renal damage requires video-urodynamic investigation, including measurement of residual urine pressure. Detrusor hyperreflexia is managed by intermittent self-catheterization and anticholinergic drugs; by sphincterotomy or urethral stents together with condom drainage in those unable to manage self-catheterization; by conduit diversion (see below); or by clam ileocystoplasty to create a low pressure bladder. Long-term suprapubic catheterization carries a significant risk of bladder cancer, and should therefore only be used as a temporary measure; urethral catheterization should be avoided. Whatever measures are used, long-term follow-up is mandatory to allow early detection of new upper tract changes.

Abnormal bladder emptying in the absence of neurological pathology has been termed non-neurogenic neurogenic bladder: synonyms include Hinman syndrome, detrusor-sphincter dyssynergia, dysfunctional lazy bladder syndrome, and occult neuropathic bladder. The syndrome is associated with a wide range of functional and psychosocial abnormalities. Progression to ESRF has been described [261,262].

Renal function following urinary diversion

Urinary diversion surgery, using an ileal or colonic conduit, has been widely used in the past for children with neurogenic bladder resulting from spina bifida and for adults with bladder malignancy. Ureterosigmoidostomy is rarely performed now, due to the associated metabolic complications [263]. Patients with ileal or colonic conduits are at remarkably high risk of progressive renal damage, by one of several mechanisms: obstruction at the ureteric anastomosis or at the stoma; reflux and infection; stone formation; or (possibly) progression as a result of previous pyelonephritic scarring. Numerous series have shown a high rate of development of abnormalities on urography in 'renal units' which were normal at the time of the initial operation [264–276]. Recurrent infection within the loop is associated with an increased risk of upper tract deterioration; absence of reflux is associated with better preservation of renal function (unless the absence of reflux is due to obstruction) [270]. In one small series of colonic conduits no 'renal unit' in which neither reflux or obstruction developed showed radiographic deterioration [274]. The putative advantage of the colonic conduit is that the thicker wall permits construction of a more successful antireflux anastomosis. However, the only randomized trial to compare ileal versus colonic conduits and antireflux versus refluxing anastomoses showed no difference in single kidney GFR between 'renal units' subjected to the various operations [276]. A non-randomized comparison of 63 patients with spina bifida managed with clean intermittent self-catheterization and 30 with urinary diversion showed a higher rate of radiographic renal deterioration, stone formation, and acute pyelonephritis in those with a diversion, in addition to adverse metabolic effects, particularly bone disease, in the diversion group [277]. For these reasons, diversion operations are now reserved for patients with malignancy and for those in whom all alternative means of urinary drainage have failed.

Analgesic nephropathy

Definition

Chronic interstitial nephritis due to analgesic ingestion was first described in the 1950s [278,279]. Analgesic related renal disease, however, remains the source of much controversy. Accordingly, the National Kidney Foundation (USA) convened a group of investigators and clinicians to develop recommendations on analgesic-related renal disease [280]. Two types of analgesic-related renal disease were identified; 'classic' AN and non-steroidal anti-inflammatory drug (NSAID)-related renal toxicity. Classic AN was defined as 'a disease resulting from the habitual consumption over several years of a mixture containing at least two antipyretic analgesics and usually codeine or caffeine. It is characterized by renal papillary necrosis and chronic interstitial nephritis that leads to the insidious onset of progressive renal failure'. NSAID-related renal toxicity was defined as 'a disorder characterized by one of several distinct presentations: acute renal failure secondary to renal vasoconstriction, interstitial nephritis often presenting as nephrotic syndrome due to minimal change glomerulopathy, hyperkalemia, sodium and water retention, and, rarely, papillary necrosis.'

Classic analgesic nephropathy

Epidemiology

The prevalence of analgesic nephropathy (AN) differs considerably between countries and has been falling significantly in the last 20 years (reviewed in [281]). Switzerland has the highest prevalence in Europe with 28% of patients accepted for renal replacement therapy having a diagnosis of classical AN in 1981 and still 12% in 1990. In contrast in the US the prevalence of AN in patients reaching ESRF less than 1%. Most countries are seeing a fall in prevalence which correlates with legislation controlling the availability of analgesics. Importantly, the Scandinavian and Australian experience emphasizes that it is legislative measures controlling over the counter sales of analgesic mixtures rather than withdrawal of a single agent which is important ([282], reviewed in [283]).

Diagnosis

The hallmark of AN is papillary necrosis and chronic interstitial nephritis [278,284,285]. As chronic interstitial nephritis is not specific for this disease, papillary necrosis may be difficult to demonstrate and reporting of analgesic intake by patients may be unreliable [286–288], the diagnosis of AN is problematic. Three prospective multicentre controlled studies have recently been undertaken to validate the criteria for diagnosis of AN ([289–291], reviewed in [292]). An initial Belgian study [289] led to the formation of the Analgesic Nephropathy Network of Europe (ANNE) specifically to evaluate more widely the criteria for diagnosis of AN [290]. Five hundred and ninety-eight patients with equivocal causes of ESRD who began dialysis between 1991 and 1992 in 23 dialysis centres in 14 European countries and Brazil were identified. Patients were evaluated using a questionnaire and sonography plus either conventional tomography or CT scan. Eighty-two patients consuming analgesic mixtures daily for at least 5 years and 495 controls were evaluated further. This study confirmed the results of the earlier study showing that renal imaging demonstrating a decrease in length of both kidneys together with either bumpy contours or papillary calcification is the only reliable method for diagnosis of AN. Although all techniques estimated renal size adequately, CT scan was significantly better than the other investigations at detecting papillary calcification (sensitivity 87%, specificity 97% in ESRD, sensitivity 92%, specificity 100% in mild to moderate renal impairment). The importance of this finding in the diagnosis of AN led this group to recommend CT scanning without contrast as the investigation of choice if considering the diagnosis of AN [291].

Pathogenesis

The National Kidney Foundation (USA) criteria specifically define AN as resulting from ingestion of analgesic mixtures. The role of analgesic mixtures as opposed to single agents remains controversial [293] and it is of interest to review the evidence for the role of individual analgesic agents. Original studies implicated phenacetin and this analgesic was subsequently removed from analgesic mixtures in much of Europe, the USA, and Australia. When reporting European Dialysis and Transplant Association–European Renal Association Registry data on the incidence of ESRD due to AN, Brunner and Selwood [281] emphasized the falling incidence across Europe since reduction in availability of phenacetin. A single case–control study reported no excess of analgesic intake in 527 patients with ESRD but defined 'abuse' as almost daily consumption for only 30 days [294]. However, a number of case–control studies [295–300] and two prospective studies [301,302] have demonstrated that removal of phenacetin from sale has not abolished AN as they reported a range of analgesic mixtures to be associated with a significantly increased risk of ESRD. Barrett has reviewed this literature pointing out methodological problems with the case–control studies [303]. However, overall these studies confirm the nephrotoxic potential of chronic analgesic intake particularly if analgesic mixtures are taken and highlight the injurious potential of acetaminophen (paracetamol). The absolute risk of developing ESRD even with prolonged daily analgesic intake is, however, low. Dubach *et al.* [301] studied 623 working women with evidence of analgesic abuse and 621 age-matched controls. They calculated an absolute risk of developing ESRF attributable to analgesic abuse of only 1.7/1000 per year.

The central role of phenacetin was first challenged on epidemiological grounds; the decrease in incidence of AN in Belgium and Australia resulted from restriction of the availability of analgesic mixtures not from withdrawal of phenacetin (reviewed in [292,304]). A role for acetaminophen is in keeping with the early reports of phenacetin-induced interstitial nephropathy and papillary necrosis as phenacetin undergoes extensive first-pass metabolism generating predominantly acetaminophen with very little phenacetin being detectable in the kidney [305–307]. Thus, although phenacetin was the first analgesic implicated in AN, these data would suggest its metabolite, acetaminophen, to be the injurious agent. This is clearly important as phenacetin was only available in combined analgesics and when it was withdrawn it was frequently replaced with acetaminophen. Furthermore, acetaminophen is consumed as a single agent in large amounts. Turning to consideration of whether chronic ingestion of single analgesics cause renal damage, animal studies show phenacetin, acetaminophen, and aspirin alone to be able to cause papillary necrosis ([308,309], reviewed in [310]). There are also case reports of AN following apparent ingestion of acetaminophen alone [311]. The case–control studies discussed above are less clear on the injurious potential of single agents, only three studies presenting relevant data [296,299,300]. In their population based study Perneger *et al.* [300] interviewed 716 patients drawn from the Mid-Atlantic Renal Coalition registry of patients with ESRD and 361 control subjects. Patients were assigned to nine groups on the basis of lifetime intake of three analgesic agents (0–999, 1000–4999, >5000 tablets for each of acetaminophen, aspirin, and NSAIDs). Odds ratios were then calculated adjusted for age, sex, race, use of other drugs included in this analysis, and possible consumption of phenacetin. No increase in odds ratio for ESRD was seen for lifetime consumption of 0–999 tablets of any of the three analgesic groups. Significantly increased odds ratios were seen for 1000–4999 (2.0, 1.3–2.2) and >5000 (2.4, 1.2–4.8) acetaminophen containing tablets and >5000 (8.8, 1.1–71.8) NSAIDs. This study challenges the suggestion that AN is seen only with combination preparations as it adjusts for ingestion of other agents in the calculation of odds ratios. Data were, however, not presented on the percentage of patients taking a single agent and adjustment cannot be made for a synergistic action as discussed below for aspirin and acetaminophen. In contrast to other single agents, large numbers of patients taking aspirin alone for prolonged periods of time have been studied and shown to have no excess of renal impairment [312–315]. Of the case–control studies discussed above three found no increased risk of ESRD with ingestion of aspirin alone and one found an odds ratio of 2.5 (CI 1.24 to 5.20) as compared with an odds ration of 19.0 for phenacetin containing analgesic mixtures. Importantly, aspirin has been suggested to increase greatly the potential for papillary necrosis following acetaminophen ingestion by depleting renal papillary glutathione, which is then not available for conjugation with the injurious metabolites of acetaminophen [316].

Given the large amount of analgesic which needs to be ingested before disease develops it is unlikely that the potential for renal injury will be manifest in humans if a single agent is ingested. However, if the potentially synergistic combination of aspirin and acetaminophen is taken, particularly in association with a substance which may be addictive, the likelihood of ingesting sufficient analgesic to cause renal injury is greatly increased.

Two aspects of chronic analgesic ingestion are of particular interest when addressing the question of progression of chronic TIN; does renal impairment progress if analgesic intake is stopped and does analgesic intake influence progression of other types of renal disease. Unfortunately, inadequate data are available to be able to provide an answer to either of these questions. Hauser *et al.* [317] followed 23 patients with AN who reported abstention from analgesic abuse. In 12 patients no deterioration in plasma creatinine was seen over 1 year. In 11 patients the mean serum creatinine rose from 3.86 ± 1.06 to 6.4 ± 3.18 mg/dl in the same time period. Blood tests for acetaminophen and salicylate were positive in two patients from the group without progression and nine patients from the group showing progression of disease. Schwarz *et al.* [318] studied 57 patients with AN concluding similarly that continued analgesic abuse was associated with a more rapid decline in renal function. However, those patients apparently abstaining from analgesic intake still showed progression of renal impairment with a loss of GFR of 4.1 ± 11.0 ml/min per year. De Broe and Elseviers reviewed the published data on the influence of analgesic ingestion on progression of renal disease [292]. Three case–control studies had claimed an increased odds ratio for development of ESRD due to renal disease other than AN if there was also a significant intake of analgesics. As discussed above these studies are methodologically flawed and no definitive conclusion can be reached.

Treatment

Management of AN may be considered under two headings: prevention of further abuse and management of complications [319]. The importance of abstention from analgesic intake is illustrated by a study of 57 patients with AN who were monitored for the presence of acetaminophen in the urine [318]. The 13 patients who continued to abuse analgesics had a mean loss of GFR of 6.9 ± 5.5 ml/min per year whereas the 44 patients who abstained from analgesic abuse had a mean rate of deterioration of 4.1 ± 11.0 ml/min per year with all nine patients showing improvement in function abstaining from analgesic intake. These findings, however, demonstrate that renal impairment in AN is progressive in most patients even following abstention from analgesic intake. Furthermore, abstention is often difficult to achieve as central to this syndrome is the addictive nature of the agents abused [320]. Thus Schwarz *et al.* [318,321] found that 21% of analgesic abusers with renal impairment and 25% on hemodialysis continued their abuse. The effect of interventions of proven benefit in other forms of chronic TIN has not been determined in AN. The essential predisposing factor in animal models is dehydration [322] and close attention should therefore be paid to fluid balance, particularly given the reduced urinary concentrating ability seen in many patients with AN. Acute deterioration in renal function may be seen secondary to obstruction caused by a sloughed papilla and appropriate investigations to exclude this most be performed. Recurrent urinary tract infection is common in patients with AN [319]. Patients with AN show actuarial survival on hemodialysis equal to that of patients with other renal diseases

[321] and recurrence following transplantation, even with continued analgesic abuse, is rare [323].

Non-steroidal anti-inflammatory drugs

A number of distinct renal syndromes attributable to NSAID use have been identified [280,324–328]. Chronic interstitial nephritis and papillary necrosis are of relevance to this discussion of chronic TIN. In their review of renal complications due to NSAIDs, Carmichael and Shankel found papillary necrosis to be the commonest defined complication occurring in 20% of cases cited in the world literature to that date [329].

Diagnosis

Although patients abusing NSAIDs do not have the characteristic psychological profile associated with classical analgesic abuse, the renal manifestations of these two syndromes are similar [330]. No studies have defined precisely the amount of NSAIDs which need to be taken in order to be at risk of chronic interstitial nephritis and papillary necrosis. Using intravenous pyelography, renal ultrasound and/or CT Segasothy *et al.* [331] identified 38 patients who had radiological evidence of papillary necrosis and had consumed at least 1000 NSAID capsules and/or tablets. Twenty-nine patients had consumed only NSAIDs and 26 of the 38 had an elevated plasma creatinine. Thus the radiological criteria defined for classical analgesic abuse would seem to be appropriate for NSAID-related disease and 1000 capsules and/or tablets are sufficient to cause disease. In a case–control study, Sandler *et al.* [298] compared 554 North Carolina residents with a new diagnosis of chronic renal dysfunction and 516 age-, race-, and sex-matched controls. The increased risk of chronic renal disease was confined to men over 65 years of age with daily NSAID use for the previous year. When corrected for ingestion of other analgesics this group had an odds ratio of 10.0 (CI, 1.2–82.7).

Pathogenesis

In experimental animals a wide range of NSAIDs have been demonstrated to cause papillary necrosis [308,325,332–334]. In the rat these effects are potentiated by caffeine [335]. In humans caffeine has been suggested to potentiate the nephrotoxicity of mefenamic acid [336] but this effect was not substantiated for unspecified NSAID use in the case–control study of Sandler *et al.* [298]. Phenylbutazone [337–339], indomethacin [338–340], naproxen [341], benoxaprofen [342], ibuprofen [338,343,344], ketoprofen [331], diclofenac sodium [331], mefenamic acid [345,346], fenoprofen [347], and piroxicam [328] have all been reported as causing papillary necrosis in humans.

Progression

Their is a paucity of data on progression of NSAID related chronic renal impairment. Four of the 26 patients reported by Nanra [330] showed a progressive decline in GFR.

Balkan nephropathy

Balkan endemic nephropathy (BEN) occurs in specific localized areas in alluvial valleys of tributaries of the Danube river in the Balkan states of south-east Europe [348,349]. It is characterized by low molecular weight proteinuria [350,351] (including increased β_2-microglobulin excretion), anemia disproportionate to the degree of renal impairment [352] and a slow progression to ESRF. It has been suggested that the low molecular weight proteinuria (and in particular β_2-microglobulinuria) is not simply a marker of tubular damage but may play a pathogenetic role [353]. The histological findings are those of TIN [354]. The prognosis is poor with relentless progression to ESRF. In areas where BEN is prevalent as many as 50% of patients on renal replacement therapy may have BEN as the cause of their renal failure. The epidemiological data argue strongly for an environmental insult as the triggering factor in BEN [355,356]. Study of patients who are exposed to this initial insult but then leave the endemic area could therefore provide useful insight into whether renal impairment secondary to tubulo-interstitial disease inevitably progresses even in the absence of the initiating factor. Although it has been reported that emigres before age 17–18 do not develop disease data on patients who emigrate after development of disease is lacking. Furthermore, few data are available on the effects of interventions shown to be useful in other types of chronic tubulo-interstitial nephropathy. Thus, consideration of BEN cannot at present shed light on whether progression is inevitable in tubulo-interstitial disease even in the absence of the initial insult.

Chinese herb nephropathy

Recently, a rapidly progressive fibrosing interstitial nephritis has been described in association with ingestion of Chinese slimming herbs [357,358], characterized by low molecular weight proteinuria [359]; quantitation of urinary neutral endopeptidase may help in predicting progression [360]. The nephrotoxic substance appears to be Aristocholic acid, resulting from the inadvertent substitution of *Aristocholia fang chi* for *Stephania tetrandra*. This condition may be associated with an increased risk of urothelial malignancy [361]. An increased incidence of cardiac valvular abnormalities has also been reported, but may have been due to concomitant ingestion of fenfluramine, dexfenfluramine, or phentermine.

Chronic renal allograft nephropathy

Definition

Although 1 year renal allograft survival has improved significantly over the last decade, the half-life of a renal transplant has changed very little [362,363]. Thus, the leading cause of graft loss, after death of the patient with a functioning graft, is now late allograft failure, often called chronic renal allograft dysfunction (CRAD). Parallels may be drawn with the graft arteriosclerosis seen in up to 60% of cardiac allografts and the bronchiolitis obliterans seen in up to 50% of lung transplants. CRAD is a useful terminology as it encompasses the numerous causes of late graft failure

Table 10.1 Pathological mechanisms causing chronic allograft dysfunction

Immunological	Non-immunological
Chronic allograft nephropathy	
Late acute rejection	Remnant nephropathy
Cyclosporin resistant T-cell responses	Recurrent disease
	De novo glomerulonephritis
	Cyclosporin toxicity
	Obstruction
	Infarction
	Infection
	Renal artery stenosis

(Table 10.1) without inferring a pathophysiological mechanism [364]. Of interest in discussion of chronic TIN is the subset of patients with CRAD who have 'chronic transplant nephropathy' [365]. This term is preferred to the more often used chronic rejection as this latter terminology implies an immunological mechanism, whereas the aetiology of chronic transplant nephropathy remains undetermined, but is clearly multifactorial with immunological and non-immunological insults contributing [366–371]. In this review the terms chronic rejection and chronic allograft nephropathy will be used interchangeably as determined by usage in the study to which reference is being made. Chronic allograft nephropathy is characterized by a slow decline in GFR usually in association with proteinuria and hypertension. Characteristic histological changes have been described. The Banff classification [365] grades 'chronic transplant nephropathy' on the basis of interstitial fibrosis, tubular atrophy and glomerular changes without reference to vascular abnormalities. Hume *et al.* [372] first described the vascular changes often considered typical of chronic rejection in a human 'homotransplant' surviving 5½ months without immunosuppression. Mihatsch *et al.* [373] included vascular and glomerular changes in their classification considering interstitial fibrosis in the absence of vascular or glomerular pathology insufficient for the diagnosis of chronic rejection. Some authors have defined separate entities of transplant glomerulopathy versus chronic tubulo-interstitial rejection with differences in risk factors and 2-year graft survival [374]. More often these diagnoses are considered together as part of the spectrum of chronic allograft nephropathy, with the glomerular changes most often being associated with vascular changes [369].

Early vascular and glomerular changes specific for chronic rejection have been described in a significant proportion of cases in the setting of apparently normal graft function (reviewed in [364,375,376]). Thus a committee convened at the 4th Alexis Carrel Conference included the Banff classification within a working definition of 'chronic rejection' which included clinical and histological criteria [377]. The severity of the histopathological findings correlates with long-term function and both the Banff classification and the classification proposed by the committee convened at the 4th Alexis Carrel Conference have been shown to be useful in prediction of graft outcome [378,379].

Incidence and natural history

Renal allograft failure is the fourth commonest cause of ESRF in the US and accounts for 11–25% of late graft loss [380–383]. In a prospective study of 128 patients carried out in Helsinki, using protocol biopsies at 2 years post-transplantation, 40% of patients had histological evidence of 'chronic rejection'. At 4–5 years 30% of the same group of patients had clinical graft dysfunction [375]. The rate of fall in GFR accelerates in most but not all patients [384,385]. From onset of fall in GFR to graft failure is typically 3–4 years [385].

Diagnosis

The triad of deteriorating graft function, hypertension, and proteinuria are typical of chronic allograft nephropathy. However, care should be exercised as many patients identified using these criteria alone have alternative causes for their graft dysfunction. Obstruction and renal artery stenosis should be excluded before proceeding to transplant biopsy to confirm the diagnosis. Importantly, this will also facilitate exclusion of overt cyclosporin toxicity. Registry data suggest that 1–2% of adult patients with CRAD will have recurrent disease [386].

Risk factors

The serum creatinine at 6 months post-transplantation has been shown to be an important predictor of long-term graft function [387]. Many risk factors have been proposed for chronic allograft graft dysfunction [371,388] including; number of episodes of acute rejection [387,389–399], 'severity' of acute rejection [395,396,400–403], HLA mismatch [394,401,403–407], delayed graft function [401,405,406,408–410], increased donor age [387,394,398,403,406,407,411–413], donor source (living related versus cadaveric) [401], female donor [394,399,413,414], increased cold ischaemic time [405,415], recipient obesity [416], infection [bacterial or viral [394]], cytomegalovirus (CMV) [403,417,418], or hypercholesterolemia [370,419–421]. A number of reports have also suggested 'low-dose' cyclosporin to be associated with a higher incidence of chronic graft loss [394,422,423]. Further analysis of the effect of cyclosporin dose suggests that a trough level lower than 100 ng/ml at 1 year may be associated with increased 'chronic rejection' [424]. As in other forms of renal disease, the effect of ACE genotype on renal allograft survival has been studied. No influence of ACE I/D polymorphisms on allograft survival could be detected in a study of 269 Caucasian patients [425]. Other authors have reported no effect of donor age [396,400], warm ischemia time [396], cold ischemia time [426], hyperlipidemia [383,427] or 'low-dose' cyclosporin (<5 mg/kg per day at 1 year [398], mean cyclosporin dose of 3.2 mg/kg (trough levels 80–120 ng/ml) from 3 months post-transplantation [428].

From this plethora of data using different immunosuppressive regimens in patient populations from widely disparate population groups which risk factors stand out as most important?

In a study of 642 patients receiving first cadaveric grafts at a single centre four variables were significantly associated with biopsy proven 'chronic rejection'; increased donor age, CMV disease, acute rejection episodes, and HLA-DR match [403]. These authors emphasized the need for care when extrapolating from the literature in general to a particular patient population.

Acute rejection

In a multivariate analysis it was concluded that acute rejection episodes are the most important risk factor for biopsy proven chronic rejection [394]. However, even this risk factor is not universally accepted [429,430]. Emphasizing the concerns about extrapolating from the literature as a whole to a particular patient population, the Finnish population studied in these latter reports may not be representative due to the high genetic homogeneity of this population. Furthermore, the latter report used a clinical definition of chronic allograft nephropathy without histopathological confirmation. Massy *et al.* [401] reported on 706 renal transplants surviving more than 6 months performed between 1976 and 1991 at Hennepin County Medical Center, Minneapolis. 84% of patients with progressive decline in renal function were biopsied, chronic rejection being diagnosed according to the description of Kasiske *et al.* [400]. This study found late (after 3 months) acute rejection to be the most important risk factor for chronic rejection. Interestingly, donor source, number of DR mismatches, and delayed graft function were all risk factors for chronic rejection on univariate analysis but these factors did not influence chronic rejection independent of acute rejection on multivariate analysis.

It is likely that acute rejection *per se* is not associated with chronic allograft nephropathy, but that the type of acute rejection is of more importance, i.e. steroid resistant acute rejection, late acute rejection (after 3 months) or acute vascular rejection [387,396,400,401,405]. This would be consistent with the findings of Isoniemi *et al.* [429] as this study only included acute rejection episodes occurring before 3 months which may not predict chronic graft loss in this scheme.

It has also been argued that it is not the severity of the rejection episode that determines long-term graft survival, but its reversibility. Thus even steroid-resistant rejection may be associated with a good prognosis if treatment achieves a plasma creatinine below 130 μmol/l [431].

Donor age

A deleterious effect of increased donor age is frequently reported. Reviewing the United Network for Organ Sharing (UNOS) data, Terasaki *et al.* [407] have argued that up to 21% of kidney allograft failures result from insufficient renal mass due to age. In this patient group the 5-year graft survival of zero HLA-A, -B, and -DR mismatched kidneys fell from 81% with donor age 21–30 to 39% with donor age greater than 60. Unfortunately, many confounding factors complicate this analysis as kidneys from older donors may differ from kidneys from younger donors in many respects (e.g. pre-existing vascular disease).

HLA mismatch

In most studies HLA mismatch is a determinant of long-term graft survival. Which loci are of most importance is less clear. In European patients HLA-A, -B, and -DR matching significantly affects long-term graft survival [432]. This benefit may be particularly marked for black kidney allograft recipients [433]. In contrast Flechner *et al.* [387] reported no effect of HLA mismatch on graft survival in 507 first renal allografts receiving cyclosporin-based immunotherapy in Cleveland, Ohio and UNOS registry data does not show a benefit of matching at DR [434]. Furthermore, detailed DNA typing can subdivide the commonly identified 'broad specificities' at the A, B, and DR loci into 'split specificities'. Matching for split specificities at the class I loci has been shown to result in improved graft survival in European populations [435,436]. The situation for splits at the DR locus is more complex with no effect seen for first cadaveric grafts but a benefit of matching for split specificities becoming apparent for regrafts [437]. Finally, matching at the DPB locus has been suggested to be beneficial also to allograft survival [438].

Cytomegalovirus

CMV infection is of clear importance in cardiac allografts [439] and in a rat model of chronic renal allograft rejection CMV infection has been shown to exacerbate graft arteriosclerosis [440]. However, the role of CMV viremia in CRAD in humans is less clear [441]. CMV infection has most often been associated with transplant glomerulopathy [442,443], although even this lesion is controversial [444]. CMV infection has been suggested as a trigger for acute rejection [445,446], which may in turn have deleterious effects on long-term graft function.

Pathophysiology

It is unlikely that, even in an individual kidney, a single mechanism is responsible for the development of chronic allograft nephropathy. A multitude of insults, both immunological and non-immunological, acute and chronic, may initiate the chain of events which ultimately brings about graft failure. The role of non-immunological factors is emphasized by the development of histopathological features similar to those of chronic rejection in experimental and human isografts [447,448] and by the 40% failure at 10 years of human grafts between identical twins [448]. Two general mechanisms have been proposed to explain the development and progression of chronic allograft nephropathy. They differ in the target for the primary insult, although both may occur in parallel. The 'response-to-injury' hypothesis considers the vascular changes to be predominant, drawing a direct parallel with atherosclerosis [449,450]. The vascular lesions typical of chronic renal allograft nephropathy are suggested to develop following repeated endothelial injury with subsequent smooth muscle cell and fibroblast proliferation and extracellular matrix deposition [370,451,452]. Many of the 'injuries' recognized as predisposing to late graft failure would impact directly on the endothelium. The second related but distinct hypothesis sees nephron underdosing as the initiating event with all other changes consequent upon this deficiency. Clearly, a graft which starts disadvantaged in terms of nephron mass is more likely, following further insults, to reach the threshold at which hyperfiltration becomes significant. In support of this hypothesis, analysis of UNOS data has suggested that kidneys predicted to have lower nephron number (female donor, donor at extremes of age range and African-American donor), have poorer graft survival (reviewed in 364, [412]) as discussed above. However, these grafts may be 'high risk' in many respects in addition to reduced nephron number and a study of 169 patients grafted between 1989 and 1994 at SUNY Health Science Center, New York, did not show any correlation between kidney volume/body surface area ratio and serum creatinine, degree of proteinuria, or graft survival up to 5 years [453]. Hyperfiltration as a mechanism of progression of tubulo-interstitial disease in general has been reviewed elsewhere in this volume. The influence of nephron mass specifically on allograft survival has been elegantly studied in the Fisher (F344) to Lewis rat model [454,455]. The F344 kidney is particularly prone to develop increased glomerular capillary pressure and proteinuria following reduction in renal mass [456]. MacKenzie *et al.* [454] transplanted F344 kidneys into unilaterally nephrectomized Lewis recipients and at day 7 manipulated nephron mass by either excising the contralateral kidney, leaving it in place or replacing it with a second F344 kidney. Rats with only one kidney developed proteinuria, segmental glomerulosclerosis, and glomerular hyperfiltration without systemic hypertension. A second native *or* allogeneic kidney protected against these changes.

The distinction between the 'response-to-injury' and 'nephron underdosing' hypotheses may be thought artificial as they most probably define ends of a spectrum with reality lying somewhere in between. Furthermore, vascular injury may of course lead to nephron loss and glomerular hyperfiltration to endothelial damage. The two hypotheses are, however, fundamentally distinct in their definition of the primary insult and this may be relevant when considering therapeutic interventions.

Of particular interest are the roles of cyclosporin A and TGF-β in development of chronic allograft nephropathy. Both may contribute to endothelial damage, nephron loss and interstitial fibrosis.

Role of cyclosporin

The history of cyclosporin-based immunosuppressive regimens has been characterized by initial enthusiasm for this agent's improved immunosuppressive effects followed by concern about its nephrotoxicity. Improved 1 year graft survival with cyclosporin has not translated into an improved graft half-life and theoretical considerations, animal studies, and some clinical observations argue for progressive loss of GFR with chronic cyclosporin usage even without overt nephrotoxicity [380,457,458]. A number of mechanisms for this have been proposed. First, cyclosporin may have deleterious effects on vascular endothelium in general [459] and graft vasculature in particular [460]. Second, cyclosporin may induce systemic hypertension and hyperlipidemia. Third, cyclosporin has been suggested to potentiate directly TGF-β release as discussed below. Finally, if cyclosporin-induced graft ischemia induces activation of the renin–angiotensin system, increased angiotensin II production may exacerbate TGF-β mediated graft fibrosis. Thus, cyclosporin itself may contribute to the progressive tubulo-interstitial disease characteristic of chronic allograft nephropathy and a balance between the deleterious effects of cyclosporin and maintenance of adequate immunosuppression was for many years the holy grail. Until recently the drugs most frequently used were cyclosporin, azathioprine, and prednisolone, and a number of studies have been undertaken to address the optimum usage of these agents. We will not consider here the benefits of continued prednisolone usage versus withdrawal as this is not directly relevant to the discussion of tubulo-interstitial nephropathies. Attempts to ameliorate the potentially deleterious effects of cyclosporin on the tubulo-interstitial compartment are, however, central to discussion of progressive graft dysfunction. Four types of study have been undertaken:

1. First, cyclosporin based immunosuppression has been compared directly with azathioprine and prednisolone from the time of transplantation. Review of published series comparing 4000 cyclosporin-treated patients with 10 000 azathioprine-treated patients [461] and Collaborative Transplant Study Data [462,463] do not support a deleterious long-term effect of cyclosporin in the transplant population as a whole. Considering the data from the Collaborative Transplant study these data are subject to all of the criticisms of retrospective analyses. However, patients receiving cyclosporin alone or cyclosporin plus steroids were receiving a higher mean cyclosporin dose than patients receiving cyclosporin as part of a triple therapy regimen. Despite this, graft survival was worse in the triple therapy group than either of the other groups. It seems unlikely that a patient selection bias explains this finding as concerns about cyclosporin toxicity not increased risk of rejection are most likely to drive use of triple therapy. Vanrenterghem and Peeters reached similar conclusions when reviewing their experience of long-term cyclosporin use on behalf of the Leuven Collaborative Group for Transplantation [464]. Thus, all other discussion must be undertaken with reference to these data showing no deleterious effect of cyclosporin use in the renal transplant population as a whole. It is tempting to speculate that the lack of improvement in graft half-life most probably represents a bimodal distribution with some patients benefiting from cyclosporin use with others being particularly sensitive to the deleterious long-term effects.
2. Before considering further the deleterious effects of cyclosporin it is important to recognize that some authors have argued that chronic allograft dysfunction is due to inadequate immunosuppression. In support of this, it has been suggested that chronic immune responses to allografts are dependent on indirect recognition of graft antigens and that the T lymphocytes mediating these responses are relatively resistant to cyclosporin. However, addition of azathioprine to cyclosporin and prednisolone does not improve graft survival. Furthermore, in studies where azathioprine was added to 'reduced dose' cyclosporin and prednisolone but in which *no* reduction in cyclosporin levels was seen, no

improvement in graft survival was demonstrated. The finding that chronic rejection is not responsive to corticosteroids and antibody treatments used in acute rejection [465,466] argues either against a significant contribution from T-cell-mediated immune responses in chronic allograft nephropathy or that the T cells involved differ in their sensitivity to these immunosuppressive agents.

3. Of more relevance to examining the potentially deleterious effects of cyclosporin are studies comparing 'full-dose' cyclosporin from the time of transplantation (either triple therapy or cyclosporin and prednisolone) with conversion at a later stage to a regimen utilizing 'reduced dose' or no cyclosporin. This conversion may be carried out as part of a routine protocol or only in those grafts showing deteriorating function. Conversion studies ask a potentially complex set of questions. If cyclosporin acts as an initiating factor in a self-perpetuating chain of events then conversion may be doomed to failure. Furthermore, if conversion substitutes an inferior immunosuppressive agent then no effect or even worse graft survival may be seen irrespective of whether cyclosporin was itself injurious to the graft. Thus, no improvement in graft survival following cyclosporin reduction does not allow the conclusion that cyclosporin is not deleterious to graft function. However, improved graft function would support the conclusion that cyclosporin is deleterious, particularly given the lack of benefit of azathioprine addition without cyclosporin reduction discussed above. Initial reports of conversion of small numbers of patients to cyclosporin sparing regimens were encouraging leading to studies of early protocol conversion (1–3 months) from cyclosporin-based to azathioprine-based regimens or of reduction in cyclosporin dose with addition of azathioprine being undertaken. In a randomized study comparing patients initially receiving cyclosporin with protocol conversion to azathioprine at 3 months with patients receiving azathioprine throughout, those initially receiving cyclosporin had higher plasma creatinine levels to 3 months than those receiving azathioprine [467,468]. However, following conversion plasma creatinine in the group initially receiving cyclosporin fell to the level of the azathioprine group and histology at 1 year was no different in kidneys of patients converted at 3 months compared with those receiving azathioprine from transplantation [469]. This study is important as it found no benefit from cyclosporin withdrawal and emphasized also that long-term graft survival, not plasma creatinine, should be used as the study end-point. A number of conversion studies emphasized this lack of improvement in long-term graft survival, even when an initial improvement in creatinine was seen following conversion [470–474]. Meta-analysis of 10 randomized trials of protocol conversion from cyclosporin and prednisolone to azathioprine and prednisolone at 3–6 months found no improvement in graft survival at a mean of 26 months after transplantation [475]. A single study of conversion at 1 year also showed no benefit [476]. Finally, the protocol conversion study of McLean *et al.* [471] again raised the spectre of under immunosuppression as a risk factor for 'chronic rejection'.

4. The final type of study is comparison of 'full-dose' cyclosporin double therapy (cyclosporin and prednisolone) with 'reduced dose' cyclosporin triple therapy (cyclosporin, azathioprine, and prednisolone) from the time of transplantation. In common with the conversion studies discussed above, these studies attempt to address the potentially deleterious effects of cyclosporin on long-term graft survival. Lindholm *et al.* [477] reported on 463 patients randomized to receive either double or triple therapy from the time of transplantation and followed up for a minimum of 4 years. The triple therapy group received significantly less cyclosporin than the double therapy group for the first year but not thereafter. Mean prednisolone doses did not differ significantly between the two groups. There was no difference in graft survival at 4 years between the two groups. Meta-analysis has been attempted to compare triple with double therapy [478]. These authors could identify only five randomized trials. In two of these, follow up was for 12 and 18 months only. Of the remaining three trials Isoniemi *et al.* [479] randomized only 128 patients in total, 32 to each of four treatment protocols (cyclosporin, azathioprine, and prednisolone; cyclosporin plus azathioprine; cyclosporin plus prednisolone; or azathioprine plus prednisolone). They used the same maintenance cyclosporin dose for double versus triple therapy making interpretation of results complicated as discussed above. Triple therapy resulted in less chronic rejection on protocol biopsy at 2 years than any of the dual agent regimens. However, graft survival at 4 years was no different between the groups. Similarly, the Lindholm study discussed above had similar cyclosporin levels in both groups beyond 1 year and only the study of Ponticelli *et al.* [480] maintained low-dose cyclosporin in the triple therapy group throughout the study. Given these fundamental differences between studies, attempts at meta-analysis must be considered folly. However, it is striking that no study has shown benefit from use of reduced dose cyclosporin.

It must remain a concern that low-dose cyclosporin regimens may provide inadequate immunosuppression even with addition of azathioprine. Furthermore, some authors have suggested that it is those patients with 'chronic rejection' who benefit least from cyclosporin reduction [481,482]. Conversely, it is the subgroup of patients developing chronic allograft nephropathy (as opposed to cyclosporin nephrotoxicity) on cyclosporin who are particularly worthy of study as they may have declared themselves as particularly sensitive to the deleterious effects of this drug. It is thus disappointing that no adequately powered studies have specifically addressed the benefits of cyclosporin reduction or withdrawal in patients with a proven diagnosis of chronic allograft nephropathy. As argued above, from a purely theoretical standpoint, the hypothesis that cyclosporin is deleterious to long-term graft survival can only be addressed by comparison of graft survival with and without cyclosporin using protocols of equivalent immunosuppressive efficacy and using agents with clearly defined effects on the multitude of interactions constituting the response of the recipient to the graft. It is thus impossible to design a clinical trial which will answer definitively whether cyclosporin is deleterious to long-term graft function. Immunotherapeutic agents with at least equivalent immunosuppressive actions to cyclosporin are now available (e.g. tacrolimus, mycophenolate mofetil) as discussed below.

Transforming growth factor-β

Interstitial macrophages are an important source of molecules capable of stimulating collagen synthesis by fibroblasts. Upregulation of a range of macrophage products has been demonstrated in chronic allograft dysfunction [483,484]. TGF-β1 has attracted much interest because of the demonstration of polymorphisms in elements of the TGF-β1 gene [485] which *may* regulate TGF-β1 production and the suggestion that analysis of these polymorphisms may guide tailored immunotherapy (*vide infra*). TGF-β is produced by a wide range of cells including all types of leucocyte, platelets, and endothelial cells. Its production may thus be initiated by antigen-specific and non-antigen-specific responses including glomerular hypertension [486]. Three closely related isoforms of TGF-β are recognized, the TGF-β1 isoform being studied most in the context of chronic allograft nephropathy. TGF-β1 is a cytokine which has multiple roles including stimulation of extracellular matrix deposition and suppression of immune responses [487–490]. A number of studies have demonstrated accumulation of extracellular matrix and either increased [491–495] or altered distribution of [496] TGF-β1 mRNA or protein in kidneys with chronic dysfunction. Conversely, in models of autoimmune disease [497] and transplantation [498] TGF-β production has been demonstrated to be associated with suppression of deleterious responses. This dual action makes it difficult to extrapolate from *in vitro* studies to the clinical setting as TGF-β can be argued to have effects both beneficial and deleterious to long-term graft survival. Importantly, it is likely to be the combination of polymorphisms in both the TGF-β and other genes (e.g. ACE) which determine overall TGF-β activity and the combination with other cytokines [e.g. interleukin (IL)-10] which determines the net effect of TGF-β production. However, the dominant feature of chronic allograft nephropathy is interstitial fibrosis suggesting that in patients developing chronic allograft nephropathy the deleterious effects of TGF-β predominate.

The TGF-β promoter region and leader sequence contains seven polymorphic residues [485]. Analysis of the structural consequences of these polymorphisms suggests that they may be of functional significance although definitive data confirming the influence of genotype on TGF-β production is lacking. Given the benefit of ACE blockade in progressive renal disease it is also of interest that angiotensin II induces smooth muscle TGF-β-mRNA [499] and increases rat mesangial cell TGF-β expression and extracellular matrix protein synthesis [500]. Furthermore, ACE inhibitor treatment reduces renal TGF-β1 mRNA expression in patients with IgA nephropathy [501]. Thus, a genotype predisposing to high levels of angiotensin II production may augment the deleterious effects of TGF-β. Finally, the effect of immunosuppressive agents on TGF-β production is of interest. *In vitro* assays of the effect of cyclosporin on human T-cell cytokine production show TGF-β production to be preserved even when IL-2 production is reduced [502] and cyclosporin elicits TGF-β release from the MVL1Lu mink lung epithelial cell line [503] and causes accumulation of TGF-β in the rat juxtaglomerular apparatus [504]. In human kidneys increased TGF-β staining has been suggested to correlate with cyclosporin toxicity [505]. This study also demonstrated strong TGF-β staining in 36% of biopsies with acute rejection. However, a further study [506] examined biopsies from 21 transplanted kidneys for TGF-β finding no difference between non-rejecting kidneys, kidneys with acute rejection and kidneys with chronic rejection. In contrast, non-transplanted kidneys showed very little TGF-β staining.

All three TGF-β isoforms are secreted as latent molecules which are activated by cleavage. Importantly, the commercially available assays for TGF-β include an acid activation step which results in cleavage of the latent molecule therefore assaying total not *in vivo* activated TGF-β. Furthermore, antibodies used for immunocytochemistry frequently do not differentiate between latent and activated forms of TGF-β. Data assaying only total TGF-β must be interpreted with caution. Cyclosporin has been demonstrated to elicit TGF-β release from a number of different cell types (see above) and patients receiving cyclosporin have been shown to have elevated plasma total TGF-β levels [507]. If plasma TGF-β levels of patients receiving cyclosporin and tacrolimus are compared using an ELISA which does not require acid activation and which therefore measures *in vivo* activated TGF-β only, patients receiving cyclosporin are found to have similar TGF-β levels to those receiving tacrolimus. Furthermore, if these samples are acid activated prior to assay total TGF-β is elevated in those patients receiving cyclosporin as previously reported (P. Brenchley, personal communication). Thus, the excess of plasma TGF-β in cyclosporin-treated patients is due to elevation of latent not activated TGF-β. Normal venepuncture elicits platelet TGF-β release. If samples are assayed also for a marker of platelet activation (e.g. β-thromboglobulin) the contribution of platelet degranulation to circulating total TGF-β levels can be corrected for. These studies demonstrate that the effect of cyclosporin on plasma TGF-β is due to a destabilizing effect on platelets promoting TGF-β release. The relevance of this to clinical disease is unclear. It could be argued that TGF-β produced *in situ* in the graft interstitium and vascular endothelium is of most importance making these observations irrelevant to development of chronic allograft nephropathy. However, platelet aggregation is seen in graft vasculature in chronic allograft nephropathy and if these platelets were to release TGF-β more readily its effects in the graft might be potentiated. Thus, although tacrolimus shares many of the nephrotoxic effects of cyclosporin [508] it may avoid the potentiation of TGF-β-mediated effects. Whether this is beneficial or detrimental to long-term graft survival remains to be determined and is likely to differ between individual patients.

Management

Diagnosis of most causes of CRAD (Table 10.1), including overt cyclosporin nephrotoxicity, is straightforward and management options, although often limited, are self-evident. Much more difficult is management of the remaining cases of chronic allograft nephropathy, which are relevant to this discussion of chronic TIN.

Hypertension

As in other forms of chronic TIN the role of hypertension in progression of graft dysfunction is of interest. Following transplantation recipient hypertension is significantly correlated with increased graft loss [509] and faster progression of graft failure has been reported in patients with a diastolic blood pressure above 90 mmHg [384,427,510]. However, as in other diseases, association does not prove causality and definitive intervention trials are lacking. Given the potential pathogenetic mechanisms of chronic allograft nephropathy and the benefits of ACE inhibition in other progressive tubulo-interstitial disease, treatment of patients with chronic allograft nephropathy with an ACE inhibitor seems a logical management strategy. In a retrospective study Barnas *et al.* [511] examined the effect of Lisinopril treatment on 40 patients with progressive allograft dysfunction. In the year prior to treatment creatinine clearance decreased by 9 ± 1.2 ml/min. In the year after starting treatment creatinine clearance decreased by 4.8 ± 1.3 ml/min. There was a significant negative correlation between the reduction in excretory function and reduction in proteinuria during the year of ACE inhibitor therapy. The authors acknowledge the methodological problems with this study arguing that the natural history of CRAD is for acceleration in the rate of decline of excretory function making it likely that these findings are reliable. However, considerable variation in the rate of progression of renal impairment has been described [384,385] with some patients showing significant slowing. Thus, these findings must be interpreted with caution. With it now being possible to block angiotensin II receptors selectively it is of interest to ask whether this strategy is equivalent to ACE inhibition in the prevention of progression of renal disease in general and allograft nephropathy in particular. It is important to reiterate that ACE has a number of substrates in addition to angiotensin I (bradykinin, substance P, neurokinins, luteinizing hormone-releasing hormone). The importance of this is demonstrated by the inability of losartan (an AT1 receptor antagonist) to prevent renal injury in the obese Zucker rat [512]. Alternatively, a number of enzymes can catalyse angiotensin II formation suggesting that receptor blockade may be beneficial. It is then important to ask whether selective blockade of AT1 versus AT2 receptors has any benefit particularly as selective blockade of AT1 receptors potentiates effects through the AT2 receptor by increased angiotensin II generation. These considerations have been debated for renal disease in general [513–515] but studies specifically in CRAD are lacking. In reviewing the treatment of hypertension in renal allograft recipients, Curtis [516] emphasizes that the studies available do not allow us to differentiate between the different antihypertensive agents available and that 'blood pressure effects on the myocardium are of greatest importance'.

Immunosuppressive regimen

The development of novel immunosuppressive drugs (e.g. tacrolimus, mycophenolate mofetil, rapamycin, anti-CD25 antibodies), with at least equivalent immunosuppressive action compared with cyclosporin widens our therapeutic options and facilitates studies of the benefit of cyclosporin withdrawal. Tacrolimus and cyclosporin both lower renal blood flow and increase vascular resistance [517,518], although tacrolimus usage may avoid effects of cyclosporin on TGF-β. Experimental data in the F344 into LEW aortic transplant model of chronic rejection suggest FK506 to be superior to cyclosporin in preventing intimal thickening and destruction of the internal elastic lamina [519]. Mycophenolate mofetil is of interest as it not only avoids the potentially deleterious effects of cyclosporin on TGF-β production, but has also been shown to inhibit smooth muscle cell proliferation thereby inhibiting the arteriosclerosis seen in the rat aortic allograft model of chronic rejection [520]. There have been a number of reports of 'cyclosporin sparing' regimens substituting tacrolimus or mycophenolate mofetil for cyclosporin in patients with chronic allograft dysfunction. To date, these studies have enrolled only small numbers of patients, have reported only short-term follow up, and have enrolled a significant proportion of patients without transplant biopsy. These 'pilot' studies have, however, suggested benefit from cyclosporin withdrawal (e.g. [521]) and the final reporting of these studies will be of great interest. Intriguingly, these initial reports suggest that only a subgroup of patients benefit from cyclosporin withdrawal. In general these findings would support a multifactorial pathogenetic mechanism, only some causes being amenable to treatment by cyclosporin withdrawal. It is therefore imperative to determine the characteristics which identify those patients who would benefit from cyclosporin withdrawal and to identify the best alternative regimen. Attempts to select patients at high risk of the deleterious effects of cyclosporin have focused on cytokine polymorphisms and in particular the TGF-β polymorphisms [485]. The dual actions of TGF-β make it difficult to predict whether high TGF-β production will be deleterious or protective and as argued above it will probably be the interaction of TGF-β with other cytokines or susceptibility determinants which ultimately decide which way the scales tip. Furthermore, there is a paucity of data correlating TGF-β genotype with levels of TGF-β production. However, the appeal of being able to select patients in whom cyclosporin should be avoided on the basis of an easily determined genotype is obvious. Thus, sufficiently powered clinical trials of conversion to novel agents are urgently required as is more information on selection of patients for conversion therapy.

Finally, a range of treatments aimed at inhibiting smooth muscle proliferation have been tried with limited success [522].

Hypercholesterolemia

Given the importance of vascular changes in chronic allograft nephropathy and the high incidence of dyslipidemia in transplant recipients [523] the role of hypercholesterolemia in progression of chronic allograft nephropathy is of interest. Hypercholesterolemia and hypertriglyceridemia have both been correlated with chronic rejection (*vide supra*) and cholesterol level has been suggested to correlate with the rate of progression of renal impairment [524]. Hydroxymethylglutaryl CoA reductase inhibitors are effective treatments for hypercholesterolemia in this population, although they may be associated with significant side-effects and care must therefore be taken with their use. A small study of renal transplant recipients has shown pravastatin administration to reduce significantly acute rejection episodes [525]. No data are available on the effect of treatment of hypercholesterolemia on long-term graft survival. Given the high risk of cardiovascular morbidity and mortality in this group of patients aggressive treatment of dyslipidemia is, however, essential, irrespective of potential benefits on graft function.

Conclusions

Although all of these conditions have in common a primary insult on the interstitial compartment of the kidney, they teach us that, as hypothesized in the introduction, all are not equal and that it is dangerous to assume that management strategies which are effective in one condition inevitably will be efficacious in another. A common theme is whether following removal of injury progression is inevitable. Again it is clear that significant differences exist between these diseases with some (e.g. ADPKD) demonstrating progression attributable to an inevitable ongoing insult, some (e.g. obstructive nephropathy) showing little or no progression once the injury is removed, even if renal impairment is marked, and others (e.g. AN) most probably showing progression even in the absence of ongoing injury. Furthermore, although therapeutic options to slow progression are clear in some of these diseases, the inability to prevent progression of ADPKD demonstrates the need for caution when extrapolating between these very different diseases, demanding randomized controlled intervention trials in individual diseases before benefit can be considered proven.

Key references

Becker GJ, Kincaid-Smith P. Reflux nephropathy: the glomerular lesion and progression of renal failure. *Pediatric Nephrology* 1993; **7**: 365–369.

Birmingham Reflux Study Group. Prospective trial of operative versus non-operative treatment of severe vesicoureteric reflux in children: five years' observation. *British Medical Journal* 1987; **295**: 237–241.

Brenner BM, Cohen RA, Milford EL. In renal transplantation, one size may not fit all. *Journal of the American Society of Nephrology* 1992; **3**: 162–169.

Curtis JJ. Treatment of hypertension in renal allograft patients: Does drug selection make a difference? *Kidney International* 1997; **52** (Suppl. 63): S75–S77.

De Broe ME, Elseviers MM. Analgesic nephropathy. *New England Journal of Medicine* 1998; **338**: 446–452.

Gabow PA. Autosomal dominant polycystic kidney disease. *New England Journal of Medicine* 1993; **329**: 332–342.

Harris PC, Watson ML. Autosomal dominant polycystic kidney disease: neoplasia in disguise? *Nephrology Dialysis Transplantation* 1997; **12**: 1089–1090.

Kasiske BL. Clinical correlates to chronic renal allograft rejection. *Kidney International* 1997; **52** (Suppl. 63): S71–S74.

Kristjansson A, Wallin L, Mansson W. Renal function up to 16 years after conduit (refluxing or anti-reflux anastomosis) or continent urinary diversion. 1. Glomerular filtration rate and patency of uretero-intestinal anastomosis. *British Journal of Urology* 1995; **76**: 539–545.

Kunz R, Neumayer HH. Maintenance therapy with triple versus double immunosuppressive regimen in renal transplantation: a meta-analysis. *Transplantation* 1997; **63**: 386–392.

Nortier JL, Deschodt-Lanckman MM, Simon S, *et al.* Proximal tubular injury in Chinese herbs nephropathy: monitoring by neutral endopeptidase enzymuria. *Kidney International* 1997; **51**: 288–293.

Paul LC, Hayry P, Foegh M, *et al.* Diagnostic criteria for chronic rejection/accelerated graft atherosclerosis in heart and kidney transplants: Joint proposals from the Fourth Alexis Carrel Conference on Chronic Rejection and Accelerated Arteriosclerosis in Transplanted Organs. *Transplantation Proceedings* 1993; **25**: 2022–2023.

Sacks SH, Aparichio SAJR, Bevan A, Oliver DO, Will EJ, Davison AM. Late renal failure due to prostatic outflow obstruction: a preventable disease. *British Medical Journal* 1989; **298**: 156–159.

Striker GE. Report on a workshop to develop management recommendations for the prevention of progression in chronic renal disease Bethesda (MA) April 1994. *Nephrology Dialysis Transplantation* 1995; **10**: 290–292.

Weiss R, Duckett J, Spitzer A. Results of a randomized clinical trial of medical versus surgical management of infants and children with grades III and IV primary vesicoureteral reflux (United States). *Journal of Urology* 1992; **148**: 1667–1673.

References

1. Risdon RA, Sloper JC, de Wardener HE. Relationship between renal function and histological changes found in renal-biopsy specimens from patients with persistent glomerular nephritis. *Lancet* 1968; **ii**: 363–366.
2. Schainuck LI. Structural-functional correlations in renal disease. Part II. *Human Pathology* 1970; **1**: 631–641.
3. Mackensen-Haen S, Bohle A, Christensen J, Wehrmann M, Kendziorra H, Kokot F. The consequences for renal function of widening of the interstitium and changes in the tubular epithelium or the renal cortex and outer medulla in various renal diseases. *Clinical Nephrology* 1992; **37**: 70–77.
4. Wehrmann M, Bohle A, Held H, Schumm G, Kendziorra H, Pressler H. Long-term prognosis of focal sclerosing glomerulonephritis an analysis of 250 cases with particular regard to tubulointerstitial changes. *Clinical Nephrology* 1990; **33**: 115–122.
5. Bogenschutz O, Bohle A, Batz C, *et al.* IgA nephritis: on the importance of morphological and clinical parameters in the long-term prognosis of 239 patients. *American Journal of Nephrology* 1990; **10**: 137–147.
6. Fine LG, Ong ACM, Norman JT. Mechanisms of tubulo-interstitial injury in progressive renal diseases. *European Journal of Clinical Investigation* 1993; **23**: 259–265.
7. Fick GM, Gabow PA. Hereditary and acquired cystic disease of the kidney. *Kidney International* 1994; **46**: 951–964.
8. Sedman A, Bell P, Manco-Johnson M, *et al.* Autosomal dominant polycystic kidney disease in childhood: A longitudinal study. *Kidney International* 1987; **31**: 1000–1005.
9. Gabow PA. Autosomal dominant polycystic kidney disease. *New England Journal of Medicine* 1993; **329**: 332–342.
10. Parfrey PS, Bear JC, Morgan J, *et al.* The diagnosis and prognosis of autosomal dominant polycystic kidney disease. *New England Journal of Medicine* 1990; **323**: 1085–1090.
11. Ravine D, Gibson RN, Walker RG, Sheffield LJ, Kincaid-Smith P. Evaluation of ultrasonographic diagnostic criteria for autosomal dominant polycystic kidney disease. *Lancet* 1994; **343**: 824–827.

12. Levine E, Grantham JJ. The role of computed tomography in the evaluation of adult polycystic kidney disease. *American Journal of Kidney Disease* 1981; **1**: 99.
13. Iglesias CG, Torres VE, Offord KP, Holley KE, Beard CM, Kurland LT. Epidemiology of adult polycystic kidney disease. Olmstead County, Minn.: 1935–1980. *American Journal of Kidney Disease* 1983; **2**: 630–639.
14. Dalgaard OZ. Bilateral polycystic kidney disease of the kidneys. A follow up of two hundred and eighty four patients and their families. *Acta Medica Scandinavica* 1957; Suppl. **328**: 1–255.
15. Zerres K, Volpel M-C, Weiss H. Cystic kidneys: Genetics, pathological anatomy, clinical picture and prenatal diagnosis. *Human Genetics* 1984; **68**: 104–135.
16. Reeders ST, Breuning MH, Davies KE, *et al.* A highly polymorphic DNA marker linked to adult polycystic kidney disease on chromosome 16. *Nature* 1985; **317**: 542–544.
17. Germino GG, Weinstat-Saslow D, Himmelbauer H, *et al.* The gene for autosomal dominant polycystic kidney disease lies in a 750 kb CpG-rich region. *Genomics* 1992; **13**: 144–151.
18. The European Polycystic Kidney Disease Consortium. The polycystic kidney disease 1 gene encodes a 14kb transcript and lies within a duplicated region on chromosome 16. *Cell* 1994; **77**: 881–894.
19. Peters DJM, Sandkuijl LA. Genetic heterogeneity of polycystic kidney disease in Europe. In: Breuning MH, Devoto M, Romeo G, eds. *Polycystic kidney disease*. Basel: Krager, 1992: 128–139.
20. The International Polycystic Kidney Disease Consortium. Polycystic kidney disease: The complete structure of the *PKD1* gene and its protein. *Cell* 1995; **81**: 289–298.
21. Romeo G, Costa G, Catizone L, *et al.* A second genetic locus for autosomal dominant polycystic kidney disease. *Lancet* 1988; **i**: 8–11.
22. Kimberling WJ, Fain PR, Kenyon JB, Goldgar D, Sujansky E, Gabow PA. Linkage heterogeneity of autosomal dominant polycystic kidney disease. *New England Journal of Medicine* 1988; **319**: 913–918.
23. Kimberling WJ, Kumar S, Gabow PA, Kenyon JB, Connolly CJ, Somlo S. Autosomal dominant polycystic kidney disease: Localization of the second gene to chromosome 4q13–q23. *Genomics* 1993; **18**: 467–472.
24. Peters DJM, Spruit L, Saris JJ, *et al.* Localization of a second gene for autosomal dominant polycystic kidney disease on chromosome 4. *Nature Genetics* 1993; **5**: 359–362.
25. Daoust MC, Reynolds DM, Bichet DG, Somlo S. Evidence for a third genetic locus for autosomal dominant polycystic kidney disease. *Genomics* 1995; **25**: 733–736.
26. Fossdal R, Bothvarsson M, Amundsson P, *et al.* Icelandic families with autosomal dominant polycystic kidney disease: families unlinked to chromosome 16p13.3 revealed by linkage analysis. *Human Genetics* 1993; **91**: 609–613.
27. Turco AE, Clementi M, Rossetti S, Tenconi R, Pignatti PF. An Italian family with autosomal dominant polycystic kidney disease unlinked to either the PKD1 or PKD2 gene. *American Journal of Kidney Disease* 1996; **28**: 759–761.
28. Hughes J, Ward CJ, Peral B, *et al.* The polycystic kidney disease 1 (*PKD1*) gene encodes a novel protein with multiple cell recognition domains. *Nature Genetics* 1995; **10**: 151–160.
29. Mochizuki T, Wu G, Hayashi T, *et al.* PKD2, a gene for polycystic kidney disease that encodes an integral membrane protein. *Science* 1996; **272**: 1339–1342.
30. Grantham JJ, Geiser JL, Evan AP. Cyst formation and growth in autosomal dominant polycystic kidney disease. *Kidney International* 1987; **31**: 1145–1152.
31. Brasier JL, Henske EP. Loss of polycystic kidney disease (*PKD1*) region of chromo-

some 16p13 in renal cyst cells supports a loss-of-function model for cyst pathogenesis. *Journal of Clinical Investigation* 1997; **99**: 194–199.

32. Qian F, Watnick TJ, Onuchic LF, Germino GG. The molecular basis of focal cyst formation in human autosomal dominant polycystic kidney disease type I. *Cell* 1996; **87**: 979–987.
33. Geberth S, Ritz E, Zeier M, Stier E. Anticipation of age at renal death in autosomal dominant polycystic kidney disease (ADPKD)? *Nephrology Dialysis Transplantation* 1995; **10**: 1603–1606.
34. Milutinovic J, Rust PF, Fialkow PJ, *et al.* Intrafamilial phenotypic expression of autosomal dominant polycystic kidney disease. *American Journal of Kidney Disease* 1992; **19**: 465–472.
35. Peral B, Ong ACM, San Millan JL, Gamble V, Rees L, Harris PC. A stable, nonsense mutation associated with a case of infantile onset polycystic kidney disease 1 (PKD1). *Human Molecular Genetics* 1996; **5**: 539–542.
36. Levy M, Duyme M, Serbelloni P, Conte F, Sessa A, Grunfeld J-P. Is progression of renal involvement similar in twins with ADPKD? A multicentric European study. In: Sessa A, Conte F, Serbelloni P, Milani S, eds. *Autosomal dominant polycystic kidney disease. Contributions to Nephrology*, Vol. 115. Basel: Karger, 1995: 97–101.
37. Watnick TJ, Piontek KB, Cordal TM, *et al.* An unusual pattern of mutation in the duplicated portion of PKD1 is revealed by use of a novel strategy for mutation detection. *Human Molecular Genetics* 1997; **6**: 1473–1481.
38. Moy GW, Mendoza LM, Schulz JR, Swanson WJ, Glabe CG, Vacquiar VD. The sea urchin sperm receptor for egg jelly is a modular protein with extensive homology to the human polycystic kidney disease protein, PKD1. *Journal of Cell Biology* 1996; **133**: 809–817.
39. Ong ACM, Harris PC. Molecular basis of renal cyst formation-one hit or two? *Lancet* 1997; **349**: 1039–1040.
40. Vorechovsky I, Luo L, Dyer MJS, *et al.* Clustering of missense mutations in the ataxia-telangiectasia gene in a sporadic T cell leukemia. *Nature Genetics* 1997; **17**: 96–99.
41. Mangoo-Karim R, Ye M, Wallace DP, Grantham JJ, Sullivan LP. Anion secretion drives fluid secretion by monolayers of cultured human polycystic cells. *American Journal of Physiology* 1995; **269**: F381–F388.
42. Wallace DP, Grantham JJ, Sullivan LP. Chloride and fluid secretion by cultured human polycystic kidney cells. *Kidney International* 1996; **50**: 1327–1336.
43. Tsiokas L, Kim E, Arnould T, Sukhatme VP, Walz G. Homo- and heterodimeric interactions between the gene products of PKD1 and PKD2. *Proceedings of the National Academy of Sciences, USA* 1997; **94**: 6965–6970.
44. Qian F, Germino FJ, Cai Y, Zhang X, Somlo S, Germino GG. PKD1 interacts with PKD2 through a probable coiled-coil domain. *Nature Genetics* 1997, **16**. 179–183.
45. Gardner Jr KD, Glew RH, Evan AP, McAteer JA, Bernstein J. Why renal cysts grow. *American Journal of Physiology* 1994; **266**: F353–F359.
46. Ye M, Grant M, Sharma M, *et al.* Cyst fluid from human autosomal dominant polycystic kidneys promotes cyst formation and expansion by renal epithelial cells in vitro. *Journal of the American Society of Nephrology* 1992; **3**: 984–994.
47. Grantham JJ, Ye M, Davidow C, Holub B, Sharma M. Evidence for a potent lipid secretagogue in the cyst fluids of patients with autosomal dominant polycystic kidney disease. *Journal of the American Society of Nephrology* 1995; **6**: 1242–1249.
48. Grantham JJ. Mechanisms of progression in autosomal dominant polycystic kidney disease. *Kidney International* 1997; **52** (Suppl. 63): S93–S97.

49. EDTA European Dialysis and Transplant Association. Demography of dialysis and transplantation in Europe, 1984. *Nephrology Dialysis Transplantation* 1989; **4** (Suppl. 4): 5–29.
50. Valderrabano F, Jones EHP, Mallick NP. Report on the management of renal failure in Europe XXIV. *Nephrology Dialysis Transplantation* 1993; **10** (Suppl. 5): 4–9.
51. US Renal Data System. Annual Report: Incidence and prevalence of ESRD. *American Journal of Kidney Disease* 1997; **30** (Suppl. 1): S40–S53.
52. Franz KA, Reubi FC. Rate of functional deterioration in polycystic kidney disease. *Kidney International* 1983; **23**: 526–529.
53. Marcelli D, Locatelli F, Alberti D, *et al.* Hypertension as a factor in chronic renal insufficiency progression in polycystic kidney disease. *Nephrology Dialysis Transplantation* 1995; **10** (Suppl. 6): 15–17.
54. Churchill DN, Bear JC, Morgan J, *et al.* Prognosis of adult onset polycystic kidney disease re-evaluated. *Kidney International* 1984; **26**: 190.
55. Choukroun G, Itakura Y, Albouze G, *et al.* Factors influencing progression of renal failure in autosomal dominant polycystic kidney disease. *Journal of the American Society of Nephrology* 1995; **6**: 1634–1642.
56. Milutinovic J, Fialkow PJ, Agodoa LY, Phillips LA, Rudd TG, Bryant JI. Autosomal dominant polycystic kidney disease: symptoms and clinical findings. *Quarterly Journal of Medicine* 1984; **53**: 511–522.
57. Gabow PA, Johnson AM, Kaehny WD, *et al.* Factors affecting progression of renal disease in autosomal dominant polycystic kidney disease. *Kidney International* 1992; **41**: 1311–1319.
58. Torra R, Darnell A, Estivill X, Botey A, Revert L. Interfamilial and intrafamilial variability of clinical expression in ADPKD. In: Sessa A, Conte F, Serbelloni P, Milani S, eds. Autosomal dominant polycystic kidney disease. *Contributions to Nephrology*, Vol. 115. Basel: Karger, 1995: 97–101.
59. Klahr S, Breyer JA, Beck GJ, *et al.* Dietary protein restriction, blood pressure control and the progression of polycystic kidney disease. *Journal of the American Society of Nephrology* 1995; **5**: 2037–2047.
60. Walser M. Progression of chronic renal failure in man. *Kidney International* 1990; **37**: 1195–1210.
61. Hannedouche T, Chauveau P, Kalou F, Albouze G, Lacour B, Jungers P. Factors affecting progression in advanced chronic renal failure. *Clinical Nephrology* 1993; **39**: 312–320.
62. Williams PS, Fass G, Bone JM. Renal pathology and proteinuria determine progression in untreated mild/moderate chronic renal failure. *Quarterly Journal of Medicine* 1988; **252**: 343–354.
63. Chapman AB, Johnson AM, Rainguet S, Hossack K, Gabow PA, Schrier RW. Left ventricular hypertrophy in autosomal dominant polycystic kidney disease. *Journal of the American Society of Nephrology* 1997; **8**: 1292–1297.
64. Ivy DD, Shaffer EM, Johnson AM, Kimberling WJ, Dobin A, Gabow PA. Cardiovascular abnormalities in children with autosomal dominant polycystic kidney disease. *Journal of the American Society of Nephrology* 1995; **5**: 2032–2036.
65. Zeier M, Geberth S, Schmidt KG, Mandelbaum A, Ritz E. Elevated blood pressure profile and left ventricular mass in children and young adults with autosomal dominant polycystic kidney disease. *Journal of the American Society of Nephrology* 1993; **3**: 1451–1457.
66. Gabow PA, Chapman AB, Johnson AM, *et al.* Renal structure and hypertension in

autosomal dominant polycystic kidney disease. *Kidney International* 1990; **38**: 1177–1180.
67. Fick GM, Duley IT, Johnson AM, Strain JD, Manco-Johnson ML, Gabow PA. The spectrum of autosomal dominant polycystic kidney disease in children. *Journal of the American Society of Nephrology* 1994; **4**: 1654–1660.
68. Delaney VB, Adler S, Bruns FJ, Licinia M, Segel DP, Fraley DS. Autosomal dominant polycystic kidney disease: presentation, complications and prognosis. *American Journal of Kidney Disease* 1985; **5**: 104–111.
69. Zeier M, Ritz E, Geberth S, Gonzalo A. Genesis and significance of hypertension in autosomal dominant polycystic kidney disease. *Nephron* 1994; **68**: 155–158.
70. Gonzalo A, Gallego A, Rivera M, Orte L, Ortuno J. Shape of the relationship between hypertension and the rate of progression of renal failure in autosomal dominant polycystic kidney disease. *Nephron* 1992; **62**: 52–57.
71. Parfrey PS, Barrett B. Hypertension in autosomal dominant polycystic kidney disease. *Current Opinion in Nephrology and Hypertension* 1995; **4**: 460–464.
72. Chapman AB, Johnson A, Gabow PA, Schrier RW. The renin angiotensin system and autosomal polycystic kidney disease. *New England Journal of Medicine* 1990; **323**: 1085–1090.
73. Watson ML, MacNicol AM, Allan PL, Wright AF. Effects of angiotensin converting enzyme inhibition in adult polycystic kidney disease. *Kidney International* 1992; **41**: 206–210.
74. Barrett BJ, Foley RN, Morgan J, Hefferton D, Parfrey P. Differences in hormonal and renal vasculature responses between normotensive patients with autosomal dominant polycystic kidney disease and unaffected family members. *Kidney International* 1994; **46**: 1118–1123.
75. Cornell SH. Angiography in polycystic disease of the kidneys. *Journal of Urology* 1970; **103**: 24–26.
76. Graham PC, Lindrop GBM. The anatomy of the renin-secreting cell in adult polycystic kidney disease. *Kidney International* 1988; **33**: 1084–1090.
77. Vlahakos DV, Hahalis G, Vassilakos P, Marathias KP, Geroulanos S. Relationship between left ventricular hypertrophy and plasma renin activity in chronic hemodialysis patients. *Journal of the American Society of Nephrology* 1997; **8**: 1764–1770.
78. Jeunmaitre X, Soubrier F, Kotelavtsev YV, *et al.* The molecular basis of human hypertension. Role of angiotensinogen. *Cell* 1992; **71**: 169–180.
79. Bonnardeux A, Davies E, Jeunmaitre X, *et al.* Angiotensin II type 1 receptor gene polymorphism in human essential hypertension. *Hypertension* 1994; **24**: 63–69.
80. Navis G, de Jong PE, de Zeeuw D. I/D polymorphism of the angiotensin converting enzyme gene: a clue to the heterogeneity in the progression of renal disease and in the renal response to therapy? *Nephrology Dialysis Transplantation* 1997; **12**: 1097–1100.
81. Rigat B, Hubert C, Alhenac Gelas F, Cambien F, Corvol P, Soubrier F. An insertion/deletion polymorphism in the angiotensin I converting enzyme gene accounting for half the variance in serum enzyme levels. *Journal of Clinical Investigation* 1990; **86**: 1343–1346.
82. Danser JAH, Schalekamp MADH, Bax WA. Angiotensin converting enzyme. Effect of the deletion/insertion polymorphism. *Circulation* 1995; **92**: 1387–1388.
83. Baboolal K, Ravine D, Daniels J, *et al.* Association of the angiotensin I converting enzyme gene deletion polymorphism with early onset of ESRF in *PKD1* adult polycystic kidney disease. *Kidney International* 1997; **52**: 607–613.
84. Murphy G, Tzamaloukas AH, Listrom MB, Gibel LJ, Smith SM, Gardner KD.

Nephrotic syndrome and rapid renal failure in autosomal dominant polycystic kidney disease. *American Journal of Nephrology* 1990; **10**: 69–72.
85. Ravine D, Walker RG, Gibson RN, *et al.* Phenotype and genotype heterogeneity in autosomal dominant polycystic kidney disease. *Lancet* 1992; **340**: 1330–1333.
86. Wright GD, Hughes AE, Larkin KA, Doherty CC, Nevin NC. Genetic linkage analysis, clinical features and prognosis of autosomal dominant polycystic kidney disease in Northern Ireland. *Quarterly Journal of Medicine* 1993; **86**: 459–463.
87. Torra R, Badenas C, Darnell A, *et al.* Linkage, clinical features and prognosis of autosomal dominant polycystic kidney diseases types 1 and 2. *Journal of the American Society of Nephrology* 1996; **7**: 2142–2151.
88. Bear JC, Parfrey PS, Morgan JM, Martin CJ, Cramer BC. Autosomal dominant polycystic kidney disease. New information for genetic counselling. *American Journal of Medical Genetics* 1992; **43**: 548–553.
89. Bozza A, Aguiari G, Scapoli C, *et al.* Autosomal dominant polycystic kidney disease linked to PKD2 locus in a family with severe extrarenal manifestations. *American Journal of Nephrology* 1997; **17**: 458–461.
90. Cairns HWB. Heredity in polycystic kidney disease of the kidneys. *Quarterly Journal of Medicine* 1925; **18**: 359–393.
91. Fick GM, Johnson AM, Strain JD, *et al.* Characteristics of very early onset autosomal dominant polycystic kidney disease. *Journal of the American Society of Nephrology* 1993; **3**: 1863–1870.
92. Brook JD, McCurrach ME, Harley HG, *et al.* Molecular basis of myotonic dystrophy: expansion of a trinucleotide (CTG) repeat at the 3' end of a transcript encoding a protein kinase family member. *Cell* 1992; **68**: 799–808.
93. Zerres K, Rudnik-Schoneborn S. On genetic heterogeneity, anticipation, and imprinting in polycystic kidney diseases. *Nephrology Dialysis Transplantation* 1995; **10**: 7–9.
94. Yium J, Gabow P, Johnson A, Kimberling W, Martinez-Maldonado M. Autosomal dominant polycystic kidney disease in blacks: Clinical course and effects of sickle-cell hemoglobin. *Journal of the American Society of Nephrology* 1994; **4**: 1670–1674.
95. Stewart JH. End-stage renal failure appears earlier in men than women with polycystic kidney disease. *American Journal of Kidney Disease* 1994; **24**: 181–188.
96. Gretz N, Zeier M, Geberth S, Strauch M, Ritz E. Is gender a determinant for evolution of renal failure? A study in autosomal dominant polycystic kidney disease. *American Journal of Kidney Disease* 1989; **14**: 178–183.
97. Gonzalo A, Rivera M, Querda C, Ortuno J. Clinical features and prognosis of adult polycystic kidney disease. *American Journal of Nephrology* 1990; **10**: 470–474.
98. Cowley Jr BD, Grantham JJ, Muessel MJ, Kraybill AL, Gattone II VH. Modification of disease progression in rats with inherited polycystic kidney disease. *American Journal of Kidney Disease* 1996; **27**: 865–879.
99. Ingelfinger J, Fon EA, Ellison KE, *et al.* Localization of the intrarenal renin angiotensin system (RAS) by in situ hybridisation of renin and angiotensin (ANG-N) mRNAs. *Kidney International* 1988; **33**: 269A.
100. Grantham JJ. Pathogenesis of renal cyst expansion: Opportunities for therapy. *American Journal of Kidney Disease* 1994; **23**: 210–218.
101. Woo DDL, Miao SYP, Pelayo JC, Woolf AS. Taxol inhibits progression of congenital polycystic kidney disease. *Nature* 1994; **368**: 750–753.
102. Schafer K, Gretz N, Bader M, *et al.* Characterization of the Han: SPRD rat model for hereditary polycystic kidney disease. *Kidney International* 1994; **46**: 134–152.
103. Nauta J, Goedbloed MA, Luider TM, Hoogeveen AT, Van den Ouweland AMW, Halley

DJJ. The Han:SPRD rat is not a genetic model of human autosomal dominant polycystic kidney disease type 1. *Laboratory Animals* 1997; **31**: 241–247.

104. Martinez JR, Cowley BDJ, Gattone II VH, *et al.* The effect of paclitaxel on the progression of polycystic kidney disease in rodents. *American Journal of Kidney Disease* 1997; **29**: 435–444.
105. Gile RD, Cowley Jr BD, Gattone II VH, O'Donnell MP, Swan SK, Grantham JJ. Effect of lovastatin on the development of polycystic kidney disease in the Han:SPRD rat. *American Journal of Kidney Disease* 1995; **26**: 501–507.
106. Elzinga LW, Barry JM, Torres VE, *et al.* Cyst decompression surgery for autosomal dominant polycystic kidney disease. *Journal of the American Society of Nephrology* 1992; **2**: 1219–1226.
107. Brown JA, Torres VE, King BF, Segura JW. Laparoscopic marsupialization of symptomatic polycystic kidney disease. *Journal of Urology* 1996; **156**: 22–27.
108. Klahr S, Levey AS, Beck GJ, *et al.* The effects of dietary protein restriction and blood-pressure control on the progression of chronic renal disease. *New England Journal of Medicine* 1994; **330**: 877–884.
109. Maschio G, Alberti D, Janin G, *et al.* Effect of the angiotensin-converting-enzyme inhibitor benazepril on the progression of chronic renal insufficiency. *New England Journal of Medicine* 1996; **334**: 939–945.
110. Hossack KF, Leddy CL, Schrier RW, Gabow PA. Incidence of cardiac abnormalities associated with autosomal dominant polycystic kidney disease (ADPKD). *Kidney International* 1987; **31**: 203.
111. Leier CV, Baker PB, Kilman JW, Wooley CF. Cardiovascular abnormalities associated with adult polycystic kidney disease. *Annals of Internal Medicine* 1984; **100**: 683–688.
112. Fick GM, Johnson AM, Hammond WS, Gabow PA. Causes of death in autosomal dominant polycystic kidney disease. *Journal of the American Society of Nephrology* 1995; **5**: 2048–2056.
113. Striker GE. Report on a workshop to develop management recommendations for the prevention of progression in chronic renal disease Bethesda (MA) April 1994. *Nephrology Dialysis Transplantation* 1995; **10**: 290–292.
114. Geberth S, Stier E, Zeier M, Mayer G, Rambausek M, Ritz E. More adverse renal prognosis of autosomal dominant polycystic kidney disease in families with primary hypertension. *Journal of the American Society of Nephrology* 1996; **6**: 1643–1648.
115. Kamper A-L, Strandgaard S, Leyssac PP. Effect of enalapril on the progression of chronic renal failure. *American Journal of Hypertension* 1992; **5**: 423–430.
116. Hannedouche T, Landais P, Goldfarb B, *et al.* Randomised controlled trial of enalapril and β blockers in non-diabetic chronic renal failure. *British Medical Journal* 1994; **309**: 833–837.
117. Becker GJ, Whitworth JA, Ihle BU, Shahinfar S, Kincaid-Smith P. Prevention of progression in non-diabetic chronic renal failure. *Kidney International* 1994; **45** (Suppl. 45): S167–S170.
118. Zucchelli P, Zuccala A, Borghi M, *et al.* Long-term comparison between captopril and nifedipine in the progression of renal insufficiency. *Kidney International* 1992; **42**: 452–458.
119. Apperloo AJ, de Zeeuw D, Sluiter HE, de Jong PE. Differential effects of enalapril and atenolol on proteinuria and renal hemodynamics in non-diabetic renal disease. *British Medical Journal* 1991; **303**: 821–824.
120. Ogborn M, Sareen S, Pinette G. Cilazipril delays progression of hypertension and

uremia in rat polycystic kidney disease. *American Journal of Kidney Disease* 1995; **26**: 942–946.

121. Williams PS, Stevens ME, Fass G, Irons L, Bone JM. Failure of dietary protein and phosphate restriction to retard the rate of progression of chronic renal failure: a prospective, randomized controlled trial. *Quarterly Journal of Medicine* 1991; **81**: 837–855.
122. Ihle BU, Becker GJ, Whitworth JA, Charlwood RA, Kincaid-Smith PS. The effect of protein restriction on the progression of renal insufficiency. *New England Journal of Medicine* 1989; **321**: 1773–1777.
123. Rosman JB, Meijer S, Sluiter WJ, ter Wee PM, Piers-Becht TPM, Donker AJM. Prospective randomised trial of early dietary protein restriction in chronic renal failure. *Lancet* 1984; **i**: 1291–1296.
124. Rosman JB, Langer K, Brandl M, *et al.* Protein-restricted diets in chronic renal failure: A four year follow-up shows limited indications. *Kidney International* 1989; **36** (Suppl. 27): S96–S102.
125. Locatelli F, Alberti D, Graziani G, Buccianti G, Redaelli B, Giangrande A. Prospective, randomised, multicentre trial of the effect of protein restriction on progression of chronic renal insufficiency. *Lancet* 1991; **337**: 1299–1304.
126. Tufveson G, Geerlings W, Brunner FP, *et al.* Combined report on regular dialysis and transplantation in Europe, XIX, 1988. *Nephrology Dialysis Transplantation* 1989; **4** (Suppl. 4): 5–29.
127. Bailey RR, Lynn KL, Robson RA. End-stage reflux nephropathy. *Renal Failure* 1994; **16**: 27–35.
128. Esjborner E, Berg U, Hansson S. Epidemiology of chronic renal failure in children: a report from Sweden 1986–1994. *Pediatric Nephrology* 1997; **11**: 438–442.
129. Jacobson SH, Eklof O, Eriksson CG, Lins L-E, Tidgren B, Winberg J. Development of hypertension and uremia after pyelonephritis in childhood: 27 year follow up. *British Medical Journal* 1989; **299**: 703–706.
130. Tamminen TE. The relation of the shape of renal papillae and of collecting duct openings to intrarenal reflux. *British Journal of Urology* 1977; **49**: 345–354.
131. Hodson CJ, Wilson S. Natural history of chronic pyelonephritic scarring. *British Medical Journal* 1965; **ii**: 191–194.
132. Ransley PG, Risdon RA. Reflux nephropathy: effects of antimicrobial therapy on the evolution of the early pyelonephritic scar. *Kidney International* 1981; **20**: 733–742.
133. Hodson CJ, Cotran RS. Vesicoureteral reflux, reflux nephropathy, and chronic pyelonephritis. In: Cotran RS, ed. *Tubulo-interstitial nephropathies. Contemporary issues in Nephrology*, Vol. 10. New York: Churchill Livingstone, 1983: 83–120.
134. Smellie JM, Poulton A, Prescod NP. Retrospective study of children with renal scarring associated with reflux and urinary infection. *British Medical Journal* 1994; **1994**: 1193–1196.
135. Risdon RA. The small scarred kidney of childhood. A congenital or acquired lesion? *Pediatric Nephrology* 1987; **1**: 632–637.
136. Risdon RA, Yeung CK, Ransley RA. Reflux nephropathy in children submitted to unilateral nephrectomy: a clinicopathological study. *Clinical Nephrology* 1993; **40**: 308–304.
137. Smellie JM, Normand ICS, Katz G. Children with urinary infection: a comparison of those with and those without vesicouretric reflux. *Kidney International* 1981; **20**: 717–722.
138. Politano VA. Vesicoureteral reflux in children. *Journal American Medical Association* 1968; **172**: 1252–1256.

139. McGovern JH. Vesicoureteral regurgitation in children. *Journal of Urology* 1960; **83**: 122–149.
140. Editorial. Screening for reflux. *Lancet* 1978; **ii**: 23–24.
141. Coulthard MG, Lambert HJ, Keir MJ. Occurrence of renal scars in children after their first referral for urinary tract infection. *British Medical Journal* 1997; **315**: 918–919.
142. Vernon SJ, Coulthard MG, Lambert HJ, Keir MJ, Matthews JNS. New renal scarring in children who at age 3 and 4 years had had normal scans with dimercaptosuccinic acid: follow-up study. *British Medical Journal* 1997; **315**: 905–908.
143. Smellie JM, Ransley PG, Normand ICS, Prescod N, Edwards D. Development of new renal scars: a collaborative study. *British Medical Journal* 1985; **290**: 1957–1960.
144. Gordon AC, Thomas DFM, Arthur RJ, Irving HC, Smith SEW. Prenatally diagnosed reflux: a follow-up study. *British Journal of Urology* 1990; **65**: 407–412.
145. de Vargas A, Evans K, Ransley P, *et al.* A family study of vesicoureteric reflux. *Journal of Medical Genetics* 1978; **15**: 85–96.
146. Chapman CJ, Bailey RR, Janus ED, Abbott GD, Lynn KL. Vesicoureteric reflux: segregation analysis. *American Journal of Medical Genetics* 1985; **20**: 577–584.
147. Aggarwal VK, Verrier Jones K. Vesicoureteric reflux: screening of first degree relatives. *Archives of Disease in Childhood* 1989; **64**: 1538–1541.
148. Feather SA, Woolf AS, Gordon I, Risdon RA, Verrier Jones K, Aynsley-Green A. Vesicoureteric reflux: all in the genes? *Lancet* 1996; **348**: 725–728.
149. Scott JES, Swallow V, Coulthard MG, Lambert H, Lee REJ. Screening of newborn babies for familial ureteric reflux. *Lancet* 1997; **350**: 396–400.
150. Goonasekera CDA, Shah V, Wade AM, Barratt TM, Dillon MJ. 15-year follow-up of renin and blood pressure in reflux nephropathy. *Lancet* 1996; **347**: 640–643.
151. Sinaiko A, Michael A. Reflux nephropathy and hypertension: more whys and wherefores. *Lancet* 1996; **347**: 633–634.
152. Wallace DMA, Rotwell DL, Williams DI. The long-term follow-up of surgically treated vesicoureteric reflux. *British Journal of Urology* 1978; **50**: 479–484.
153. Report of a working group of the research unit, Royal College of Physicians. Guidelines for the management of acute urinary tract infection in childhood. *Journal of the Royal College of Physicians* 1991; **25**: 36–42.
154. Verrier Jones K. Screening babies for vesicoureteric reflux. *Lancet* 1997; **350**: 380–381.
155. Craig JC, Knight JF, Sureshkumar P, Lam A, Onikul E, Roy LP. Vesicoureteric reflux and timing of micturating cystourethrography after urinary tract infection. *Archives of Disease in Childhood* 1997; **76**: 275–277.
156. Marshall JL, Johnson ND, de Campo MP. Vesicoureteric reflux in children: prediction with Colour Doppler imaging. *Radiology* 1990; **175**: 355–358.
157. Risdon RA. The small scarred kidney in childhood. *Pediatric Nephrology* 1993; **7**: 361–364.
158. Hinchcliffe SA, Chan Y-F, Jones H, Chan N, Kreczy A, van Velzen D. Renal hypoplasia and postnatally acquired cortical loss in children with vesicouretral reflux. *Pediatric Nephrology* 1992; **6**: 439–444.
159. Stutley JE, Gordon I. Vesico-ureteric reflux in the damaged non-scarred kidney. *Pediatric Nephrology* 1992; **6**: 25–29.
160. Hiraoka M, Hori C, Tsukahara H, Kasuga K, Ishihara Y, Sudo M. Congenitally small kidneys with reflux as a common cause of nephropathy in boys. *Kidney International* 1997; **52**: 811–816.
161. Atiyeh B, Husmann D, Baum M. Contralateral renal abnormalities in patients with renal agenesis and noncystic renal dysplasia. *Pediatrics* 1993; **91**: 812–815.

162. Chrispin AR. Medullary necrosis in infancy. *British Medical Bulletin* 1972; **28**: 233–236.
163. Oldrizzi L, Rugiu C, Valvo E, *et al.* Progression of renal failure in patients with renal disease of diverse etiology on protein-restricted diet. *Kidney International* 1985; **27**: 553–557.
164. Hannedouche T, Albouze G, Chauveau P, Lacour B, Jungers P. Effects of blood pressure and antihypertensive treatment on progression of advanced chronic renal failure. *American Journal of Kidney Disease* 1993; **21** (Suppl. 2): 131–137.
165. Jungers P, Hannedouche T, Itakura Y, Albouze G, Descamps-Latscha B, Man NK. Progression rate to end-stage renal failure in non-diabetic kidney diseases: a multivariate analysis of determinant factors. *Nephrology Dialysis Transplantation* 1995; **10**: 1353–1360.
166. Locatelli F, Marcelli D, Comelli M, *et al.* Proteinuria and blood pressure as causal components of progression to end-stage renal failure. *Nephrology Dialysis Transplantation* 1996; **11**: 461–467.
167. Tomlinson PA, Smellie JM, Prescod N, Dalton RN, Chantler C. Differential excretion of urinary proteins in children with vesicoureteric reflux and reflux nephropathy. *Pediatric Nephrology* 1994; **8**: 21–25.
168. Konda R, Sakai K, Ota S, Takeda A, Orikasa S. Followup study of renal function in children with reflux nephropathy after resolution of vesicoureteral reflux. *Journal of Urology* 1997; **157**: 975–979.
169. Arze RS, Ramos JM, Owen JP, *et al.* The natural history of chronic pyelonephritis in the adult. *Quarterly Journal of Medicine* 1982; **51**: 396–410.
170. Delano BG, Goodwin NJ, Thomson GE, Minkowitz S, Friedman EA. 'Chronic pyelonephritis' as a cause of massive proteinuria (?nephrotic syndrome). *Archives of Internal Medicine* 1972; **129**: 73–76.
171. Dayan S, Smith EC. Nephrotic syndrome secondary to chronic pyelonephritis and ureterovesical reflux. *Journal of Urology* 1976; **115**: 108–109.
172. Woods HF, Walls J. Nephrotic syndrome in vesicoureteric reflux. *British Medical Journal* 1976; **ii**: 917–918.
173. Bhathena DB, Weiss JH, Holland NH, *et al.* Focal and segmental glomerular sclerosis in reflux nephropathy. *American Journal of Medicine* 1980; **68**: 886–892.
174. Torres VE, Velosa JA, Holley KE, Kelalis PP, Stickler GB, Kurtz SB. The progression of vesicoureteral reflux nephropathy. *Annals of Internal Medicine* 1980; **92**: 776–784.
175. El-Khatib M, Becker G, Kincaid-Smith P. Morphometric aspects of reflux nephropathy. *Kidney International* 1987; **32**: 261–266.
176. Cotran RS. Glomerulosclerosis in reflux nephropathy. *Kidney International* 1982; **21**: 528–534.
177. Yoshiara S, White RHR, Raafat R, Smith NC, Shah KJ. Glomerular morphology in reflux nephropathy: functional and radiological correlations. *Pediatric Nephrology* 1993; **7**: 15–22.
178. Becker GJ, Kincaid-Smith P. Reflux nephropathy: the glomerular lesion and progression of renal failure. *Pediatric Nephrology* 1993; **7**: 365–369.
179. El-Khatib MT, Becker GJ, Kincaid-Smith PS. Reflux nephropathy and primary vesicoureteric reflux in adults. *Quarterly Journal of Medicine* 1990; **77**: 1241–1253.
180. Yoshida Y, Fogo A, Shiraga H, Glick AD, Ichikawa I. Serial micropuncture analysis of single nephron function in subtotal renal ablation. *Kidney International* 1988; **33**: 855–867.
181. Yoshida Y, Fogo A, Ichikawa I. Effects of antihypertensive drugs on glomerular morphology. *Kidney International* 1989; **36**: 626–635.

182. Yoshida Y, Fogo A, Ichikawa I. Glomerular hemodynamic changes vs hypertrophy in experimental glomerular sclerosis. *Kidney International* 1989; **35**: 654–660.
183. Fogo A, Yoshida Y, Glick AD, Homma T, Ichikawa I. Serial micropuncture analysis of glomerular function in two rat models of glomerulosclerosis. *Journal of Clinical Investigation* 1988; **82**: 322–330.
184. Fries JWU, Sandstrom DJ, Meyer TW, Rennke HG. Glomerular hypertrophy and epithelial cell injury modulate progressive glomerulosclerosis in the rat. *Laboratory Investigation* 1989; **60**: 205–218.
185. Newbold KM, Howie AJ, Koram A, Adu D, Michael J. Assessment of glomerular size in renal biopsies including minimal change nephropathy and single kidneys. *Journal of Pathology* 1990; **160**: 255–258.
186. Fogo A, Hawkins EP, Berry PL, *et al.* Glomerular hypertrophy in minimal change disease predicts subsequent progression to focal glomerular sclerosis. *Kidney International* 1990; **38**: 114–123.
187. Howie AJ, Lee SJ, Green NJ, *et al.* Different clinicopathological types of segmental sclerosing glomerular lesions in adults. *Nephrology Dialysis Transplantation* 1993; **8**: 590–599.
188. Hinchcliffe SA, Kreczy A, Ciftci AO, Chan YF, Judd BA, van Velzen D. Focal and segmental glomerulosclerosis in children with reflux nephropathy. *Pediatric Pathology* 1994; **14**: 327–338.
189. D'Souza RCM, Kotre CJ, Owen JP, Keir MJ, Ward MK, Wilkinson R. Computed tomography evaluation of renal parenchymal volume in patients with chronic pyelonephritis and its relationship to glomerular filtration rate. *British Journal of Radiology* 1995; **68**: 130–133.
190. Jacobson SH. A five-year prospective follow-up of women with non-obstructive pyelonephritic renal scarring. *Scandinavian Journal of Urology and Nephrology* 1991; **25**: 151–157.
191. Martinell J, Claesson I, Lidin-Janson G, Jodal U. Urinary infection, reflux and renal scarring in females continuously followed for 13–38 years. *Pediatric Nephrology* 1995; **9**: 131–136.
192. Cardiff-Oxford Bacteriuria Study Group. Sequelae of covert bacteriuria in schoolgirls. *Lancet* 1978; **i**: 889–893.
193. Newcastle Covert Bacteriuria Research Group. Covert bacteriuria in schoolgirls in Newcastle upon Tyne. a 5-year follow-up. *Archives of Disease in Childhood* 1981; **56**: 585–592.
194. Davison JM, Sprott MS, Selkon JB. The effect of covert bacteriuria in schoolgirls on renal function at 18 years and during pregnancy. *Lancet* 1984; **ii**: 651–655.
195. Ozen S, Alikasifoglu M, Tuncbilek E, *et al.* Genetic predisposition to scar formation in reflux nephropathy: evidence for a role of angiotensin converting enzyme gene polymorphism. *Pediatric Nephrology* 1997; **11**: C26.
196. Cheong HI, Park HW, Choi Y. Role of the angiotensin converting enzyme gene polymorphism in the development of reflux nephropathy in children with vesicoureteric reflux. *Journal of the American Society of Nephrology* 1996; **7**: 1383.
197. Report of the International Reflux Study Committee. Medical versus surgical treatment of primary vesicoureteral reflux. *Pediatrics* 1981; **67**: 392–400.
198. Weiss R, Duckett J, Spitzer A. Results of a randomized clinical trial of medical versus surgical management of infants and children with grades III and IV primary vesicoureteral reflux (United States). *Journal of Urology* 1992; **148**: 1667–1673.
199. Smellie JM, Tamminen-Mobius T, Olbing H, *et al.* Five-year study of medical or

surgical treatment in children with severe reflux: radiological renal findings. The International Reflux Study in Children. *Pediatric Nephrology* 1992; **6**: 223–230.

200. Birmingham Reflux Study Group. Prospective trial of operative versus non-operative treatment of severe vesicoureteric reflux in children: five years' observation. *British Medical Journal* 1987; **295**: 237–241.
201. El Nahas AM, Masters-Thomas A, Brady SA, *et al*. Selective effect of low protein diets in chronic renal diseases. *British Medical Journal* 1984; **289**: 1337–1341.
202. Feest TG, Round A, Hamad S. Incidence of severe acute renal failure in adults: results of a community based study. *British Medical Journal* 1993; **306**: 481–483.
203. Sacks SH, Aparichio SAJR, Bevan A, Oliver DO, Will EJ, Davison AM. Late renal failure due to prostatic outflow obstruction: a preventable disease. *British Medical Journal* 1989; **298**: 156–159.
204. Greig JD, Raine PAM, Young DG, *et al*. Value of antenatal diagnosis of abnormalities of the urinary tract. *British Medical Journal* 1989; **298**: 1417–1419.
205. White RHR. Fetal uropathy. Conservative management is best. *British Medical Journal* 1989; **298**: 1408–1409.
206. Arthur RJ, irving HC, Thomas DFM, Watters JK. Bilateral fetal uropathy; what is the outlook? *British Medical Journal* 1989; **298**: 1419–1420.
207. Livera LN, Brookfield DSK, Egginton JA, Hawnaur JM. Antenatal ultrasonography to detect fetal renal abnormalities: a prospective screening programme. *British Medical Journal* 1989; **298**: 1421–1423.
208. Dudley JA, Haworth JM, McGraw ME, Frank JD, Tizard EJ. Clinical relevance and implications of antenatal hydronephrosis. *Archives of Disease in Childhood* 1997; **76**: F31–F34.
209. Atwell JD. Posterior urethral valves in the British Isles: a multicenter B.A.P.S. Review. *Journal of Pediatric Surgery* 1983; **18**: 70–74.
210. Warshaw BL, Edelbrock HH, Ettenger RB, *et al*. Progression to end-stage renal disease in children with obstructive uropathy. *Journal of Pediatrics* 1982; **100**: 183–187.
211. Chevalier RL. Effects of ureteral obstruction on renal growth. *Seminars in Nephrology* 1995; **15**: 353–360.
212. Abrams P. New words for old: lower urinary tract symptoms for 'prostatism'. *British Medical Journal* 1994; **308**: 929–930.
213. George NJ, O'Reilly PH, Barnard RJ, Blacklock NJ. High pressure chronic retention. *British Medical Journal* 1983; **286**: 1780–1783.
214. Jones DA, George NJR, O'Reilly PH, Barnard RJ. Reversible hypertension associated with unrecognised high pressure chronic retention of urine. *Lancet* 1987; **i**: 1052–1054.
215. Styles RA, Ramsden PD, Neal DE. Chronic retention of urine. The relationship between upper tract dilatation and bladder pressure. *British Journal of Urology* 1986; **58**: 647–651.
216. George NJR, Feneley RCL, Roberts JBM. Identification of the poor risk patient with 'prostatism' and detrusor failure. *British Journal of Urology* 1986; **58**: 290–295.
217. Hill AM, Philpott N, Kay JDS, Smith JC, Fellows GJ, Sacks SH. Prevalence and outcome of renal impairment at prostatectomy. *British Journal of Urology* 1993; **71**: 464–468.
218. Baker LRI, Mallinson JW, Gregory MC, *et al*. Idiopathic retroperitoneal fibrosis: a retrospective analysis of 60 cases. *British Journal of Urology* 1988; **60**: 497–503.
219. Lalli AF. Retroperitoneal fibrosis and inapparent obstructive uropathy. *Radiology* 1977; **122**: 339–342.

220. Webb JAW. Ultrasonography in the diagnosis of renal obstruction. *British Medical Journal* 1990; **301**: 944–946.
221. Bullock N. Idiopathic retroperitoneal fibrosis. *British Medical Journal* 1988; **297**: 240–241.
222. Keith DS, Larson TS. Idiopathic retroperitoneal fibrosis. *Journal of the American Society of Nephrology* 1993; **3**: 1748–1752.
223. Higgins PM, Bennett-Jones DN, Naish PF, Aber GM. Non-operative management of retroperitoneal fibrosis. *British Journal Surgery* 1988; **75**: 573–577.
224. Lyons K, Matthews P, Evans C. Obstructive uropathy without dilatation: a potential diagnostic pitfall. *British Medical Journal* 1988; **296**: 1517–1518.
225. O'Reilly P, Aureall M, Britton K, Kletter K, Rosenthal L, Testa T. Consensus on diuresis renography for investigating the dilated upper urinary tract. *Journal of Nuclear Medicine* 1996; **37**: 1872–1876.
226. Whitaker RH, Buxton-Thomas MS. A comparison of pressure flow studies and renography in equivocal upper urinary tract obstruction. *Journal of Urology* 1984; **131**: 446–449.
227. Bullock KN, Whitaker RH. Does good upper tract compliance preserve renal function. *Journal of Urology* 1984; **131**: 914–916.
228. Shokeir AA, Provost AP, Nijman RJM. Resistive index in obstructive uropathy. *British Journal of Urology* 1997; **80**: 195–200.
229. Klahr S, Purkerson ML. The pathophysiology of obstructive nephropathy: the role of vasoactive compounds in the hemodynamic and structural abnormalities of the obstructed kidney. *American Journal of Kidney Disease* 1994; **34**: 219–223.
230. Harris KPG, Klahr S, Schreiner G. Obstructive nephropathy: from mechanical disturbance to immune activation? *Experimental Nephrology* 1993; **1**: 198–204.
231. Harris RC, Martinez-Maldonado M. Angiotensin II-mediated renal injury. *Mineral and Electrolyte Metabolism* 1995; **1995**: 328–335.
232. Ishidoya S, Morrissey J, McCracken R, Klahr S. Delayed treatment with enalapril halts tubulointerstitial fibrosis in rats with obstructive nephropathy. *Kidney International* 1996; **49**: 1110–1119.
233. Rinder CA, Halushka PV, Sens MA, Ploth DW. Thromboxane A_2 receptor blockage improves renal function and histopathology in the post-obstructive kidney. *Kidney International* 1994; **45**: 185–192.
234. Wilson B, Reisman D, Moyer CA. Fluid balance in the urological patient: disturbances in the renal regulation of the excretion of water and sodium salts following decompression of the urinary bladder. *Journal of Urology* 1951; **66**: 805–815.
235. Bricker NS, Shwayri EI, Reardan JB, Kellog D, Merrill JP, Holmes JH. An abnormality in renal function resulting from urinary tract obstruction. *American Journal Medicine* 1957; **23**: 554–564.
236. Peterson LJ, Yarger WE, Schocken DD, Glenn JF. Post-obstructive diuresis: a varied syndrome. *Journal of Urology* 1975; **113**: 190–194.
237. Huland H, Gonnermann D, Werner B, Possin U. A new test to predict reversibility of hydronephrotic atrophy after stable partial unilateral ureteral obstruction. *Journal of Urology* 1988; **140**: 1591–1594.
238. Carr MC, Peters CA, Retik AB, Mandell J. Urinary levels of the renal tubular enzyme N-acetyl-β-D-glucosaminidase in unilateral obstructive uropathy. *Journal of Urology* 1994; **151**: 442–445.
239. Bishop MC. Diuresis and renal functional recovery in chronic retention. *British Journal of Urology* 1985; **57**: 1–5.

240. Woolf AS. Clinical impact and biological basis of renal malformations. *Seminars in Nephrology* 1995; **15**: 361–372.
241. Rodby RA, Schwartz MM. Nephrotic syndrome in a patient with unilateral renal dysplasia. *American Journal of Kidney Disease* 1995; **25**: 88–95.
242. Case Records of the Massachusetts General Hospital. Case 17–1985. *New England Journal of Medicine* 1985; **312**: 1111–1119.
243. Solomon LR, Mallick NP, Lawler W. Progressive renal failure in a remnant kidney. *British Medical Journal* 1985; **291**: 1610–1611.
244. Reinberg Y, Manivel JC, Pettinato G, Gonzalez R. Development of renal failure in children with the prune belly syndrome. *Journal of Urology* 1991; **145**: 1017–1019.
245. Rittenberg MH, Hulbert WC, Snyder HM, Duckett JW. Protective factors in posterior urethral valves. *Journal of Urology* 1988; **140**: 993–996.
246. Sarmina I, Resnick MI. Obstructive uropathy in patients with benign prostatic hyperplasia. *Journal of Urology* 1989; **141**: 866–869.
247. Lewis HY, Pierce JM. Return of function after relief of complete ureteral obstruction of 69 days' duration. *Journal of Urology* 1962; **88**: 377–379.
248. Shapiro SR, Bennett AH. Recovery of renal function after prolonged unilateral ureteral obstruction. *Journal of Urology* 1976; **115**: 136–140.
249. Ibrahim A, Fahal AH. Recovery of radiologically functionless obstructed kidneys. *British Journal of Urology* 1984; **56**: 113–115.
250. Ghose RR. Prolonged recovery of renal function after prostatectomy for prostatic outflow obstruction. *British Medical Journal* 1990; **300**: 1376–1377.
251. Bander SJ, Buerkert JE, Martin D, Klahr S. Long-term effects of 24-hr unilateral ureteral obstruction on renal function in the rat. *Kidney International* 1985; **28**: 614–620.
252. Steinhardt GF, Ramon G, Salinas-Madrigal L. Glomerulosclerosis in obstructive uropathy. *Journal of Urology* 1988; **140**: 1316–1318.
253. Schiller B, Moran J. Focal glomerulosclerosis in the remnant kidney model—an inflammatory disease mediated by cytokines. *Nephrology Dialysis Transplantation* 1997; **12**: 430–437.
254. Teichman JMH, Long RD, Hulbert JC. Long-term renal fate and prognosis after staghorn calculus management. *Journal of Urology* 1995; **153**: 1403–1407.
255. Nygaard IE, Kreder KJ. Urological management in patients with spinal cord injuries. *Spine* 1996; **21**: 128–132.
256. Foley SJ, McFarlane JP, Shah PJR. Vesico-ureteric reflux in adult patients with spinal injury. *British Journal of Urology* 1997; **79**: 888–891.
257. Silveri M, Capitanucci ML, Capozza N, Mosiello G, Silvano A, Gennaro MD. Occult spinal dysraphism: neurogenic voiding dysfunction and long-term urologic follow-up. *Pediatric Surgery International* 1997; **12**: 148–150.
258. Capitanucci ML, Iacobelli BD, Silveri M, Mosiello G, De-Gennaro M. Long-term urological follow-up of occult spinal dysraphism in children. *European Journal of Pediatric Surgery* 1996; **6** (Suppl. 1): 25–26.
259. Greig JD, Young DG, Azmy AF. Follow-up of spina bifida children with and without upper renal tract changes at birth. *European Journal of Pediatric Surgery* 1991; **1**: 5–9.
260. Lewis MA, Webb NJ, Stellman-Ward GR, Bannister CM. Investigative techniques and renal parenchymal damage in children with spina bifida. *European Journal of Pediatric Surgery* 1994; **4** (Suppl. 1): 29–31.
261. Kaneti J, Sober I, Gradus D. Fate of non-neurogenic neurogenic bladder—end-stage renal failure. *European Journal of Urology* 1988; **14**: 422–425.

262. Varlam DE, Dippell J. Non-neurogenic bladder and chronic renal insufficiency in childhood. *Pediatric Nephrology* 1995; **9**: 1–5.
263. McDougal WS. Metabolic complications of urinary intestinal diversion. *Journal of Urology* 1992; **147**: 1199–1209.
264. Schmidt JD, Hawtrey CE, Flocks RH, Culp DA. Complications, results and problems of ileal conduit diversions. *Journal of Urology* 1973; **109**: 210–216.
265. Richie JP. Intestinal loop diversion in children. *Journal of Urology* 1974; **111**: 687–689.
266. Schwartz GR, Jeffs RD. Ileal conduit urinary diversion in children: computer analysis of follow-up from 2 to 16 years. *Journal of Urology* 1975; **114**: 285–288.
267. Shapiro SR, Lebowitz R, Colodny AH. Fate of 90 children with ileal conduit urinary diversion a decade later: analysis of complications, pyelography, renal function, and bacteriology. *Journal of Urology* 1975; **114**: 289–295.
268. Altwein JE, Jonas U, Hohenfellner R. Long-term follow up of children with colon conduit urinary diversion and ureterosigmoidostomy. *Journal of Urology* 1977; **118**: 832–836.
269. Dunn M, Roberts JBM, Smith PJB, Slade N. The long-term results of ileal conduit urinary diversion in children. *British Journal of Urology* 1979; **51**: 458–461.
270. Elder DD, Moisey CU, Rees RWM. A long-term follow-up of the colonic conduit operation in children. *British Journal of Urology* 1979; **51**: 462–465.
271. Pitts WR, Muecke EC. A 20-year experience with ileal conduits: the fate of the kidneys. *Journal of Urology* 1979; **122**: 154–157.
272. Neal D. Complications of ileal conduit diversion in adults with cancer followed up for at least five years. *British Medical Journal* 1985; **290**: 1695–1697.
273. Akerlund S, Delin K, Kock NG, Lycke G, Philipson BM, Volkmann R. Renal function and upper urinary tract configuration following urinary diversion to a continent ileal reservoir (Kock pouch): a prospective 5 to 11 year follow-up after reservoir. *Journal of Urology* 1989; **142**: 964–968.
274. Husmann DA, McLorie GA, Churchill BM. Nonrefluxing colonic conduits: a long-term life-table analysis. *Journal of Urology* 1989; **142**: 1201–1203.
275. Kristjansson A, Bajc M, Wallin L, Willner J, Mansson W. Renal function up to 16 years after conduit (refluxing or anti-reflux anastomosis) or continent urinary diversion. 2. Renal scarring and location of bacteriuria. *British Journal of Urology* 1995; **76**: 546–550.
276. Kristjansson A, Wallin L, Mansson W. Renal function up to 16 years after conduit (refluxing or anti-reflux anastomosis) or continent urinary diversion. 1. Glomerular filtration rate and patency of uretero-intestinal anastomosis. *British Journal of Urology* 1995; **76**: 539–545.
277. Koch MO, McDougal WS, Hall MC, Hill DE, Braren HV, Donofrio MN. Long-term metabolic effects of urinary diversion: a comparison of meningomyelocele patients managed by clean intermittent catheterization and urinary diversion. *Journal of Urology* 1992; **147**: 1343–1347.
278. Spuhler O, Zollinger HU. Die chronisch-interstitielle Nephritis. *Zeitschrift für Klinische Medizin* 1953; **151**: 1–50.
279. Zollinger HU. Chronische interstitielle Nephritis bei Abusus von phenacetinhaltigen Analgetica (Saridon usw). *Scweizerische Medizinische Wochenschrift* 1955; **85**: 746.
280. Henrich WL, Agodoa LE, Barrett B, *et al.* Analgesics and the kidney: Summary and recommendations to the scientific advisory board of the National Kidney Foundation from an ad hoc committee of the National Kidney Foundation. *American Journal of Kidney Diseases* 1996; **27**: 162–165.
281. Brunner FP, Selwood NH. End-stage renal failure due to analgesic nephropathy, its

changing pattern and cardiovascular mortality. *Nephrology Dialysis Transplantation* 1994; **9**: 1371–1376.

282. Noels LM, Elseviers MM, de Broe ME. Impact of legislative measures on the sales of analgesics and the subsequent prevalence of analgesic nephropathy: a comparative study in France, Sweden and Belgium. *Nephrology Dialysis Transplantation* 1995; **10**: 167–174.
283. De Broe ME, Elseviers MM. Analgesic nephropathy—Still a problem? *Nephron* 1993; **64**: 505–513.
284. Kincaid-Smith P. Pathogenesis of the renal lesion associate with the abuse of analgesics. *Lancet* 1967; **i**: 859–862.
285. Burry AF, de Jersey P, Weedon D. Phenacetin and renal papillary necrosis: results of a prospective autopsy investigation. *Medical Journal of Australia* 1966; **53**: 873–879.
286. Murray TG, Goldberg M. Analgesic associated nephropathy in the USA. Epidemiological, clinical and pathogenetic features. *Kidney International* 1978; **13**: 64–71.
287. Schwarz A, Faber U, Borner K, Keller F, Offermann G, Molzahn M. Reliability of drug history in analgesic users. *Lancet* 1984; **ii**: 1163–1164.
288. Finnigan D, Burry AF, Smith IDB. Analgesic consumption in an antenatal clinic survey. *Medical Journal of Australia* 1974; **1**: 761–762.
289. Elseviers MM, Bosteels V, Cambier P, *et al.* Diagnostic criteria of analgesic nephropathy in patients with end-stage renal failure: Results of the Belgian study. *Nephrology Dialysis Transplantation* 1992; **7**: 479–486.
290. Elseviers MM, Waller I, Nenov D, *et al.* Evaluation of diagnostic criteria for analgesic nephropathy in patients with end-stage renal failure: Results of the ANNE study. *Nephrology Dialysis Transplantation* 1995; **10**: 808–814.
291. Elseviers MM, De Schepper A, Corthouts R, *et al.* High diagnostic performance of CT scan for analgesic nephropathy in patients with incipient to severe renal failure. *Kidney International* 1995; **48**: 1316–1323.
292. De Broe ME, Elseviers MM. Analgesic nephropathy. *New England Journal of Medicine* 1998; **338**: 446–452.
293. Fox JM, Menges K, Coper H, *et al.* No proof for a particular role of combination analgesics causing end-stage renal failure [1]. *Nephrology Dialysis Transplantation* 1996; **11**: 2519–2520.
294. Murray TG, Stolley PD, Anthony JC, Schinnar R, Hepler-Smith E, Jeffreys JL. Epidemiologic study of regular analgesic use and end-stage renal disease. *Archives of Internal Medicine* 1983; **143**: 1687–1693.
295. McCredie M, Ford JM, Taylor JS, Stewart JH. Analgesics and cancer of the renal pelvis in New South Wales. *Cancer* 1982; **49**: 2617–2625.
296. Morlans M, Laporte JR, Vidal X, Cabeza D, Stolley PD. End-stage renal disease and non-narcotic analgesics: a case-control study. *British Journal of Clinical Pharmacology* 1990; **30**: 717–723.
297. Pommer W, Bronder E, Greiser E, *et al.* Regular analgesic intake and the risk of end-stage renal failure. *American Journal of Nephrology* 1989; **9**: 403–412.
298. Sandler DP, Burr FR, Weinberg CR. Nonsteroidal anti-inflammatory drugs and the risk of chronic renal disease. *Annals of Internal Medicine* 1991; **115**: 165–172.
299. Sandler DP, Smith JC, Weinberg CR. Analgesic use and chronic renal disease. *New England Journal of Medicine* 1989; **320**: 1238–1243.
300. Perneger TV, Whelton PK, Klag MJ. Risk of kidney failure associated with the use of acetaminophen, aspirin, and non-steroidal antiinflammatory agents. *New England Journal of Medicine* 1994; **331**: 1675–1679.
301. Dubach UC, Rosner B, Pfister E. Epidemiologic study of abuse of analgesics contain-

ing phenacetin: renal morbidity and mortality. *New England Journal of Medicine* 1983; **308**: 357–362.

302. Elseviers MM, De Broe ME. A long-term prospective study of analgesic abuse in Belgium. *Kidney International* 1995; **48**: 1912–1919.
303. Barrett BJ. Acetaminophen and adverse chronic renal outcomes: An appraisal of the epidemiologic evidence. *American Journal of Kidney Disease* 1996; **28** (Suppl. 1): S14–S19.
304. Molzahn M, Pommer W. Analgesic nephropathy. In: Cameron JS, Davison AM, Grunfeld J-P, Kerr D, Ritz E, eds. *Oxford Textbook of Clinical Nephrology*, Vol. 2. Oxford University Press, 1992: 803–819.
305. Raaflaub J, Dubach UC. Dose-dependent changes in the pattern of phenacetin metabolism in man and its possible significance in analgesic nephropathy. *Klinische Wochenschrift* 1969; **23**: 1286–1287.
306. Bluemle LWJ, Goldberg M. Renal accumulation of salicylate and phenacetin: possible mechanisms in the nephropathy of analgesic abuse. *Journal of Clinical Investigation* 1969; **47**: 2507–2514.
307. Shelley JH. Pharmacological mechanisms of analgesic nephropathy. *Kidney International* 1978; **13**: 15–26.
308. Prescott LF. Analgesic nephropathy: a reassessment of the role of phenacetin and other analgesics. *Drugs* 1982; **23**: 75–149.
309. Nanra RS, Kincaid-Smith P. Papillary necrosis in rats caused by aspirin and aspirin-containing mixtures. *British Medical Journal* 1970; **3**: 559–561.
310. D'Agati V. Does aspirin cause acute or chronic renal failure in experimental animals and in humans? *American Journal of Kidney Disease* 1996; **28** (Suppl. 1): S24–S29.
311. Segasothy M, Kong Chiew Tong B, Kamal A, Murad Z, Suleiman AB. Analgesic nephropathy associated with paracetamol. *Australia and New Zealand Journal of Medicine* 1984; **14**: 23–26.
312. Bonney SL, Northington RS, Hedrich DA, Walker BR. Renal safety of two analgesics used over the counter: Ibuprofen and aspirin. *Clinical Pharmacology and Therapeutics* 1986; **40**: 373–377.
313. Emkey RD, Mills JA. Aspirin and analgesic nephropathy. *Journal of the American Medical Association* 1982; **247**: 55–57.
314. Akyol SM, Thompson M, Kerr DNS. Renal function after prolonged consumption of aspirin. *British Medical Journal* 1982; **284**: 631–632.
315. Burry HC, Dieppe PA. Renal function after prolonged consumption of aspirin. *British Medical Journal* 1982; **284**: 1117–1118.
316. Duggin GG. Combination analgesic-induced kidney disease: the Australian experience. *American Journal of Kidney Disease* 1996; **28** (Suppl. 1): S39–S47.
317. Hauser AC, Derfler K, Balcke P. Progression of renal insufficiency in analgesic nephropathy: Impact of continuous drug abuse. *Journal of Clinical Epidemiology* 1991; **44**: 53–56.
318. Schwarz A, Kunzendorf U, Keller F, Offermann G. Progression of renal failure in analgesic-associated nephropathy. *Nephron* 1989; **53**: 244–249.
319. Schwarz A. Treatment of renal failure due to analgesics. In: Stewart JH, ed. *Analgesic and NSAID-induced kidney disease. Oxford Monographs on Clinical Nephrology*, Vol. 2. Oxford: Oxford University Press, 1993: 119–132.
320. Maruta T, Swanson DW, Finlayson RE. Drug use and dependency in patients with chronic pain. *Mayo Clinic Proceedings* 1970; **54**: 241–244.
321. Schwarz A, Keller F, Kunzendorf U, *et al.* Characteristics and clinical course of

hemodialysis patients with analgesic associated nephropathy. *Clinical Nephrology* 1988; **29**: 299–306.

322. Molland EA. Experimental renal papillary necrosis. *Kidney International* 1978; **13**: 5–14.
323. Cameron JS. Effect of the recipient's renal disease on the results of transplantation (other than diabetes mellitus). *Kidney International* 1983; **23** (Suppl. 14): S24–S33.
324. Clive DM, Stoff JS. Renal syndromes associated with nonsteroidal antiinflammatory drugs. *New England Journal of Medicine* 1984; **310**: 563–572.
325. Wiseman EH, Reinert H. Anti-inflammatory drugs and renal papillary necrosis. *Agents and Actions* 1975; **5**: 322–325.
326. Nanra RS, Stuart-Taylor J, de Leon AH, White KH. Analgesic nephropathy: etiology, clinical syndrome, and clinicopathologic correlates in Australia. *Kidney International* 1978; **13**: 79–92.
327. Adam O, Vetter-Kerkhoff C, Schlondorff D. Renal side effects of non-steroidal anti-inflammatory drugs. *Medizinische Klinik* 1994; **89**: 305–311.
328. Adams DH, Howie AJ, Michael J, McConkey B, Bacon PA, Adu D. Non-steroidal anti-inflamatory drugs and renal failure. *Lancet* 1986; **i**: 57–59.
329. Carmichael J, Shankel SW. Effects of non-steroidal anti-inflammatory drugs on prostaglandins and renal function. *American Journal of Medicine* 1985; **78**: 992–1000.
330. Nanra RS. Renal papillary necrosis (RPN) and chronic interstitial nephritis (CIN) with non-steroidal anti-inflammatory drugs (NSAIDs)—Comparison with the analgesic syndrome. *Kidney International* 1989; **33**: 572.
331. Segasothy M, Samad SA, Zulfigar A, Bennett WM. Chronic renal disease and papillary necrosis associated with the long-term use of non-steroidal anti-inflammatory drugs as the sole or predominant analgesic. *American Journal of Kidney Disease* 1994; **24**: 17–24.
332. Brown DM, Hardy TL. Short-term study of the effect of phenacetin, phenazone and aminopyrine on the rat kidney. *British Journal of Pharmacology and Chemotherapy* 1968; **32**: 17–24.
333. Kaump DH. Pharmacology of the fenamates II. Toxicology in animals. *Annals of Physical Medicine* 1966; **9**: 16–23.
334. Nanra RS, Kincaid-Smith P. Experimental evidence for nephrotoxicity of analgesics. In: Stewart JH, ed. *Analgesic and NSAID-induced kidney disease. Oxford Monographs on Clinical Nephrology*, Vol. 2. Oxford: Oxford University Press, 1993: 17–31.
335. De Crespigny P, Hewitson T, Birchall I, Kincaid-Smith P. Caffeine potentiates the nephrotoxicity of mefenamic acid on the rat renal papilla. *American Journal of Nephrology* 1983; **10**: 311–315.
336. De Crespigny PJ, Kincaid-Smith PS. Caffeine aggravates mefenamic acid-associated renal papillary damage. *Kidney International* 1988; **33**: 135–136.
337. Morales A, Steyn J. Papillary necrosis following phenylbutazone ingestion. *Archives of Surgery* 1971; **103**: 420–421.
338. Lourie SH, Denman SJ, Schroeder ET. Association of renal papillary necrosis and ankylosing spondylitis. *Arthritis and Rheumatism* 1977; **20**: 917–921.
339. Jackson B, Lawrence JR. Renal papillary necrosis associated with indomethacin and phenylbutazone treated rheumatoid arthritis. *Australia and New Zealand Journal of Medicine* 1978; **8**: 165–167.
340. Mitchell H, Muirden KD, Kincaid-Smith P. Indomethacin-induced renal papillary necrosis in juvenile chronic arthritis. *Lancet* 1982; **ii**: 558–559.
341. Caruana RJ, Semble E. Renal papillary necrosis due to naproxen. *Journal of Rheumatology* 1984; **11**: 90–91.

342. Erwin L, Boulton Jones JM. Benoxaprofen and papillary necrosis. *British Medical Journal* 1982; **285**: 694–695.
343. Shah GM, Muhalwas KK, Winer RL. Renal papillary necrosis due to ibuprofen. *Arthritis and Rheumatism* 1981; **24**: 1208–1210.
344. Rossi E, Menta R, Cambi V. Partially reversible chronic renal failure due to long-term use of non-steroidal antiinflammatory drugs. *Nephrology Dialysis Transplantation* 1988; **3**: 469–470.
345. Segasothy M, Thyaparan A, Kamal A. Mefenamic acid nephropathy. *Nephron* 1987; **45**: 156–157.
346. Robertson CE, Ford MJ, Van Someren V, Dlugolecka M, Prescott LF. Mefenamic acid nephropathy. *Lancet* 1980; **ii**: 232–233.
347. Husserl FE, Lange RK, Kantrow CM. Renal papillary necrosis and pyelonephritis accompanying fenoprofen therapy. *Journal of the American Medical Association* 1979; **242**: 1896–1898.
348. Feder GL, Radovanovic Z, Finkelman RB. Relationship between weathered coal deposits and the etiology of Balkan endemic nephropathy. *Kidney International* 1991; **40** (Suppl. 34): S9–S11.
349. Weeden RP. Environmental renal disease: Lead, cadmium and Balkan endemic nephropathy. *Kidney International* 1991; **40** (Suppl. 34): S4–S8.
350. Raicevic S, Trnacevic S, Hranisavljevic J, Vucelic D. Renal function, protein excretion, and pathology of Balkan endemic nephropathy. II. Protein excretion. *Kidney International* 1991; **40** (Suppl. 34): S52–S56.
351. Hrabar A, Aleraj B, Ceovic S, Cvoriscec D, Vacca C, Hall III P. beta2-microglobulin studies in endemic Balkan nephropathy. *Kidney International* 1991; **40** (Suppl. 34): S38–S40.
352. Pavlovic-Kentera V, Djukanovic L, Clemons GK, Trbojevic S, Dimkovic N, Slavkovic A. Anemia in Balkan endemic nephropathy. *Kidney International* 1991; **40** (Suppl. 34): S46–S48.
353. Batuman V. Possible pathogenetic role of low-molecular-weight proteins in Balkan nephropathy. *Kidney International* 1991; **40** (Suppl. 34): S89–S92.
354. Ferluga D, Hvala A, Vizjak A, Trnacevic S, Halilbasic A. Renal function, protein excretion, and pathology of Balkan endemic nephropathy. III. Light and electron microscope studies. *Kidney International* 1991; **40** (Suppl. 34): S57–S67.
355. Ceovic S, Hrabar A, Radonic M. An etiological approach to Balkan endemic nephropathy based on the investigation of two genetically different populations. *Nephron* 1985; **40**: 175–179.
356. Radovanovic Z. Aetiology of Balkan nephropathy: A reappraisal after 30 years. *European Journal of Epidemiology* 1989; **5**: 372–377.
357. Vanherweghem JL, Depierreux M, Tielemans C, *et al.* Rapidly progressive interstitial renal fibrosis in young women: association with slimming regimen including Chinese herbs. *Lancet* 1993; **341**: 387–391.
358. van Ypersele de Strihou C, Vanherweghem JL. The tragic paradigm of Chinese herbs nephropathy. *Nephrology Dialysis Transplantation* 1995; **10**: 157–160.
359. Kabanda A, Jadoul M, Lauwerys R, Bernard A, van Ypersele de Strihou C. Low molecular weight proteinuria in Chinese herbs nephropathy. *Kidney International* 1995; **48**: 1571–1576.
360. Nortier JL, Deschodt-Lanckman MM, Simon S, *et al.* Proximal tubular injury in Chinese herbs nephropathy: monitoring by neutral endopeptidase enzymuria. *Kidney International* 1997; **51**: 288–293.
361. Vanherweghem J-L, Tielemans C, Simon J, Depierreux M. Chinese herbs

nephropathy and renal pelvic carcinoma. *Nephrology Dialysis Transplantation* 1995; **10**: 270–273.

362. Cho YW, Terasaki PI. Long-term survival. In: Terasaki P, ed. *Clinical transplants*. Los Angeles: UCLA Tissue Typing Laboratory, 1988: 277–282.
363. Schweitzer EJ, Matas AJ, Gillingham KJ, *et al*. Causes of renal allograft loss. *Annals of Surgery* 1991; **214**: 679–688.
364. Paul LC. Chronic renal transplant loss. *Kidney International* 1995; **47**: 1491–1499.
365. Solez K, Axelsen RA, Benediktsson H, *et al*. International standardization of criteria for the histologic diagnosis of renal allograft rejection: The Banff working classification of kidney transplant pathology. *Kidney International* 1993; **44**: 411–422.
366. Feehally J, Harris KPG, Bennett SE, Walls J. Is chronic renal transplant rejection a non-immunological phenomenon? *Lancet* 1986; **ii**: 486–488.
367. Azuma H, Nadeau K, Takada M, Mackenzie HS, Tilney NL. Cellular and molecular predictors of chronic renal dysfunction after initial ischemia/reperfusion injury of a single kidney. *Transplantation* 1997; **64**: 190–197.
368. Paul LC. Functional and histologic characteristics of chronic renal allograft rejection. *Clinical Transplantation* 1994; **8**: 319–323.
369. Laine J, Holmberg C, Hayry P. Chronic rejection and late renal allograft dysfunction. *Pediatric Nephrology* 1996; **10**: 221–229.
370. Fellstrom B. Immune injury—Is it all there is to chronic graft rejection? *Nephrology Dialysis Transplantation* 1995; **10**: 149–151.
371. Hostetter TH. Chronic transplant rejection. *Kidney International* 1994; **46**: 266–279.
372. Hume DM, Merrill JP, Miller BF, Thorn GW. Experiences with renal homotransplantation in the human: Report of nine cases. *Journal of Clinical Investigation* 1955; **34**: 327–328.
373. Mihatsch MJ, Ryffel B, Gudat F. Morphological criteria of chronic rejection: Differential diagnosis including cyclosporin-nephropathy. *Transplantation Proceedings* 1993; **25**: 2031–2037.
374. Kupin W, Nakhleh R, Lee M, *et al*. Separate risk factors for the development of transplant glomerulopathy vs chronic tubulointerstitial rejection. *Transplantation Proceedings* 1997; **29**: 245–246.
375. Isoniemi H, Krogerus L, Von Willebrand E, Taskinen E, Ahonen J, Hayry P. Histopathological findings in well-functioning long-term renal allografts. *Kidney International* 1992; **41**: 155–160.
376. Rush DN, Henry SF, Jeffery JR, Schroeder TJ, Cough J. Histological findings in early routine biopsies of stable renal allograft recipients. *Transplantation* 1994; **57**: 208–211.
377. Paul LC, Hayry P, Foegh M, *et al*. Diagnostic criteria for chronic rejection/accelerated graft atherosclerosis in heart and kidney transplants: Joint proposals from the Fourth Alexis Carrel Conference on Chronic Rejection and Accelerated Arteriosclerosis in Transplanted Organs. *Transplantation Proceedings* 1993; **25**: 2022–2023.
378. Oh CK, Jeong HJ, Kim YS, *et al*. Clinical validity of Banff grading of chronic rejection in renal transplantation. *Transplantation Proceedings* 1996; **28**: 1441–1442.
379. Isoniemi H, Taskinen E, Hayry P. Histological chronic allograft damage index accurately predicts chronic renal allograft rejection. *Transplantation* 1994; **58**: 1195–1198.
380. Salaman J. Chronic rejection as a cause of graft failure: Introduction. *Round Table Series Royal Society of Medicine Issue* 1994; **34**: 1–5.

381. Kasiske BL, Massy ZA, Guijarro C, Ma JZ. Chronic renal allograft rejection and clinical trial design. *Kidney International* 1995; **48** (Suppl. 52): S116–S119.
382. Beckingham IJ, O'Rourke JS, Stubington SR, Hinwood M, Bishop MC, Rigg KM. Impact of cyclosporin on the incidence and prevalence of chronic rejection in renal transplants. *Annals of the Royal College of Surgeons of England* 1997; **79**: 138–142.
383. Knight RJ, Kerman RH, Welsh M, *et al.* Chronic rejection in primary renal allograft recipients under cyclosporine-prednisone immunosuppressive therapy. *Transplantation* 1991; **51**: 355–359.
384. Modena FM, Hostetter TH, Salahudeen AK, Najarian JS, Matas AJ, Rosenberg ME. Progression of kidney disease in chronic renal transplant rejection. *Transplantation* 1991; **52**: 239–244.
385. Kasiske BL, Heim-Duthoy KL, Tortorice KL, Rao KV. The variable nature of chronic declines in renal allograft function. *Transplantation* 1991; **51**: 330–334.
386. Mathew TH. Recurrence of disease following renal transplantation. *American Journal of Kidney Disease* 1988; **12**: 85–96.
387. Flechner SM, Modlin CS, Serrano DP, *et al.* Determinants of chronic renal allograft rejection in cyclosporine-treated recipients. *Transplantation* 1996; **62**: 1235–1241.
388. Naimark DMJ, Cole E. Determinants of long-term renal allograft survival. *Transplant Reviews* 1994; **8**: 93–113.
389. Shaikewitz ST, Chan L. Chronic renal transplant rejection. *American Journal of Kidney Diseases* 1994; **23**: 884–893.
390. Ferguson R. Acute rejection episodes—Best predictor of long-term primary cadaveric renal transplant survival. *Clinical Transplantation* 1994; **8**: 328–331.
391. Matas AJ, Gillingham KJ, Payne WD, Najarian JS. The impact of an acute rejection episode on long-term renal allograft survival (t1/2). *Transplantation* 1994; **57**: 857–859.
392. Tesi RJ, Elkhammas EA, Henry ML, Davies EA, Salazar A, Ferguson RM. Acute rejection episodes: best predictor of long-term primary cadaveric renal transplant survival. *Transplantation Proceedings* 1993; **25**: 901.
393. Basadonna GP, Matas AJ, Gillingham KJ, *et al.* Relationship between early vs late acute rejection and onset of chronic rejection in kidney transplantation. *Transplantation Proceedings* 1993; **25** (Suppl. 1): 910–911.
394. Almond PS, Matas AJ, Gillingham K, *et al.* Risk factors for chronic rejection in renal transplant recipients. *Transplantation* 1993; **55**: 752–757.
395. Gulanikar AC, MacDonald AS, Sugurtekin U, Belitsky P. The incidence and impact of early rejection episodes on graft outcome in recipients of first cadaver kidney transplants. *Transplantation* 1992; **53**: 323.
396. Foster MC, Rowe PA, Dennis MJ, Morgan AG, Burden RP, Blamey RW. Characteristics of cadaveric renal allograft recipients developing chronic rejection. *Annals of the Royal College of Surgeons of England* 1990; **72**: 23–26.
397. Lindholm A, Ohlman S, Albrechtsen D, Tufveson G, Persson H, Persson NH. The impact of acute rejection episodes on long-term graft function and outcome in 1347 primary renal transplants treated by 3 cyclosporine regimens. *Transplantation* 1993; **56**: 307.
398. Kim HC, Suk J, Joo I, *et al.* Risk factors for chronic rejection in renal allograft recipients. *Transplantation Proceedings* 1996; **28**: 1456–1457.
399. Pallardo LM, Sanchez J, Puig N, *et al.* Chronic rejection in 500 kidney transplant patients treated with cyclosporine: Incidence and risk factors. *Transplantation Proceedings* 1995; **27**: 2215–2216.

400. Kasiske BL, Kalil RSN, Lee HS, Rao KV. Histopathologic findings associated with a chronic progressive decline in renal allograft function. *Kidney International* 1991; **40**: 514–524.
401. Massy ZA, Guijarro C, Kasiske BL. Clinical predictors of chronic renal allograft rejection. *Kidney International* 1995; **48** (Suppl. 52): S85–88.
402. Baltzan MA, Shoker AS, Baltzan RB, George D. HLA-identity-long-term renal graft survival, acute vascular, chronic vascular, and acute interstitial rejection. *Transplantation* 1996; **61**: 881–885.
403. Kapsner T, Schneeberger H, Land W. How valid are risk factors for chronic transplant failure in renal transplant patients found in the literature with regard to our patients: Results of a multivariate analysis. *Transplantation Proceedings* 1995; **27**: 878–880.
404. Opelz G, For the collaborative transplant study. Strength of HLA-A, HLA-B, and HLA-DR mismatches in relation to short- and long-term kidney graft survival. *Transplant International* 1991; **5** (Suppl. 1): S621–S624.
405. van Saase J, Van der Woude FJ, Thorogood J, *et al*. The relation between acute vascular and interstitial renal allograft rejection and subsequent chronic rejection. *Transplantation* 1995; **59**: 1280–1285.
406. Hofmann GO, Schneeberger H, Land W. Risk factors for chronic transplant failure after kidney transplantation. *Transplantation Proceedings* 1995; **27**: 2031–2032.
407. Terasaki PI, Gjertson DW, Cecka JM, Takemoto S, Cho YW. Significance of the donor age effect on kidney transplants. *Clinical Transplantation* 1997; **11**: 366–372.
408. Sanfilippo F, Vaughn WK, Spees EK, Lucas BA. The detrimental effects of delayed graft function in cadaver donor renal transplantation. *Transplantation* 1984; **38**: 643–648.
409. Halloran PF, Aprile MA, Farewell V, *et al*. Early function as the principal correlate of graft survival. *Transplantation* 1988; **46**: 223–228.
410. Cacciarelli T, Sumrani N, Delaney V, Hong JH, Di Benedetto A, Somner BG. The influence of delayed renal allograft function on long-term outcome in the cyclosporine era. *Clinical Nephrology* 1993; **39**: 335–339.
411. Yuge J, Cecka JM. Sex and age effects in renal transplantation. In: Terasaki P, ed. *Clinical transplants*. Los Angeles: UCLA Tissue Typing Laboratory, 1991: 257–267.
412. Chertow GM, Brenner BM, MacKenzie HS, Milford EL. Non-immunologic predictors of chronic renal allograft failure: data from the United Network of Organ Sharing. *Kidney International* 1995; **48** (Suppl. 52): S48–S51.
413. Brenner BM, Cohen RA, Milford EL. In renal transplantation, one size may not fit all. *Journal of the American Society of Nephrology* 1992; **3**: 162–169.
414. Odland MD, Kasiske BL. Kidneys from female donors are at increased risk for chronic allograft rejection. *Transplantation Proceedings* 1993; **25**: 912.
415. Cho YW, Terasaki PI, Graver B. Fifteen year kidney graft survival. In: Terasaki P, ed. *Clinical transplants*, 1988. Los Angeles: UCLA Tissue Typing Laboratory, 1989: 325–334.
416. Terasaki PI, Koyama H, Cecka JM, Gjertson DW. The hyperfiltration hypothesis in human renal transplantation. *Transplantation* 1994; **57**: 1450–1454.
417. Rubin R, Tolkoff-Rubin N, Oliver D, *et al*. Multicenter ser-epidemiologic study of the impact of cytomegalovirus infection on renal transplantation. *Transplantation* 1985; **40**: 243–249.
418. Yilmaz S, Koskinen PK, Kallio E, Bruggeman CA, Hayry PJ, Lemstrom KB. Cytomegalovirus infection-enhanced chronic kidney allograft rejection is linked with intercellular adhesion molecule-1 expression. *Kidney International* 1996; **50**: 526–537.

419. Guijarro C, Massy ZA, Kasiske BL. Clinical correlation between renal allograft failure and hyperlipidemia. *Kidney Internatonal* 1995; **48** (Suppl. 52): S56–S59.
420. Isoniemi H, Nurminen M, Tikkanen M, *et al.* Risk factors predicting chronic rejection of renal allograft. *Transplantation* 1994; **57**: 68–72.
421. Dimeny E, Fellstrom B, Larsson E, Tufveson G, Lithell H. Chronic vascular rejection and hyperlipoproteinemia in renal transplant patients. *Clinical Transplantation* 1993; **7**: 482–490.
422. Burke JF, Pirsch JD, Ramos EL, *et al.* Long-term efficacy and safety of cyclosporine in renal-transplant patients. *New England Journal of Medicine* 1994; **331**: 358–363.
423. Matas AJ, Burke JFJ, DeVault GAJ, Monaco A, Pirsch JD. Chronic rejection. *Journal of the American Society of Nephrology* 1994; **4**: S23.
424. Matas A, Sells RA, Johnson RWG, *et al.* Trend towards long-term reduction in cyclosporin levels: A risk factor for chronic graft rejection? *Round Table Series Royal Society of Medicine Issue* 1994; **34**: 11–21.
425. Beige J, Scherer S, Weber A, *et al.* Angiotensin-converting enzyme genotype and renal allograft survival. *Journal of the American Society of Nephrology* 1997; **8**: 1319–1323.
426. Peters TG, Shaver TR, Ames JE, *et al.* Cold ischemia and outcome in 17 937 cadaveric kidney transplants. *Transplantation* 1995; **59**: 191.
427. Brazy PC, Pirsch JD, Belzer FO. Factors affecting renal allograft function in long term recipients. *American Journal of Kidney Disease* 1992; **19**: 558–566.
428. Uchida K, Orihara A, Yamada N, *et al.* Two immunosuppressive drug regimens after renal transplantation: low dose cyclosporine adjusted on the basis of high-performance liquid chromatography whole blood levels and prednisone. *Transplantation Proceedings* 1988; **20** (Suppl. 1): 401–405.
429. Isoniemi H, Kyllonen L, Eklund B, *et al.* Acute rejection under triple immunosuppressive therapy does not increase the risk of late first cadaveric renal allograft loss. *Transplantation Proceedings* 1995; **27**: 875–877.
430. Lehtonen RKS, Isoniemi MH, Salmela TK, Taskinen IE, von Willebrand OE, Ahonen PJ. Long-term graft outcome is not necessarily affected by delayed onset of graft function and early acute rejection. *Transplantation* 1997; **64**: 103–107.
431. Opelz G. Critical evaluation of the association of acute with chronic graft rejection in kidney and heart transplant recipients. *Transplantation Proceedings* 1997; **29**: 73 76.
432. Opelz G, For the collaborative transplant study group. Collaborative transplant study-10 year report. *Transplantation Proceedings* 1992; **24**: 2342–2355.
433. Opelz G, Mytilineos J, Scherer S, Wujciak T. Influence of HLA matching and DNA typing on kidney and heart transplant survival in black recipients. *Transplantation Proceedings* 1997; **29**: 3333–3335.
434. Cecka JM, Terasaki PJ. The UNOS Scientific renal transplant registry. In: Terasaki PI, Cecka JM, eds. *Clinical transplants*, 1992. Los Angeles: UCLA Tissue Typing Laboratory, 1993: 1–16.
435. Opelz G. Importance of HLA antigen splits for kidney transplant matching. *Lancet* 1988; **ii**: 61–64.
436. Gore SM, Gilks WR, Opelz G. HLA antigen splits for kidney matching. *Lancet* 1988; **ii**: 632.
437. Opelz G, Scherer S, Mytilineos J. Analysis of HLA-DR split-specificity matching in cadaver kidney transplantation. *Transplantation* 1997; **63**: 57–59.
438. Mytilineos J, Deufel A, Opelz G. Clinical relevance of HLA-DPB locus matching for cadaver kidney transplants. *Transplantation* 1997; **63**: 1351–1354.

439. Grattan MT, Moreno-Cabral CE, Starnes VA, Oyer PE, Stinson EB, Shumway NE. Cytomegalovirus infection is associated with cardiac allograft rejection and atherosclerosis. *Journal of the American Medical Association* 1989; **261**: 3561–3566.
440. Lautenschlager I, Soots A, Krogerus L, *et al.* Effect of cytomegalovirus on an experimental model of chronic renal allograft rejection under triple-drug treatment in the rat. *Transplantation* 1997; **64**: 391–398.
441. Koskinen PK, Lemstrom KB, Hayry PJ. Cytomegalovirus infection and its role in the development of clinical and experimental allograft arteriosclerosis. In: Tilney NL, Strom TB, Paul LC, eds. *Transplantation biology cellular and molecular aspects.* Philadelphia: Lippincott Raven, 1996: 601–618.
442. Richardson WP, Colvin RB, Cheeseman SK, *et al.* Glomerulopathy associated with cytomegalovirus viremia in renal allografts. *New England Journal of Medicine* 1981; **305**: 57–63.
443. Tuazon TV, Schneeberger EE, Bahn AK, *et al.* Mononuclear cells in acute allograft glomerulopathy. *American Journal of Pathology* 1987; **129**: 119–132.
444. Herrera GA, Alexander RW, Cooley CF, *et al.* Cytomegalovirus glomerulopathy: A controversial lesion. *Kidney International* 1986; **29**: 725–733.
445. Lopez C, Simmons RL, Mauer SM, Najarian JS, Good RA. Association of renal allograft rejection with virus infections. *American Journal of Medicine* 1974; **56**: 280.
446. Reinke P, Fiestze E, Ode-Hakim S, *et al.* Late renal acute allograft rejection and symptomless cytomegalovirus infection. *Lancet* 1994; **344**: 1737.
447. Tullius SG, Heemann UW, Hancock WW, Azuma H, Tilney NL. Long-term kidney isografts develop functional and morphological changes that mimic those of chronic allograft rejection. *Annals of Surgery* 1994; **220**: 425–435.
448. Glassock RJ, Feldman D, Reynolds EG, Dammin G, Merrill J. Human renal isografts: a clinical and pathological analysis. *Medicine (Baltimore)* 1968; **47**: 411–454.
449. Brenchley PEC, Short CD, Roberts ISD. Is persistent TGFβ1 expression the mechanism responsible for chronic renal allograft loss? *Nephrology Dialysis Transplantation* 1998; **13**: 548–551.
450. Ross R. The pathogenesis of atherosclerosis: a perspective for the 1990's. *Nature* 1993; **362**: 801–809.
451. Fellstrom B, Larsson E, Tufveson G. Strategies in chronic rejection of transplanted organs: a current view of pathogenesis, diagnosis and treatment. *Transplantation Proceedings* 1989; **21**: 1435–1439.
452. Foegh ML. Chronic rejection-graft arteriosclerosis. *Transplantation Proceedings* 1990; **22**: 119–122.
453. Miles AMV, Sumrani N, John S, *et al.* The effect of kidney size on cadaveric renal allograft outcome. *Transplantation* 1996; **61**: 894–897.
454. Mackenzie HS, Azuma H, Rennke HG, Tilney NL, Brenner BM. Renal mass as a determinant of late allograft outcome: Insights from experimental studies in rats. *Kidney International* 1995; **48** (Suppl. 52): S38–42.
455. Mackenzie HS, Tullius SG, Heemann UW, *et al.* Nephron supply is a major determinant of long-term renal allograft outcome in rats. *Journal of Clinical Investigation* 1994; **94**: 2148–2152.
456. Kingma I, Chea R, Davidhoff A, Benediktsson H, Paul LC. Glomerular capillary pressure in long-surviving rat renal allografts. *Transplantation* 1993; **56**: 53–60.
457. Myers BD, Newton L. Cyclosporine induced chronic nephropathy: An obliterative microvascular renal injury. *Journal of the American Society of Nephrology* 1995; **2**: S45–S52.

458. Remuzzi G, Perico N. Cyclosporine-induced renal dysfunction in experimental animals and humans. *Kidney International* 1995; **48** (Suppl. 52): S70–S74.
459. Singh N, Gayowski T, Marino IR. Hemolytic uraemic syndrome in solid-organ transplant recipients. *Transplant International* 1996; **9**: 68.
460. Van Buren DH, Burke JF, Lewis RM. Renal function in patients receiving long-term cyclosporine therapy. *Journal of the American Society of Nephrology* 1994; **4**: S17.
461. Lewis RM. Long-term use of cyclosporine A does not adversely impact on clinical outcomes following renal transplantation. *Kidney International* 1995; **48** (Suppl. 52): S75–S78.
462. Opelz G. Effect of maintenance immunosuppressive drug regimen on kidney transplant outcome. *Transplantation* 1994; **58**: 443–446.
463. Opelz G. Influence of treatment with cyclosporine, azathioprine and steroids on chronic allograft failure. *Kidney International* 1995; **48** (Suppl. 52): S89–S92.
464. Vanrenterghem Y, Peeters J. Chronic renal allograft function under cyclosporin treatment. *Transplantation Proceedings* 1996; **28**: 2097–2099.
465. Cheigh JS, Stenzel KH, Susin M, Rubin AL, Riggio RR, Whitsell JC. Kidney transplant nephrotic syndrome. *American Journal of Medicine* 1974; **57**: 730–740.
466. Paul LC, Fellstrom B. Chronic vascular rejection of the heart and kidney-Have rational treatment options emerged? *Transplantation* 1992; **53**: 1169–1179.
467. Morris PJ, French ME, Dunnill MS, *et al.* A controlled trial of cyclosporine in renal transplantation with conversion to azathioprine and prednisolone after three months. *Transplantation* 1983; **36**: 273–277.
468. Chapman JR, Griffiths D, Harding NG, Morris PJ. Reversibility of cyclosporin nephrotoxicity after three months treatment. *Lancet* 1985; **i**: 128–130.
469. d'Ardenne AJ, Dunnill MS, Thompson JF, McWhinnie D, Wood RF, Morris PJ. Cyclosporin and renal graft histology. *Journal of Clinical Pathology* 1986; **39**: 145–151.
470. Hollander AAMJ, van Saase JLCM, Kootte AMM, *et al.* Beneficial effects of conversion from cyclosporin to azathioprine after kidney transplantation. *Lancet* 1995; **345**: 610–614.
471. McLean A, Fernando O, Varghese Z, Sweny P. Conversion of stable renal allografts from CyA to azathioprine: A five year follow up. *Transplantation Proceedings* 1997; **29**: 285.
472. Thiel G, Bock A, Spondlin M, *et al.* Long-term benefits and risks of cyclosporin A (Sandimmun)-an analysis at 10 years. *Transplantation Proceedings* 1994; **26**: 2493–2498.
473. Hall BM, Tiller DJ, Hardie I, *et al.* Comparison of three immunosuppressive regimens in cadaveric renal transplantation: long term cyclosporine, short term cyclosporine followed by azathioprine and prednisolone, and azathioprine and prednisolone without cyclosporine. *New England Journal of Medicine* 1988; **318**: 1499–1507.
474. Hoitsma AJ, van Lier HJJ, Wetzels JFM, Berden JHM, Koene RAP. Cyclosporin treatment with conversion after three months versus conventional immunosuppression in renal allograft recipients. *Lancet* 1987; **i**: 584–586.
475. Kasiske BL, Heim-Duthoy K, Ma JZ. Elective cyclosporine withdrawal after renal transplantation. A meta-analysis. *Journal of the American Medical Association* 1993; **269**: 395–400.
476. Pederson EB, Hansen HE, Kornerup HJ, Madsen S, Sorensen AW. Long-term graft survival after conversion from cyclosporin to azathioprine 1 year after renal transplantation. A prospective, randomized study from 1 to 6 years after transplantation. *Nephrology Dialysis Transplantation* 1993; **8**: 250–254.

477. Lindholm A, Albrechtsen D, Tufveson G, Karlberg I, Persson NH, Groth C-G. A randomized trial of cyclosporine, azathioprine, and prednisone in primary cadaveric renal transplantation. *Transplantation* 1992: 54.
478. Kunz R, Neumayer HH. Maintenance therapy with triple versus double immunosuppressive regimen in renal transplantation: a meta-analysis. *Transplantation* 1997; **63**: 386–392.
479. Isoniemi HM, Ahonen J, Tikkanen MJ, *et al.* Long-term consequences of different immunosuppressive regimens for renal allografts. *Transplantation* 1993; **55**: 494–499.
480. Ponticelli C, Tarantino A, Montagnino G, *et al.* A randomized trial comparing triple-drug and double-drug therapy in renal transplantation. *Transplantation* 1988; **45**: 913–918.
481. Castelao AM, Grino JM, Sabate I, *et al.* Cyclosporin A (CSA)–azathioprine (AZA) overlap in renal transplants with chronic rejection (CR) or CSA nephrotoxicity. *Kidney International* 1990; **37**: 1601.
482. Lorber MI, Flechner SM, van Buren CT, Sorensen K, Kerman RH, Kahan BD. Management of immunosuppressive problems in renal allograft recipients. *Transplantation Proceedings* 1987; **19**: 1951–1954.
483. Heemann UW, Tullius SG, Tamatami T, Miyasaka M, Milford E, Tilney NL. Infiltration patterns of macrophages and lymphocytes in chronically rejecting rat kidney allografts. *Transplantation International* 1994; **7**: 349–355.
484. Paul LC, Grothman GT, Benediktsson H, Davidoff A. Macrophage subpopulations that infiltrate normal and rejecting heart and kidney grafts in the rat. *Transplantation* 1992; **53**: 157.
485. Cambien F, Ricard S, Troesch A, *et al.* Polymorphisms of the transforming growth factor-β1 gene in relation to myocardial infarction and blood pressure. *Hypertension* 1996; **28**: 881–887.
486. Shankland SJ, Ly H, Thai K, Scholey JW. Increased glomerular capillary pressure alters glomerular cytokine expression. *Circulation Research* 1994; **75**: 844–853.
487. Waltenberger J, Miyazono K, Funa K, Wanders A, Fellstrom B, Heldin C-H. Transforming growth factor-β and organ transplantation. *Transplantation Proceedings* 1993; **25**: 2038–2040.
488. Lawrence DA. Transforming growth factor-β: An overview. *Kidney International* 1995; **47** (Suppl. 49): S19–S23.
489. Verbanac KM, Carver FM, Haisch CE, Thomas JM. A role for transforming growth factor-beta in the veto mechanism in transplant tolerance. *Transplantation* 1994; **57**: 893–900.
490. Yamamoto T, Noble NA, Miller DE, Border WA. Sustained expression of TGF-β1 underlies development of progressive kidney fibrosis. *Kidney International* 1994; **45**: 916–927.
491. Border WA, Noble NA. TGF-beta in kidney fibrosis: A target for gene therapy. *Kidney International* 1997; **51**: 1388–1396.
492. Noronha IL, Weis H, Hartley B, Wallach D, Cameron SJ, Waldherr R. Expression of cytokines, growth factors and their receptors in renal allograft biopsies. *Transplantation Proceedings* 1993; **25**: 917–918.
493. Shihab F, Yamamoto T, Nast C, *et al.* Acute and chronic allograft rejection in human kidney correlate with the expression of TGF-β and extracellular matrix proteins. *Journal of the American Society of Nephrology* 1993; **4**: 918.
494. Gould VE, Martinez-Lacabe V, Virtanen I, Sahlin KM, Schwartz MM. Differential distribution of tenascin and cellular fibronectins in acute and chronic renal allograft rejection. *Laboratory Investigation* 1992; **67**: 71–79.

495. Sharma VK, Bologa RM, Xu G-P, *et al.* Intragraft TGF-beta1 mRNA: A correlate of interstitial fibrosis and chronic allograft nephropathy. *Kidney International* 1996; **49**: 1297–1303.
496. Horvath LZ, Friess H, Schilling M, *et al.* Altered expression of transforming growth factor-βs in chronic renal rejection. *Kidney International* 1996; **50**: 489–498.
497. Santambrogio L, Hochwald GM, Saxena B, *et al.* Studies on the mechanism by which transforming growth factor-β (TGF-β) protects against allergic encephalomyelitis. *Journal of Immunology* 1993; **151**: 1116–1127.
498. Hewitt CW, Strande L, Santos M, *et al.* Rat renal allograft tolerance is associated with local TGF-beta and absence of IL-2r expression within chimeric immunocytic foci. *Transplantation Proceedings* 1997; **29**: 2183–2184.
499. Gibbons GH, Pratt RE, Dzau VJ. Vascular smooth muscle cell hypertrophy vs. hyperplasia. *Journal of Clinical Investigation* 1992; **90**: 456–461.
500. Kagami S, Border WA, Miller DA, Noble NA. Angiotensin II stimulates extracellular matrix protein synthesis through induction of transforming growth factor-b expression in rat glomerular mesangial cells. *Journal of Clinical Investigation* 1994; **93**: 2431–2437.
501. Nishimura M, Okamura M, Konishi Y, *et al.* Effect of treatment with ACE inhibitor (ACEI) on TGF-beta gene expressions in renal biopsy from patients with IgA nephropathy. *Journal of the American Society of Nephrology* 1995; **6**: 397.
502. Li B, Sehajpal PK, Khanna A, *et al.* Differential regulation of transforming growth factor β and interleukin 2 genes in human T cells: Demonstration by usage of novel competitor DNA constructs in the quantitative polymerase chain reaction. *Journal of Experimental Medicine* 1991; **174**: 1259–1262.
503. Khanna A, Suthanthiran M. New insight into the anti-proliferative activity of cyclosporine: Inhibition of DNA synthesis by a transforming growth factor β dependent mechanism. *Molecular Biology of the Cell* 1992; **3**: 27A.
504. Shehata M, Cope GH, Johnson TS, Raftery AT, El Nahas AM. Cyclosporine enhances the expression of TGF-beta in the juxtaglomerular cells of the rat kidney. *Kidney International* 1995; **48**: 1487–1496.
505. Pankewycz OG, Miao L, Isaacs R, *et al.* Increased renal tubular expression of transforming growth factor beta in human allografts correlates with cyclosporine toxicity. *Kidney International* 1996; **50**: 1634–1640.
506. Lantz I, Dimeny E, Larsson E, Fellstrom B, Funa K. Increased immunoreactivity of transforming growth factor-beta in human kidney transplants. *Transplant Immunology* 1996; **4**: 209–214.
507. Shin G-T, Khanna A, Sharma VK, *et al.* In vivo hyperexpression of transforming growth factor-β1 in humans: Stimulation by cyclosporine. *Transplantation Proceedings* 1997; **29**: 284.
508. Bennett WM. Immunosuppressive drug nephrotoxicity. In: Tilney NL, Strom TB, Paul LC, eds. *Transplantation biology cellular and molecular aspects*. Philadelphia: Lippincott Raven, 1996: 587–600.
509. Opelz G, Wujciak T, Ritz E. Association of chronic kidney graft failure with recipient blood pressure. *Kidney International* 1998; **53**: 217–222.
510. Cheigh JS, Haschemeyer RH, Wang JCL. Hypertension in kidney transplant recipients-effect on long term renal allograft survival. *American Journal of Hypertension* 1989; **2**: 341.
511. Barnas U, Schmidt A, Haas M, Oberbauer R, Mayer G. The effects of prolonged angiotensin-converting enzyme inhibition on excretory kidney function and proteinuria in renal allograft recipients with chronic progressive transplant failure. *Nephrology Dialysis Transplantation* 1996; **11**: 1822–1824.

512. Crary GS, Swan SK, O'Donnell MP, Kasiske BL, Katz SA, Keane WF. The angiotensin II receptor antagonist losartan reduces blood pressure but not renal injury in obese Zucker rats. *Journal of the American Society of Nephrology* 1995; **6**: 1295–1299.
513. Hollenberg NK. ACE inhibitors, AT1 receptor blockers, and the kidney. *Nephrology Dialysis Transplantation* 1997; **12**: 381–383.
514. Ichikawa I. Will Ang II A1 antagonists be renoprotective in humans? *Kidney International* 1996; **50**: 684–692.
515. Geiger H. Are angiotensin II receptor blockers superior to angiotensin converting enzyme inhibitors with regard to their renoprotective effect? *Nephrology Dialysis Transplantation* 1997; **12**: 640–642.
516. Curtis JJ. Treatment of hypertension in renal allograft patients: Does drug selection make a difference? *Kidney International* 1997; **52** (Suppl. 63): S75–S77.
517. Klintmalm G. FK506: An update. *Clinical Transplantation* 1994; **8**: 207–210.
518. Randhawa P, Shapiro R, Jordan M, Starzl T, Demetris A. The histopathological changes associated with allograft rejection and drug toxicity in renal transplant recipients maintained on FK 506—Clinical significance and comparison with cyclosporine. *American Journal of Surgical Pathology* 1993; **17**: 60–68.
519. Cole OJ, Stubington SR, Shehata M, Rigg KM. The effect of different immunosuppressants on the development of chronic rejection in the rat aortic model. *International Conference on New Trends in Clinical and Experimental Immunosuppression*. Geneva, 1998.
520. Raisanen-Sokolowski A, Vuoristo P, Myllarniemi M, Yilmaz S, Kallio E, Hayry P. Mycophenolate mofetil (MMF, RS-61443) inhibits inflammation and smooth muscle cell proliferation in rat aortic allografts. *Transplant Immunology* 1995; **3**: 342–351.
521. Weir M, Anderson L, Fink JC, *et al.* A novel approach to the treatment of chronic allograft nephropathy. *Transplantation* 1997; **64**: 1706–1710.
522. Lee HM. Chronic rejection: Pathogenesis and treatment. *Transplantation Proceedings* 1996; **28**: 1146–1147.
523. Satterthwaite R, Aswad S, Sunga V, *et al.* Incidence of new-onset hypercholesterolemia in renal transplant patients treated with FK506 or cyclosporine. *Transplantation* 1998; **65**: 446–449.
524. Washio M, Okuda S, Ikeda M, *et al.* Hypercholesterolemia and the progression of the renal dysfunction in chronic renal failure patients. *Journal of Epidemiology* 1996; **6**: 172–177.
525. Katznelson S, Wilkinson AH, Kobashigawa JA, *et al.* The effect of pravastatin on acute rejection after kidney transplantation—A pilot study. *Transplantation* 1996; **61**: 1469–1474.
526. Kasiske BL. Clinical correlates to chronic renal allograft rejection. *Kidney International* 1997; **52** (Suppl. 63): S71–S74.

11

The kidney in tropical infections

Rashad S. Barsoum

Introduction

The 'tropical zone' is classically defined as that lying within 10° on either side of the Equator. However, the term is conventionally applied to a wider range extending from the Cancer to the Capricorn orbits, thereby including the whole of South-east Asia and Central America, most of Africa, Arabia, India, and significant parts of Australia, South America, and Mexico (Fig. 11.1).

The tropical warm and humid climate modifies the prevalence and clinical patterns of different diseases in the domain of nephrology. This is largely attributed to its influence on tropical bio-ecology, which eventually echoes on the kidneys. Warmth and humidity support vectors and reservoirs of many microbial agents, hence the high environmental pollution with parasites (Fig. 11.2), bacteria, viruses, fungi, and fungal toxins. Some of these are entertained in the rest of the world, while many are almost specific to the tropics. The latter are conventionally called 'endemic tropical infections'.

For socio-political reasons, most tropical countries have stumbled in their industrial development, and subsequently became economically underdeveloped. This misfortune reflects on many aspects of life, including modest educational standards and poor health services. Inadequate control of the spread of infections, lack of knowledge about their renal manifestations and delay in their diagnosis, the inadvertent use of medications, and the wide implementation of 'traditional medicine' are the major ingredients that generate the scenario of 'tropical nephrology'.

For many decades, infection has been held responsible for the extremely high prevalence of both acute and chronic renal failure in the tropics [1]. In a recent review, it was estimated to account for up to 42.5% of ARF in Thailand, compared with a contemporary figure of 7.3% in the United Kingdom [2]. The incidence of chronic renal failure in the tropical zone ranges between about 100 and 200 new patients per million population every year [3], which is many folds that reported in the developed world. Infection is the major player in this drama, being responsible for a considerable proportion of glomerulonephritis, interstitial nephritis, urinary obstruction, urolithiasis, amyloidosis, vasculitis, and even renovascular hypertension.

Recent years have witnessed the spread of tropical infections outside the tropics. With the enormous expansion of globetrotting, patients, carriers, and vectors

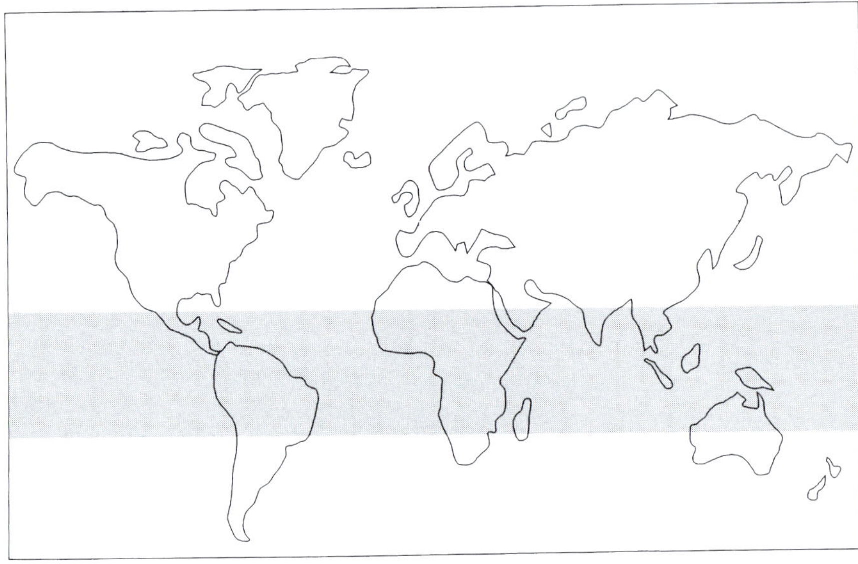

Fig. 11.1 Map of the world showing the 'tropical zone'.

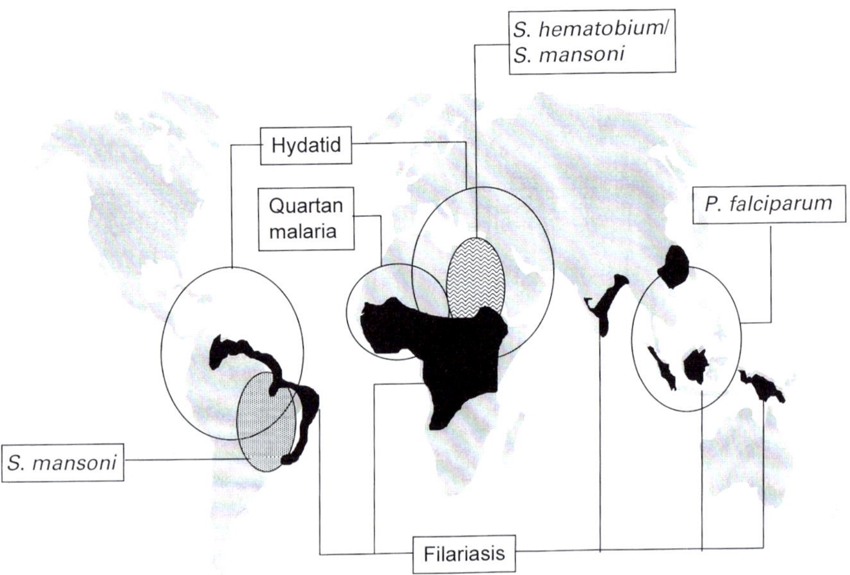

Fig. 11.2 Global distribution of parasitic diseases, also shown are the territories where renal complications have been reported.

conveyed tropical infections to the north, while tourists, troops, and experts acquired the endemic infections of the south. The targets of the initial impact were immunocompromised patients whose lives were threatened by such infections as salmonellosis [4], cryptosporidosis [5], toxoplasmosi [6], leishmaniasis [7], trypanosomiasis [8], strongyloidiasis [9], malaria [10], and schistosomiasis [1]. These infections were either acquired *de novo* (e.g. toxoplasmosis, malaria), or activated as a consequence of immunosuppression (e.g. cryptosporidosis, strongyloidiasis).

It was soon realized that even the immunocompetent non-tropical inhabitant was also at risk. Patients were reported to have acquired severe malaria by expo-sure to infected mosquitoes in Paris airport [12]. Schistosomiasis was reported in Netherlands hospitals [13], filariasis in Texas [14], strongyloidiasis in Montreal [15], cysticercosis in New York schools [16], and Kala-azar in British children [17].

Facing this demographic and ecological evolution, renal physicians worldwide have no choice but to get acquainted with the impact of tropical infection on the kidneys. Not only is this important for the bedside diagnosis and management of patients with kidney disease, but there is also a lot to learn from the relevant pathophysiological mechanisms, which may add to their insight into other areas of nephrology.

The spectrum of infection-associated tropical nephropathies

The clinical spectrum of tropical nephropathies may be categorized into three groups: (a) acute renal failure (ARF) complicating the severe systemic illness associated with a tropical infection; (b) subclinical or mild self-limited glomerular or tubulo-interstitial disease, and (c) chronic and progressive renal disease which may lead to end-stage.

Acute renal failure

A long list of tropical infections may be associated with ARF (Table 11.1). Those of considerable *epidemiological* importance are falciparum malaria [27], leptospirosis [18], septicemic melioidosis [19], shigellosis [20], and AIDS [30].

Falciparum malaria is responsible for a considerable sector of ARF in South-east Asia [27], Vietnam [36], the Indian peninsula [37,38], and Africa [39,40,41]. Infection is associated with acute tubular necrosis in 1–4% of cases; the incidence being as high as 60% in 'malignant malaria' [42]. The reported mortality ranges from 15 to 30% [43]. In severe cases associated with 'black water fever', a fatal outcome is almost the rule. Intravascular red cell sludging, hemolysis, and massive monocyte activation are the main pathogenetic mechanisms (Fig. 11.3). Rhabdomyolysis and fluid and electrolyte loss via the gastrointestinal tract are additional factors in some cases. Patients with Falciparum-associated ARF usually have jaundice, hyponatremia, acidosis, and may become hypoglycemic or hypoxic [27]. Coma eventually supervenes due to these metabolic perturbations, or due to clogging of the cerebral circulation by clumps of merozoites (cerebral malaria) [44].

Table 11.1 Tropical infections frequently associated with acute renal failure

	Ref.	Crescentic GN	AIN	ATN	HUS	Hemolysis	DIC	Jaundice	Commonly associated features
Bacterial									
Leptospirosis	18		++	++++	+	+	+	++++	Hemorrhagic tendency
Melioidosis	19		+++	++					Hyponatremia
Shigellosis	20			+	++	+	+	+	Neurological complications
Salmonellosis	21		++	+	+	+	+	+	Gastrointestinal manifestations
Cholera	22			+					Hypokalemia, acidosis
Tetanus	23			+++					Convulsions
Scrub typhus	24		+	+		+		+	
Diphtheria	25		++	+					Myocarditis, Polyneuritis
Leprosy	26	+		+					Lepromatous features
Lepromatous				+++					
Other				+					
Parasitic									
Malignant malaria	27		+	++++		+++	+	++	Coma, hypoxia, hypoglycemia
Babessjosis	28		+	+++					
Kala-azar	29		+++	+					
Viral									
AIDS	30	+	+	++++					Diarrhoea, concomitant infections
Dengue	31		+	++					
Hanta virus disease	32		+++						
Infectious mononucleosis	33		+						
Hepatitis A	34	+							
Hepatitis C	35	+	+	+					Polyuria

AGN = Acute glomerulonephritis; AIN = acute interstitial nephritis; ATN = acute tubular necrosis; HUS = hemolytic uremic syndrome; DIC = disseminated intravascular coagulation.
+, <10%; ++, 10–24%; +++, 25–49%; ++++, 50–80%.

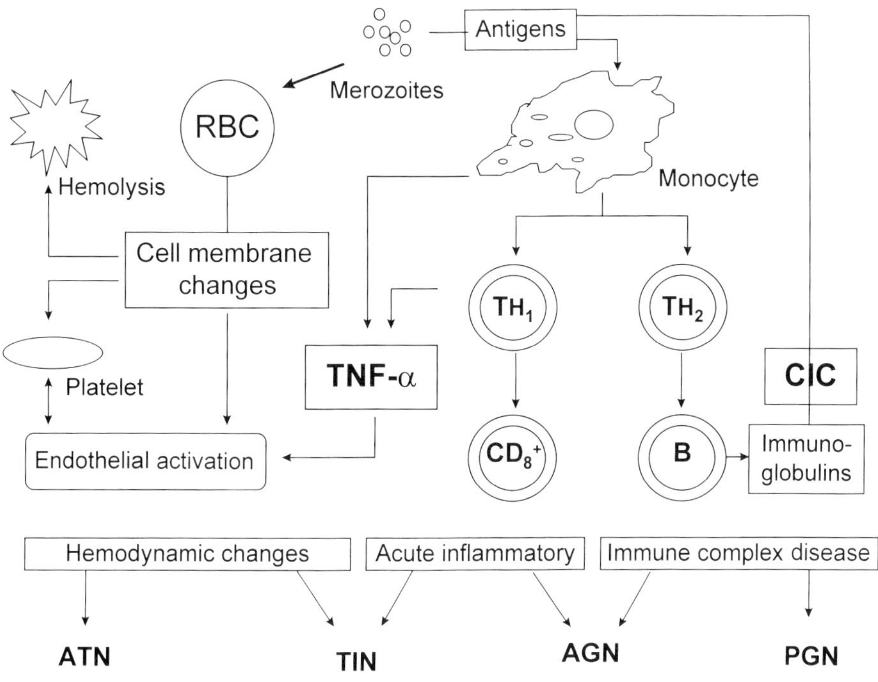

Fig. 11.3 Principal pathogenetic mechanisms in falciparum malarial infection.

Leptospirosis is a major cause of ARF in South-east Asia, India, and Sri Lanka, accounting for one-fourth to one-third of all reported ARF [18]. The kidney is invariably involved in leptospirosis, both by direct invasion of the interstitium by leptospires, the immune response to the infection, the effects of endotoxemia, and rhabdomyolysis [45]. Hepatic involvement and thrombocytopenia are common leading, in severe cases, to a hemorrhagic hepatorenal syndrome often called 'Weil's disease'. This condition may be confused with Hanta virus infection [32], yet hepatic involvement in unusual with Hanta. Renal recovery is the rule in patients who survive the acute extrarenal manifestations of both conditions.

Melioidosis is a community acquired infection, endemic in South-east Asia. Infection may be subclinical, but it often leads to a rapidly fatal septicemia [19]. Acute renal failure is reported in up to 35% of case [46]. Severe hyponatremia is characteristic, being encountered in more than 90% of cases, presumably an expression of a 'sick cell' syndrome.

Shigella infections are particularly alarming in communities with poor hygienic standards. In a study from India, up to 26% of patients with shigella-induced dysentery developed ARF either due to fluid depletion or to the development of hemolytic uremic syndrome (HUS) [47]. The latter was reported to be responsible for 34% of all ARF in another study from the same country [20], which is attributed to the massive endothelial injury induced by shigella endotoxin.

Of *pathogenetic* interest, although of less clinical and epidemiological concern, is the ARF complicating tetanus. The clinical picture is dominated by the convulsions; ARF being often overlooked and is seldom the cause of death. However, its occurrence is of particular pathogenetic interest, being one of the unusual conditions in which renal failure seems to be induced by catecholamine overshoot [48]. In this respect, it mimics the renal failure encountered with the prolonged use of vasopressor agents, and that complicating head injury. Rhabdomyolysis is extremely common in tetanus, and may contribute to ARF, although the latter does not necessarily correlate with creatine phosphokinase levels [23]. No direct effect of tetanus exotoxin has been demonstrated on the kidneys.

Reversible renal disease

This category includes a large number of tropical infections (Table 11.2), in which renal involvement is noted by accidental urine analysis or by minimal symptoms and signs that are often over-ridden by the manifestations of the primary infection. Renal involvement in readily reversible by merely controlling the infection.

Glomerulonephritis

The mesangium is the principal target in all these infections, being essentially the front-line of glomerular defense. Activated by antigens, immune complexes, and/or complement, they proliferate and increase matrix deposition. Proliferative glomerulonephritis is, therefore, the prototype lesion seen in most of these infections. Transit cells, comprising lymphocytes and neutrophils are often seen, reflecting the systemic immune activation. Immune complexes are detected by electron microscopy as dense mesangial and subendothelial deposits. By immunofluorescence, IgM and C3 are detected in virtually all cases, microbial antigens in most, and IgG, IgA, and fibrinogen in variable combinations in some (see Fig. 11.4).

Although some of these glomerular lesions may be modified by specific features of the immune kinetics of a particular agent, they remain essentially self-limited. They tend to resolve spontaneously upon successful treatment of the infection, and often remain stationary even without treatment of a parasitic infection. This feature is attributed to three main mechanisms:

1. Antigen modulation, which includes frequent modification of the antigenic molecular structure as with malaria [69] or concealing with host's antigens (e.g. H blood group substance, or HLA antigens) as with schistosomiasis [70]. Induction of the antigen clearance mechanisms [71] or conversely, the development of antigen excess [72] may also be involved in certain situations.
2. Switching to Th2 predominance (Fig. 11.5), which is characteristic of many infections particularly the helminthic. This tends to constrain the intensity of the immune response at the cellular as well as the humoral level. Although the switch supports B-lymphocyte proliferation, it selectively promotes inhibitory immunoglobulins as IgM and IgG4 [73].
3. Macrophage/monocyte inhibition by parasitic products [74] and Th2 cytokines as interleukin (IL −10) [75]. This hits a key position in the immune response

Table 11.2 Tropical infections frequently associated with self-limited renal pathology

	Ref.	Glomerulonephritis		Interstitial nephritis	Vasculitis
		Proliferation	IC deposits		
Bacterial					
Streptococcal skin infection [*]	49	+++	M,G,C3,Ag	+	+
Salmonellosis	50	++	M,G,C3,Ag	++	+
Leptospirosis	45	+	M,C3	++	++
Melioidosis	46	+		+++	
Scrub typhus	51	+		+	+
Diphtheria	52			+++	+
Leprosy	53				
Lepromatous [*]		+++	M,G,C3,Ag	+++	
Other		+		+	
Protozoal					
Falciparum malaria	27	+	M,G,C3,Ag	++	
Visceral leishmaniasis	53	+	M,G,C3,Ag	+++	
Trypanosomiasis [**]	54	+	M,C3		
Toxoplasmosis	55	+	M,C3,	+	
Cestodal					
Ecchinococcosis [*]	56	++	M,G,C3	+	
Trematodal					
Schistosomiasis					
Hematobium [*]	57	++	M,G,C3,Ag	++	
Mansoni [*]	58	+++	M,G,C3,Ag	+	
Japonicum	59	+	M,G,C3,Ag		
Mekongi	60			+++	
Nematodal					
Filariasis					
W. bancrofti [*]	61	+	M,G,C3	+	
O. volvulus	62	+++	M,G,C3,Ag	+	
L. ioa [*]	63	+	M,G,C3,Ag	+	
Strongyloidiasis	64	+	M,G,C3,Ag		
Trichinosis	65	+	M,G,C3		+
Viral					
Dengue	66	+	G,M,C3,		
HBV [*]	67				+++
HCV [*]	68	++	Cryos, G,M,C3,		++

* May also cause ovent glomerular disease.
** Based on experimental data.

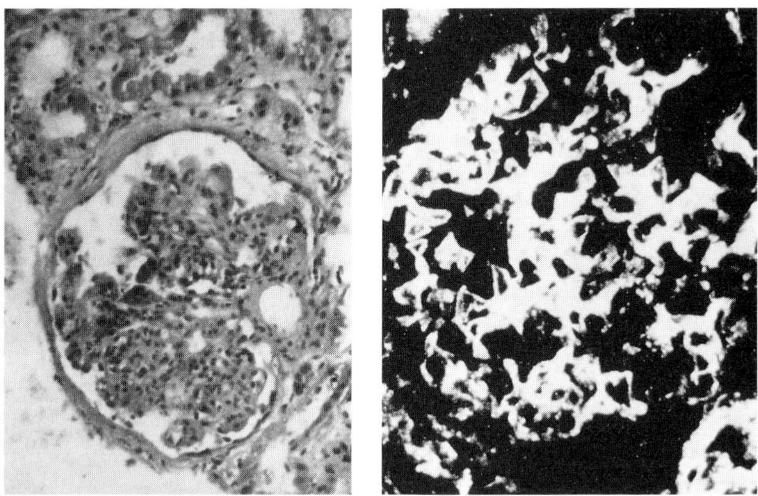

Fig. 11.4 Mesangial proliferation (left) with IgM deposits (right), the typical glomerular lesion associated with most tropical infections.

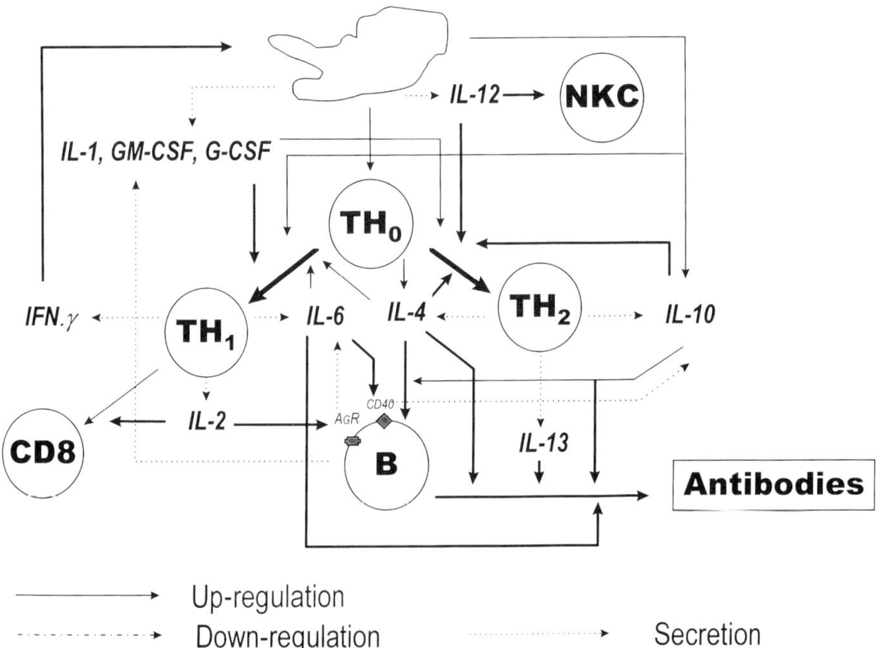

Fig. 11.5 Principal pathways of immune activation in tropical infections. Explanation in text.

cascade, in addition to reflecting on the proliferative potential of mesangial cells.

Interstitial nephritis

Interstitial nephritis is a frequent complication of many infections either due to direct invasion by the infective agent or to the relevant immune response. Acute suppurative interstitial nephritis may lead to the formation of microabscesses (e.g. typhoid) or even well defined renal abscess (e.g. septicemic melioidosis). On the other hand, the immune-mediated interstitial infiltrates are mainly composed of lymphocytes and plasma cells, and are often associated with a lot of edema. In severe cases, such as with Hanta viral infection [32] and Kala-azar [29] (Fig. 11.6) this may present with ARF.

Like the glomerular lesions, infection-associated interstitial nephritis tends to regress without sequelae upon the eradication of the cause, or even without as in Kala-azar. This course reflects the late inhibition of the host's immune response in parasitic infections (*vide supra*).

Progressive renal disease

Contrary to the general trend, the renal lesions associated with certain infections tend to progress, even after successful extermination of the original disease. In endemic areas, such diseases may amount to an epidemiologically significant issue, in addition to being interesting models that may shed a lot of light on the mechanisms of progression in general. For the purpose of systematized clinical approach, these disorders shall be classified according to the predominant pattern of renal injury.

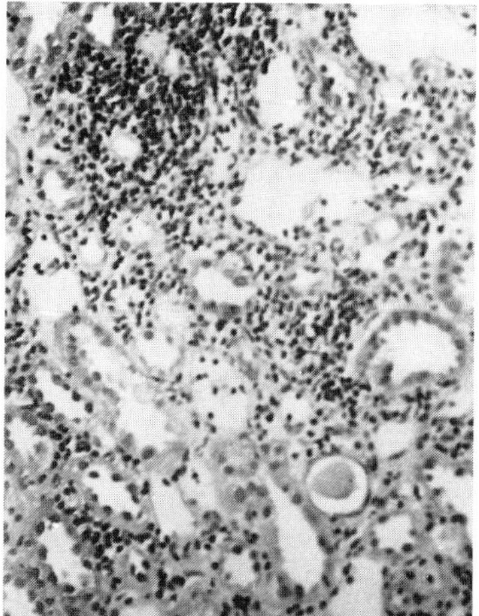

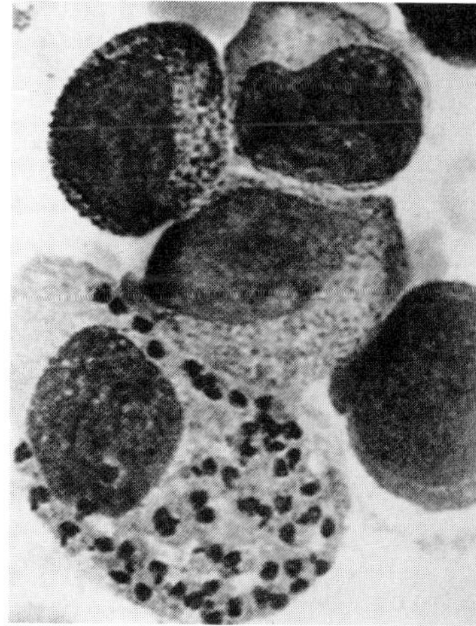

Fig. 11.6 Kala-azar nephropathy. Left: Interstitial edema and round cellular infiltration; right: live and intact amastigotes in a macrophage.

Glomerulonephritis

Schistosomal glomerulopathy As with other infection-associated glomerulopathies, mesangial cellular proliferation is the hallmark of glomerular injury in schistosomiasis, being associated with infections with all three major human pathogenetic strains, namely *Schistosomiasis mansoni* [57], *S. hematobium* [58], and *S. japonicum* [59]. It is also consistently induced in many experimental models infected with these parasitic specie [76].

The majority of patients, particularly those with *S. hematobium* and *S. japonicum* infections, remain asymptomatic with little evidence of any disease progression. Microalbuminuria or mild dipstick detectable proteinuria may be the only clinical expression of renal involvement. However, an occasional patient may present with overt nephrotic syndrome with or without hypertension, but renal function is usually preserved. The factors which identify this subset of patients are not understood. Differences in parasitic strains, intensity of infection, and host genetic factors have been blamed [60]. The effect of anti-schistosomal therapy is controversial, largely due to the heterogeneity of reported cases. In our experience, patients with pure mesangial proliferation usually respond to such treatment.

On the other hand, the lesions tend to progress to renal failure in about 15% of patients with *S. mansoni*-induced hepatic fibrosis [77]. In those cases mesangial matrix expands and may lead to secondary focal or global glomerulosclerosis (Fig. 11.7). Parasitic antigens, usually of gut origin [78], along with IgM and C3, are detected by immunofluorescence in early glomerular lesion. IgG and IgA deposits

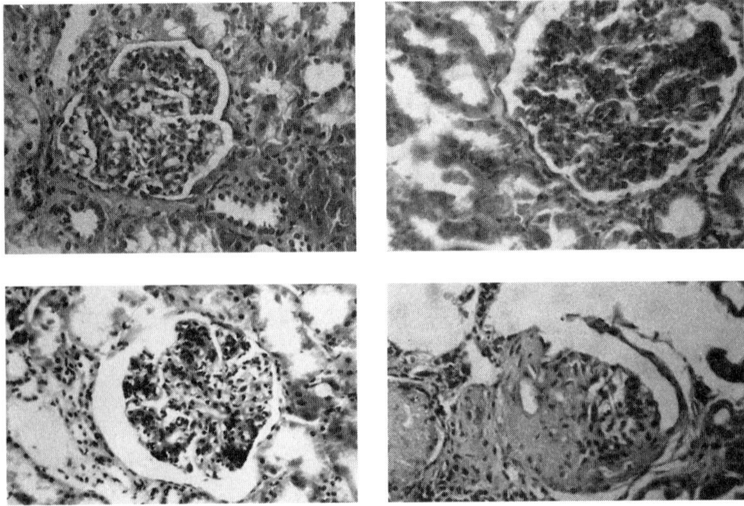

Fig. 11.7 Schistosomal glomerulopathy. Top left: axial mesangial proliferation (class I); top right: exudative glomerulonephritis in the presence of concomitant salmonella infection (class II); bottom left: mesangiocapillary glomerulonephritis (class III); bottom right: focal and segmental glomerulosclerosis (class IV).

are detected with increasing frequency as the disease progresses [79]. Electron microscopic localization shows that the deposits are essentially mesangial, subendothelial, and occasionally subepithelial [58].

This category is characterized by the association of hepatosplenomegaly and the nephrotic syndrome in a patient with present or past evidence of *S. mansoni* infection [80,81]. Most patients are malnourished due to associated endemic infestations. Younger patients acquiring the infection during their first decade are often stunted or even infantile. Blood pressure is elevated in 50% of patients. The liver is palpable and firm, often shrunken due to extensive fibrosis. The spleen is enlarged, usually pushing down towards the left iliac fossa, but rarely crossing the middle line being anchored by adhesions to the abdominal wall. Portal hypertension is common, leading to the formation of lower esophageal and gastric fundal varices, as well as secondary hemorrhoids. Abdominal wall collaterals may be visible, particularly around the umbilicus (caput medusae). A venous hum of rapid and turbulent blood flow in those veins may be auscultated at the lower sternal end (Cruvilhier–Baumgarten sign). Ascites invariably precedes peripheral edema, due to the favorable hemodynamic milieu generated by portal hypertension. Many patients display evidence of schistosomal involvement of other organs as the colon (pericolic masses), lungs (cor pulmonale), lower urinary tract (hydronephrosis), and less often the genitals, skin, nervous system, and conjunctivae.

Urinary protein excretion is usually in the nephrotic range, and the sediment shows increased red and white cells and different types of casts. Serum albumin is often very low, due to the association of hepatocellular impairment and nutritional deficiency with proteinuria. In contrast, all globulin fractions are increased particularly, α_2–β being associated with the nephrotic syndrome and γ-globulins as a response to chronic granulomatous infection. Rheumatoid factor and other serological markers of an autoimmune reaction are often detected. Blood cholesterol is seldom significantly elevated presumably due to the impaired hepatic synthesis. Overt renal involvement of this kind in Manson's schistosomiasis does not respond to treatment by antiparasitic agents, steroids, or immunosuppression.

An interesting variant is encountered in patients co-infected with *S. mansoni* and one or another of different strains of *Salmonella*, usually *S. parathyphi-A* [82]. The association does not occur by mere co-incidence; various studies have shown that salmonella gets shelter from the host's immune response by hiding within the cuticle of schistosome [83]. In such cases, the glomerular lesion is exudative (Fig. 11.7), with plenty of neutrophils infiltrating the mesangium as well as the renal interstitium [82].

Patients with concomitant salmonella infection are febrile, severely anemic, and develop a characteristic vasculitic skin eruption. They become acutely nephrotic and rapidly hypoproteinemic. If untreated, they may die of severe emaciation or endotoxemia, yet they respond very well to combined antiparasitic and antibiotic therapy.

Quartan malarial nephropathy The glomerular lesion is dominated by subendothelial deposits [84], seen by light microscopy (Fig. 11.8) as thickening of the capillary walls, giving a double contour appearance to the basement membrane. Mesangial

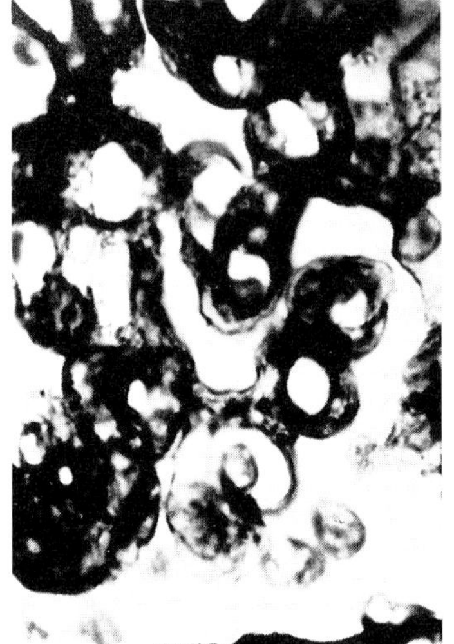
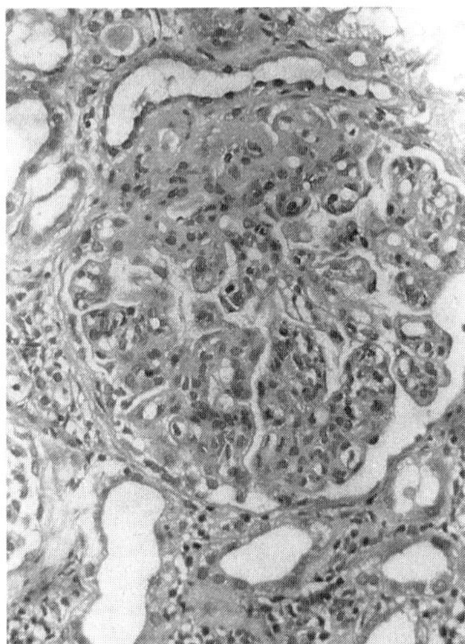

Fig. 11.8 Quartan malarial nephropathy. Mesangial proliferation with apparent basement membrane thickening due to subendothelial deposits, which are shown to the left by silver stain and higher magnification.

proliferation is rare, being encountered mainly in adults. By immunofluorescence the deposits usually exhibit a coarsely granular pattern containing IgG (most commonly IgG3), IgM, C3, and malarial antigens in early cases. Electron microscopy shows subendothelial deposits of electron-dense or basement membrane-like material, associated with the formation of intra-membranous lacunae.

Quartan malarial nephropathy is a disease of children, usually becoming manifest at the age of 5 years. It ushers in as a steroid-resistant nephrotic syndrome that often progresses to end-stage renal disease in a few years, even after successful parasitological cure by adequate antimalarial chemotherapy.

Filarial nephropathy Although glomerular lesions have been described with many filarial infections [61–63], clinically significant renal disease is usually associated with *Onchocerca volvulus* [62]. Mesangiocapillary (Fig. 11.9) and chronic sclerosing glomerulonephritis are the lesions most often reported. Subendothelial and mesangial immune complexes containing IgM, IgG, C3, and *Onchocerca* antigens are detected by immunofluorescence and mesangial electron-dense deposits by electron microscopy.

Renal involvement usually manifests by nephrotic-range proteinuria and hypertension in young adults, and soon progresses to chronic renal failure despite treatment. Most patients have features of associated autoimmune disorders as polyarthritis and chorioretinitis.

Hepatitis C-associated glomerulopathies Although hepatitis C is not strictly a tropical infection, its prevalence in tropical countries is extremely high. Part of this is

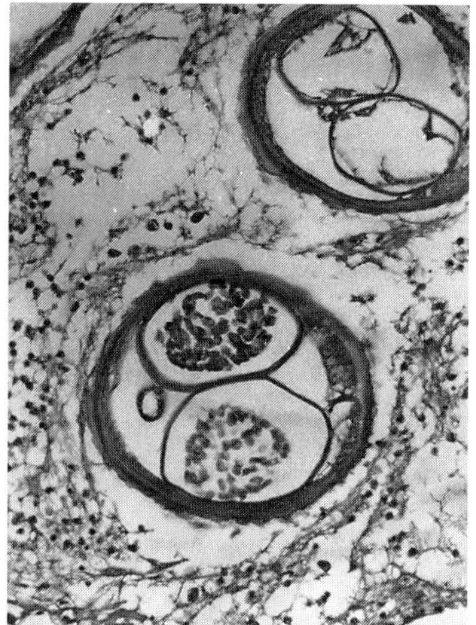
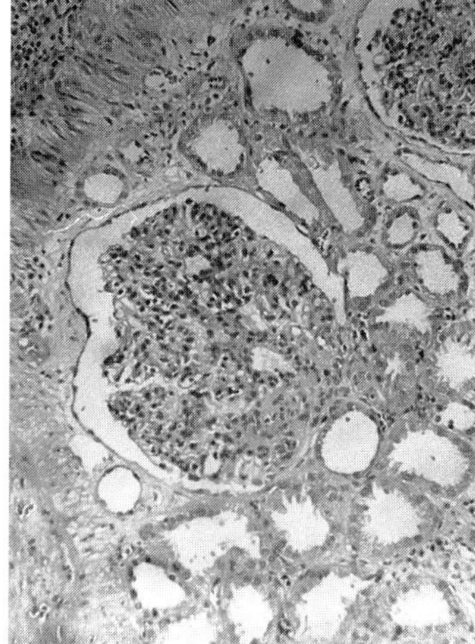

Fig. 11.9 Filarial nephropathy. Left: *Onchocerca volvulus* deposits in tissues; Right: marked mesangioproliferative glomerulonephritis.

explained by its close association with schistosomiasis, but also by the prevailing poor sanitary standards and other, unknown community-related factors. Hepatitis C virus (HCV) is classically associated with mesangiocapillary glomerulonephritis [85], less often with membranous nephropathy [86] and IgA nephropathy when there is significant hepatic disease. Many patients also have circulating cryoglobulins, which infer certain histopathological features.

Interstitial nephritis

Progressive interstitial nephropathy accounts for at least one-third of chronic renal failures in many tropical countries [1]. In addition to infection, this has been also attributed to environmental pollution [2], the abuse of drugs, herbs [87], and other traditional medications [2].

'Non-specific' organisms causing acute or chronic interstitial nephritis are rarely blamed in the pathogenesis of progressive renal disease, unless associated with obstruction, reflux, or a co-morbid renal condition. On the other hand, certain 'specific' infections may lead to progressive fibrosis, ending up with renal failure. In the tropics, such infections include tuberculosis and leprosy. In experimental animals, certain strains of schistosomes may lead to the same end.

Tuberculosis is alarmingly spreading in the tropics, even out of proportion of the worldwide trend. Renal involvement is characterized by the formation of interstitial granulomas containing the characteristic Langhan's cells (Fig. 11.10). Interstitial caseation may lead to multiple large cavities in the kidneys, and may obstruct calyces leading to characteristic radiological findings. Diffuse interstitial renal tuberculosis is increasingly reported as a cause of obscure anemia, pyrexia, acquired tubular defects, and progressive renal failure. Involvement of the lower urinary tract leads

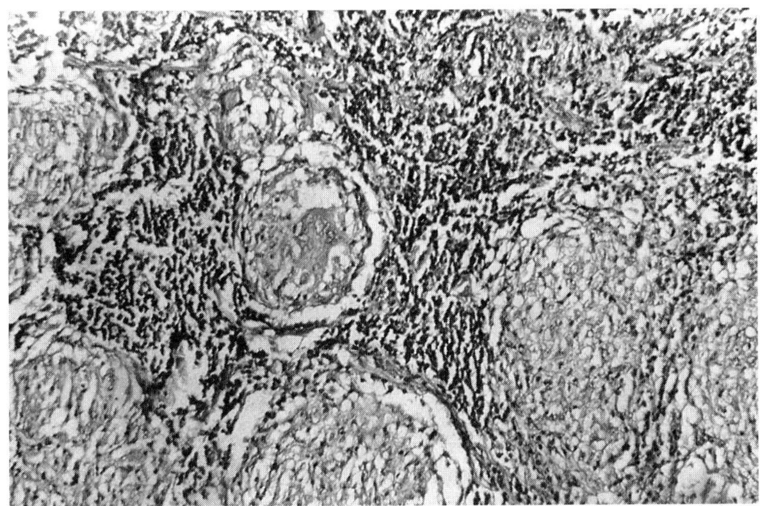

Fig. 11.10 Renal tuberculosis. Note the extensive interstitial round cellular infiltration and the granulomas containing epithelioid cells and Langhan's giant cells.

to bladder ulcers, ureteric strictures, and back pressure. Tuberculosis remains on top of the list of tropical amyloidosis [88]. Tuberculosis is a considerable problem in tropical dialysis units and a threat to renal transplant recipients.

Although a variety of glomerular lesions are associated with leprosy, interstitial nephritis is the most common cause of renal failure in those patients [26,89]. This may be attributed to the immune response to infection, yet the use of drugs, such as Dapsone, Rifampicin, and non-steroidal anti-inflammatory drugs may play a major part. Co-infection with tuberculosis has been reported in up to 25% of patients from Malaysia [89].

Although fungal infections are often reported to affect the renal interstitium in autopsy studies, progressive interstitial disease is quite rare. Papillary necrosis has been reported with candidiasis and cryptococcosis. However, antifungal drug nephrotoxicity is more notorious in this respect.

On the other hand, fungal toxins have been blamed in the pathogenesis of interstitial nephritis. Most famous is the Balkan nephropathy, attributed to ochratoxin (Fig. 11.11). The latter has been recently detected in patients with progressive interstitial nephropathy of obscure etiology in tropical countries as Tunisia [90] and Egypt [91]. It is noteworthy that the related aflatoxin has been widely incriminated in the hepatic morbidity in east and southern Africa.

Obstructive nephropathy

Tropical infections associated with urinary obstruction include tuberculosis (*vide supra*), *S. hematobium*, and occasionally, hydatid disease (echinococcosis).

Schistosoma hematobium This parasite is endemic and highly prevalent in Africa. However, prevalence does not reflect morbidity, which is widely variable according

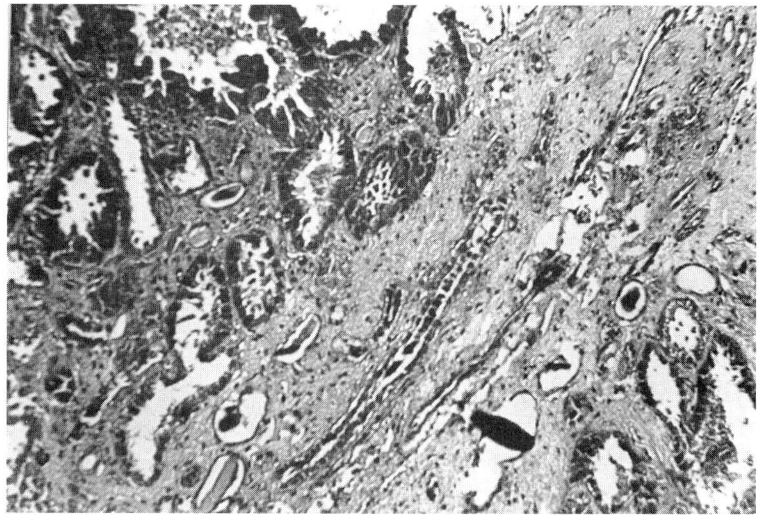

Fig. 11.11 Ochratoxin-associated interstitial fibrosis (kindly provided by Saadi *et al.* Ref. 91).

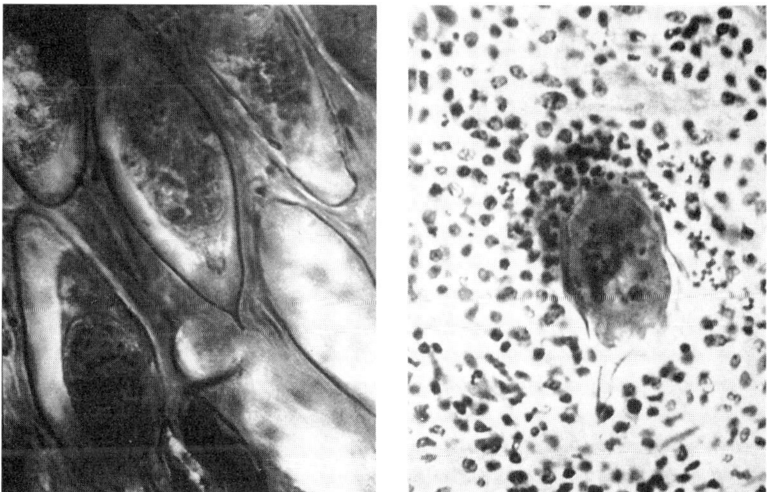

Fig. 11.12 *Schistosoma hematobium*. Left: Sheet of ova; right: granuloma around a partially disrupted ovum.

to the infective strains, intensity of infection, repeated infections, and host susceptibility [60].

Infection is acquired by contact with freshwater rivers and canals. The infective agent, the cercaria, matures into schistosomulae, which migrate to settle ultimately in the perivesical plexus of veins. The mature worms lay eggs with terminal spikes (Fig. 11.12), which find their way to the exterior via the mucosa of the lower urinary tract. A very small fraction of those eggs is trapped in the submucosa, where they excite an immune reaction leading to the formation of 'pseudotubercles', that coalesce to form nodules, ulcerate, and ultimately heal by fibrosis (Fig. 11.13). Although the early lesions may be associated with a lot of symptoms, they hardly reflect on the renal structure or function. It is in the late stages of cicatricial narrowing of the ureters that back pressure affects the kidneys (Fig. 11.14). Many functional consequences are reported including tubular defects in salt and water handling, tubular acidosis, and finally impairment of the glomerular filtration rate. Superimposed infection leads to progressive interstitial nephritis, which progresses to end-stage renal failure.

Renal amyloidosis

The high prevalence of amyloidosis in the tropics has been reported in the sixties, and was attributed to the 'associated bacterial and parasitic infections'. Tuberculosis and leprosy were counted as the principal tropical infections associated with this condition, and indeed remain so in many tropical territories. Evidence was presented in the mid-seventies by Sudanese nephrologists, that schistosomiasis was responsible for renal amyloidosis in four patients [92]. This relation was firmly established by subsequent clinical [93] and experimental [94] evidence, and was shown not to be species-specific [93]. Other tropical infections also associated with amyloidosis include leishmaniasis [29], filariasis [95], and echinococcosis [96].

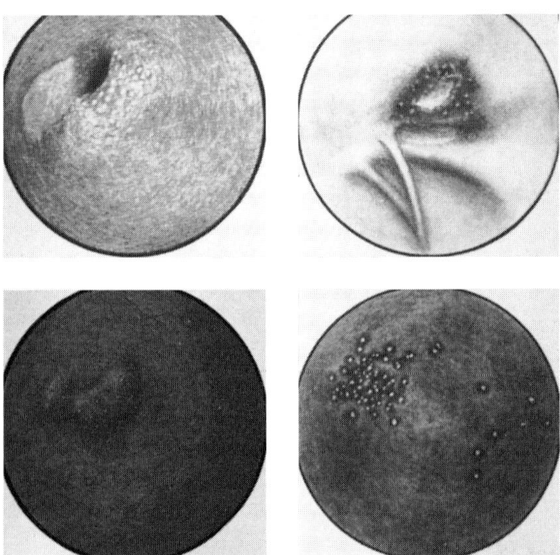

Fig. 11.13 Cystoscopic appearances in *S. hematobium* infection. Bottom right: Pseudotubercles; bottom left: Sessile mass covered by pseudotubercles in a congested mucosa; top right: Ulcer surrounded by pale mucosa containing a few pseudotubercles; top left: healed lesion with a pale mucosa containing calcified tubercles 'sandy patches'.

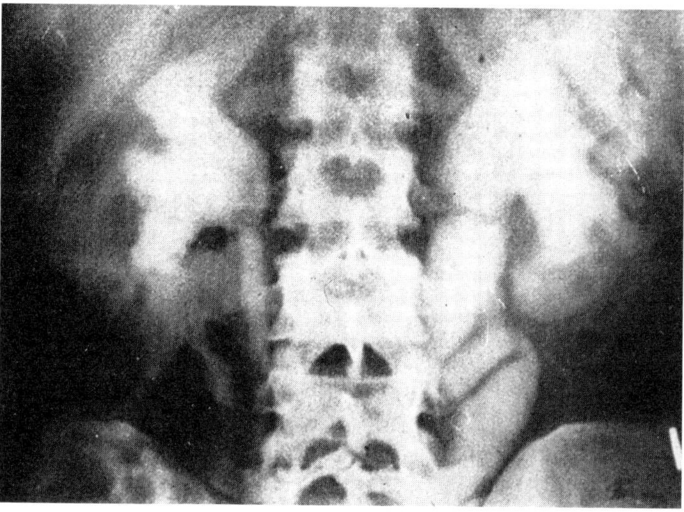

Fig. 11.14 Intravenous urography showing severe hydronephrosis associated with bilharzial (schistosomal) ureteric strictures.

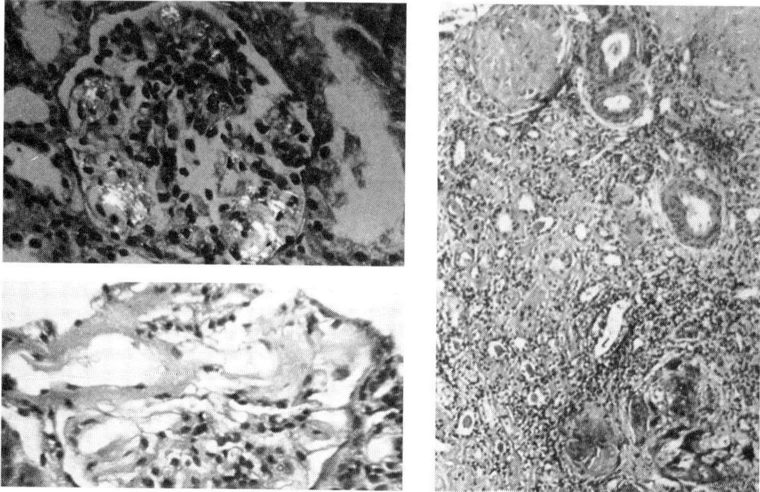

Fig. 11.15 Schistosoma-associated amyloidosis (class V). *Top left*: green birefringence of early amyloid glomerular deposits, stained by Congo-Red/hematoxylin. *Bottom left*: glomerular amyloid deposits at the vascular pole, associated with mesangial proliferation. *Right*: total replacement of the glomerular structure by amyloid deposits, amidst extensive interstitial fibrosis and inflammatory cellular infiltration cellular infiltration. Note the schistosomal granuloma at the right lower corner.

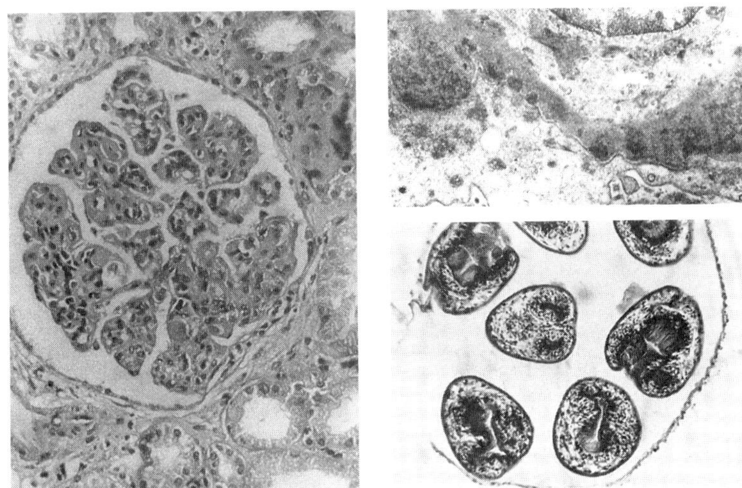

Fig. 11.16 *In-situ* immune complex deposition. Extramembranous electron-dense deposits (top right) in a case of echinococcosis (daughter scolices shown bottom right), associated with mesangiocapillary (type III) glomerulonephritis (left).

In all reports, the amyloid deposits were mostly renal (Fig. 11.15), with occasional hepatic and splenic involvement. Their distribution was mainly peri-reticulin, and whenever reported the fibrils were composed of AA protein. Many patients were asymptomatic [93] but the majority presented with the nephrotic syndrome and progressed to chronic renal failure.

Renal vasculitis

Although vasculitis is a fairly common feature of many tropical infections as salmonellosis, brucellosis, leptospirosis, and others, clinically significant renal vasculitis is only seen with human immunodeficiency virus (HIV), hepatitis B virus (HBV), HCV-associated cryoglobulinemia, and cytomegalovirus infections in the immunocompromised.

Of particular interest is 'tropical vasculitis' which affects the aorta and large and medium-sized arteries. Although often referred to as tropical Takayasu disease, it differs from classical Takayasu in affecting the lower part of the body with equal or even higher frequency than the upper. It has been frequently incriminated in renovascular hypertension in the tropics. Recent evidence suggests a causal relation between tropical vasculitis and tuberculosis [97].

Mechanisms of progression

From the foregoing display, it can be seen that progression is the exception rather than the rule in infection-associated nephropathies. At this point, it would be interesting to examine critically the immune response profiles associated with progression, that seem to intercept the natural tendency to reversibility.

Immune complexes

Glomerular immune deposits are characteristic of the renal involvement in most infective tropical glomerulopathies. They are classically seen in post-streptococcal glomerulonephritis, as well as in the nephropathies associated with typhoid [50], leptospirosis [45], leprosy [52], schistosomiasis [58], malaria [84], filariasis [62], leishmaniasis [53], trichinosis [65], echinococcosis [56], trypanosomiasis [54], toxoplasmosis [55], hepatitis viral infection [68], dengue [66], EBV [98], and others. Infective agent antigens have been identified in the glomerular deposits in most of the mentioned conditions, particularly by the use of sensitive techniques as immunoelectron microscopy [99], enzyme histochemistry, *in-situ* hybridization, and countercurrent electrophoresis of renal tissue eluates. As a general rule, specific antigens tend to disappear with progression of the glomerular pathology.

In the majority of those conditions, agent-specific circulating immune complexes have been simultaneously identified, often associated with activation of the classical complement pathway. They tend to follow the density of the glomerular deposits on a quantitative basis, and to decline with progression of renal pathology. In a few instances, usually those associated with subepithelial deposits, circulating complexes could not be detected and complement was not consumed, suggestive of *in-situ* immune complex formation. This has been reported with HCV, schistosomiasis, echinococcosis, and others.

As mentioned earlier, IgM is the most prominent immunoglobulin detected in the glomerular deposits as well as the circulating complexes. IgE has been also reported in a number of experimental studies [100], but has been skimpily looked for in clinical material. The potential role of the latter immunoglobulin in inducing the glomerular pathology [101] or at least paving the way for IgM deposition may turn out to be crucial.

The subsequent immunoglobulin profile seems to be the bottleneck in progression, as superimposition or replacement of IgM or by IgG or IgA deposits hallmark all infection-associated progressive glomerulopathies.

Serum IgG levels start to rise shortly following the establishment of infection. Both the magnitude and IgG class specificity seem to reflect on progression. Too much, as well as too sparse IgG may be associated with progression. IgG2 is an early bird that has been associated with most of the initial glomerular deposits, as in malaria [102] and leishmaniasis [103]. Its pathogenetic role is suggested by its ability to induce apoptosis in mesangial cell cultures [104]. IgG3 appears in the scene a little later, as confirmed by an elegant longitudinal study in shigellosis [105]. IgG3 deposits tend to predominate in quartan malarial nephropathy (Fig. 11.8), being mostly seen near the glomerular capillaries [103]. Based on this information, as well as the recent evidence incriminating IgG3 cryoglobulins in the pathogenesis of 'wire loop' lesions in lupus nephritis [106], IgG_3 tends to be the main constituent of sub-endothcliel glomerular deposite. IgG1 and IgG4 appear even later, being associated with a predominantly Th2 cell response. IgG_4, in particular, is a suppressor of the immune reaction. It seems to have a paradoxical effect to that of IgE in determining the persistence of parasitic infection as seen, for example, in schistosomiasis [107], malaria [108], and others. IL-12, a late cytokine supervening with Th2 supremacy, has been shown to switch the peripheral blood mononuclear cells away from IgE synthesis [109], in favor of IgG4. Glomerular deposits of the latter immunoglobulin have been often linked with fibrillary [110] and membranous [111] nephropathies.

IgA is also a late player, gaining particular importance in mucosal infections. Its role in parasitic glomerulopathies has been explored mainly with schistosomiasis [112–114]. Studies on hamsters have shown IgA glomerular deposits 18 weeks after experimental infection with *S. japonicum* or *S. mansoni*. Such deposits correlated with the progression and severity of glomerular pathology in experimental models [114] as well as in humans [112], High serum IgA levels have been observed in patients with schistosomal glomerulopathy [83,113]. Although the associated hepatic fibrosis may be partly responsible through inhibition of macrophage function [112], increased mucosal synthesis is confirmed by the disproportionate increase in antigliadin IgA antibodies [113]. Recent data have shown a several-fold increase in IgA-bearing peripheral blood mononuclear (PBMN) cells in patients with progressive schistosomal glomerulopathy, suggestive of a switch at the expense of IgM [Barsoum R, Saleh E, Abdel-Badie I, unpublished data, 1998]. It is probable that such switching may be an expression of an IL-10 [115] effect, which predominates in late colonic schistosomal granulomas [75].

While the impact of these immunoglobulin changes seems to be fairly clear, very little is known about the mechanisms underlying the predominance of one or another in a particular infection. Specific features about the microbial antigen may be involved, as suggested by the tendency of certain species and strains of the same agent to be more nephritogenic. An interesting example is the ability of certain strains of *S. hematobium* to induce glomerular lesions as compared with others [60].

Co-infection may have an important impact, as suggested in an animal model where the renal pathogenicity of *Plasmodium brasilanum* was augmented by concomitant infection with EBV [116]. As mentioned earlier on, the pathogenicity of *S. mansoni* is quantitatively and qualitatively modified by associated salmonella or HCV infection. The pathogenicity of malaria in rodents is considerably modified by associated strongyloides infection [117]. These associations lead to striking modification of the serum immunoglobulin profiles, which seem to be crucial in inducing morbidity.

Auto-immunity may also be involved in modifying the immunoglobulin response. Clinical manifestations of auto-immunity are often observed in conjunction with infection-associated progressive renal disease. Vasculitis, chorioretinitis arthritis, and erythema nodosum in leprosy [118] are typical examples. Serum levels of rheumatoid factor are significantly increased in many patients with bacterial, viral, and parasitic nephropathies. It has been suggested to interact with immune complexes, as an immunoabsorbant, in the pathogenesis of glomerular pathology [119]. Anti-DNA antibody [120], antiphospholipid antibody [121], antineutrophil cytotoxic antibodies [122], and several anti-idiotypic antibodies [123] have also been reported.

Complement activation

As complement activation is crucial for the induction of morbidity, it is understandable that differences in the pathogenicity of immune complexes may be related to their ability to interact with complement. Such variations may be an expression of antigenic differences, immunoglobulin diversity, or genetically determined host differences.

It is noteworthy that certain microbial products may directly activate complement via the alternative pathway, without the intervention of immune complexes. This has been incriminated in the pathogenesis of glomerular lesions in salmonellosis [82], leprosy [124], malaria [125], and other infections. Direct complement activation is usually blamed when the glomerular lesions are more florid, with a lot of transit cells, and no or scanty immune complex deposits. Subendothelial granular C3 deposits, on the other hand are characteristically abundant.

Cellular mechanisms

It has been clearly shown, in recent years, that while the initial renal lesions associated with infection occur during the Th1 predominance phase, progression paradoxically occurs when the Th2 phase supervenes. This implies that the late cytokines IL-4, IL-5, and IL-10, which are responsible for the self-limited nature of most infection-associated nephropathies, may, under certain conditions, be involved in a different scenario.

It has been shown that, with the exception of mycobacterial infections, co-morbidity is essential for infection-associated nephropathies to progress. As displayed earlier, this may be a concomitant infection or an autoimmune reaction, which may maintain a critical level of Th1 activation that modifies the effects of Th2 cytokines. Indeed, it has been shown both in experimental and human models, that Th1 and Th2 cytokines interact at the level of the C-gene [115], where they switch the emerging B-lymphocyte clones to a particular immunoglobulin or another (see Fig. 11.5).

A different profile is generated when the monocytes rather than Th1 cells are persistently co-activated during the Th2 phase of infection. Monocyte activation involves different functions differently. Under certain conditions, this perturbation may disturb the rate of generation of amyloid A protein in relation to that of its uptake, leading to accumulation and tissue deposition [126]. This mechanism is generally accepted to explain the amyloidosis complicating many chronic tropical infections where antigen release continues at a low rate for many years (*vide supra*).

Management

The past few decades have witnessed revolutionary development of antimicrobial chemotherapy against most tropical infections. Viral infections remain as a major cosmopolitan challenge. The emergence of resistant strains of tuberculosis, malaria, schistosomes, salmonella, and others, is a serious threat, particularly in the immunocompromised. Fortunately, the control of the causative infection usually cures the renal complications. However, active nephrological intervention is needed in patients who develop ARF and those with progressive renal disease.

Management of acute renal failure:

Patients who develop ARF are those with the worst infections, who are often neglected, dehydrated, and hyperpyrexial. Owing to the restricted renal services in the tropics, patients may not be referred until they have become shocked, jaundiced, and bleeding. Hyperkalemia is usually severe, due to the associated rhabdomyolysis, hemolysis, gastrointestinal bleeding, or acidosis.

With this scenario, there is little room for conservative treatment. Hemodialysis is often impossible or extremely risky owing to the circulatory instability and hemorrhagic tendency. Let alone the lack of equipment and trained personnel. Peritoneal dialysis is a fair alternative, easily available in distant territories. However, it is often inadequate in shocked patients, and is not very effective in the control of hyperkalemia. In well-equipped centers, continuous arteriovenous hemofilration (CAVH) has been offered as a much more efficient modality. Exchange transfusions, in vogue several decades ago, are no longer used in malignant malaria. Plasma exchange has a distinct place in the treatment of HUS.

Management of progressive renal disease

As the mechanisms of progression are not necessarily, not even frequently related to the persistence of infection, specific antimicrobial therapy may be ineffective. This has been shown with schistosomiasis [127], quartan malaria [84], and filariasis [62]. At a certain point, even mycobacterial diseases continue to deteriorate after the control of infection, largely due to hemodynamic and immunological mechanisms. Steroids and immunosuppressive agents have not been successful. Recent experimental data suggest that the induction of antigen excess in schistosomiasis may be helpful [72].

Management of end-stage renal disease

Patients who reach end-stage require renal replacement therapy. Late referral, comorbid conditions, and undernutrition are major obstacles to an efficient therapy. The lack of funds reflects on the quality of dialysis, inter-dialytic patient care, supplementary therapy with erythropoietin, active vitamin D, etc. Poor hygienic conditions favor the spread of dialysis-associated infections as HBV, HCV, and HIV [3]. They also stun the efforts to establish Continuous Ambulatory Peritoneal Dialysis (CAPD) as a first-line RRT in most tropical countries. Mexico and South-east Asian countries, however, have overcome this obstacle and established excellent widely spread CAPD [3].

About 10% of the global transplant activity is performed in tropical countries. The results are generally matching with international standards, as this line of treatment is focused in the larger units, that are privileged by well trained staff and good equipment. Infection remains, however, as the major cause of graft failure as well as patients death.

Key references

Barsoum R, Sitprija V. Tropical nephrology. In *Diseases of the Kidney* (eds RW Schrier and CW Gottaschalk ed.), Vol. VI. Little Brown & Co, Boston, 1996: 2221–2268.

Barsoum RS. Dialysis in developing countries. In: *Replacement of Renal Function by Dialysis* (eds IVC Jacobs, CM Kjellstrand, KM Koch, JF Winchester). Kluwer Inc, ed IV Dordsecht: Boston 1996: 1433–1442.

Barsoum RS. Schistosomal glomerulopathies. *Kidney Int* 1993; **44**: 1–12.

Sitprija V. Nephrology Forum: Nephropathy in falciparum malaria. *Kidney Int* 1988; **34**: 866.

References

1. Barsoum R. Nephrology and African ecology. An overview. *Artif Organs* 1991; **14**: 235.
2. Barsoum R, Sitprija V. Tropical nephrology. In *Diseases of the Kidney* (eds RW Schrier and CW Gottaschalk ed.), Vol. VI. Little Brown & Co, Boston, 1996: 2221–2268.
3. Barsoum RS. Dialysis in developing countries. In: *Replacement of Renal Function by Dialysis* (eds IVC Jacobs, CM Kjellstrand, KM Koch, JF Winchester). Kluwer Inc, Ed IV Dordsecht: Boston 1996: 1433–1442.
4. Saady MG, *et al.* Salmonella associated rejection in renal transplant recipients. Abstract: XI International Congress of Nephrology, Tokyo, Japan, 1990.
5. Crawford FG, Vermund SH. Human cryptosporidosis. *CRC Crit Rev Microbiol* 1988; **16**: 113–159.
6. Renoult E, Georges E, Biava MF, *et al.* Toxoplasmosis in kidney transplant recipients: a life-threatening but treatable disease. *Transplant Proc* 1997; **29**: 821–822.
7. Portoles J, Prats D, Torralbo A, *et al.* Visceral leishmaniasis: a cause of opportunistic infection in renal transplant patients in endemic areas. *Transplant* 1994; **57**: 1677–1679.
8. Lopez Blanco OA, Cavalli NH, Jasovich A, *et al.* Chagas' disease and kidney transplantation—follow-up of nine patients for 11 years. *Transplant Proc* 1992; **24**: 3089–3090.
9. DeVault GA Jr, King JW, Rohr MS, *et al.* Opportunistic infection with *Strongyloides stercoralis* in renal transplantation. *Rev Infect Dis* 1990; **12**: 653–671.
10. Sever MS, Ecder T, Aydin AE, *et al.* Living unrelated (paid) kidney transplantation in Third-World countries: high risk of complications besides the ethical problem. *Nephrol Dial Transplant* 1994; **9**: 350–354.
11. Azevedo LS, de Paula FJ, Ianhez LE, *et al.* Renal transplantation and *Schistosomiasis mansoni*. *Transplantation* 1987; **44**: 795–798.
12. Giacomini T, Toledano D, Baledent F. The severity of airport malaria. *Bull Soc Pathol Exot Faliales* 1988; **81** (3): 345–350.
13. Visser LG, Polderman AM, Stuiver PC. Outbreak of schistosomiasis among travelers returning from Mali, West Africa. *Clin Infect Dis* 1995; **20** (2): 280–285.
14. Rakita RM, White AC Jr, Kielhofner MA. Loa loa infection as a cause of migratory angioedema: report of three cases from the Texas Medical Center. *Clin Infect Dis* 1993; **17** (4): 691–694.
15. Libman MD, MacLean JD, Gyorkos TW. Screening for schistosomiasis, filariasis, and strongyloidiasis among expatriates returning from the tropics. *Clin Infect Dis* 1993; **17** (3): 353–359.

16. Schantz PM, Moore AC, Munoz JL, *et al.* Neurocysticercosis in an Orthodox Jewish community in New York City. *N Engl J Med* 1992; **327** (10): 692–695.
17. Smith OP, Hann IM, Cox H, *et al.* Visceral leishmaniasis: rapid response to AmBisome treatment. *Arch Dis Child* 1995; **73** (2): 157–159.
18. Lai KN, Aarons I, Woodroffe AJ, *et al.* Renal lesions in leptospirosis. *Aust N Z J Med*, 1982; **12**: 276.
19. Susaengrat W, Dhiensiri T, Sinavatana P, *et al.* Renal failure in melioidosis. *Nephron* 1987; **46**: 167.
20. Srivastava RN, Mocedgil A, Bagga A, *et al.* Hemolytic uremic syndrome in children in northern India. *Pediatr Nephrol* 1991; **5**: 284.
21. Glover SC, Smith CC, Porter IA. Fatal salmonella septicemia with disseminated intravascular coagulation and renal failure. *J Med Microbiol* 1982; **15**: 117.
22. Benyajali C, Keoplung M, Beisel WR, *et al.* Acute renal failure in Asiatic cholera: Clinicopathologic correlations with acute tubular necrosis and hypokalemic correlations with acute tubular necrosis and hypokalemic nephropathy. *Ann Intern Med* 1960; **52**: 960.
23. Martinelli R, Matos CM, Rocha H. Tetanus as a cause of acute renal failure: possible role of rhabdomyolysis. *Rev Soc Brasileira Med Trop* 1993; **26**: 1.
24. Hsu GJ, Young T, Peng MY, *et al.* Acute renal failure associated with scrub typhus. report of a case. *J Formosan Med Ass* 1993; **92**: 475.
25. Singh M, Saidali A, Bakhtiar A, *et al.* Diphtheria in Afghanistan: review of 155 cases. *J Trop Med Hyg* 1985; **88**: 373.
26. Singhal PC, Chugh KS, Kaur S, *et al.* Acute renal failure in leprosy. *Int J Lepr* 1977; **45**: 171.
27. Sitprija V. Nephrology Forum: Nephropathy in falciparum malaria. *Kidney Int* 1988; **34**: 866.
28. Vargas Pabon M, Roson Porto C, Lopez Ponga B, *et al.* Hemolytic anemia and kidney failure in a female splenectomy patient. *Rev Clin Esp* 1996; **196** (5): 335–336.
29. Caravaca F, Munoz A, Pizarro, *et al.* Acute renal failure in visceral leishmaniasis. *Am J Nephrol* 1991; **11** (4): 350–352.
30. Rao TK, Friedman EA. Outcome of severe acute renal failure in patients with acquired immunodeficiency syndrome. *Am J Kidney Dis* 1995; **25** (3): 390–398.
31. Jatanasen S. DHF in the Southeast Asia Region. *Dengue Newslett* 1992; **17**: 1.
32. Tkachenko EA, Lee HW. Etiology and epidemiology of hemorrhagic fever with renal syndrome. *Kidney Int* 1991; **40**: 54.
33. Mayer HB, Wanke CA, Williams M, *et al.* Epstein-Barr virus-induced infectious mononucleosis complicated by acute renal failure: case report and review. *Clin Infect Dis* 1996; **22** (6): 1009–1018.
34. Mattoo TK, Mahmood MA, al Sowailem AM. Acute renal failure in nonfulminant hepatitis A infection. *Ann Trop Paediatr* 1991; **11**: 213.
35. Coroneos E, Petrusevska G, Varghese F, *et al.* Focal segmental glomerulosclerosis with acute renal failure associated with alpha-interferon therapy. *Am J Kidney Dis* 1996; **28** (6): 888–892.
36. Trang TT, Phu NH, Vinh H, *et al.* Acute renal failure in patients with severe falciparum malaria. *Clin Infect Dis* 1992; **15** (5): 874–880.
37. Prakash J, Gupta A, Kumar O, *et al.* Acute renal failure in falciparum malaria-increasing prevalence in some areas of India—a need for awareness. *Nephrol Dial Transplant*, 1996; **11** (12): 2414–2416.
38. Naqvi R, Ahmed E, Akhtar F, *et al.* Analysis of factors causing acute renal failure. *J Pak Med Assoc* 1996; **46** (2): 29–30.

39. Mate-Kole MO, Yeboah ED, Affram RK, Adu D. Blackwater fever and acute renal failure in expatriates in Africa. *Ren Fail* 1996 **18** (3): 525–531.
40. Lalloo DG, Trevett AJ, Paul M, *et al.* Severe and complicated falciparum malaria in Melanesian adults in Papua New Guinea. *Am J Trop Med Hyg* 1996; **55** (2): 119–124.
41. Loban KM, Popova SP. The characteristics of the clinical course of malaria in Ethiopia. *Med Parasitol* 1996; **2**: 10–13.
42. Boonpucknaving V, Sitprija V. Renal disease in acute *Plasmodium falciparum* infection in man. *Kidney Int* 1979; **16**: 44.
43. Barsoum R. Malarial nephropathies. *Nephrol Dial Transplant*, 1998; **13**: 1588–1597.
44. Miller LH, Good MF, Milon G. Malaria pathogenesis. *Science* 1994: **264**: 1878–1883.
45. Sitprija V, Pipatanagul V, Mertowidjojo K, *et al.* Pathogenesis of renal disease in leptospirosis. *Kidney Int* 1980; **17**: 827.
46. Susaengrat W, Dhiensiri T, Sinavatana P, *et al.* Renal failure in melioidosis. *Nephron* 1987; **46** (2): 167–169.
47. Bennish ML, Harris JR, Wojtyniak BJ, *et al.* Death in shigellosis: incidence and risk factors in hospitalized patients. *J Infect Dis* 1990; **161**: 500.
48. Daher EF, Abdulkader RC, Motti E, *et al.* Prospective study of tetanus-induced acute renal dysfunction: role of adrenergic overactivity. *Am J Trop Med Hyg* 1997; **57** (5): 610–614.
49. Reid HF, Bassett DC, Gaworzewska E, *et al.* Streptococcal serotypes newly associated with epidemic post-streptococcal acute glomerulonephritis. *J Med Microbiol* 1990; **32** (2): 111–114.
50. Khajehdehi P, Rastegar A, Kharazmi A. Immunological and clinical aspects of kidney disease in typhoid fever in Iran. *Q J Med* 1984; **53**: 209.
51. Sitprija V. Interstitial nephritis in infection. *J Med Assoc Thai* 1974; **57**: 517.
52. Chugh KS, Damle PB, Kaur S. Renal lesions in leprosy amongst north Indian patients. *Postgrad Med J* 1983; **59**: 707.
53. Duarte MIS, Silva MRR, Goto H, *et al.* Interstitial nephritis in human kala-azar. *Trans R Soc Trop Med Hyg* 1983; **77**: 531.
54. Nagle RB, Ward PA, Lindsky HB, *et al.* Experimental infections with African trypanosomiasis. *Am J Trop Med Hyg* 1974; **23**: 15.
55. Ginsburg BE, Wasserman J, Huldt G, *et al.* A. Case of glomerulonephrits associated with acute toxoplasmosis. *Br Med J* 1974; **3**: 664.
56. Okelo GBA, Kyobe J. A three year review of human hydatid disease seen at Kenyata National Hospital. *East Afr Med J* 1981; **58**: 695.
57. Ezzat E, Osman R, Ahmed KY, *et al.* The association between *Schistosoma haematobium* infection and heavy proteinuria. *Trans R Soc Trop Med Hyg* 1974; **68**: 315 317.
58. Barsoum RS. Schistosomal glomerulopathies. *Kidney Int* 1993; **44**: 1–12.
59. Watt G, Long GW, Calubaquib C, *et al.* Prevalence of renal involvement in *Schistosoma japonicum* infection. *Trans R Soc Trop Med Hyg* 1987; **81**: 339.
60. Barsoum RS. Schistosomal glomerulopathy: selection factors. *Nephrol Dialysis Transplant* 1987; **2**: 488–497.
61. Date A, Gunasekaran V, Kirubakaran MG, *et al.* Acute eosinophilic glomerulonephritis with *Bancroftian filariasis*. *Postgrad Med J* 1979; **55**: 905.
62. Ngu JL, Chatelanat F, Leke R, *et al.* Nephropathy in Cameroon: evidence for filarial derived immune complex pathogenesis in some cases. *Clin Nephrol* 1985; **24**: 128.
63. Pillay VKG, Kirch E, Kurtzman NA. Glomerulopathy associated with filarial loiasis (letter). *JAMA* 1973; **255**: 179.

64. Genta RM. Global prevalence of strongyloidiasis. Critical review with epidemiologic insights into the prevention of disseminated disease. *Rev Infect Dis* 1989; **11**: 755.
65. Sitprija V, Keoplung M, Boonpucknaving V, *et al.* Renal involvement in human trichinosis. *Arch Intern Med* 1980; **140**: 544.
66. Boonpucknavig V, Bhamarapravati N, Boonpucknavig S, *et al.* Glomerular changes in dengue hemorrhagic fever. *Arch Pathol Lab Med* 1976; **100**: 206.
67. Nityanand S, *et al.* Immune complex mediated vasculitis in hepatitis B and C infections and the effect of antiviral therapy. *Clin Immunol Immunopathol*, 1997; **82** (3): 250–257.
68. Horikoshi S, Okada T, Shirato I, *et al.* Diffuse proliferative glomerulonephritis with hepatitis C virus-like particles in paramesangial dense deposits in a patient with chronic hepatitis C virus hepatitis. *Nephron* 1993; **64**: 462.
69. Borst P, Bitter W, McCulloch R, *et al.* Antigenic variation in malaria. *Cell* 1995; **82**: 1–4.
70. McLaren DJ, Terry RJ. The protective role of acquired host antigens during schistosome maturation. *Parasite Immunol* 1982; **4**: 129–148.
71. Cantor HM, Dumont AE. Hepatic suppression of sensitisation to antigen absorbed into the portal system. *Nature* 1967; **215**: 744–745.
72. Sobh M, Moustafa F, Hamid S, *et al.* Schistosomal-specific nephropathy in Syrian golden hamsters: treatment by induction of antigen excess. *Nephrol Dial Transplant* 1996; **11**: 2178–2184.
73. Khalife J, *et al.* Immunity in human *Schistosomiasis mansoni*. Regulation of protective immune mechanisms by IgM blocking antibodies. *J Exp Med* 1986; **164**: 1626–1640.
74. Prina E, Lang T, Glaichenhaus N, *et al.* Presentation of the protective parasite antigen LACK by Leishmania-infected macrophages. *J Immunol* 1996; **156**: 4318–4327.
75. King CL, Medhat A, Malhorta I, *et al.* Cytokine control of parasite-specific anergy in human urinary schistosomiasis. IL-10 modulates lymphocyte reactivity. *J Immunol* 1996; **156**: 4715–4721.
76. Houba V. Experimental renal disease due to schistosomiasis. *Kidney Int* 1979; **16**: 30–43.
77. Sobh MA, Moustafa F, Basta M, *et al.* Schistosomal-specific nephropathy leading to end-stage renal failure. *Kidney Int* 1987; **31**: 1006–1011.
78. de Water R, Marck EA, Fransen JA, *et al. Schistosoma mansoni*: ultrastructual localization of the circulating anodic antigen and the circulating cathodic antigen in the mouse kidney glomerulus. *Am J Trop Med Hyg* 1988; **38**: 118–124.
79. Hillyer GV, Liwert RM. Studies on renal pathology in hamsters infected with *S. mansoni* and *S. japonicum*. *Am J Trop Med Hygiene* 1979; **23**: 404–411.
80. Andrade ZA, Rocha H. Schistosomal glomerulopathy. *Kidney Int* 1979; **16**: 23–29.
81. Barsoum RS, Bassily S, Baligh O, *et al.* Renal disease in hepatosplenic schistosomiasis: a clinicopathological study. *Trans R Soc Trop Med Hyg* 1977; **71**: 387.
82. Bassily S, Farid Z, Barsoum RS, *et al.* Renal biopsy in schistosoma-salmonella associated nephrotic syndrome. *J Trop Med Hygiene* 1976; **79**: 256–258.
83. Young SW, Higashi G, Kamel R. Interaction of salmonella and schistosomes in host-parasite relations. *Trans R Soc Trop Med Hyg* 1973; **67**: 797–802.
84. Houba V, Lambert RG, Adeniyi A. Quartan malarial nephrotic syndrome in children. *Kidney Int* 1979; **16**: 64.
85. Burstein DM, Rodby RA. Membranoproliferative glomerulonephritis associated with hepatitis C virus infection. *J Am Soc Nephrol* 1993; **4**: 1288.
86. Davda R, Peterson J, Weiner R, *et al.* Membranous glomerulonephritis in association with hepatitis C virus infection. *Am J Kidney Dis* 1993; **22**: 452.
87. van Ypersele de Strihou C, Vanherweghem JL. The tragic paradigm of Chinese herbs nephropathy editorial. *Nephrol Dialysis Transplant* 1995; **10** (2): 157–160.

88. Ben-Moussa F, Abdrrahim E, Kaaroud H, *et al.* Renal amyloidosis: Etiological aspects. Study of 350 cases Abstract 4th AFRAN/ASNRT joint meeting, Tunis, Tunisia 188, 1995.
89. Jayalakshmi P, Looi LM, Lim KJ, *et al.* Autopsy findings in 35 cases of leprosy in Malaysia. *Int J Lepr Other Mycobact Dis* 1987; **55** (3): 510–514.
90. Achour A, Maaroufi K, Hammami M, *et al.* Chronic interstitial nephritis and Ochratoxin. A. Abstract II Int Congr Geog Nephrol Hurghada Egypt, 1993: 52.
91. Saadi MG, Abdulla E, Fadel F, *et al.* Prevalence of Ochratoxin. A (OT.A) among Egyptian children and adults with different renal diseases. Abstract II Int Congr Geog Nephrol Hurghada Egypt, 1993: 22.
92. Omer HO, Wahab SMA. Secondary amyloidosis due to schistosomiasis mansoni infection. *Br Med J* 1976; **1**: 375–377.
93. Barsoum RS, Bassily S, Soliman MM, *et al.* Renal amyloidosis and schistosomiasis. *Trans Rl Soc Trop Med Hyg* 1979; **73**: 367–374.
94. Luty AJ, Mackenzie CD, Moloney NA. Secondary amyloidosis in normal and immunocompromised mice infected with *Schistosoma japonicum. Br J Exp Pathol* 1987; **68**: 825–838.
95. Crowell WA, Votava CI. Amyloidosis induced in hamsters by a filarid parasite (*Dipetalonema vitae*). *Vet Pathol* 1975; **12**: 178–185.
96. Ali-Khan Z, Sipe JD, Du T, *et al.* Echinococcus multilocularis: relationship between persistent inflammation, serum amyloid A protein response and amyloidosis in four mouse strains. *Exp Parasitol* 1988; **67**: 334–345.
97. Singarayar J, Umerah B. Tropical vasculitis and tuberculosis. *Med J Zambia* 1978; **12** (3): 74–76.
98. Nadasdy T, Park CS, Peiper SC, *et al.* Epstein-Barr virus infection-associated renal disease: diagnostic use of molecular hybridization technology in patients with negative serology. *J Am Soc Nephrol* 1992; **2** (12): 1734–1742.
99. van Velthuysen ML, Mayen AE, Prins FA, *et al.* Phagocytosis by glomerular endothelial cells in infection-related glomerulopathy. *Nephrol Dial Transplant* 1994; **9** (8): 1077–1083.
100. Capron A, Dessaint JP, Capron M, *et al.* Specific IgE antibodies in immune adherence of normal macrophages to *Schistosoma mansoni* schistosomules. *Nature* 1975; **253**: 474–475.
101. Shu KH, Lian JD, Lu YS, *et al.* Immuno-globulin-E-specific suppressor factors in primary glomerulonephritis with nephrotic syndrome. *Nephron* 1992; **60** (4): 432–435.
102. Houba V, Lambert RG. Immunological studies on tropical nephropathies. *Adv Biosci* 1973; **12**: 617.
103. Sartori A, Roque-Barreira MC, Coe J, *et al.* Immune complex glomerulonephritis in experimental kala-azar. II. Detection and characterization of parasite antigens and antibodies eluted from kidneys of *Leishmania donovani*-infected hamsters. *Clin Exp Immunol* 1992; **87** (3): 386–392.
104. Sato T, Dixhoorn MG, Schroeijers WE, *et al.* Apoptosis of cultured rat glomerular mesangial cells induced by IgG2a monoclonal anti-Thy-1 antibodies. *Kidney Int* 1996; **49** (2): 403–412.
105. Islam D, Wretlind B, Ryd M, *et al.* Immunoglobulin subclass distribution and dynamics of Shigella-specific antibody responses in serum and stool samples in shigellosis. *Infect Immun* 1995; **63** (5): 2054–2061.
106. Lemoine R, Berney T, Shibata T, *et al.* Induction of 'wire-loop' lesions by murine monoclonal IgG3 cryoglobulins. *Kidney Int* 1992; **41**: 65–72.
107. Demeure CE, Rihet P, Abel L, *et al.* Resistance to *Schistosoma mansoni* in humans:

influence of the IgE/IgG4 balance and IgG2 in immunity to reinfection after chemotherapy. *J Infect Dis* 1993; **168** (4): 1000–1008.

108. Elghazali G, Perlmann H, Rutta AS, *et al.* Elevated plasma levels of IgE in *Plasmodium falciparum*-primed individuals reflect an increased ratio of IL-4 to interferon-gamma (IFN-gamma) -producing cells. *Clin Exp Immunol* 1997; **109**: 84–89.
109. Kiniwa M, Gately M, Gubler U, *et al.* Recombinant interleukin-12 suppresses the synthesis of immunoglobulin E by interleukin-4 stimulated human lymphocytes. *J Clin Invest* 1992; 90: 262–266.
110. Iskandar SS, Falk RJ, Jennette JC. Clinical and pathologic features of fibrillary glomerulonephritis. *Kidney Int* 1992; **42** (6): 1401–1407.
111. Imai H, Hamai K, Komatsuda A, *et al.* IgG subclasses in patients with membranoproliferative glomerulonephritis, membranous nephropathy, and lupus nephritis. *Kidney Int* 1997; **51**: 270–276.
112. Barsoum RS, *et al.* Hepatic macrophage function in schistosomal glomerulopathy. *Nephrol Dialysis Transplant* 1988; **3**: 612–616.
113. Barsoum RS, Nabil M, Saady G, *et al.* Immunoglobulin A and the pathogenesis of schistosomal glomerulopathy. *Kidney Int* 1996; **50**: 920–928.
114. El Sherif A, Befus D. Redominance of IgA deposits in glomeruli of schistosomal *mansoni*-infected mice. *Clin Exp Immunol* 1988; **71**: 39–44.
115. Burdin N, Kooten C, Galibert L, *et al.* Endogenous IL-6 and IL-10 contribute to the differentiation of CD40-activated human B-lymphocytes. *J Immunol* 1995; **154**: 2533–2544.
116. Wedderburn N, Ochs HD, Clark EA, *et al.* Glomerulonephritis in common marmosets infected with *Plasmodium brasilianum* and Epstein–Barr virus *J Infect Dis* 1988; **148**: 289.
117. Bailenger J, Guy M. Interactions of 2 associated parasitoses in the rat: *Plasmodium berghei* and *Strongyloides ratti.* (In French.) *Ann Parasitol Hum Comp* 1982; **57** (6): 513–526.
118. Drutz DJ, Gutman RA. Renal mainifestations of leprosy: Glomerulonephritis, a complication of erythema nodosum leprosum. *Am J Trop Med Hyg* 1973; **22**: 496.
119. Ford PM. Interaction of rheumatoid factor with immune complexes in experimental glomerulonephritis-possible role of antiglobulins in chronicity. *J Rheumatol* 1983; **11** (Suppl.): 81–84.
120. Natali PG, Cioli D. Immune complex nephritis in mice infected with *S. mansoni*. *Fed Proc* 1974; **33**: 757.
121. Jakobsen PH, Morris-Jones SD, Hviid L, *et al.* Anti-phospholipid antibodies in patients with *Plasmodium falciparum* malaria. *Immunology* 1993; **79** (4): 653–657.
122. Yahya TM, Benedict S, Shalabi A, *et al.* Antineutrophil cytoplasmic antibody (ANCA) in malaria is directed against cathepsin G. *Clin Exp Immunol* 1997; **110**: 41–44.
123. Thomas MA, Frampton G, Isenberg DA, *et al.* A common anti. DNA antibody idiotype and anti.phospholipid antibodies in sera from patients with schistosomiasis and filariasis with and without nephritis. *J Autoimmun* 1989; **2**: 803.
124. Shwe T. Serum complement (C3) in leprosy. *Lepr Rev* 1972; **42**: 268.
125. Srichaikul T, Puwastien P, Karnjanajetanee J, *et al.* Complement changes and disseminated intravascular coagulation in *P. falciparum* malaria. *Lancet* 1975; **i**: 770.
126. Smith JW, McDonald TL. Production of serum amyloid A and C-reactive protein by HepG2 cells stimulated with combinations of cytokines or monocyte cionditioned media: the effects of prednisolone. *Clin Exp Immunol* 1992; **90**: 293–299.
127. Sobh MA, Moustafa FE, Sally SM, *et al.* Effect of antischistosomal treatment on schistosoma-specific nephropathy. *Nephrol Dialysis Transplant* 1988; **3**: 744–751.

12
Clinical interventions in chronic renal failure

G. A. Coles and A. M. El Nahas

Definition

Chronic renal failure (CRF) may be defined as the presence of permanent impairment of renal function, usually judged by the finding of a persistently raised plasma creatinine and depressed creatinine clearance [glomerular filtration rate (GFR)]. Progressive renal failure is diagnosed when there is a continuing decline in renal function, usually recognized by the patient having a progressive increase in plasma creatinine (or a decline in creatinine clearance). The distinction between these two definitions is important because some patients may have impaired but stable renal function for many years. Such individuals will make any supposed treatment for progression appear effective unless the therapy is evaluated by a proper controlled trial including a run-in period to establish the nature (progressive or stable) of their CRF. All too often, clinical trials have failed to take this factor into consideration assuming that all patients with CRF have a progressive decline in renal function leading to the inclusion of patients with stable, albeit impaired renal function, thus confounding the outcome and interpretation of these studies.

Diagnosis

The starting point for managing CRF must be an attempt to make a specific diagnosis as some causes are potentially treatable (Table 12.1) (see previous chapters). Diagnosis is made in the time-honoured manner using history, examination, and then tests. Where applicable, specific therapy should be given. Unfortunately, for the majority of patients the condition is too advanced to be clearly identified or to respond to treatment. Often, there is no proven treatment. There is thus a continuing need for one or more therapies which will slow, halt, or better still, reverse the progression of CRF. This chapter will attempt to critically evaluate available therapies.

Factors affecting progression

Although a large number of different therapies are of proven value in slowing progression in various experimental models of CRF (see Chapters 3 and 4), it has so far proven difficult to translate this success into clinical practice. A major problem

Table 12.1 Common causes of chronic renal failure and potential treatment

Cause	Potential specific treatment
Chronic glomerulonephritis	?Immunosuppression
Hypertensive nephrosclerosis	Control of hypertension
Diabetic nephropathy	Early control of hyperglycemia
Reflux nephropathy	None
Analgesic nephropathy	?Discontinuation of analgesics
Renovascular disease	?Angioplasty/reconstructive surgery
Obstructive uropathy	Relief of obstruction
Polycystic kidney disease	None

?, Not always successful at restoring renal function or preventing its decline.

Table 12.2 Factors affecting progression of human chronic renal disease (see chapter 2)

Age	In general faster in the elderly
Gender	In general faster in males
Race	Faster in Afro-Americans and Native Americans
Genetic factors	PKD1, ACE gene, and other polymorphisms?
Primary renal disease	Faster in PKD and CGN
Hypertension	Poor control
Proteinuria	>1–3 g/24 h
Renal function at presentation	Impaired

PKD, polycystic kidney disease; CGN, chronic glomerulonephritis; ACE, angiotensin-converting enzyme.

in assessing the benefit of any treatment for patients, is the number of factors that are known to influence the progression of human renal diseases. These are discussed in detail in Chapter 2 and are listed in Table 12.2. Of these, there is little doubt that systemic hypertension and the level of proteinuria are among the most important prognostic factors. A further consideration is the variable natural history, even for the same condition. For instance, membranous glomerulonephritis may remit or progress (see Chapter 8) and some patients with autosomal dominant polycystic kidney disease (PKD) may reach end-stage renal failure by the age of 30 years, whereas other individuals can survive to 70 years without significant impairment of renal function. The latter may be affected by genetic influences with PKD1 patients having a worse prognosis [1]. As a result, the only way to ensure all these variables do not inadvertently bias the results of a study, is to assess a potential therapy by a very large randomly allocated prospective trial involving several hundred patients. Unfortunately, this has seldom been the case in clinical trials on the progression of CRF where the small number of patients studied and their heterogeneous nature have often confounded the interpretation of the data.

Problems in performing a controlled trial

Ideally, one should investigate each condition separately. This has been done extensively for diabetic nephropathy (see Chapter 7) and to a more limited extent for certain types of glomerulonephritis (see Chapter 8). A few reports have commented on autosomal dominant PKD [2–5], but there appear to be no studies on the treatment of progression specifically looking at other causes of CRF such as chronic pyelonephritis. The inclusion of a heterogeneous population of patients, including for instance a large number with PKD who may not respond to a given intervention, has in the past affected the interpretation of some clinical trials [6]. A major difficulty is, of course, that no single centre is likely to have sufficient patients with any particular disease to perform a satisfactory investigation of a single disease entity. Thus, to ensure adequate numbers, studies will probably have to be multicentre, and as human renal disease progresses relatively slowly they will have to be conducted over a long period of time. Short follow-up periods may lead to optimistic interpretations and premature conclusions of clinical trials. These may be contradicted by a longer follow-up. This has been the case with a large study on dietary protein restriction [7] and another study on the effects of antiplatelet agents on the progression of mesangiocapillary glomerulonephritis [8]. In both studies, the early optimistic reports were not confirmed by a longer follow up [9,10]. Attention should also be paid when evaluating the result of clinical trials to the number of individuals remaining within the trial when the data are analysed; as all too often the number is small favouring a false positive interpretation of the results (type II statistical error) [11]. Finally, clinical trials based on historical controls are difficult to interpret and may give the misleading impression of benefits of more recent interventions [11]. This fails to take into account the fact that the natural history of chronic nephropathies has improved with time [10].

The next consideration when assessing the management of CRF is how should progression be assessed. The best way would undoubtedly be to have as a trial end-point so called renal death, i.e. death from uremia or the commencement of long-term dialysis. As noted previously, this would mean trials of 5–10 years duration so that sufficient numbers of patients had reached the end-point to give a meaningful result. Such a study is in practice difficult to perform, not only because of the impatience of the investigators and the difficulties with patients' compliance but also the near impossibility of obtaining funding for such an extended period. As a consequence, a number of other markers of progression have been suggested and are listed in Table 12.3. The simplest and the most practical test for routine clinical use is the plasma creatinine. If the plasma creatinine concentration doubles, then it is clear that a significant deterioration in renal function has occurred. How much is less certain for each individual, as it is well known that if there is a constant rate of decline in the GFR the plasma creatinine rises exponentially. Some studies in the literature have, however, used an increase of less than twice the starting value of plasma creatinine. As will be discussed later, lesser degrees of change may not always reflect a true change in GFR.

The reciprocal of the plasma creatinine concentration has also been used. The

Table 12.3 Possible methods of measuring progressive renal failure

Plasma creatinine
Reciprocal of serum creatinine
Creatinine clearance
Inulin clearance
Radiocontrast (iothalamate, Iohexol) clearance
Isotope clearance (^{51}Chromium-ethylenediamine tetra-acetic acid, ^{99}Tc-diethylenetriaminepenta-acetic acid)

resultant number is usually plotted on a semi-logarithmic scale against time. If the values fall on a straight line, then this implies renal function is declining at a constant rate. Unfortunately, this does not occur in all patients [12,13]. In addition, changes in the slope are not always due to changes in the rate of decline in GFR [14].

Creatinine clearance has been utilized as a marker of progression. It is well known to be an inaccurate marker of GFR, partly because errors in urine collection are relatively common and also because of increasing deviation from true GFR as renal failure advances. Once again, a reduction by 50% or more probably means a significant decline in renal function but lesser changes may not represent true alterations in GFR. GFR estimations have been derived from measurements of plasma creatinine (Pcr) and its mathematical conversion according to Cockcroft and Gault [15]: $\text{GFR ml/min} = 1.2 \times [140 - \text{age (years)} \times \text{wt (kg)}] \div \text{Pcr}\,\mu\text{mol/l}$. Such a formulation has been used to serially monitor changes in GFR in response to clinical interventions in trials on progression [16]. Another GFR prediction equation has been put forward recently by the investigators of the Modification of Diet in Renal Disease (MDRD) study where $\text{GFR}/1.73\,\text{m}^2 = 223 \times [\text{Pcr}]^{-0.999} \times [\text{age}]^{-0.176} \times [0.762$ if female$] \times 1.180$ if black$] \times [\text{SUN}]^{-0.170} \times [\text{Alb}]^{+0.318}$ [17].

Isotope methods of measuring GFR (^{51}Chromium ethylenediamine tetraacetic acid or ^{99}Tc-diethylenetriaminepentaacetic acid clearances) have been well validated against inulin clearance, the gold standard, particularly if renal clearance is measured with a constant infusion and urine collection. Somewhat simpler is to measure plasma clearance after a single shot of the isotopically labelled marker. This technique, although more practical for mass usage, is less accurate. This also applies to methods based on the measurement of the clearance of radiocontrast material such as iothalamate and iohexol [18].

The reference for all other methods is inulin clearance. Although widely used in small physiological studies, the need for a constant infusion and chemical analysis of the samples, makes it more difficult to employ in a multicentre trial.

A further consideration when choosing the best method for assessing progression, is whether or not the therapy will affect the actual measurement independently of changes in GFR thereby giving a false impression as to efficacy or the converse. In the recent MDRD study the investigators reported that both a low protein diet and low blood pressure affected the tubular secretion of creatinine [14]. Furthermore, a low protein intake also affected creatinine excretion. As a result, there were changes in creatinine clearance and reciprocal creatinine which were not due to parallel alterations in GFR as judged by an isotopically labelled marker. Thus, those studies which have investigated either protein restriction or blood pressure control and have used either of these methods for assessing progression, should be viewed with some circumspection.

In the absence of long-term follow-up and hard end-points relating to the progression of CRF such as changes in the rate of decline of renal function or time to end-stage renal insufficiency (renal death), investigators have considered surrogate end-points. These may consist of changes in microalbuminuria, proteinuria, or renal histological parameters. This assumes that the earlier changes observed to take place in the surrogate end-points reflect the longer-term changes in renal function. Unfortunately, such an assumption cannot always be made as for instance a reduction in proteinuria may not invariably lead to the slowing of the progression of the underlying nephropathy.

It is important when assessing the evidence from controlled trials, to ask whether each study has sufficient power to determine if any therapy was beneficial. The size of the trial should be determined by the magnitude of the expected or required effect. If, for instance, during a fixed period of time, 50% of the control group will reach a predetermined end-point and one wishes to reduce this proportion to 25%, then to have a 95% chance of being sure such a difference is significant with $p < 0.05$, a total of 182 individuals must complete the study. On the other hand, if the aim is to reduce the chances of reaching the end-point from 10% to 5%, then 1438 subjects will be needed. These numbers fall to 110 and 858, respectively, if one is satisfied with only an 80% chance of finding a real difference. It is important to realize that these are minimum estimates for trial size as they do not allow for drop-outs for another reason, e.g. heart attacks, road accidents, etc. In the context of renal failure, the longer the length of the trial, the lower the number of patients required but the higher the allowance for unrelated drop-out. Care should also be taken in the interpretation of clinical trials where a high drop-out rate leads to a small number of patients remaining under investigation when the data are analysed. This can lead to a type II statistical error with a false positive result [10]. This has been a weakness of numerous clinical trials on progression where statistical significance between groups is only reached when the number of patients under evaluation falls and becomes too small for statistical scrutiny [19,20].

Trial design must also allow for the relatively slow progression of human renal disease. This is of some importance because the therapies most widely studied, namely a blood pressure reduction or a low protein diet, will actually cause a small decrease in GFR within the first 4 months of implementation [21]. Furthermore, starting or stopping certain classes of hypotensive drugs will also be followed by a mild reduction or increase in GFR, respectively [21]. As a consequence, any trial on the progression of renal failure will have to be extended probably more than 3 years to be sure these short-term presumed hemodynamic alterations do not affect the assessment of long-term benefit or otherwise of any proposed therapy [21]. In addition, early apparent benefits are not always translated into long-term gain. For

Table 12.4 Characteristics of an ideal trial to assess treatment of progressive renal failure

Single nephropathy
Measurement of progression by isotope glomerular filtration rate
Long follow-up (at least 4 years)
Several hundred patients studied (number needed depends on magnitude of therapeutic effect)
Confounding variables such as diet, blood pressure, antihypertensive drugs should be controlled throughout the study

instance, a study from the Netherlands suggested that a low protein diet was beneficial when introduced early in the course of CRF [7], until a subsequent analysis after 4 years showed only limited indications for this therapy [9]. A similar over-optimistic conclusion was drawn in a 2-year study on the effects of antiplatelet agents on the progression of mesangiocapillary glomerulonephritis [8]. This was subsequently refuted by a longer follow-up of the same patients [10].

As a result of this critique, it is possible to draw up a list of the characteristics of an ideal trial in this field. These are highlighted in Table 12.4. Realizing these aims is difficult if not impossible at times. Clearly, if one wishes to control blood pressure at some pre-determined level, it will not be practical to confine oneself to only one or two classes of hypotensive agents. It is therefore not surprising that the studies that are available for review are far from perfect but may be the best that can be achieved at the present time.

Non-diabetic renal disease

Diet trials

Because of the strong evidence for benefit from animal studies (see Chapter 3), low protein diets have been advocated for slowing the progression of human CRF. Unfortunately, many of the published studies are seriously flawed and have not used proper controls [22]. There are only six randomly allocated prospective controlled trials available with a mean follow up of more than 1 year. The main features of these studies are shown in Table 12.5.

The first prospective trial of a low protein diet was performed by Rosman and colleagues with a total of 228 patients studied [7]. Patients were stratified according to sex, age (more or less than 40 years old) and creatinine clearance (more or less than 30 ml/min) giving eight groups. Each group was then randomized to a normal or low protein diet. Those whose creatinine clearance was greater than 30 ml/min received 0.6 g protein/kg body weight per day and if the value was less than 30 ml/min, a 0.4 g protein/kg body weight per day diet was prescribed. Subsequently, data for age and sex were pooled. The follow up was variable; a total of 149 patients reached at least 18 months. The main outcome measures were a 10% increase in plasma creatinine and the slope of the reciprocal creatinine. Blood pressure was said

Table 12.5 Low protein diets in chronic renal failure: randomly allocated prospective trials and meta-analyses

Authors	Patients (*n*)	Diet (g/kg/day)	Parameter	Duration (months)	Outcome
Rosman *et al.* (1984)	228	0.4 or 0.6 versus normal	Serum creatinine	Variable	+
Rosman *et al.* (1989)	248	0.4 or 0.6 versus normal	Creatinine clearance	>36	±
Ihle *et al.* (1989)	64	0.4 versus 0.75	Isotope GFR	18	+
Locatelli *et al.* (1991)	456	0.6 versus 1	Serum creatinine	24	–
Williams *et al.* (1991)	60	0.6 versus > 0.8	Creatinine clearance	18	–
Klahr/MDRD (1994)	585	0.58 versus 1.3	Isotope GFR	26	–
Klahr *et al.* (1994)	255	0.28 versus 0.58	Isotope GFR	26	–
D'Amico *et al.* (1994)	128	0.6 versus 1	Creatinine clearance	27	±
Fouque *et al.* (1992)	890	0.3–0.6	Variable	12–24	+
Pendrini *et al.* (1996)	1413	0.4–0.6	Variable	18–36	+
Kasiske *et al.* (1998)	2248	0.68 versus 1.01	Variable	6–36	±

+, Positive outcome; –, negative outcome; ±, borderline effect; GFR, glomerular filtration rate.

to be equal in all groups. The authors reported a slowing of progression claiming benefit. The data are, however, difficult to interpret and it is not clear what numbers were available for analysis at each time point. Furthermore, the use of two different diets and the problems already noted of using these particular outcome measures, makes any conclusions of benefit suspect. Subsequently, the authors published a follow up with 153 patients having been observed for more than 36 months [9]. This time a persistent 50% reduction in creatinine clearance was used as the outcome measure. There was no difference in subjects with a starting clearance greater than 30 ml/min but an apparent slowing of progression with a low protein diet if the initial value was lower. Further analysis suggested any benefit was most likely to occur in males with glomerulonephritis. The next published study by Ihle *et al.* [23] looked at the effect of a normal or a 0.4 g/kg per day low protein diet in 64 patients over 18 months. Renal function was assessed by isotope GFR. It is noteworthy that patients had a starting serum creatinine of between 350 and 1000 μmol/l, i.e. they all had more advanced renal failure than the majority of patients in the other studies.

The authors report an apparent benefit both in GFR and number of patients reaching end-stage renal failure.

The largest trial to date where only one variable has been tested is that of Locatelli *et al.* [24]. They enrolled 456 patients whose plasma creatinine was between 119 and 619 µmol/l and whose creatinine clearance was less than 60 ml/min. Subjects were randomly assigned to 1 g/kg body weight/day of protein or 0.6 g/kg per day. Patients were followed for 2 years or until they reached the end-points of either a doubling of the plasma creatinine or the need for dialysis. Overall, the difference between the outcome for the two groups was borderline ($p < 0.06$). Subgroup analysis suggested benefit for patients whose starting plasma creatinine lay between 222 and 442 µmol/l but not higher or lower. The authors concluded that any benefit from the diet would be marginal. It is worth noting that compliance was not as good as desired so that judging from urinary urea excretion, the difference in protein catabolic rate was 0.16 g/kg per day and not 0.4 g/kg per day as planned. It is therefore possible this is too small a difference to show a positive effect.

Williams *et al.* [25] studied 60 patients with CRF and a plasma creatinine of >150 µmol/l for males and >130 µmol/l for females and evidence of deteriorating renal function. After randomization, 31 patients received 0.6 g/kg per day of protein and 29 control subjects received at least 0.8 g/kg per day. The mean difference in protein intake was calculated to be 0.45 g/kg per day. There was no difference in the rate of decline of creatinine clearance or reciprocal plasma creatinine with an average follow up of 18 months. They concluded that there was no benefit from a low protein diet.

The largest study to date is the MDRD trial [6] involving 840 patients. This investigation, however, looked at the effect of three types of diet and also two levels of blood pressure control. A total of 585 patients with a GFR between 25 and 55 ml/min per 1.73 m^2 surface area were randomly assigned to 1.3 g/kg per day protein or 0.58 g/kg per day and to a mean arterial pressure of 107 or 92 mmHg. The remaining 255 patients had a GFR of 13–24 ml/min per 1.73 m^2 surface area and were randomly assigned to 0.58 g/kg per day protein or 0.28 g/kg per day supplemented with a keto acid—essential amino acid mixture as well as the same two levels of blood pressure control as in the group with a higher GFR. Renal function was measured using an isotope GFR technique. The mean follow-up was 2.2 years. For those subjects with a higher starting GFR there was no apparent benefit of the low protein diet with results projected up to 3 years. Similarly, in the lower GFR group there was no apparent benefit of the very low protein intake. The patients in the higher GFR group who received 0.6 g/kg per day of protein had an initial drop in renal function during the first 4 months of therapy. Subsequently, the mean GFR declined more slowly than in the normal protein intake group.

The last controlled trial published to date is that presented by D'Amico *et al.* [26]. They studied 128 patients with a creatinine clearance between 15 and 70 ml/min. They were randomly assigned to 1 g/kg per day protein or 0.6 g/kg per day with a mean follow up for 27 months. The end-point, defined as halving of the creatinine clearance, was reached by 40% of the controls and 28.6% of the low protein group. This was statistically significant by life table analysis ($p = 0.038$). This study also showed that the factors determining progression in this study were primarily the level of renal insufficiency and the severity of proteinuria [26].

Subsequent to the original publication, the MDRD study was re-analysed looking at the effect of the actual protein intake during the trial rather than on an intention to treat basis. For patients in the higher GFR group there was no significant correlation between GFR decline and achieved protein intake over 3 years [27]. In contrast, when the results from the lower GFR group were re-analysed, a 0.2 g/kg per day lower achieved protein intake was associated with a 1.15 ml/min per year slower mean decline in GFR ($p = 0.011$) [27]. The authors suggested this represented 29% of the mean decline in GFR and would lead to a 41% prolongation in the time to renal failure.

In an attempt to establish the efficacy or otherwise of a low protein diet, Pendrini *et al.* [28] performed a meta-analysis using data from Rosman [7], Ihle [23], Locatelli [24], Williams [25], and the higher GFR group in the MDRD study [6]. This gave a total of 1413 subjects for a pooled analysis. The study of D'Amico was not included, presumably because it did not give information on the number of patients who reached end-stage renal failure or died. Pendrini *et al.* concluded that the relative risk of renal failure or death was 0.67 (CI 0.5–0.89, $p = 0.007$) in favour of a low protein diet. This was despite the varying lengths of follow up, different outcome measures and different diets used in these studies. The authors state there were no statistically significant differences in the relative risk of renal failure or death between the five studies. It was calculated that a trial of 1000 or more patients was needed to detect a 33% risk reduction with a low protein diet. Assuming a low protein diet does reduce progression, the actual benefit to a patient would depend on the previous rate of decline of renal function. Other meta-analyses showed conflicting results, with one showing undoubted benefit (odds ratio for renal death on low protein diet compared with control of 0.54) [29] while the other, more recent and comprehensive, showed little benefit [30]. The latter included 13 randomized and 11 other trials including a total of 2248 patients and showed a marginal benefit for dietary protein restriction with patients treated having a slower decline in GFR of 0.53 ml/min per year. This means that starting from a GFR of 30 ml/min a low protein diet would gain a patient 1 extra year before reaching 6 ml/min. The authors concluded that other therapies are needed to slow the progression of CRF [30].

The concern with the use of these diets is that they might produce malnutrition. The authors of the studies quoted in this chapter claim no serious side-effects occurred. The patients were all, however, in a trial situation with close supervision by a trained dietician. Levey *et al.* [31] comment that frequent monitoring of protein and energy intake as well as nutritional status, are necessary to assure the safety of patients using a low protein diet. It is probably that in routine clinical practice, it would not be possible to provide as intensive supervision as occurs in trials. It is worth noting therefore, the natural history of food intake during progression renal failure. Two studies have shown that there is a spontaneous reduction of protein intake with falling GFR. In the report by Ikizler *et al.* [32], protein intake declined by 0.06 g/kg per day for each 10 ml decline in GFR. Pollock *et al.* [33] suggest protein intake falls from about 1.1 g/kg per day when creatinine clearance is 100 ml/min to about 0.75 g/kg per day when dialysis commences. Furthermore, despite being urged to increase food consumption, the patients did not eat significantly more protein 3 months after starting dialysis. The increase eventually occurred after 6–9 months [33]. If a diet were to be prescribed, then a value of 0.6 g/kg per day of protein would be the most likely choice [28]. This would mean, however, a lower total protein consumption during the period of progression than occurs naturally. Thus, there is a real risk that malnutrition could occur with widespread use of a low protein diet. Protein–calorie depletion at the start of dialysis is well known to be an adverse risk factor for subsequent morbidity and survival [34]. The full nutritional consequences of the MDRD study have recently been analysed [35]. This report shows that male patients receiving a low protein diet had a significantly lower energy intake, weight, percentage body fat, arm muscle area, and urinary creatinine excretion compared with those taking a more normal diet. Female subjects also consumed less energy and had lower creatinine excretion. Though the differences were relatively small, they occurred despite close supervision by full-time research dieticians. In routine clinical practice it is therefore likely the nutritional consequences would be worse.

Pollock *et al.* [33] have commented that there are no follow up data relating to outcome of patients deliberately prescribed a low protein diet in an attempt to slow progression once they subsequently start dialysis. Thus, there is the possibility that a patient might gain more time off dialysis at the price of less time on this therapy. In other words, there is no evidence to date that a low protein diet increases a patient's total life span. It might even reduce it. It should be pointed out, however, that Walser *et al.* have claimed that a properly prescribed low protein diet may actually help to maintain nutrition [36]. This may well be true when a patient is cared for in a centre with a special research interest in this topic but at this point in time, we do not feel able to recommend the routine use of a low protein diet. It is up to the individual clinician to decide whether to prescribe such a regimen to a highly motivated fully informed patient when excellent dietetic supervision is available. Finally, it is worth noting that a large European multicentre trial of a low protein diet in children failed to show any benefit in terms of slowing progression [37]. This study, like many others, stressed the impact of proteinuria and hypertension on progression [37].

Other diets

Despite some experimental evidence for possible benefit, there has been only one controlled trial in patients of a low phosphate diet. This was performed by Williams *et al.* [25], who randomly assigned 29 patients to the diet with at least 3 months follow up, the average being 19 months. The same 29 controls were used as for the comparison with a low protein diet. As before, no blood pressure differences were noted and there was no benefit as judged by creatinine clearance.

The only other diet to be tested in a randomly allocated prospective fashion, is that of a fish oil supplement in patients with IgA nephropathy. There have been five such studies (only three of which were randomized) which came to opposite conclusions as two showed some benefit and three did not [38–42]. The two largest studies were conflicting. Bennett *et al.* [39] studied 37 patients with biopsy proven IgA nephropathy. Patients either had a creatinine of 120–400 μmol/l or <120 μmol/l but active disease as judged by proteinuria, urinary red blood cells 200 000/ml or 10% crescents in the biopsy [39]. Seventeen patients received 1.8 g of eicosapentaenoic acid and 1.2 g of docosahexaenoic acid daily. The remaining 20 subjects acted as controls. At the end of the 2-year follow up, there was an equal decline in overall renal function and no benefit was seen. Donadio *et al.* [42] also studied 106 patients with biopsy proven IgA nephropathy who in addition had >1 g of proteinuria per 24 h or whose serum creatinine had increased by 25% or more during the preceding 6 months. Fifty-five patients received 1.87 g of eicosapentaenoic acid and 1.36 g of docosahexaenoic acid per day and 51 subjects were controls. The follow up was 2 years. The main end-point was a 50% increase in serum creatinine which occurred in three patients in the fish oil group and 14 in the placebo group ($p = 0.002$). Subsequently, more patients died or developed end-stage renal disease in the placebo group ($p = 0.006$). There were apparently no differences in blood pressure. In both studies, the fish oil was apparently well tolerated but it is difficult to disguise the taste. It is worth noting that in the report by Donadio *et al.* [42] the source of the fish oil changed during the investigation so that the daily dose of the acids decreased to 1.68 g and 0.97 g respectively. The reason for the different outcomes in these studies is not clear. It is noteworthy, however, that the report by Bennett *et al.* [39] may have had too few patients to show an effect. In addition, not all patients had significant proteinuria or impaired function and thus the outcome may have been biased by the inclusion of individuals who were not going to have progressive renal failure. The study of Donadio *et al.* [42] suggests possible benefit in those who are in a higher risk group for progression. However, this study was criticized in view of the unusually fast rate of decline of the renal function of the placebo-treated group [43]. The majority of these patients with IgA nephropathy reached end-stage renal insufficiency within the 3 years observation time; a most unusual course for this type of chronic glomerulonephritis. Recently, a meta-analysis of the results of the published studies on the efficacy of fish oil in IgA nephropathy has been performed by Dillon [44]. Although the calculated mean effect was positive, i.e. in the direction of benefit from the intervention, this was not statistically significant. This conclusion was the same whether all five studies or only the three randomized trials were included. Assuming the true benefit of fish oil was the same as the calculated mean effect for the five studies, it was estimated that a trial of 251 patients per group would be needed to have an 80% probability of detecting this difference with $p = 0.05$ [44].

Pharmacological treatment

Blood pressure control

There is no hard evidence that lowering blood pressure slows progression of renal failure, as there are no trials which have included as controls, patients with untreated hypertension. In view of the known reduction in risk of other end-points, e.g. cerebrovascular accident, such a study would, of course, be unethical. There is, however, evidence of benefit from a number of sources. Klag *et al.* [45] in the Multiple Risk Factor Intervention Trial, studied 332 544 middle-aged men and found that during an average 16-year follow up, there was a strong graded relation between systolic and diastolic blood pressure and end-stage renal disease. This does not prove cause and effect but is certainly justification for trials of lowering blood pressure to normal or near normal values. Brazy *et al.* [46] observed that the rate of decline of renal function was twice as fast in patients with diastolic blood pressure values higher than 90 mmHg. Alvestrand *et al.* [47] followed a group of patients with declining renal function and then tried to lower the blood pressure by the addition of one or more hypotensive agents. There was a correlation between the change in blood pressure and the change in the slope of the creatinine clearance. In other words, the more the blood pressure fell, the slower became the rate of decline of renal function and vice versa. In the MDRD trial as already noted, two target mean arterial blood pressures (MAP) were studied, namely 107 and 92 mmHg. There was no significant difference between the groups in the rate of decline of renal function when analysed on an intention to treat basis [27]. It is understood that the actual achieved mean pressures were in fact 97 and 92 mmHg and thus it is possible this much lower than planned difference may have been too small to show an influence on outcome. Subsequent subgroup analysis, although to be treated with caution, does show an interesting trend [48]. Patients with proteinuria of more than 1 g per day had a significantly slower decline in GFR if they were in the low pressure group (MAP = 92 mmHg). Furthermore, the loss of renal function was faster the higher the actual level of blood pressure during follow up if the patient had significant proteinuria. It should be noted that as already emphasized, proteinuria is a significant adverse risk factor and lowering blood pressure, while slowing progression, does not usually improve prognosis to that of subjects with no proteinuria. The authors conclude that if proteinuria is >1 g/day, target mean blood pressure should be 92 mmHg, for levels between 0.25 and 1 g/day, the value should be 98 mmHg and for no proteinuria levels below 107 mmHg have no proven advantage [48].

Toto *et al.* [49] reported that the decline in GFR in patients with hypertensive nephrosclerosis was not significantly different if they had a mean diastolic blood pressure of 81 mmHg as compared with 86.7 mmHg. It should be noted, however, that most of these patients had little or no proteinuria. The authors comment that the very slow deterioration in renal function seen in both patient groups was comparable to that of normotensive white males with age, suggesting but not proving, that treatment of hypertension in this condition can virtually halt disease-induced progression.

The next consideration is which hypotensive agent is best (Table 12.6). Several studies have compared angiotensin-converting enzyme (ACE) inhibitors with other agents. Kamper *et al.* [50] studied 70 patients who were randomly allocated to the enalapril or alternative therapy, but not a calcium channel blocker. After a mean 7-year follow up, 66% of the enalapril group, as compared with 86% of the controls, were alive without renal replacement therapy. There was no difference in blood pressure control. Hannedouche *et al.* [51] randomly allocated 100 hypertensive

Table 12.6 Angiotensin-converting enzyme (ACE) inhibition: clinical trials and meta-analysis in non-diabetic chronic renal failure

Authors	Patient (*n*)	Drugs	Duration (years)	Outcome
Kamper *et al.* (1995)	70	Enalapril versus others	7	+
Hannedouche (1996)	100	Enalapril versus β-blocker	2	+
Maschio *et al.* (1996)	583	Benazepril versus placebo	3	+
GISEN group (1997)	166	Ramipril versus placebo	2.5	+
Zuchelli *et al.* (1992)	142	Captopril versus Nifedipine	3	–
Kanno *et al.* (1996)	26	Captopril versus Nifedipine	2	–
Gansevoort (1995)	558	41 studies	0.3–2	+*
Giatras *et al.* (1997)	806	11 studies	1–4	RR = 0.70

+, ACE inhibitor superior to other antihypertensive agents; –, no difference between ACE inhibitor and other agents; RR, relative risk; *, beneficial antiproteinuric effect for ACE inhibitors.

patients with CRF again to enalapril or a beta-blocker. A diuretic and then a dihydropyridine calcium channel blocker or a centrally acting drug were then added stepwise if necessary. There was no difference in blood pressure but cumulative renal survival was significantly better in the enalapril group. Ihle *et al.* [52] studied 70 hypertensive patients with a plasma creatinine between 2.8 and 6.8 mg/dl. Subjects were randomly assigned to enalapril or placebo. Both groups received various combinations of other hypotensive agents as necessary to control blood pressure. After 2 years follow up there was no difference in the incidence of end-stage renal failure. Analysis using a mixed effects linear model, however, indicated that the rate of decline of GFR was slower with enalapril. This appeared to be in addition to its antihypertensive action.

These studies should be contrasted with that of Zuchelli *et al.* [53] who randomly allocated 142 hypertensive patients with CRF to captopril or nifedipine, which were added to their current antihypertensive regimen. Blood pressure fell by the same amount in both groups, but up to 3 years later there was no significant difference in the rate of decline of GFR or renal survival. In both groups the progression of the renal failure was slower than prior to the trial. A similar conclusion was reached by a Japanese study of patients with PKD who showed no therapeutic advantage of captopril over nifedipine on the rate of progression of CRF as the level of blood pressure control was comparable in both groups [3]. More recently, the Mayo nephrology collaborative trial of enalapril compared with diltiazem in patients with progressive membranous nephropathy failed to show a specific protective role for ACE inhibition and concluded that regardless of the antihypertensive agent used, the control of hypertension was the critical factor in maintaining stable renal function [54].

Maschio *et al.* [55] have reported on a large multicentre study evaluating the efficacy of another ACE inhibitor, benazepril. A total of 583 patients were studied; 300 receiving benazepril and 283 placebo. This report included 21 subjects with diabetic nephropathy. The primary end-point was doubling of the serum creatinine or the need for dialysis. After 3 years follow up, significantly fewer patients in the benazepril group had reached the end-point. Blood pressure, both systolic and diastolic, decreased in the benazepril group as compared with controls. It was claimed that even when allowance was made for this difference, the reduction in risk caused by the ACE inhibitor, was 39% (CI –5–61). Benefit was greater for patients with proteinuria more than 1 g/24 h [55].

A comparison of ramipril versus placebo has also been published [56]. A total of 166 patients with chronic renal disease and proteinuria of 3 g or more per 24 h were randomized to ramipril or placebo and then followed with serial measurements of GFR. An interim analysis suggested benefit so the code was broken. Patients receiving ramipril had a significantly slower decline in GFR than those taking placebo. There were no differences in blood pressure during the study and when the results were controlled for the level of hypertension, ramipril appeared to give additional benefit. In addition, the greater the reduction in proteinuria, the slower the decline in GFR. In this study, as with the benazapril described above, it cannot be excluded that the small differences in blood pressure control favouring treatment with the ACE inhibitor while not statistically sufficient to explain the differences in outcome could be biologically meaningful. Subsequently, Ruggenenti *et al.* [57] published a follow up of this trial reporting that after 3 years no further cases of end-stage renal failure occurred in patients originally assigned to ramipril.

In order to try and resolve the question of whether or not ACE inhibitors are more effective or safer than other hypotensive drugs, Giatras *et al.* [58] have performed a meta-analysis on 11 studies, nine of which have now been published, looking at the hard end-points of end-stage renal disease or death. The relative risk of end-stage renal disease was 0.70 (CI 0.51–0.97) suggesting benefit. The relative risk of death was 1.24 (CI 0.55–2.83) implying no excess mortality with the use of this type of drug. Blood pressure was lower in the ACE inhibitor group but due to the heterogeneous nature of the studies it was not possible to determine whether the suggested benefit was solely due to better blood pressure control or some other effect. It should be noted that blood pressure measurement in most of the studies described above was taken casually with no consideration given to blood pressure peak/trough ratio or 24-h blood pressure control. It cannot be excluded that the overall quality of the blood pressure control achieved with the ACE inhibitor may be superior to conventional agents and that whatever difference obtained may have a significant biological impact. This proved to be the case in animal experimentation where the continuous monitoring of blood pressure proved that the renal functional outcome depended primarily on the quality of blood pressure control regardless of the agent used [59].

One further factor that may influence the decision to use an ACE inhibitor in preference to other drugs, is the meta analysis performed by Gansevoort *et al.* [60]. They looked at 41 studies comprising 1124 patients (558 with non-diabetic renal disease) which had compared the antiproteinuric action of different antihypertensive agents. The reduction in proteinuria was greater than 24% when using an ACE inhibitor, compared with all other classes of blood pressure lowering drugs, but the control of hypertension was the same. Proteinuria is a significant risk factor for progression. It is not known whether reduction in proteinuria *per se* in the absence of reduced blood pressure will be protective but the possibility would favour the use of an ACE inhibitor. There are no comparative data to determine which one of this class of drugs is best. It should be noted that there is some evidence that ACE inhibitors have no special advantage in patients with autosomal dominant PKD and some have even suggested that they may be detrimental [61]. Kanno *et al.* [3] found no difference comparing this class of drug with calcium channel blockers. Maschio *et al.* [55] also commented that benazepril had no benefit in patients with this condition. Similarly, although the MDRD study was not designed to compare different antihypertensive agents, the authors did report that an ACE inhibitor had no special benefit for subjects with polycystic kidneys [5,6]. It should be noted that there may be other non-renal factors that influence the response to blood pressure reduction. A report from Van Essen *et al.* [62] showed that subjects with a DD genotype for the insertion/deletion ACE gene polymorphism, had a faster rate of decline of renal function irrespective of good blood pressure control or the use of enalapril or atenolol compared with patients with the II or ID genotypes. Finally, it is of interest to note the report by Apperloo *et al.* [63] suggesting that those patients who have an initial fall (at 12 weeks) in GFR when given an antihypertensive drug, are more likely to have stable renal function during follow up compared with those who have no initial response. This finding implies it might be possible to predict those likely to benefit from blood pressure reduction early on. It should be noted, however, that the mean fall in GFR during the first 12 weeks in the so-called responders was only 3.7 ml/min. This would only be detectable by an accurate measurement technique which is unlikely to be used in routine practice. Furthermore the analysis was based on a total of only 40 patients. Further studies are required to verify these findings.

Other pharmacological agents

Antiplatelet and anticoagulant agents

There is no good evidence that antiplatelet or anticoagulant agents slow the progression of CRF. Early data suggested a beneficial effect in a small number of patients with mesangiocapillary glomerulonephritis (MCGN) treated with aspirin and dipyridamole over a 2-year period [8]. However, a longer follow up of these patients over 5–9 years failed to confirm the initial impression [10], thus highlighting the importance of long follow ups. A more recent study showed that aspirin and dipyridamole reduces proteinuria in patients with chronic MCGN without affecting renal function [64]. While the combination of antiplatelet agents and anticoagulants have been reported to improve renal function in one study [65], larger clinical trials of anticoagulation in chronic glomerulonephritis failed to confirm such findings [66]. Anticoagulation was associated with significant morbidity and mortality in patients with progressive renal insufficiency [66]. There is, therefore, no indication for anti-coagulation in patients with progressive CRF.

Lipid lowering

There is a growing body of evidence that a wide range of lipid-lowering agents are effective in reducing the hyperlipidemia or CRF. However, there is so far no convincing evidence that such a reduction of circulating lipids levels affects the rate of decline in renal function. A study by Thomas *et al.* [67] showed that simvastatin, an 3-hydroxy-3-methylglutaryl coenzyme A reductase inhibitor, was effective in correcting the hyperlipidemia of a small group patients with CRF, without significantly affecting proteinuria or the rate of decline in renal function over a 2-year period [67]. Once more, the small number of patients studied and the relative short follow up preclude any meaningful conclusions.

Dopaminergic agents

As dopamine improves renal blood flow in the normal subject, there has been interest that this agent might be beneficial in renal failure. Stefone *et al.* [68] reported on the use of ibopamine, an orally active dopamine analogue. A total of 189 patients with a plasma creatinine of 1.5–4.0 mg/dl were studied. After randomization, 96 received 100 mg/day of ibopamine and 93 were controls. After a 2-year follow up, significantly fewer subjects receiving the test drug had reached the end-point of either a 20% or a 40% increase in plasma creatinine. There was no difference in mean blood pressure and no ACE inhibitors were used. This study contrasts with another unpublished study showing no effect of a similar dopaminergic agent (fenoldapam) on the progression of CRF (A. Nathwani, personal communication).

Prostaglandin manipulations

A small study suggested that the administration of prostaglandin E_1 to patients with progressive CRF reverses this trend; an effect which appeared to be sustained even after the prostaglandin administration was discontinued [69]. The small nature of this study and its short observation time preclude any meaningful conclusions.

Growth factor administration

It has been demonstrated that the parenteral administration of recombinant human insulin-like growth factor-I (IGF-I) to patients with moderate to severe chronic renal insufficiency leads to a transient but significant improvement in renal function [70]. In these patients, the administration of IGF-I led to a substantial increase in both GFR and renal blood flow [70]. Unfortunately, the transient nature of the response with tachyphylaxis to the IGF-I makes this form of treatment of limited long-term value. However, a better understanding of the pharmacokinetics of IGF-I in patients with CRF may lead to different administration schedules, including intermittent administration, aimed at obtaining a sustained response with prolonged improvement in renal function [71]. This form of treatment holds great promise for the future as it highlights the fact that there is a residual renal functional reserve even in patients with GFR as low as 10–15 ml/min [70].

Miscellaneous

A range of clinical interventions have been promoted to slow the progression of CRF. Many of these are based on the adsorption within the gut of potential uraemic toxins such as indoxyl sulphate by oral sorbents. These studies have been performed primarily in Japan where the oral administration of the sorbent (AST-120) [72] or extracts of Chinese herbs (EJM) [73] have been tested. The small number of the patients studied and the anecdotal nature of these reports preclude any meaningful conclusion.

Studies have also been performed in China with traditional herbal remedies suggesting that these, alone or in combination with immunosuppressive agents, may have a beneficial effect on the progression of CRF [74]. The potential of these remedies remain to be explored and validated.

Other non-pharmacological therapies

Besides pharmacological agents, the only therapy subjected to a controlled trial is exercise. This may have been prompted by the observations made in uraemic rats that exercise slows the rate of decline of their renal function [75]. Eidemak *et al.* [76] reported on a prospective randomized study of exercise. Thirty patients received either an exercise training programme or no intervention. Follow up was a median of 20 months. There was no difference in isotope GFR but the maximal work capacity increased significantly in the exercise group. This study, although interesting, may well have been too small to show any significant effect. At face value, it would seem that jogging may be good for the heart but not necessarily for the kidneys!

General conclusions and recommendations

In our opinion, the evidence for a beneficial effect of lowering blood pressure is strong particularly in subjects with proteinuria. There may be some slowing of progression with a low protein diet but in the absence of long-term follow-up data after dialysis commences, we remain cautious about this therapy because of potential risks. Thus at present we would recommend that hypertension should always be treated with a target mean arterial pressure of 98–107 mmHg (130/85–140/90 mmHg) if there is no proteinuria and 92 mmHg (116/80 mmHg) if proteinuria is more than 1 g per 24 h. As regards choice of drug, ACE inhibitors are clearly effective and may have some added non-hypotensive beneficial effect. If a cough proves troublesome, angiotensin II receptor blocking agents should be of value but we know of no published controlled trials related to progression. It is clearly important to monitor serially renal function in case renal arterial disease is present and ACE inhibition induces a deterioration in renal function [77]. As noted previously, ACE inhibitors are not of any extra value for PKD and some have even suggested that they may be deleterious in these patients [61]. It should be recognized that it may not be possible to achieve these targets in every patient despite use of multiple agents without serious side-effects. This should not deter the clinician, as even if some patients can be treated effectively there will be benefit. Finally, and possibly even more important, is the close observation and monitoring of the patients. Bergström *et al.* [78] showed that by increasing the frequency of follow-up visits without altering therapy, the rate of decline of renal function became slower. This was in part due to better blood pressure control. The reasons are fairly clear. The more interest a clinician takes in his/her patients, the more likely they are to listen and to heed the advice being given. As a result, they are more likely to comply with the prescribed regimen.

Future directions

Although dialysis and transplantation are effective modes of treatment, they are strictly speaking palliative and their cost makes them unavailable to about two-thirds of the world's population. Even in the richer countries, renal replacement therapy is causing financial strain on the various health-care systems. There is thus an urgent need to prevent terminal renal failure occurring.

As can be seen from the above, although it is possible to slow progression of CRF in some patients, there is still no therapy which is effective in all and which also completely halts or even reverses deterioration in renal function. This should be the long-term goal, although clearly this is not achievable at present.

Various treatments are showing promise in experimental models of chronic uremia (see Chapters 3 and 4) but the problem will be to prove their efficacy in human disease. As noted previously, renal function takes several years, often 10 or more, to decline to end-stage. Thus unless some therapy completely halts progression, trials that will show real benefit will need to be as large as the MDRD study, and last several years. Unfortunately, the expense of such studies may mean they will not take place unless some pharmaceutical manufacturer feels there will be a significant profit if their product seems effective. It is unlikely governments will fund such an investigation.

A further issue is that as detailed in Chapters 3 and 4, progression is probably due to the interaction of a multiplicity of mechanisms. Effective therapy might well mean a combination of different agents blocking or enhancing different pathways. A study of a single drug is difficult enough to perform but the numbers needed to prove that one particular mixture of therapies was the best, would be a logistical nightmare.

We do not wish to appear nihilistic but raise these issues as it is important that would-be investigators do not waste their own and the patients' time on fruitless exercises. Future trials must be carefully planned to ensure they have sufficient power for the result to be clinically meaningful despite all the confounding variables found in human renal disease.

Key references

El Nahas AM, Coles GA. Dietary treatment of chronic renal failure: ten unanswered questions. *Lancet* 1986; **i**: 597–600.

Klahr S, Levey AS, Beck GJ, Caggiula AW, Hunsicker L, Kusek JW, Striker G. The effects of dietary protein restriction and blood pressure control on the progression of chronic renal disease. *N Engl J Med* 1994; **330**: 877–884.

Kline Bolton W. The nature of clinical trials in nephrology. *Kidney Int* 1992; **42**: 1061–1069.

Maschio G, Alberti D, Janin G, Locatelli F, Mann JFE, Motolese M, Ponticelli C, Ritz E, Zucchelli P and the Angiotensin-converting Enzyme Inhibition in Progressive Renal Insufficiency Study Group. Effect of angiotensin-converting-enzyme inhibitor benazepril on the progression of chronic renal insufficiency. *N Engl J Med* 1996; **334**: 939–945.

The GISEN Group (Gruppo Italiano di Studi Epidemiologici in Nefrologia). Randomised placebo-controlled trial of effect of ramipril on decline in glomerular filtration rate and risk of terminal renal failure in proteinuric, non-diabetic nephropathy. *Lancet* 1997; **349**: 1857–1863.

References

1. Hateboer N, Torra R, Estivill E, Bogdanova N, Davies F, Lazarou L, v. Dijk M, Breuning M, Saggar-Malik A, Jeffery S, San Millan JL, Martinez I, Walker R, Holmans P, Ravine D. PKD2: the phenotype defined. *Kidney Int*, 1997; **52**: 1122.
2. Franz KA, Reubi FC. Rate of functional deterioration of polycystic disease. *Kidney Int* 1983; **23**: 526–529.
3. Kanno Y, Suzuki H, Okada H, Takenaka T, Saruta T. Calcium channel blockers versus ACE inhibitors as antihypertensives in polycystic kidney disease. *Q J Med* 1996; **89**: 65–70.
4. Johnson AM, Gabow PA. Identification of patients with autosomal dominant polycystic kidney disease at highest risk for end-stage renal disease. *J Am Soc Nephrol* 1997; **8**: 1560–1567.
5. Klahr S, Breyer JA, Beck GJ, Dennis VW, *et al.* Dietary protein restriction, blood pressure control and the progression of polycystic kidney disease. Modification of Diet in Renal Disease Study Group. *J Am Soc Nephrol* 1995; **5**: 2037–2047.
6. Klahr S, Levey AS, Beck GJ, Caggiula AW, Hunsicker L, Kusek JW, Striker G. The effects of dietary protein restriction and blood pressure control on the progression of chronic renal disease. *N Engl J Med* 1994; **330**: 877–884.
7. Rosman JB, ter Wee PM, Meijer S, Piers-Brecht TPN, Sluiter WJ, Donker AJM. Prospective randomised trial of early protein restriction in chronic renal failure. *Lancet* 1984; **2**: 1291–1296.
8. Donadio JV, Anderson CF, Mitchell JC, Holley KE, Ilstrup DM, Fuster V, Chesebro JH. Membranoproliferative glomerulonephritis. A prospective clinical trial of platelet-inhibitor therapy. *N Engl J Med* 1984; **310**: 1421–1426.
9. Rosman JB, Langer K, Brandl M, Piers-Brecht TPM, van der Hem GK, ter Wee PM, Donker AJM. Protein-restricted diets in chronic renal failure: four year follow up shows limited indications. *Kidney Int* 1989; **36** (Suppl. 27): S96–S102.
10. Donadio JV, Offord KP. Reassessment of treatment results in membranoproliferative glomerulonephritis. *Am J Kidney Dis* 1989; **14**: 445–451.
11. Kline Bolton W. The nature of clinical trials in nephrology. *Kidney Int* 1992; **42**: 1061–1069.

12. Rutherford WE, Blondin J, Miller JP, Greenwalt AS, Vavra JD. Chronic progressive renal disease: rate of change of serum creatinine concentration. *Kidney Int* 1977; **11**: 62–70.
13. Zoccali C, Postorino M, Martorano C, Salnitro F, Maggiore Q. The 'breakpoint' test, a new statistical method for studying progressive chronic renal failure. *Nephrol Dial Transpl* 1989; **4**: 101–104.
14. Modification of Diet in Renal Disease Study Group. Effects of diet and antihypertensive therapy on creatinine clearance and serum creatinine concentration in the modification of diet in renal disease study. *J Am Soc Nephrol* 1996; **7**: 556–565.
15. Cockroft D, Gault MH. Prediction of creatinine clearance from serum creatinine. *Nephron* 1976; **16**: 31–41.
16. van Essen GG, Stegeman CA, Aperloo AJ, Rensma D, de Zeeuw D, de Jong PE. Serum cystatin C is not superior to creatinine-based methods to estimate GFR during long term followup. *J Am Soc Nephrol* 1997; **8**: 79A.
17. Levey AS, Bosch JP, Breyer JA, Greene T, Rogers N, Roth D. Predicting GFR from serum creatinine in the MDRD study. *J Am Soc Nephrol* 1997; **8**: 141A.
18. Gaspari F, Perico N, Matalone M, Signorini O, Azzolini N, Mister M, Remuzzi G. Precision of iohexol plasma clearance for GFR estimation in patients with renal disease. *J Am Soc Nephrol* 1997; **8**: 69A.
19. Donadio JV, Glassock RJ. Immunosuppressive drug therapy in lupus nephritis. *Am J Kidney Dis* 1993; **21**: 229–250.
20. Peto R, Pike MC, Armitage P, Brestlow NE, Cox DR, *et al.* Design and analysis of randomised clinical trials requiring prolonged observation of each patient. II Analysis and examples. *Br J Cancer* 1977; **35**: 1–39.
21. Modification of Diet in Renal Disease Study Group. Short-term effects of protein intake, blood pressure and antihypertensive therapy on glomerular filtration rate in the modification of diet in renal disease study. *J Am Soc Nephrol* 1996; **7**: 2097–2109.
22. El Nahas AM, Coles GA. Dietary treatment of chronic renal failure: ten unanswered questions. *Lancet* 1986; **i**: 597–600.
23. Ihle BU, Becker GJ, Whitworth JA, Charlwood RA, Kincaid-Smith PS. The effect of protein restriction on the progression of renal insufficiency. *N Engl J Med* 1989; **321**: 1773–1777.
24. Locatelli F, Alberti D, Graziani G, Buccianti G, Redaelli B, Giangrande A and the Northern Italian Cooperative Group. Prospective, randomised, mulitcentre trial of effect of protein restriction on progression of chronic renal insufficiency. *Lancet* 1991; **337**: 1299–1304.
25. Williams PS, Stevens ME, Fass G, Irons L, Bone JM. Failure of dietary protein and phosphate restriction to retard the progression of chronic renal failure: a prospective, randomized, controlled trial. *Q J Med* 1991; **81**: 837–855.
26. D'Amico G, Gentile MG, Fellin G, Manna G, Cofano F. Effect of dietary protein restriction on the progression of renal failure: a prospective controlled trial. *Nephrol Dial Transpl* 1994; **9**: 1590–1594.
27. Modification of Diet in Renal Disease Study Group. Effects of dietary protein restriction on the progression of moderate renal disease in the modification of diet in renal disease study. *J Am Soc Nephrol* 1996; **7**: 2616–2626.
28. Pendrini MT, Levey AS, Lau J, Chalmers TC, Wang PH. The effect of dietary protein restriction on the progression of diabetic and non-diabetic renal disease: a meta-analysis. *Ann Intern Med* 1996; **124**: 627–632.
29. Fouque D, Laville M, Boissel JP, Chiflet R, Labeeuw M, Zech PY. Controlled trials of

low protein diets in chronic renal insufficiency. Meta-analysis. *Br Med J* 1992; **304**: 216–220.

30. Kasiske BL, Lakatua JDA, Ma JZ, Louis TA. A meta-analysis of the effects of dietary protein restriction on the rate of decline in renal function. *Am J Kidney Dis* 1998; **31**: 954–961.
31. Levey AS, Adler S, Caggiula AW, England BK, Greene T, Hunsicker LG, Kusek JW, Rogers NL, Teschan PE. Effects of dietary protein restriction on the progression of advanced renal disease in the modification of diet in renal disease study. *Am J Kidney Dis* 1996; **27**: 652–663.
32. Ikizler TA, Greene JH, Wingard RL, Parker RA, Hakin RM. Spontaneous dietary protein intake during progression of chronic renal failure. *J Am Soc Nephrol* 1995; **6**: 1386–1391.
33. Pollock CA, Ibels LS, Zhu F-Y, Warnant M, Caterson RJ, Waugh DA, Mahony JF. Protein intake in renal disease. *J Am Soc Nephrol* 1997; **8**: 777–783.
34. Acchiardo SR, Moore LW, Latour PA. Malnutrition as the main factor in morbidity and mortality of hemodialysis patients. *Kidney Int* 1983; **16** (Suppl.): S199–S203.
35. Modification of Diet in Renal Disease Study Group, Kopple J, Levey AS, Greene T, *et al.* Effect of dietary protein restriction on nutritional status in the modification of diet in renal disease study. *Kidney Int* 1997; **52**: 778–791.
36. Walser M, Mitch WE, Maroni BJ, Kopple JD. Should protein intake be restricted in pre-dialysis patients? *Kidney Int* 1999; **55**: 771–777.
37. Wingen AM, Fabian-Bach C, Schaeffer F, Mehls O. Randomised multicentre study of a low protein diet on the progression of chronic renal failure in children. European Study Group of Nutritional Treatment of Chronic Renal Failure in Childhood. *Lancet* 1997; **349**: 1117–1123.
38. Hamazaki T, Tateno S, Shishido H. Eicosapentaenoic acid and IgA nephropathy. *Lancet*, 1984; **i**: 1017–1018.
39. Bennett WW, Walker RG, Kincaid-Smith P. Treatment of IgA nephropathy with eicosapentaenoic acid (EPA): a two-year prospective trial. *Clin Nephrol* 1989; **31**: 128–131.
40. Cheng IKP, Chan PCK, Chan MK. The effect of fish-oil dietary supplement on the progression of mesangial IgA glomerulonephritis. *Nephrol Dial Transplant* 1990; **5**: 241–246.
41. Pettersson EE, Rekola S, Berglund L, Sundqvist KG, Angelin B, Diczfalusy U, Bjorkhem L, Bergström J. Treatment of IgA nephropathy with omega-3-polyunsaturated fatty acids: a prospective, double blind, randomized study. *Clin Nephrol* 1994; **41**: 183–190.
42. Donadio JV, Bergstralh EJ, Offord KP, Spencer DC, Holley KE. A controlled trial of fish oil in IgA nephropathy. *N Engl J Med* 1994; **331**: 1194–1199.
43. Van Ipersele de Strihou C. Fish oil for IgA nephropathy? *N Engl J Med* 1994; **331**: 1227–1228.
44. Dillon JJ. Fish oil therapy for IgA nephropathy; efficacy and inter study variability. *J Am Soc Nephrol* 1997; **8**: 1739–1744.
45. Klag MJ, Whelton PK, Randell BL, Neaton JD, Brancati FL, Ford CE, Shulman NB, Stamler J. Blood pressure and end-stage renal disease in men. *N Engl J Med* 1996; **334**: 13–18.
46. Brazy PC, Stead WW, Fitzwilliam JF. Progression of renal insufficiency: role of blood pressure. *Kidney Int* 1989; **35**: 670–674.
47. Alvestrand A, Gutierrez A, Bucht H, Bergstrom J. Reduction of blood pressure retards the progression of chronic renal failure in man. *Nephrol Dial Transpl* 1988; **3**: 624–631.
48. Peterson JC, Adler S, Burkart JM, Greene T, Hebert LA, Hunsicker LG, King AJ, Klahr S, Massry SG, Seifer JL for the Modification of Diet in Renal Disease (MDRD) Study

Group. Blood pressure control, proteinuria, and the progression of renal disease. The Modification of Diet in Renal Disease study. *Ann Intern Med* 1995; **123**: 754–762.

49. Toto RD, Mitchell RC, Smith RD, Lee H-C, McIntyre D, Pettinger WA. 'Strict' blood pressure control and the progression of renal disease in hypertensive nephrosclerosis. *Kidney Int* 1995; **48**: 851–859.
50. Kamper A-L, Strandgaard S, Leyssac PP. Late outcome of a controlled trial of enalapril treatment in progressive chronic renal failure. Hard end-points and influence of proteinuria. *Nephrol Dial Transpl* 1995; **10**: 1182–1188.
51. Hannedouche T, Landais P, Goldfarb B, El Esper N, Fournier A, Godin M, Durand D, Chanard J, Mignon F, Suc J-M, Grunfeld J-P. Randomised controlled trial of enalapril and blockers in non-diabetic chronic renal failure. *Br J Med* 1996; **309**: 833–837.
52. Ihle BU, Whitworth JA, Shahinfar S, Cnaan A, Kincaid-Smith PS, Becker GJ. Angiotensin-converting enzyme inhibition in non-diabetic progressive renal insufficiency: a controlled double-blind trial. *Am J Kidney Dis* 1996; **27**: 489–495.
53. Zucchelli P, Zuccala A, Borghi M, Fusaroli M, Sasdelli M, Stallone C, Sanna G, Gaggi R. Long-term comparison between captopril and nifedipine in the progression of renal insufficiency. *Kidney Int* 1992; **42**: 452–458.
54. Donadio JV, Grande JP, Bergstralk EJ, Spencer DC. The Mayo nephrology collaborative trial of an angiotensin converting enzyme inhibitor (ACEi) versus a calcium antagonist (CA) in idiopathic membranous nephropathy (IMN) with nephrotic syndrome in adults. *J Am Soc Nephrol* 1997; **8**: 85A.
55. Maschio G, Alberti D, Janin G, Locatelli F, Mann JFE, Motolese M, Ponticelli C, Ritz E, Zucchelli P and the Angiotensin-converting Enzyme Inhibition in Progressive Renal Insufficiency Study Group. Effect of angiotensin-converting-enzyme inhibitor benazepril on the progression of chronic renal insufficiency. *N Engl J Med* 1996; **334**: 939–945.
56. The GISEN Group (Gruppo Italiano di Studi Epidemiologici in Nefrologia). Randomised placebo-controlled trial of effect of ramipril on decline in glomerular filtration rate and risk of terminal renal failure in proteinuric, non-diabetic nephropathy. *Lancet* 1997; **349**: 1857–1863.
57. Ruggenenti P, Perna A, Gherardi G, Gaspari F, Benini R, Remuzzi G on behalf of Gruppo Italiano di Studi Epidemiologici in Nefrologia (GISEN). Renal function and requirements for dialysis in chrone nephropathy patients on long term ramipril: REIN follow-up tual. *Lancet* 1998; **352**: 1252–1256.
58. Giatras J, Lau J, Levey AS. Effect of angiotensin-converting-enzyme inhibitors on the progression of non-diabetic renal disease: a meta-analysis of randomized trials. *Ann Intern Med* 1997; **127**: 337–345.
59. Griffin KA, Picken M, Bidani AK. Radiotelemetric BP monitoring, antihypertensives and glomeruloprotection in remnant kidney model. *Kidney Int* 1994; **46**: 1010–1018.
60. Gansevoort RT, Sluiter WJ, Hemmelder MH, de Zeeuw D, de Jong PE. Antiproteinuric effect of blood-pressure-lowering agents: a meta-analysis of comparative trials. *Nephrol Dial Transpl* 1995; **10**: 1963–1974.
61. Chapman AB, Gabow PA, Schrier RW. Reversible renal failure associated with angiotensin-converting enzyme inhibitors in polycystic kidney disease. *Ann Intern Med* 1991; **115**: 769–773.
62. van Essen GG, Rensma PL, de Zeeuw D, Sluiter WJ, Scheffer H, Apperloo AJ, de Jong PE. Association between angiotensin-converting-enzyme gene polymorphism and failure of renoprotective therapy. *Lancet* 1996; **347**: 94–95.
63. Apperloo AJ, de Zeeuw D, de Jong PE. A short term antihypertensive treatment-induced

fall in glomerular filtration rate predicts long-term stability of renal function. *Kidney Int* 1997; **51**: 793–797.

64. Zauner I, *et al.* Effect of aspirin and dipyridamole on proteinuria in idiopathic membranoproliferative glomerulonephritis; a multicentre prospective trial. *Nephrol Dial Transpl* 1994; **9**: 619–622.
65. Zimmerman SW, *et al.* Prospective trial of warfarin and dipyridamole in patients with membranoproliferative nephritis. *Am J Med* 1983; **75**: 920–927.
66. Cattran DC, *et al.* Results of a controlled drug trial in membranoproliferative glomerulonephritis. *Kidney Int* 1985; **27**: 265–280.
67. Thomas ME, Harris KP, Ramaswamy C, Hattersley JM, Wheeler DC, Varghese Z, Williams JD, Walls J, Moorhead JF. Simvastatin therapy for hypercholesterolaemic patients with nephrotic syndrome or significant proteinuria. *Kidney Int* 1993; **44**: 1124–1129.
68. Stefoni S, Mosconi G, LaManna G, Bonomini V, Mioli V, *et al.* Low-dosage ibopamine treatment in progressive renal failure: a long-term multicentre trial. *Am J Nephrol* 1996; **16**: 489–499.
69. Niwa T, Asada H, Yamada K. Prostaglandin E1 infusion therapy in chronic glomerulonephritis—a double blind crossover trial. *Prostagl Leukotr Med* 1985; **19**: 227–233.
70. Miller SB, Moulton M, O'Shea M, Hammerman MR. Effects of IGF-I on renal function in end-stage chronic renal failure. *Kidney Int* 1994; **46**: 201–207.
71. Ike JO, Fervenza FC, Hoffman AR, Yeh I, Hintz RL, Liu F, Rabkin R. Early experience with extended use of insulin-like growth factor-1 in advanced chronic renal failure. *Kidney Int* 1997; **51**: 840–849.
72. Owada A, Nakao M, Koike J, Ujiie K, Tomita K, Shiigai T. Effects of oral adsorbent AST-120 on the progression of chronic renal failure: a randomized controlled study. *Kidney Int*, 1997; **52** (Suppl. 63): S188–S190.
73. Sanaka T, Kihara T, Shinobe M, *et al.* Suppressive effect on progression of chronic renal failure (CRF) by decreasing intestinal levels of indoxyl sulfate (IS). *J Am Soc Nephrol* 1997; **8**: 75A.
74. Zhang JH, Li L-S, Zhang M. Clinical effects of rheum and captopril on progression of chronic renal failure. *Chin Med* 1990; **103**: 788–793.
75 Heifets M, Davis TA, Tegtmeyer E, Klahr S. Exercise training ameliorates progressive renal disease in rats with subtotal nephrectomy. *Kidney Int* 1987; **32**: 815–820.
76. Eidemark I, Haaber AB, Feldt-Rasmussen B, Kanstrup I-L, Strandgaard S. Exercise training and the progression of chronic renal failure. *Nephron* 1997; **75**: 36–40.
77. Devoy MAB, Tomson CRV, Edmunds ME, Feehally J, Walls J. Deterioration of renal function associated with angiotensin converting enzyme inhibitor therapy is not always reversible. *J Int Med* 1992; **232**: 493–498.
78. Bergström J, Alvestrand A, Bucht H, Guiterrez A. Progression of chronic renal failure in man is retarded with more frequent follow-ups and better blood pressure control. *Clin Nephrol* 1986; **25**: 1–6.

13

Outcome and interventions in chronic renal disease: evidence from adequately designed clinical trials and meta-analysis

Suzanne K. Swan and Bertram L. Kasiske

Treatment of glomerular diseases constitutes a significant portion of the practice of clinical nephrology. Yet, a paucity of knowledge and experience concerning the treatment of glomerular diseases often results in a confused therapeutic decision-making process. Conducting clinical trials in patients with primary glomerular disease, however, has become increasingly difficult in recent years. Nephrology practice has been steadily moving from tertiary care centers into private, multi-specialty, outpatient clinics. As a result, within a given practice, it is no longer possible to identify adequate numbers of patients with a specific renal disease for which experimental protocols can be applied. Further, clinical trials conducted in tertiary care centers or government-funded research institutions in the past often used protocols that would be difficult to implement in community-based practice today. Additionally, the natural history of a specific glomerular disease may be so variable that formulation of a rational therapeutic approach is precluded. This is particularly true when the only published data are from small, short-term studies that are neither randomized nor controlled, and did not carry out risk stratification. The relative absence of sound risk/benefit data from long-term trials has only served to widen the gap between therapeutic 'nihilists' and 'enthusiasts' as described in a recent editorial [1].

Approaches to the assessment of the effects of treatment of renal diseases

The randomized, controlled trial is the gold standard for determining whether medical therapy is effective. Occasionally, a therapy is so obviously effective (when compared with historical controls) that a randomized, controlled trial is not necessary, and may be unethical. For example, it would be unethical to study the effects of insulin in diabetic ketoacidosis using a randomized, placebo-controlled trial. However, great care must be used before deciding that a therapy is so effective that it need not, or cannot, be tested in a well-designed clinical trial. Frequently, the severity of a disease appears to change over time, due in part to a decreasing threshold for diagnosis as the disease becomes better known; a newly described disease may at first be diagnosed only when it is severe and obvious. Over time, as awareness and understanding of the disease increases, it may be diagnosed more often at an earlier, milder stage. As treatment of earlier, milder disease is usually more effective than treatment of more advanced and more severe disease, a reliance on historical controls may make a therapy appear to be more effective than it actually is.

There are few therapies for glomerular diseases that are so obviously effective that they can be accepted without properly designed, clinical trials. We will discuss these instances, but we will otherwise emphasize therapies for glomerular diseases that have been subjected to the scrutiny of at least one randomized, controlled trial. The fact that a therapy has not been tested with an appropriate clinical trial does not mean that it should not be used in individual patients. For some diseases there may be no therapy that has been studied in a randomized trial, but this does not mean that a patient with that disease should receive no treatment! However, it probably does mean that any new treatment for that disease needs to be studied before it is accepted as being effective.

We will present evidence from adequately designed, clinical trials, as well as published meta-analyses on the outcomes of therapeutic interventions in selected glomerular diseases. Membranous nephropathy, FSGS, minimal change disease or nil lesion, membranoproliferative glomerulonephritis, IgA nephropathy, antiglomerular basement membrane disease, pauci-immune rapidly progressive glomerulonephritis, thrombotic thrombocytopenic purpura, hemolytic uremic syndrome, and lupus nephritis will be included. It is beyond the scope of this chapter to provide detailed discussions of the specific pathophysiologic mechanisms underlying each glomerular lesion. Such discussions can be found elsewhere.

Meta-analysis is a type of systematic review that uses quantitative methods to combine data from separate studies in order to address a specific clinical question. In contrast to narrative reviews, in which an expert in a particular field reviews the published literature on a given topic, systematic reviews attempt to eliminate the inherent bias of such reviews by applying scientific method to critically asses published data. The reasons to perform a meta-analysis include the ability to collate a large number of studies, increase the statistical power of these studies and test hypotheses, define etiologies of study differences which may then be used to generate hypotheses, determine the need for additional trials and calculate the sample sizes for such trials, and reduce bias inherent to narrative reviews. A number of threats to the validity of meta-analysis exist and include publication bias in which journal editors favor publication of 'positive' trials as well as file-drawer bias in which investigators are reluctant to submit 'negative' studies, assuming journal rejection. Like all scientific studies meta-analysis should be reproducible. As such, one should look for quality characteristics when reviewing meta-analyses which include a statement of purpose, the author's search strategy (i.e., database and key words used), the inclusion and exclusion criteria utilized to accept or reject a study from the meta-analysis, the methods used for data extraction, the approach used to combining treatment effects, an assessment of a particular study's quality as well as the homogeneity between all studies analyzed, providing reasons for differences between studies, and the weighting of studies based upon the quality of results. In general, meta-analysis should assist clinicians in judging the strengths and weaknesses of evidence generated by clinical trials. As the number of trials increases and the medical literature expands exponentially, clinicians should develop a working knowledge of meta-analysis techniques and how to interpret their results. Comprehensive reviews on this topic can be found elsewhere in the literature.

Membranous nephropathy

Idiopathic membranous nephropathy is the most common cause of the nephrotic syndrome in adults [2,3] but its treatment remains controversial. Such controversy stems, in part, from the fact that the 10-year renal survival rate is approximately 70%, and a spontaneous remission occurs 10–30% of the time [3,4]. Thus, the majority of patients with truly *idiopathic* membranous nephropathy (as opposed to *secondary* forms associated with infectious entities such as hepatitis B or solid organ tumors) do well without aggressive treatment. It is a minority of patients, often categorized by specific risk factors, who develop progressive disease and may benefit from more aggressive therapy.

Pharmacologic therapy of idiopathic membranous nephropathy has changed its focus over time, beginning with corticosteroid therapy, followed by the addition of alkylating agents, and most recently cyclosporine A. The results of several prospective, randomized trials utilizing various pharmacologic interventions are summarized in Table 13.1. An early report by the US Collaborative Study of the Adult Idiopathic Nephrotic Syndrome concluded that immunosuppressive therapy with corticosteroids alone was beneficial when compared with placebo [5], but the average duration of follow-up was less than 24 months, only two of 34 treated patients had sustained complete remission of proteinuria, and the number of control patients with declining renal function was greater than expected based upon the natural course of the disease. Conversely, 10 years later, two trials failed to demonstrate efficacy of corticosteroid therapy when compared with placebo [6,7]. These studies involved larger numbers of patients, used a more sensitive marker of renal function in the form of creatinine clearance, and had more prolonged follow-up durations. Thus, the effectiveness of corticosteroids is questionable.

The addition of alkylating agents to the treatment regimens of membranous nephropathy has also provided mixed results. Murphy *et al.* [8], demonstrated a reduction in proteinuria, but no preservation of renal function in patients treated with oral cyclophosphamide for 6 months plus dipyridamole and warfarin therapy for 2 years compared with symptomatic therapy. Similarly, Donadio *et al.* [9]. did not find a 2-year course of oral cyclophosphamide superior to symptomatic treatment. The Medical Research Council Working Party [10] found no benefit when azathioprine was added to corticosteroid therapy. In the case of the latter trial, however, only 14 patients were treated. This underscores the fact that many published results stem from underpowered studies, potentially leading to invalid conclusions. Conversely, preservation of renal function and remission of proteinuria were noted by Ponticelli *et al.* [11] when the alkylating agent chlorambucil was combined with corticosteroid therapy compared with symptomatic treatment. For the past 14 years,

Table 13.1 Randomized, controlled trials in membranous glomerulonephritis

Trial	Treatment	Sample size	Follow-up (months)	Outcome
Collaborative Study [5]	Prednisone vs placebo	72	32 (4–52)	Renal preservation
Cattran *et al.* [7]	Prednisone vs symptomatic treatment	158	48 ± 3 (6–96)	No benefit
Cameron/MRC [6]	Prednisone vs placebo	103	36	No benefit
Murphy *et al.* [8]	Cyclophosphamide, dipyridamole, warfarin vs symptomatic treatment	40	24	Reduction in proteinuria; renal function unchanged
Donadio *et al.* [9]	Cyclophosphamide vs symptomatic treatment	22	12	No benefit
Ponticelli *et al.* [11,12]	Chlorambucil alternating with MP* monthly vs symptomatic treatment	62	120	Renal preservation; reduction in proteinuria
Falk *et al.*** [15]	Cyclophosphamide, MP, prednisone vs prednisone	26	29 ± 17	No benefit
Ponticelli *et al.*** [16]	Chlorambucil alternating with MP* monthly vs MP*	92	54 ± 17	No benefit
Cattran *et al.* [19]	Cyclosporine A vs placebo	17	21	Renal preservation; reduction in proteinuria

* MP, methylprednisolone, given as a 1 g dose intravenously for 3 days followed by 0.4 mg/kg per day orally for 27 days; ** no placebo controls.

these investigators have treated membranous nephropathy patients with a monthly alternating course of chlorambucil and corticosteroids for 6 months, and compared this regimen with symptomatic treatment. A 10-year follow-up report [12] revealed 92% renal survival in the treatment group compared with only 60% in controls which like the US Collaborative Trial discussed above, suggests that the natural history of the disease was more severe than expected. Additionally, patients enrolled in the study had relatively normal renal function at the time of entry. This is the only long-term follow-up report of any membranous nephropathy trial; again, highlighting the need for additional long-term studies.

Given its somewhat indolent course and spontaneous remission rate, clinicians have attempted to identify prospectively patients with membranous nephropathy at risk for developing a more progressive course, and treat such 'high risk' patients more aggressively. Patients who present with or develop impaired renal function have poor long-term renal survival [13,14]. Proteinuria greater than 8–10 g/24 h, male gender, advanced age, and significant renal fibrosis/sclerosis have also been reported to be negative prognostic signs, but these risk factors have not been extensively studied in prospective trials. Few prospective, randomized, controlled intervention trials have been performed in this subpopulation of patients, although many agents have been identified as 'effective'. Falk *et al.* [15] did not find any benefit from the addition of intravenous ('pulse') cyclophosphamide to corticosteroid therapy compared with prednisone alone in a prospective, randomized, controlled study. Interestingly, Ponticelli *et al.* [16] found no sustained benefit from the addition of chlorambucil to methylprednisolone when compared with methylprednisolone alone, but patients with impaired renal function (so-called 'high-risk') as well as patients with normal renal function were enrolled in the study.

Recently, cyclosporine A has been reported to induce partial or complete remissions in patients with progressive membranous nephropathy [17,18]. In the only prospective, randomized, placebo-controlled trial involving patients with progressive membranous nephropathy (impaired renal function and average protein excretion over 10 g/24 h). Cattran *et al.* [19] found cyclosporine A beneficial in reducing the rate of renal deterioration and proteinuria. Clearly, additional trials with larger numbers of patients and longer durations of follow-up are warranted before it can be concluded that cyclosporine A is effective in membranous nephropathy.

As stated in the introduction, meta-analysis has become increasingly popular as a tool to analyze data from a large number of trials to arrive at a statistically adequate sample size ('*n*'). Despite such advantages, meta-analysis has failed to clarify the issue of treatment in membranous nephropathy. Three meta-analyses [20–22] arrived at different conclusions regarding the benefit of alkylating agents in membranous patients, despite the fact that the three analyses included many of the same trials. Some of the differences in the results of these meta-analyses likely resulted from differences in the definition of end-points. Studies using 'reduction of proteinuria' tended to be positive while those using 'remission of proteinuria' were not.

In summary, mounting evidence from long-term follow-up trials would indicate that no specific immunosuppressive therapy be undertaken in patients with *non-progressive* membranous disease (i.e., normal glomerular filtration rate, proteinuria less than 8 g/24 h, absence of thromboembolic events). Conversely, patients with *progressive* membranous nephropathy may benefit from corticosteroids, cytotoxic agents, or cyclosporine A.

Membranoproliferative Glomerulonephritis

In contrast to membranous nephropathy, membranoproliferative (MPGN) or mesangiocapillary glomerulonephritis is much less common, accounting for less than

10% of histologically proven primary glomerulonephritis [23]. Although three distinct histologic categories have been described [type I, type II (dense deposit disease), and type III] clinical presentation, prognosis, and response to treatment lend little support to the clinical relevance of these categorical distinctions. Like membranous nephropathy, an idiopathic form as well as secondary forms of MPGN exist, with the majority of cases falling under the latter heading. A lengthy list of disorders associated with secondary MPGN includes infection, autoimmune disorders, liver disease, malignancy, and systemic illnesses, and are discussed elsewhere. Although spontaneous remission can occur (<10%), chronic renal failure and persistent nephrotic-range proteinuria are the rule [24]; calculated actuarial renal survival at 10 years from renal biopsy is approximately 60% [25,26].

In secondary forms of MPGN, successful treatment of underlying disorders known to be associated with MPGN such as infection (hepatitis C for example) or malignancy, may lead to the resolution of renal impairment. Treatment of *idiopathic* MPGN, on the other hand, remains controversial. Five randomized, controlled trials (Table 13.2) in both children and adults have been published [27–31], but fail to provide convincing evidence that treatment with immunomodulating compounds or antiplatelet agents are efficacious [32]. Specifically, Donadio *et al.* [30] reported in

Table 13.2 Randomized, controlled trials in membranoproliferative glomerulonephritis

Trial	Treatment	Sample size	Follow-up (months)	Outcome
Cattran *et al.* [27]	Cyclophosphamide, warfarin, dipyridamole vs placebo	59	18	No benefit
Tiller *et al.* [28]	Cyclophosphamide, warfarin, dipyridamole vs placebo	37	Not reported	No benefit
Zimmerman *et al.* [29]	Dipyridamole, warfarin vs placebo	18	12	Renal preservation
Donadio and Offord [32]	Dipyridamole, aspirin vs placebo (based on life-table analysis)	21	48	No benefit
International Study of Kidney Disease in Children [49]	Prednisone vs placebo	37	38	No benefit

1984 that antiplatelet therapy was beneficial compared with placebo. Zimmerman *et al.* [29] published similar findings in 1983. Subsequently in 1989, Donadio and Offord [32] reassessed treatment results for MPGN using life-table analyses and found no long-term benefit. A recent report by Zäuner *et al.* [33] demonstrated a significant reduction in proteinuria with aspirin and dipyridamole therapy, but no change in serum creatinine after 36 months of treatment. No post-treatment follow-up was available, however, and sample size was small. Additionally, three long-term, *uncontrolled* therapeutic trials have reported improved 10-year renal survival rates (70–85%), but had no control group with which to compare outcomes [34–36]. Use of cyclosporine A may be beneficial either by a direct disease-modifying mechanism or as a corticosteroid-sparing agent as suggested by several case reports [37]. Caution, however, is warranted given the risks associated with this drug. Prospective, randomized, controlled trials with long-term follow-up are needed to assess adequately the risk/benefit ratio and the cost-effectiveness of cyclosporine A.

Focal segmental glomerulosclerosis

Focal segmental glomerulosclerosis (FSGS) or FSGS with hyalinosis, accounts for approximately 10% of glomerular lesions among pediatric and adult patients with proteinuria [38], but is much more common in adults. As with membranous nephropathy and MPGN, both idiopathic and secondary forms of FSGS exist, with a long list of associated disorders such as infections (HIV), obesity, heroin exposure, and malignancy. Unlike other glomerular lesions, however, *no* therapeutic intervention has been shown safely to preserve renal function for adults in prospective, randomized, controlled trials with adequate follow-up duration. Corticosteroids, however, when administered for *more* than 3 months, reduced proteinuria, often resulting in complete remission, although complete remission was more common in pediatric patients [39,40]. More recently, a report by the International Study of Kidney Disease in Children found that the addition of a 90-day course of oral cyclophosphamide to a 12-month course of alternate-day prednisone was detrimental compared with prednisone therapy alone [41].

Cyclosporine A has been evaluated in both pediatric as well as adult populations. In an uncontrolled study, Ingulli *et al.* [42] gave high-dose cyclosporine A (7 mg/kg per day) to steroid and cyclophosphamide-resistant pediatric patients for an average of 2 years. After a mean duration of follow-up of 8 years, proteinuria was significantly reduced as well as serum cholesterol levels. Although 24% of the patients progressed to end-stage renal disease, this was considered significantly improved when compared with historical controls. The observation that cyclosporine A may be more effective in steroid-resistant cases as compared with alkylating agents such as cyclophosphamide has been noted by other investigators [43]. In a randomized, placebo-controlled, double-blind study, Lieberman and Tejani noted significant reductions in proteinuria, but no change in renal function, when a 6-month course of cyclosporine A was compared with placebo treatment in pediatric patients [44]. Similarly, Walker and Kincaid-Smith [45] found cyclosporine A reduced proteinuria, but did not affect renal function in adults with steroid-resistant nephrotic syndrome. Thus, no definitive treatment regimen for FSGS currently exists which can safely achieve long-term preservation of renal function.

In a comprehensive review by Korbet *et al.* [43], the authors point out that 49 years after the description of FSGS first appeared, essentially all of the published therapeutic data are based on retrospective analyses. Although important insights into treatment of FSGS have been gained by retrospective studies over time, these authors conclude that such insight merely emphasizes the need for controlled prospective randomized trials with long follow-up periods [43].

Minimal change disease

Minimal change disease, often referred to as nil lesion, is the most common cause of nephrotic syndrome in children. Initial presentation of the disease tends to be very corticosteroid responsive in children, but occasional relapses occur in 25–30%, and frequent relapses (more than two to three relapses in a 6-month period or five in an 18-month period) occur in 40–50% of patients [46,47]. Interestingly, prior to the availability of corticosteroids treatment regimens, cytotoxic therapy, and cyclosporine A, a spontaneous remission rate of 25% in children with idiopathic nephrotic syndrome was observed [48]. The dramatic response to corticosteroids makes the adoption of this therapy for childhood minimal change disease warranted, even in the absence of a randomized, controlled trial. Indeed, it would now be considered unethical to withhold this therapy in a randomized trial. The initial episode of minimal change disease should be treated with the classic regimen of 60 mg/m^2 prednisone orally daily for 4 weeks followed by alternate-day prednisone of 40 mg/m^2 for 4 weeks [49–51]. Frequent relapses (see above), or steroid-dependency to control nephrotic-range proteinuria, can be treated with cyclophosphamide or chlorambucil, generally in conjunction with corticosteroid therapy. Ueda *et al.* [52] found that 8 weeks of oral cyclophosphamide (2 mg/kg per day) was as effective as 12 weeks of therapy in maintaining a relapse-free period. Established treatment regimens are available in numerous references as well as textbooks and will not be discussed further in this section.

More recent attention has focused on the therapeutic role of cyclosporine A, but frequent relapses with cessation of the drug suggest it may only be useful in combination with other immunosuppressive agents, perhaps for dose-sparing purposes [53]. Ponticelli and Rivolta [54] reviewed several reports, as well as an ongoing Italian trial in which cyclosporine A was used either to maintain a remission or induce a remission in steroid-resistant nephrotic patients. Compilation of all the trials revealed that approximately 40% of steroid-resistant patients achieved a partial or complete remission with cyclosporine A. However, it is important to note that the patient population was quite heterogeneous, with adult, pediatric, FSGS, minimal change, IgM nephropathy, and mesangial proliferative glomerulonephritis patients combined in the analysis. Garin *et al.* [55] randomly allocated eight pediatric patients with steroid-resistant nephrotic syndrome (four with minimal change and four with FSGS) to cyclosporine A (5 mg/kg per day) or placebo for 8 weeks, then crossed each subject over to the alternate therapy. No significant change in proteinuria was noted during cyclosporine A therapy. Similarly, Tejani *et al.* [56] randomly allocated *steroid-sensitive* children to either low-dose prednisone (20 mg/m^2 per day for 4 weeks, 10 mg/m^2 every other day for 4 weeks) plus cyclosporine A (7 mg/kg per day) or high-dose prednisone therapy (60 mg/m^2 per for 4 weeks, 40 mg/m^2 every other day for 4 weeks) for 8 weeks. The cyclosporine A-treated group experienced a higher rate of remission of proteinuria, and the duration of remission did not differ between groups. Long-term, randomized, controlled trials with cyclosporine A in the treatment of minimal change disease have yet to be performed, and will likely enroll only patients with steroid resistance or frequent relapses.

IgA nephropathy

Effective treatment of IgA nephropathy, the most common glomerular disease in the world [57,58], remains ill-defined. Chronic, progressive renal failure develops in 20–40% of patients 5–25 years after diagnosis. Poor prognostic indicators include older age, male gender, heavy proteinuria, hypertension, renal impairment at the time of diagnosis, glomerular sclerosis, and interstitial fibrosis [59–61]. A number of therapeutic interventions have failed to provide convincing evidence of efficacy including corticosteroids, cytotoxic agents, antiplatelet and other anticoagulant agents. Fish oil has been used in a number of trials with mixed outcomes as detailed in Table 13.3. Dillon reviewed five trials in a recent meta-analysis of fish oil therapy for IgA nephropathy and found it not to be significantly better than placebo (Fig. 13.1) [62]. A trend, however, toward beneficial effect (75% probability) was noted with fish oil, particularly in patients with heavier proteinuria. He concluded that any future, placebo-controlled, randomized trials will require a larger sample size than previously reported studies in order to detect a beneficial effect, a longer duration of therapy/follow-up, and enrollment of patients with more severe proteinuria. Lastly, Neng Lai *et al.* [63] randomized 19 patients with IgA nephropathy and urinary protein excretion exceeding 1.5 g/day to receive either cyclosporine A ($n = 9$) or placebo ($n = 10$) for 12 weeks. Creatinine clearance transiently declined in the cyclosporine A-treated group but returned to baseline after discontinuation of therapy. After a 12-week follow-up period, proteinuria did not differ between groups.

Table 13.3 Fish oil trials in IgA nephropathy

Trial	Double-blind	Placebo	Sample size	Duration (years)	Outcome
Donadio *et al.* [94]	Yes	Olive oil	102	1.7	Renal preservation
Pettersson *et al.* [95]	Yes	Corn oil	32	0.5	No benefit
Cheng *et al.** [96]	No	None	11	0.8	No benefit
Bennett *et al.* [97]	No	None	37	2	No benefit
Hamazaki *et al.* [98]	Not reported	None	20	1	Renal preservation

* Paired observations.

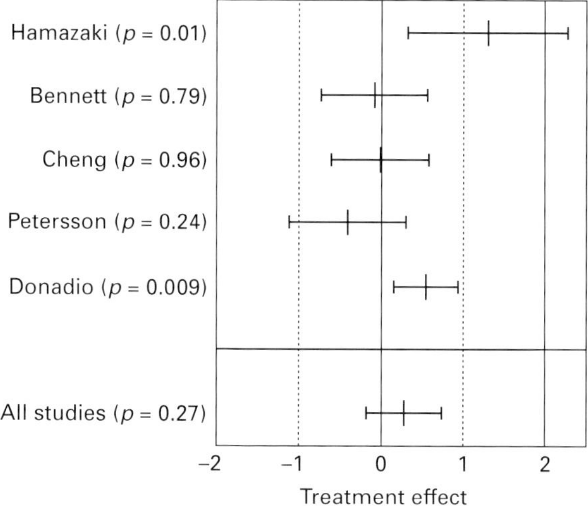

Fig. 13.1 Treatment effect sizes. Individual study outcomes and the combined outcome for all studies are presented. Positive values indicate that treatment was superior to control. Studies are identified by first author. The numbers in parentheses are two-tailed p-values calculated under a null hypothesis of no treatment effect. The error bars represent 95% confidence intervals. Reprinted with permission, Dillon [62].

Anti-glomerular basement membrane antibody nephritis

Anti-glomerular basement membrane antibody (anti-GBM) nephritis, with or without the pulmonary hemorrhage of Goodpasture's syndrome, was once associated with a very poor prognosis. Almost 90% of patients progressed to end-stage renal disease or death within 5 years, despite treatment with corticosteroids and cytotoxic agents [64]. In 1975 Lockwood and co-workers reported a patient with Goodpasture's syndrome who recovered after treatment with cyclophosphamide, corticosteroids, and plasma exchange [65]. Thereafter, a number of uncontrolled studies reported recovery with plasma exchange in a high proportion of cases. Plasma exchange, used in conjunction with immunosuppression, is now generally accepted as first-line therapy for anti-GBM nephritis, with or without pulmonary hemorrhage.

Only one, small, randomized, controlled trial has been carried out. Johnson and co-workers randomly allocated 17 patients with anti-GBM nephritis to pulse methylprednisolone or pulse methylprednisolone and plasma exchange [66]. The rate of disappearance of antibody was more rapid, and the serum creatinine at the end of therapy was lower with plasma exchange. Otherwise, there were no significant differences in results between the two groups. Indeed, outcome correlated better with the severity of disease at presentation than with the type of therapy used.

In several uncontrolled series, patients with mild disease responded to either immunosuppressive agents or plasma exchange, but patients with more severe disease responded to neither. The combined data from four series showed that among patients with serum creatinine less than 5 mg/dl and a biopsy showing fewer than 50% crescents, 11 of 14 responded to immunosuppression and 11 of 11 responded to immunosuppression plus plasma exchange [67]. On the other hand, among those with more severe disease, none of 36 patients responded to immunosuppression and none of five responded to plasma exchange. In one of these non-randomized studies the outcome among 12 patients treated symptomatically or with immunosuppression, i.e., without plasma exchange, was better than what was previously described in the literature [68]. This demonstrates the difficulty in using historical controls from the literature to conclude that recent therapies are effective. Thus, despite its general acceptance, it is not absolutely clear that plasma exchange is more effective than immunosuppression alone in anti-GBM nephritis. If it is to be effective, any therapy probably needs to be instituted before patients are oliguric.

Several other therapies have been suggested for anti-GBM nephritis. Heparin, warfarin, and ancrod have been used in experimental models, but have not been tested in clinical trials. The risk of anticoagulation in patients with pulmonary hemorrhage would, of course, increase the risk of anticoagulation. Experimental data suggest that interleukin-1 receptor antagonists, tumor necrosis factor-α receptor protein, antibodies to adhesion molecules, and even the use of the Goodpasture's epitope to remove circulating antibodies may be worthy of clinical trials in the future. Pulmonary hemorrhage in Goodpasture's syndrome, which responds more readily to treatment than anti-GBM nephritis, will not be reviewed in this chapter.

Pauci-immune, rapidly progressive glomerulonephritis

There is probably considerable overlap between vasculitis caused by Wegener's granulomatosis, polyarteritis nodosa, and renal-limited, pauci-immune, rapidly progressive, glomerulonephritis. Many of these patients have circulating antineutrophil cytoplasmic antibodies. It is not clear whether response to treatment differs substantially in patients across this clinical spectrum. Most data on treatment of vasculitis have come from trials in patients with Wegener's granulomatosis, where up to 80% eventually develop signs of renal involvement. The cornerstone of treatment for Wegener's granulomatosis is the use of alkylating agents, particularly cyclophosphamide (Table 13.4). Acceptance of this therapy has occurred in the absence of placebo-controlled, randomized trials. This is because data collected more than 40 years ago suggested that mean survival in untreated Wegener's granulomatosis was only 5 months, with 82% of patients dying by 1 year [69]. The use of cyclophosphamide for Wegener's granulomatosis was described in 1971 [70]. It was subsequently reported that cyclophosphamide produced complete remission in 79 of 85 (93%) patients [71]. It is possible that patients in earlier series had more severe disease than patients in more recent trials, as an increasing awareness of Wegener's granulomatosis may have led clinicians to make the diagnosis more often and earlier than in the past. However, the apparent dramatic improvement in survival has created an ethical imperative that no patient with Wegener's granulomatosis be left

Table 13.4 Randomized trials in patients with pauci-immune, rapidly progressive glomerulonephritis

Trial	Treatment	Sample size	Follow-up (months)	Outcome
Adu *et al.* [73]	Cyclophosphamide iv, prednisolone iv vs cyclophosphamide po, prednisolone po, azathioprine po	54	3 (1.5–10)	No benefit
Guillevin *et al.* [74]	Cyclophosphamide iv, prednisolone po vs Cyclophosphamide po, prednisolone po	50	12	More relapses; less toxicity
Rifle *et al.* [99]	Cyclophosphamide iv, methylprednisolone, plasma exchange, calcium heparinate vs methylprednisolone, plasma exchange, calcium heparinate	13*	12	Trend to improvement (not significant)
Glöckner *et al.* [75]	Plasma exchange, prednisone, cyclophosphamide, azathioprine vs prednisone, cyclophosphamide, azathioprine	26	6	No benefit
Cole *et al.* [76]	Plasma exchange, prednisolone iv, prednisone po, azathioprine po vs prednisolone iv, prednisone po, azathioprine	32	12	No benefit
Pusey *et al.* [77]	Plasma exchange, prednisone po, cyclophosphamide po, azathioprine po vs prednisone po, cyclophosphamide po, azathioprine po	48**	1	Improved (if already on dialysis)*
Rifle *et al.* [78]	Plasma exchange, methylprednisolone, immunosuppressive	14	22	Improved

Table 13.4 *(Continued)*

Trial	Treatment	Sample size	Follow-up (months)	Outcome
	agents, anticoagulants vs methylprednisolone, immunosuppressive agents, anticoagulants			
Mauri *et al.* [78]	Plasma exchange, prednisone, cyclophosphamide vs prednisone, cyclosphosphamide	22	36	Improved
Stegeman *et al.* [79]	Co-trimoxazole vs placebo	18	24	Fewer relapses
de Groot *et al.* [80]	Methotrexate vs co-trimoxazole vs prednisone, co-trimoxazole	65	20 (3–58)	Methotrexate—fewer relapses; Prednisone—no benefit

* Excluded eight patients initially enrolled: three due to lack of information and five due to failure to meet entrance criteria.
** Excluded four patients who died within 4 weeks; results were based on a *post hoc* analysis.

untreated in any clinical trial. Nevertheless, many remaining questions can be answered by randomized trials that compare the effectiveness of different therapeutic strategies. In addition, more recent long-term follow-up data have suggested that the combination of daily oral cyclophosphamide and prednisone, which became the mainstay of therapy for Wegener's granulomatosis, is associated with significant toxicity [72].

A key question is whether intravenous pulse cyclophosphamide might be equally effective, but less toxic than oral cyclophosphamide (Table 13.4). Adu and coworkers randomly allocated 54 patients with systemic vasculitis (29 had Wegener's granulomatosis) to either pulse cyclophosphamide plus prednisolone vs. oral cyclophosphamide plus oral prednisolone followed by azathioprine after 3 months [72]. There were no differences between the two groups in mortality, relapses, or treatment failures, but there was a tendency for more toxicity with continuous oral cyclophosphamide. In a randomized trial of 50 patients with Wegener's granulomatosis, Guillevin and coworkers found that prednisone plus pulse intravenous cyclophosphamide was associated with more relapses than prednisone plus oral cyclophosphamide, although the latter therapy was associated with more toxicity [73]. Thus, it appears that pulse cyclophosphamide may be both less toxic and less efficacious than continuous oral cyclophosphamide used for maintaining remission.

Several small, randomized trials have examined the use of plasma exchange as an adjunct to other therapies for the treatment of pauci-immune glomerulonephritis (Table 13.4). Studies by Glöckner *et al.* and Cole *et al.* failed to find any benefit from plasma exchange [75,76]. On the other hand, Pusey *et al.* found that in the subgroup of patients who were dialysis dependent there appeared to be some benefit [77]. Two other trials appeared to confirm this observation [74,78]. Thus, these data suggest that plasma exchange has little role in milder forms of pauci-immune glomerulonephritis, but may be of some benefit in patients who present with severe renal dysfunction. Additional randomized trials are needed to confirm the benefit in this important subgroup of patients.

In search of less toxic therapies to prevent relapses of Wegener's granulomatosis, Stegeman and coworkers randomly allocated 81 patients in remission to receive cotrimoxazole or placebo for 24 months [79]. There were significantly fewer relapses (18%) in the cotrimoxazole group compared with the placebo group (40%). Although the mechanism for the reduced rate of relapse is unclear, there were significantly fewer upper respiratory infections in the cotrimoxazole group.

Methotrexate has also been suggested as a less toxic alternative to long-term cyclophosphamide for maintenance of remissions. De Groot and coworkers randomly allocated 65 patients with Wegener's granulomatosis in remission to either methotrexate (0.3 mg/kg weekly) or cotrimoxazole twice daily [80]. Two smaller groups also received these agents in combination with prednisone. The maintenance of remission was significantly better with methotrexate.

Other therapies have been tried, but as yet have not been confirmed to be effective in controlled trials. These include the use of high-dose, pooled, intravenous immunoglobulin, cyclosporine A, anti-T-cell monoclonal antibodies, and antithymocyte globulin. Azathioprine has been used to maintain remission and reduce the toxicity of long-term cyclophosphamide, but needs additional testing in large, controlled, trials [73].

In summary, cyclophosphamide (used in combination with corticosteroids) is indicated for initial treatment of pauci-immune, rapidly progressive, glomerulonephritis. Plasma exchange may have a role in patients who present with marked renal impairment, but needs further study. The best regimen to prevent relapse is unclear. Continued oral cyclophosphamide appears to be more efficacious and more toxic than pulse cyclophosphamide. Methotrexate and/or azathioprine may be effective alternatives to long-term cyclophosphamide for maintenance of remission and deserve additional study. Cotrimoxazole can prevent relapse in some patients and deserves further study as an adjunct to other therapies. Other promising induction and maintenance therapies have yet to be tested in randomized trials.

Thrombotic, thrombocytopenic purpura, and hemolytic uremic syndrome

Idiopathic, thrombotic, thrombocytopenic purpura (TTP), and hemolytic uremic syndrome (HUS) have many similarities, but even more differences. HUS more often occurs in children and is more often preceded by diarrhea. TTP more often occurs in adults, has an insidious onset, is usually not associated with bloody diarrhea, and is frequently accompanied by neurologic manifestations. More importantly, treatment with plasma infusion or plasma exchange appears to be effective in TTP, while it is not effective in HUS.

Older literature suggests that untreated TTP was almost always fatal [81]. In the 1960s and 1970s there were anecdotal reports of treatment with corticosteroids, heparin, antiplatelet agents, vincristine, and splenectomy. In the 1980s a number of reports suggested that plasma infusion or plasma exchange induced a remission in 75% or more of cases. Given the dismal outcome without treatment that had previously been observed, it became accepted that plasma infusion or exchange is effective in TTP, even though this was never confirmed in a randomized, controlled trial.

More controversial was whether plasma exchange is superior to plasma infusion (Table 13.5). Rock and co-workers randomly allocated 102 adults with TTP to receive plasma exchange or plasma infusion [82]. After 6 months, 40 of 51 patients had responded to plasma exchange compared with 25 of 51 treated with plasma infusion ($p = 0.036$). However, patients treated with plasma exchange received three times more plasma than patients treated with infusion. Henon randomly allocated 40 adults to plasma exchange or plasma infusion and reported a trend to more remissions (80%) with plasma exchange vs. plasma infusion (52%), although these differences were not statistically significant [83]. In both of these studies patients in both groups received aspirin and dipyridamole. The role of adjunctive therapies is unclear. In the Italian Cooperative Group trial 72 patients treated with plasma exchange and corticosteroids were randomly allocated to receive either no antiplatelet therapy or aspirin and dipyridamole followed by long-term ticlopidine [84]. Although antiplatelet therapy failed significantly to alter the response rate at 15 days

Table 13.5 Randomized trials in adults with thrombotic thrombocytopenic purpura

Trial	Treat ment size	Sample	Follow-up (months)	Outcome
Rock *et al.* [82]	Plasma exchange vs plasma infusion	102	6	Improved (platelet count)
Henon *et al.* [83]	Plasma exchange, aspirin, dipyridamole vs plasma infusion, aspirin, dipyridamole	40	Not reported	No benefit
Bobbio-Pallavicini *et al.* [84]	Aspirin, dipyridamole, ticlopidine, plasma exchange, prednisone vs plasma exchange, prednisone	72	12	No benefit

(91.4% in treated patients vs. 75.6% in controls), the relapse rate by 1 year was higher in non-treated (21.4%) vs. treated (6.3%, $p = 0.02$) patients. The authors concluded that antiplatelet therapy was a beneficial adjunct to plasma exchange.

Thus, available data supports plasma exchange as a beneficial treatment in TTP. Less clear is whether plasma exchange or an equal volume of plasma infusion differ in efficacy. From a practical standpoint, it is often difficult to infuse safely large amounts of plasma to patients with renal failure, so the debate may be moot. Antiplatelet agents appear to be useful adjuncts for preventing relapses. The safety and efficacy of other therapies, including corticosteroids, vincristine, and splenectomy, are controversial and have not been tested in controlled trials.

There are no convincing data that any treatment for typical childhood HUS (other than symptomatic support) is effective (Table 13.6). Loirat and co-workers randomly allocated 79 children with HUS to either plasma infusion or conservative management [85]. At 1 and 6 months, patients in the plasma exchange group had lower serum creatinine and less proteinuria. However, at 1 year there were no significant differences in renal function or proteinuria between the two groups. Rizzoni and co-workers randomly allocated 32 children with HUS to either plasma infusion or symptomatic therapy [86]. They found no differences between the two groups in proteinuria or in renal histology. Thus, these two studies suggest that plasma infusion adds little to the symptomatic management of HUS in children. Van Damme-Lombaerts and co-workers randomly allocated 58 children with HUS to supportive management or heparin and dipyridamole, and found no substantive differences in outcomes between the two groups [86]. Thus, treatment of typical, childhood HUS should probably be limited to aggressive, symptomatic measures.

Table 13.6 Randomized trials in children with hemolytic uremic syndrome

Trial	Treatment size	Sample	Follow-up (months)	Outcome
Loirat *et al.* [85]	Plasma exchange vs plasma infusion	79	12	Improved at 1 month and 6 months, but no benefit at 12 months
Rizzoni *et al.* [86]	Plasma exchange vs plasma infusion	32	16	No benefit
Van Damme *et al.* [87]	Aspirin, dipyridamole, ticlopidine, plasma exchange, prednisone vs plasma exchange, prednisone	58	60	No benefit

Lupus nephritis

Systemic lupus erythematosus (SLE) is an autoimmune disease of unknown etiology characterized by multiple organ system involvement and a variable clinical course. Glomerulonephritis is a common complication and its presence influences long-term outcomes in SLE patients. The World Health Organization (WHO) has categorized renal involvement histologically in SLE into five major categories including: normal histology (class I), mesangial expansion (class II), focal proliferative glomerulonephritis (class III), diffuse proliferative glomerulonephritis (class IV), and membranous nephropathy (class V). Although treatment of renal involvement and renal survival in SLE have improved over time, controversy surrounds optimal therapeutic intervention [87]. The reason for this is a lack of prospective, randomized, controlled trials of adequate size. Additionally, the clinical course of SLE, in general, and lupus nephritis, in particular, varies greatly. Renal histology can change from one WHO class to another in a given patient and years of quiescent disease can be interrupted with exacerbations. Despite a plethora of retrospective studies, uncontrolled trials, and case reports, definitive conclusions regarding treatment remain elusive. As such, choosing between corticosteroids, immunosuppressive agents such as cyclophosphamide and azathioprine, and more recently, cyclosporine A, presents a daunting therapeutic dilemma for the clinician.

Recently Bansal and Beto [88] reported a meta-analysis of 19 clinical trials in lupus nephritis patients performed over a 25-year period (1970–1995). Only prospective, randomized, controlled trials were included in this analysis and the end-points of renal death (reaching end-stage renal disease) and total mortality were used to assess treatment efficacy. Renal histology, renal function, clinical severity, and activity/chronicity index scores were not used to categorize studies nor entered into the analysis itself as such information was not consistently available in all studies. The meta-analysis was used to determine whether immunosuppressive agents plus oral prednisone therapy was superior to oral prednisone alone and, if so, whether one immunosuppressive regimen was better than any other. Table 13.7 summarizes the different treatment regimens analyzed and the number of patients treated. Immunosuppressive therapy plus prednisone was found to be superior to treatment with prednisone alone for total mortality and development of end-stage renal disease [absolute risk differences, 13.2% and 12.9%, respectively (Fig. 13.2)]. Specifically, intravenous cyclophosphamide plus oral prednisone was significantly more effective than oral prednisone alone for total mortality and renal survival (absolute risk differences, 19.9% and 16.2%, respectively). Similarly, oral cyclophosphamide combined with azathioprine and prednisone was 16.9% better than oral prednisone alone in reducing the incidence of end-stage renal disease but did not significantly reduce the total mortality compared with prednisone alone. Interestingly, no immunosuppressive agent combined with prednisone was superior to any other. Likewise, the route of administration, intravenous versus oral, had no impact on efficacy. Based on these findings, the authors concluded that assessment of the individual patient and consideration of side effects for each treatment regimen will dictate, to a large extent, the clinician's therapeutic choices. The fact that this meta-

Table 13.7 Summary of randomized, controlled lupus nephritis trials based on therapeutic regimens

Treatment	Patients treated
Prednisone alone	105
Oral A + prednisone	99
Oral C + prednisone	128
Oral C + A + prednisone	30
Intravenous C + prednisone	78

A, Azathioprine; C, cyclophosphamide.
Dose ranges:
Prednisone = 0.5–1.0 mg/kg per day orally
Azathioprine = 1.0–4.0 mg/kg per day orally
Cyclophosphamide = 1.0–4.0 mg/kg per day orally
Combined A + C = 1.0–1.25 mg/kg per day orally for each agent
Intravenous C = 0.5–1.0 g/m^2 body surface area
Modified with permission [89].
For details regarding individual trials, see references Austin *et al.* 1986 [100], Boumpas *et al.* 1992 [101], Cade *et al.* 1973 [102], Carette *et al.* 1983 [103], Decker *et al.* 1975 [104], Dinant *et al.* 1989 [105], Donadio *et al.* 1972 [106], Donadio *et al.* 1974 [9], Donadio *et al.* 1976 [107], Donadio *et al.* 1978 [108], Ginzler *et al.* 1976 [109], Hahn *et al.* 1975 [110], Levey *et al.* 1992 [111], Lewis *et al.* 1992 [89], Steinberg *et al.* 1971 [112], Steinberg and Decker 1974 [113], Steinberg and Steinberg 1991 [114], Sztejnbok *et al.* 1971 [115], Valeri *et al.* 1994 [116].

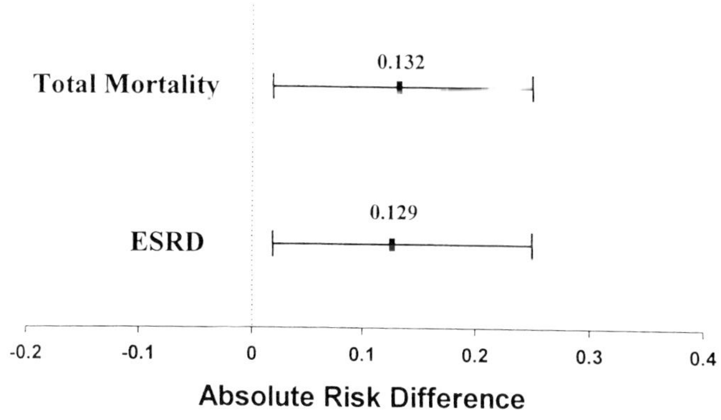

Fig. 13.2 Absolute risk differences with 95% confidence intervals for oral prednisone alone compared with all oral and intravenous immunosuppressive agents in conjunction with oral prednisone for outcome measures of total mortality and end-stage renal disease. The dotted vertical line (0.0) is the line of identity (i.e., no difference); data points are shown as decimals (e.g., 0.132 or 13.2%). Treatment is statistically significant at 0.05 level if confidence intervals do not intersect zero (indicated by *). Direction of positive risk reduction is for immunosuppression with prednisone. Reprinted with permission, Bansal and Beto [88].

analysis did not identify a definitive optimal treatment for lupus nephritis suggests the need for additional prospective, randomized, controlled trials of adequate sample size involving patients with similar clinical and histologic characteristics.

A number of prospective, randomized, controlled trials do not support a role for plasma exchange in routine lupus nephritis management [78,90–92]. Randomized controlled trials with cyclosporine A for membranous nephropathy (class V) in SLE patients are currently underway.

In 1979, the Canadian Task Force on the Periodic Health Examination reported its recommendations considering the inclusion or exclusion of specific medical conditions in screening periodic health examinations [93]. These recommendations were assigned 'grades' A–E denoting whether good evidence existed to support inclusion of a specific medical condition in the periodic health exam ('A') or good evidence indicating a specific disease should be excluded ('E') from consideration in a periodic health exam. A grade of 'C' indicated little or no evidence existed for inclusion or exclusion of a medical condition on the screening health exam. This grading system has been modified to indicate whether disease-specific treatment for various glomerular diseases is supported by evidence-based data in the literature. We have divided this 'report card' into two sections in which disease-specific treatment indications are graded for both proteinuria as well as preservation of renal function (Table 13.8). *These recommendations are not evaluations of individual treatment regimens.* Rather, they are intended to indicate whether evidence-based data exist supporting the use of treatment in a specific disease ('A') or data exist which support no treatment is beneficial ('E').

It is important to recognize that each patient must be evaluated individually and treatment may or may not be indicated for that specific patient.

Table 13.8 Evidence-based recommendations for glomerular disease-specific treatment

	Proteinuria remission	Renal function preservation
Membranous nephropathy	A	C
Membranoproliferative glomerulonephritis	B	C
Focal segmental glomerulosclerosis	B	C
Minimal change disease	A	A
IgA nephropathy	C	C
Anti-glomerular basement membrane antibody nephritis*	N/A	B/E**
Pauci-immune, rapidly progressive glomerulonephritis	N/A	A
Hemolytic uremic syndrome	N/A	E
Thrombotic, thrombocytopenic purpura	N/A	B
Lupus nephritis*	N/A	A

* Renal disease only.
** If greater than 50% sclerotic glomeruli/oligoanuric.

Key references

Brodehl J. The treatment of minimal change nephrotic syndrome: Lessons learned from multicentre co-operative studies. *Eur J Pediatr* 1991; **150**: 380–387.

Dillon JJ. Fish oil therapy for IgA nephropathy: efficacy and interstudy variability. *J Am Soc Nephrol* 1997; 8: 1739–1744.

Donadio JV Jr, Glassock RJ. Immunosuppressive drug therapy in lupus nephritis. *Am J Kidney Dis* 1993; **21** (3): 239–250.

Donadio JV Jr, Offord KP. Reassessment of treatment results in membranoproliferative glomerulonephritis, with emphasis on life-table analysis. *Am J Kidney Dis* 1989; **14** (6): 445–451.

Glassock RJ, Adler SG, Ward HJ, *et al.* Primary glomerular disease. In Brenner BM, Rector FC (eds). *The Kidney*, 4th edn, pp. 1182–1279. Philadelphia: WB Saunders, 1991.

Imperiale TF, Goldfarb S, Berns JS. Are cytotoxic agents beneficial in idiopathic membranous nephropathy? A meta-analysis of the controlled trials. *J Am Soc Nephrol* 1995; **5**: 1553–1558.

References

1. Glassock RJ. Therapy of idiopathic nephrotic syndrome in adults. *Am J Nephrol* 1993; **13**: 422–428.
2. Donadio JV Jr, Torres VE, Velosa JA, Wagoner RD, Holley KE, Okuda M, Ilstrup DM, Chu C-P. Idiopathic membranous nephropathy: the natural history of untreated patients. *Kidney Int* 1988; **33**: 708–715.
3. Glassock RJ, Adler SG, Ward HJ, *et al.* Primary glomerular disease. In Brenner BM, Rector FC (eds). *The Kidney*, 4th edn, pp. 1182–1279. Philadelphia: WB Saunders, 1991.
4. Schieppati A, Mosconi L, Perna A, Mecca G, Bertani T, Garattini S, Remuzzi G. Prognosis of untreated patients with idiopathic membranous nephropathy. *N Engl J Med* 1993; **329**: 85–89.
5. Coggins CH for the Collaborative Study of the Adult Idiopathic Nephrotic Syndrome. A controlled study of short-term prednisone treatment in adults with membranous nephropathy. *N Engl J Med* 1979; **301** (24): 1301–1306.
6. Cameron JS, Healy MJR, Adu D. The Medical Research Council Trial of short-term high-dose alternate day prednisolone in idiopathic membranous nephropathy with nephrotic syndrome in adults. *Q J Med* 1990; **74** (274): 133–156.
7. Cattran DC, Delmore T, Roscoe J, Cole E, Cardella C, Charron R, Ritchie S and the Toronto Glomerulonephritis Study Group. A randomized controlled trial of prednisone in patients with idiopathic membranous nephropathy. *N Engl J Med* 1989; **320** (4): 210–215.
8. Murphy BF, McDonald I, Fairley KF, Kincaid-Smith PS. Randomized controlled trial of cyclophosphamide, warfarin and dipyridamole in idiopathic membranous glomerulonephritis. *Clin Nephrol* 1992; **37** (5): 229–234.
9. Donadio JV Jr, Holley KE, Anderson CF, Taylor JW. Controlled trial of cyclophosphamide in idiopathic membranous nephropathy. *Kidney Int* 1974; **6**: 431–439.
10. Medical Research Council Working Party. Controlled trial of azathioprine and prednisone in chronic renal disease. *Br Med J* 1971; **2**: 239–241.
11. Ponticelli C, Zucchelli P, Imbasciati E, Cagnoli L, Pozzi C, Passerini P, Grassi C, Limido D, Pasquali S, Volpini T, *et al.* Controlled trial of methylprednisolone and chlorambucil in idiopathic membranous nephropathy. *N Engl J Med* 1984; **310** (15): 946–950.

12. Ponticelli C, Zucchelli P, Passerini P, Cesana B, Locatelli F, Pasquali S, Sasdelli M, Redaelli B, Grassi C, Pozzi C, *et al.* A 10-year follow-up of a randomized study with methylprednisolone and chlorambucil in membranous nephropathy. *Kidney Int* 1995; **48**: 1600–1604.
13. Davison AM, Cameron JS, Kerr N, Ogg CS, Wilkinson RW. The natural history of renal function in untreated idiopathic membranous glomerulonephritis in adults. *Clin Nephrol* 1984; **22** (2): 61–67.
14. Pei Y, Cattran D, Greenwood C. Predicting chronic renal insufficiency in idiopathic membranous glomerulonephritis. *Kidney Int* 1992; **42**: 960–966.
15. Falk RJ, Hogan SL, Muller KE, Jennette JC, the Glomerular Disease Collaborative Network. Treatment of progressive membranous glomerulopathy: a randomized trial comparing cyclophosphamide and corticosteroids with corticosteroids alone. *Ann Intern Med* 1992; **116**: 438–445.
16. Ponticelli C, Zucchelli P, Passerini P, Cesana B and the Italian Idiopathic Membranous Nephropathy Treatment Study Group. Methylprednisolone plus chlorambucil as compared with methlyprednisolone alone for the treatment of idiopathic membranous nephropathy. *N Engl J Med* 1992; **327** (9): 599–603.
17. DeSanto NG, Capodicasa G, Giordano C. Treatment of idiopathic membranous nephropathy unresponsive to methylprednisolone and chlorambucil with cyclosporin. *Am J Nephrol* 1987; **7**: 74–76.
18. Rostoker G, Belghiti D, Maadi AB, Rémy P, Lang P, Weil B, Lagrue G. Long-term cyclosporin A therapy for severe idiopathic membranous nephropathy. *Nephron* 1993; **63**: 335–341.
19. Cattran DC, Greenwood C, Ritchie S, Bernstein K, Churchill DN, Clark WF, Morrin PA, Lavoie S. A controlled trial of cyclosporine in patients with progressive membranous nephropathy. *Kidney Int* 1995; **47**: 1130–1135.
20. Hogan SL, Muller KE, Jennette JC, Falk RJ. A review of therapeutic studies of idiopathic membranous glomerulopathy. *Am J Kidney Dis* 1995; **25** (6): 862–875.
21. Imperiale TF, Goldfarb S, Berns JS. Are cytotoxic agents beneficial in idiopathic membranous nephropathy? A meta-analysis of the controlled trials. *J Am Soc Nephrol* 1995; **5**: 1553–1558.
22. Couchoud C, Laville M, Boissel JP. Treatment of membranous nephropathy: a meta-analysis. *Nephrol Dialysis Transplant* 1994; **9**: 469–470.
23. Simon P, Ramée M-P, Autuly V, Laruelle E, Charasse C, Cam G, Ang KS. Epidemiology of primary glomerular diseases in a French region. Variations according to period and age. *Kidney Int* 1994; **46**: 1192–1198.
24. Cameron JS, Turner DR, Heaton J, Williams DG, Ogg CS, Chantler C, Haycock GB, Hicks J. Idiopathic mesangiocapillary glomerulonephritis. *Am J Med* 1983; **74**: 175–192.
25. Schmitt H, Bohle A, Reineke T, Mayer-Eichberger D, Vogl W. Long-term prognosis of membranoproliferative glomerulonephritis type I. *Nephron* 1990; **55**: 242–250.
26. D'Amico G, Ferrario F. Mesangiocapillary glomerulonephritis. *J Am Soc Nephrol* 1992; **2**: S159–S166.
27. Cattran D, Cardella C, Roscoe J, Charron R, Rance PC, Ritchie S, Corey PN. Results of a controlled drug trial in membranoproliferative glomerulonephritis. *Kidney Int* 1985; **27**: 436–441.
28. Tiller DJ, Clarkson AR, Mathew T, *et al.* A prospective randomized trial in the use of cyclophosphamide, dipyridamole and warfarin in membranous and mesangiocapillary glomerulonephritis. In Zurukzoglu W, Papadimitriou M, Sion M, *et al.* (eds). *Eighth*

International Congress of Nephrology: Advances in Basic and Clinical Nephrology, pp. 345–351. Basel: Karger, 1981.
29. Zimmerman SW, Moorthy AV, Dreher WH, Friedman A, Varanasi U. Prospective trial of warfarin and dipyridamole in patients with membranoproliferative glomerulonephritis. *Am J Med* 1983; **75**: 920–927.
30. Donadio JV Jr, Anderson CF, Mitchell JC III, Holley KE, Ilstrup DM, Fuster V, Chesebro JH. Membranoproliferative glomerulonephritis. *N Engl J Med* 1984; **310** (22): 1421–1426.
31. International Study of Kidney Disease in Children. Report. Alternate-day steroid therapy in membranoproliferative glomerulonephritis: a randomized controlled clinical trial. *Kidney Int* 1982; **21**: 150.
32. Donadio JV Jr, Offord KP. Reassessment of treatment results in membranoproliferative glomerulonephritis, with emphasis on life-table analysis. *Am J Kidney Dis* 1989; **14** (6): 445–451.
33. Zäuner I, Böhler J, Braun N, Grupp C, Heering P, Schollmeyer P. Effect of aspirin and dipyridamole on proteinuria in idiopathic membranoproliferative glomerulonephritis: a multicentre prospective clinical trial. *Nephrol Dialysis Transplant* 1994; **9**: 619–622.
34. McEnery PT, McAdams AJ, West CD. The effect of prednisone in a high-dose, alternate-day regimen on the natural history of idiopathic membranoproliferative glomerulonephritis. *Medicine* 1986; **64** (6): 401–424.
35. Narita M, Koyama A. Therapeutic and prognostic studies in renal disease, part 2. In 1987 Annual Report of Progressive Renal Lesions, p. 244. Tokyo: Japanese Ministry of Health and Welfare 1988.
36. Lagrue G, Laurent J, Belghiti D. Renal survival in membranoproliferative glomerulonephritis (MPGN): Role of long-term treatment with nonsteroidal antiinflammatory drugs (NSAID). *Int Urol Nephrol* 1988; **20** (6): 669–677.
37. Cattran DC. Current status of cyclosporin A in the treatment of membranous, IgA and membranoproliferative glomerulonephritis. *Clin Nephrol* 1991; **35** (Suppl. 1): S43–S47.
38. Beaufils H, Alphonse JC, Guedon J, Legrain M. Focal glomerulosclerosis: natural history and treatment. *Nephron* 1978; **21**: 75–85.
39. Pei Y, Cattran D, Delmore T, Katz A, Lang A, Rance PC. Evidence suggesting under-treatment in adults with idiopathic focal segmental glomerulosclerosis. *Am J Med* 1987; **82**: 938–944.
40. Banfi G, Moriggi M, Sabadini E, Fellin G, D'Amico G, Ponticelli C. The impact of prolonged immunosuppression on the outcome of idiopathic focal-segmental glomerulosclerosis with nephrotic syndrome in adults. A collaborative retrospective study. *Clin Nephrol* 1991; **36** (2): 53–59.
41. Tarshish P, Tobin JN, Bernstein J, Edelmann CM Jr. Cyclophosphamide does not benefit patients with focal segmental glomerulosclerosis. A report of the International Study of Kidney Disease in Children. *Pediatr Nephrol* 1996; **10**: 590–193.
42. Ingulli E, Singh A, Baqi N, Ahmad H, Moazami S, Tejani A. Aggressive, long-term cyclosporine therapy for steroid-resistant focal segmental glomerulosclerosis. *J Am Soc Nephrol* 1995; **5**: 1820–1825.
43. Korbet SM, Schwartz MM, Lewis EJ. Primary focal segmental glomerulosclerosis: clinical course and response to therapy. *Am J Kidney Dis* 1994; **23** (6): 773–783.
44. Lieberman KV, Tejani A. A randomized double-blind placebo-controlled trial of cyclosporine in steroid-resistant idiopathic focal segmental glomerulosclerosis in children. *J Am Soc Nephrol* 1996; **7**: 56–63.
45. Walker RG, Kincaid-Smith P. The effect of treatment of corticosteroid-resistant

idiopathic (primary) focal and segmental hyalinosis and sclerosis (focal glomerulosclerosis) with ciclosporin. *Nephron* 1990; **54**: 117–121.

46. Grupe WE. Childhood nephrotic syndrome. Clinical associations and response to therapy. *Postgrad Med* 1979; **65** (15): 229–236.
47. Hoyer JR, Brenner BM, Stein JH, eds. Idiopathic nephrotic syndrome with minimal glomerular changes. *Contemporary Issues in Nephrology: Nephrotic Syndrome*, p. 145. New York: Churchill Livingstone, 1982.
48. Cornfeld D, Schwartz MW. Nephrosis: a long-term study of children treated with corticosteroids. *J Pediatr* 1966; **68** (4): 507–515.
49. International Study of Kidney Disease in Children. The primary nephrotic syndrome in children. Identification of patients with minimal change nephrotic syndrome from initial response to prednisone. *J Pediatr* 1981; **98** (4): 561–564.
50. Madore F, Lazarus JM, Brady HR. Therapeutic plasma exchange in renal diseases. *J Am Soc Nephrol* 1996; **7**: 367–386.
51. Brodehl J, Ehrich JHH. Short versus standard prednisone therapy for initial treatment of idiopathic nephrotic syndrome in children. *Lancet*, 1988; **1**: 380–383.
52. Ueda N, Kuno K, Ito S. Eight and 12 week courses of cyclophosphamide in nephrotic syndrome. *Arch Dis Child* 1990; **65**: 1147–1150.
53. Brodehl J. The treatment of minimal change nephrotic syndrome: Lessons learned from multicentre co-operative studies. *Eur J Pediatr* 1991; **150**: 380–387.
54. Ponticelli C, Rivolta E. Ciclosporin in minimal-change glomerulopathy and in focal segmental glomerular sclerosis. *Am J Nephrol* 1990; **10** (Suppl. 1): 105–109.
55. Garin EH, Orak JK, Hiott KL, Sutherland SE. Cyclosporine therapy for steriod-resistant nephrotic syndrome. *Am J Dis Childhood* 1988; **142**: 985–988.
56. Tejani A, Suthanthiran M, Pomrantz A. A randomized controlled trial of low-dose prednisone and ciclosporin versus high-dose prednisone in nephrotic syndrome of children. *Nephron* 1991; **59**: 96–99.
57. D'Amico G. The commonest glomerulonephritis in the world: IgA nephropathy. *Q J Med* 1987; **645**: 709–727.
58. Julian BA, Waldo FB, Rifal A, Mestecky J. IgA nephropathy, the most common glomerulonephritis worldwide: a neglected disease in the United States? *Am J Med* 1988; **84**: 129–132.
59. Hood SA, Velosa JA, Holley KE, Donadio JV Jr. IgA-IgG nephropathy: predictive indices of progressive disease. *Clin Nephrol* 1981; **16** (2): 55–62.
60. Droz D, Kramar A, Nawar T, Nöel LH. Primary IgA nephropathy: prognostic factors. *Contr Nephrol* 1984; **40**: 202–207.
61. Emancipator SN, Lamm ME. IgA nephropathy: pathogenesis of the most common form of glomerulonephritis. *Lab Invest* 1989; **60** (2): 168–183.
62. Dillon JJ. Fish oil therapy for IgA nephropathy: efficacy and interstudy variability. *J Am Soc Nephrol* 1997; **8**: 1739–1744.
63. Neng Lai K, Mac-Moune Lai F, Li PKT, Vallance-Owen J. Cyclosporin treatment of IgA nephropathy: a short term controlled trial. *Br Med J* 1987; **295**: 1165–1168.
64. Wilson CB, Dixon FJ. Anti-glomerular basement membrane antibody-induced glomerulonephritis. *Kidney Int* 1973; **3** (2): 74–89.
65. Lockwood CM, Boulton-Jones JM, Lowenthal RM, Simpson IJ, Peters DK, Wilson CB. Recovery from Goodpasture's syndrome after immunosuppressive treatment and plasmapheresis. *Br Med J* 1975; **2** (5965): 252–254.
66. Johnson JP, Moore J Jr, Austin HA, Balow JE, Antonovych TT, Wilson CB. Therapy of anti-glomerular basement membrane antibody disease: analysis of prognostic

significance of clinical, pathologic and treatment factors. *Medicine* 1985; **64** (4): 219–227.

67. Bolton WK. Goodpasture's syndrome. *Kidney Int* 1996; **50**: 1753–1766.
68. Simpson IJ, Doak PB, Williams LC, Blacklock HA, Hill RS, Teague CA, Herdson PB, Wilson CB. Plasma exchange in Goodpasture's syndrome. *Am J Nephrol* 1982; **2** (6): 301–311.
69. Wallon EW. Giant-cell granuloma of the respiratory tract (Wenger's granulomatosis). *Br Med J* 1958; **2**: 265–270.
70. Novack SN, Pearson CM. Cyclophosphamide therapy in Wegener's granulomatosis. *N Engl J Med* 1971; **284** (17): 938–942.
71. Fauci AS, Haynes BF, Katz P, Wolff SM. Wegener's granulomatosis: Prospective clinical and therapeutic experience with 85 patients for 21 years. *Ann Intern Med* 1983; **98**: 76–85.
72. Hoffman GS, Kerr GS, Leavitt RY, Hallahan CW, Lebovics RS, Travis WD, Rottem M, Fauci AS. Wegener granulomatosis: an analysis of 158 patients. *Ann Intern Med* 1992; **116** (6): 488–498.
73. Adu D, Pall A, Luqmani RA, Richards NT, Howie AJ, Emery P, Michael J, Savage CO, Bacon PA. Controlled trial of pulse versus continuous prednisolone and cyclophosphamide in the treatment of systemic vasculitis. *Q J Med* 1997; **90** (6): 401–409.
74. Guillevin L, Cordier JF, Lhote F, Cohen P, Jarrousse B, Royer I, Lesavre P, Jacquot C, Bindi P, Bielefeld P, *et al.* A prospective, multicenter, randomized trial comparing steroids and pulse cyclophosphamide versus steroids and oral cyclophosphamide in the treatment of generalized Wegener's granulomatosis. *Arthritis Rheum* 1997; **40** (12): 2187–2198.
75. Glöckner WM, Sieberth HG, Wichmann HE, Backes E, Bambauer R, Boesken WH, Bohle A, Daul A, Graben N, Keller F, *et al.* Plasma exchange and immunosuppression in rapidly progressive glomerulonephritis: a controlled, multi-center study. *Clin Nephrol* 1988; **29** (1): 1–8.
76. Cole E, Cattran D, Magil A, Greenwood C, Churchill DN, Sutton D, Clark WF, Morrin PA, Posen G, Bernstein K, *et al.* A prospective randomized trial of plasma exchange as additive therapy in idiopathic crescentic glomerulonephritis. *Am J Kidney Dis* 1992; **20** (3): 261–269.
77. Pusey CD, Rees AJ, Evans DJ, Peters DK, Lockwood CM. Plasma exchange in focal necrotizing glomerulonephritis without anti-GMB antibodies. *Kidney Int* 1991; **40**: 757–763.
78. Mauri JM, Gonzalez MT, Poveda R, Seron D, Torras J, Andujar J, Andres E, Alsina J. Therapeutic plasma exchange in the treatment of rapidly progressive glomerulonephritis. *Plasma Ther Transfus Technol* 1985; **6** (3): 587–591.
79. Stegeman CA, Tervaert JWC, de Jong PE, Kallenberg CGM. Trimethoprim-sulfamethoxazole (co-trimoxazole) for the prevention of relapses of Wegener's granulomatosis. *N Engl J Med* 1996; **335**: 16–20.
80. de Groot K, Reinhold-Keller E, Tatsis E, Paulsen J, Heller M, Nolle B, Gross WL. Therapy for the maintenance of remission in sixty-five patients with generalized Wegener's granulomatosis. Methotrexate versus trimethoprim/sulfamethoxazole. *Arthritis Rheum* 1996; **39** (12): 2052–2061.
81. Amorosi EL, Ultmann JE. Thrombotic thrombocytopenic purpura: report of 16 cases and review of the literature. *Med* 1966; **45**: 139–159.
82. Rock GA, Shumak KH, Buskard NA, Blanchette VS, Kelton JG, Nair RC, Spasoff RA.

Comparison of plasma exchange with plasma infusion in the treatment of thrombotic thrombocytopenic purpura. *N Engl J Med* 1991; **325** (6): 393–397.

83. Henon P. Treatment of thrombotic thrombocytopenic purpura. Results of a multicenter randomized clinical study. *Presse Med* 1761; 1991; **20** (36): –7.
84. Bobbio-Pallavicini E, Gugliotta L, Centurioni R, Porta C, Vianelli N, Billio A, Tacconi F, Ascari E. Antiplatelet agents in thrombotic thrombocytopenic purpura (TTP). Results of a randomized multicenter trial by the Italian Cooperative Group for TTP. *Haematologica* 1997; **82** (4): 429–435.
85. Loirat C, Sonsino E, Hinglais N, Jais JP, Landais P, Fermanian J. Treatment of the childhood hemolytic uraemic syndrome with plasma. A multicentre randomized controlled trial. The French Society of Pediatric Nephrology. *Pediatr Nephrol* 1988; **2** (3): 279–285.
86. Rizzoni G, Claris-Appiani A, Edefonti A, Facchin P, Franchini F, Gusmano R, Imbasciati E, Pavanello L, Perfumo F, Remuzzi G. Plasma infusion for hemolytic–uremic syndrome in children: results of a multicenter controlled trial. *J Pediatr* 1988; **112** (2): 284–290.
87. Van Damme-Lombaerts R, Van Proesmans W, Damme B, Eeckels R, Binda ki Muaka P, Mercieca V, Vlietinck R, Vermylen J. Heparin plus dipyridamole in childhood hemolytic–uremic syndrome: a prospective, randomized study. *J Pediatr* 1988; **113** (5): 913–918.
88. Donadio JV Jr, Glassock RJ. Immunosuppressive drug therapy in lupus nephritis. *Am J Kidney Dis* 1993; **21** (3): 239–250.
89. Bansal VK, Beto JA. Treatment of lupus nephritis: a meta-analysis of clinical trials. *Am J Kidney Dis* 1997; **29** (2): 193–199.
90. Lewis EJ, Hunsicker LG, Lan S-P, Rohde RD, Lachin JM. A controlled trial of plasmapheresis therapy in severe lupus nephritis. *N Engl J Med* 1992; **326**: 1373–1379.
91. Wei N, Lawley TJ, Steinberg AD, Klippel JH, Hall RP, Balow JE, Decker JL. Randomised trial of plasma exchange in mild systemic lupus erythematosus. *Lancet*, 1983; **1**: 17–22.
92. Clark WF, Cattran DC, Balfe JW, Williams W, Lindsay RM, Linton AL. Chronic plasma exchange in systemic lupus erythematosus nephritis. *Proc Eur Dial Transplant Assoc* 1983; **20**: 629–635.
93. Canadian Task Force on the Periodic Health Examination. Task Force Report on the Periodic Health Examination. *Can Med Assoc J* 1979; **121**: 1193–1254.
94. Donadio JV Jr, Bergstralh EJ, Offord KP, Spencer DC, Holley KE. A controlled trial of fish oil in IgA nephropathy. *N Engl J Med* 1994; **331**: 1194–1199.
95. Pettersson EE, Rekola S, Berglund L, Sundquist KG, Angelin B, Diczfalusy U, Björkhem I, Bergström J. Treatment of IgA nephropathy with omega-3-polyunsaturated fatty acids: a prospective, double blind, randomized study. *Clin Nephrol* 1994; **41** (4): 183–190.
96. Cheng IKP, Chan PCK, Chan MK. The effect of fish-oil dietary supplement on the progression of mesangial IgA glomerulonephritis. *Nephrol Dial Transplant* 1990; **5**: 241–246.
97. Bennett WM, Walker RG, Kincaid-Smith P. Treatment of IgA nephropathy with eicosapentaenoic acid (EPA): a two-year prospective trial. *Clin Nephrol* 1989; **31** (3): 128–131.
98. Hamazaki T, Tateno S, Shisido H. Eicosapentaenoic acid and IgA nephropathy. *Lancet*, 1984: 1017–1018.
99. Rifle G, Dechelette E. Treatment of rapidly progressive glomerulonephritis by plasma

exchange and methylprednisolone pulses. A prospective randomized trial of cyclophosphamide. Interim analysis. French Cooperative Group. *Prog Clin Biol Res* 1990; **337**: 263–267.

100. Austin HA III, Klippel JH, Balow JE, le Riche NGH, Steinberg AD, Plotz PH, Decker JL. Therapy of lupus nephritis: controlled trial of prednisone and cytotoxic drugs. *N Engl J Med* 1986; **314**: 614–619.
101. Boumpas DT, Austin HA III, Vaughn EM, Klippel JH, Steinberg AD, Yarboro CH, Balow JE. Controlled trial of pulse methylprednisolone versus two regimens of pulse cyclophosphamide in severe lupus nephritis. *Lancet* 1992; **340** (8822): 741–745.
102. Cade R, Spooner G, Schlein E, Pickering M, deQuesada A, Holcomb A, Juncos L, Richard G, Shires D, Levin D, *et al.* Comparison of azathioprine, prednisone, and heparin alone or combined in treating lupus nephritis. *Nephron* 1973; **10**: 37–56.
103. Carette S, Klippel JH, Decker JL, Austin HA, Plotz PH, Steinberg AD, Balow JE. Controlled studies of oral immunosuppressive drugs in lupus nephritis. A long-term followup. *Ann Intern Med* 1983; **99** (1): 1–8.
104. Decker JL, Klippel JH, Plotz PH, Steinberg AD. Cyclophosphamide or azathioprine in lupus glomerulonephritis. A controlled trial: Results at 28 months. *Ann Intern Med* 1975; **83** (5): 606–615.
105. Dinant HJ, Decker JL, Klippel JH, Balow JE, Plotz PH, Steinberg AD. Alternative modes of cyclophosphamide and azathioprine therapy in lupus nephritis. *Ann Intern Med* 1982; **96**: 728–736.
106. Donadio JV, Holley KE, Wagoner RD, Ferguson RH, McDuffie FC. Treatment of lupus nephritis with prednisone and combined prednisone and azathioprine. *Ann Intern Med* 1972; **77**: 829–835.
107. Donadio JV Jr, Holley KE, Ferguson RH, Ilstrup DM. Progressive lupus glomerulonephritis. Treatment with prednisone and combined prednisone and cyclophosphamide. *Mayo Clin Proc* 1976; **51**: 484–494.
108. Donadio JV Jr, Holley JL, Ferguson RH, Ilstrup DM. Treatment of diffuse proliferative lupus nephritis with prednisone and combined prednisone and cyclophosphamide. *N Engl J Med* 1978; **299** (21): 1151–1155.
109. Ginzler E, Diamond H, Guttadauria M, Kaplan D. Prednisone and azathioprine compared to prednisone plus low-dose azathioprine and cyclophosphamide in the treatment of diffuse lupus nephritis. *Arthritis Rheum* 1976; **19** (4): 693–699.
110. Hahn BH, Kantor OS, Osterland CK. Azathioprine plus prednisone compared with prednisone alone in the treatment of systemic lupus erythematosus. Report of a prospective controlled trial in 24 patients. *Ann Intern Med* 1975; **83** (5): 597–605.
111. Levey AS, Lan S-P, Corwin HL, Kasinath BS, Lachin J, Neilson EG, Hunsicker LG, Lewis EJ. Progression and remission of renal disease in the Lupus Nephritis Collaborative Study. Results of treatment with prednisone and short-term oral cyclophosphamide. *Ann Intern Med* 1992; **116** (2): 114–123.
112. Steinberg AD, Kaltreider HB, Staples PJ, Goetzl EJ, Talal N, Decker JL. Cyclophosphamide in lupus nephritis: a controlled trial. *Ann Intern Med* 1971; **75**: 165–171.
113. Steinberg AD, Decker JL. Double-blind controlled trial comparing cyclophosphamide, azathioprine and placebo in the treatment of lupus glomerulonephritis. *Arthritis Rheum* 1974; **17** (6): 923–937.
114. Steinberg AD, Steinberg SC. Long-term preservation of renal function in patients with lupus nephritis receiving treatment that includes cyclosphosphamide versus those treated with prednisone only. *Arthritis Rheum* 1991; **34** (8): 945–950.

115. Sztejnbok M, Stewart A, Diamond H, Kaplan D. Azathioprine in the treatment of systemic lupus erythematosus. *Arthritis Rheum* 1971; **14** (5): 639–645.
116. Valeri A, Radhakrishnan J, Estes D, D'Agati V, Kopelman R, Pernis A, Flis R, Pirani C, Appel GB. Intravenous pulse cyclophosphamide treatment of severe lupus nephritis: a prospective five-year study. *Clin Nephrol* 1994; **42** (2): 71–78.

INDEX